Mental Health Atlas

2005

Mental Health: Evidence and Research
Department of Mental Health and Substance Abuse
World Health Organization

Geneva

WHO Library Cataloguing-in-Publication Data

World Health Organization.
Mental health atlas : 2005.

1.Mental health services - statistics 2.Mental health services - atlases 3.Health policy - trends
4.Health personnel - statistics 5.World health

ISBN 92 4 156296 X (NLM classification: WM 17)

Designed by Tushita Graphic Vision Sàrl, Thônex, Switzerland

Printed in Singapore

The information provided in the profiles should be viewed as the best information available with WHO from all sources combined and not as the official viewpoint of the Member States.

For further information, please contact:

Shekhar Saxena
Coordinator
Mental Health: Evidence and Research
Department of Mental Health and Substance Abuse
World Health Organization
Avenue Appia 20, CH-1211 Geneva 27, Switzerland
Tel: +41 22 791 21 11, Fax: +41 22 791 4160, Email: saxenas@who.int

Contents

SECTION III

The Project Team and Partners

Atlas is a project of WHO Headquarters, Geneva, supervised and coordinated by Dr Shekhar Saxena. Dr Benedetto Saraceno provided vision and guidance to this project. The first set of publications from this project appeared in 2001. The Mental Health Atlas-2005 represents the project's updated and revised edition.

Key collaborators from WHO Regional Offices include: Dr Therese Agossou, African Regional Office; Dr Caldas de Almeida and Dr Claudio Miranda, Regional Office for the Americas; Dr Ahmad Mohit and Dr R. S. Murthy, Eastern Mediterranean Regional Office; Dr Matthijs Muijen and Dr Wolfgang Rutz, European Regional Office; Dr Vijay Chandra, South-East Asia Regional Office; and Dr Xiangdong Wang, Western Pacific Regional Office. They have contributed to planning the project, obtaining and validating the information from Member States and reviewing the results.

WHO Representatives and Liaison Officers in WHO Country Offices were responsible for collecting and validating the information received from Governments.

Ministry of Health officials in Member States provided the information and responded to the many requests for clarification that arose from the data.

The World Psychiatric Association provided data from some countries through their member associations.

A number of experts in countries assisted the Ministries in obtaining and providing information. They also provided relevant literature and reports to support the data.

In the course of the project, a number of colleagues at WHO provided advice and guidance. Significant among them are: Dr Tom Barrett, Dr Myron Belfer, Dr José Bertolote, Dr Dan Chisholm, Dr Michelle Funk, Dr Itzhak Levav, Dr Vladimir Poznyak, Dr Leonid Prilipko and Dr Mark van Ommeren.

Dr Pratap Sharan was the overall project manager for the Mental Health Atlas-2005. Ms Sogol Noorani assisted with completing the project beginning in September 2004. Dr Sujatha Chandrasekaran, Dr Emily Daley, Dr David Hong, Ms Olga Kupcova, Ms Yen-Ying Liu, and Ms Christina Westhoff assisted in updating the database and in its validation during their internship in the Department. Ms Maria Villenueva and Ms Elmira Adenova assisted with the translation of material. Ms Grazia Motturi and Ms Rosemary Westermeyer provided administrative support; in addition Ms Rosemary Westermeyer assisted with proofreading and overall production. The contribution of each of these team members and partners, along with the input of many other unnamed people, has been vital to the success of this project.

The graphic design of this volume has been done by Ms Tushita Bosonet.

Preface

We are pleased to present Mental Health Atlas-2005.

The primary responsibility of the World Health Organization is to provide technical assistance to its Member States in matters related to health. However, this responsibility cannot be fulfilled satisfactorily if the Organization lacks basic information about the existing infrastructure and resources available for health care within countries. Unfortunately, until recently, this has been the case with mental health. Although substantial information was available about the burden that mental and behavioural disorders place on society, very little was known about the resources on hand in different countries to alleviate these problems. Most of the information available about mental health resources is related to a few high-income countries. For the vast majority of countries, there was almost no information available. Furthermore, because available studies had used different units of measurement, the information that was accessible was not comparable across different countries or over time.

In 2000, the World Health Organization launched Project Atlas to address this gap. The objectives of this project include the collection, compilation and dissemination of relevant information about mental health resources in different countries.

The first set of publications from the project appeared in October 2001 and was titled, Atlas: Mental Health Resources in the World, 2001 and Atlas: Country Profiles on Mental Health Resources in the World, 2001. The Mental Health Atlas-2005 is the second edition from the project, and it provides aggregate results as well as country profiles on mental health. Atlas 2005 is the result of complete updating of information from countries, supplemented by a search of relevant literature and reports of WHO and other international and national organizations. One significant addition is the inclusion of information on epidemiology of mental disorders for all low and middle income countries; this is likely to enhance the usefulness of the Mental Health Atlas-2005 as the most comprehensive reference source for global mental health information.

The country profiles confirm what mental health professionals working in these countries have known for a long time: that mental health services are grossly inadequate when compared to the needs for mental health care. The value of the Atlas therefore is that it replaces impressions and opinions with facts and figures. The profiles attempt to give a clear picture of existing resources and crucial needs in countries around the world. They also provide a baseline for monitoring changes over time. By using uniform definitions and units of measurement they encourage consistency of reporting.

A note of caution! Although great care has been taken to ensure the reliability of the data presented in the country profiles, it is possible that some errors may have crept in. We see Project Atlas as an ongoing activity of WHO, where more accurate information will become available as the concepts and definitions of resources become more refined and data sources become more organized and reliable.

Overall, we hope that the Mental Health Atlas-2005 will assist health planners and policy-makers within countries to identify areas that need urgent attention. The profiles can also help to set realistic targets by enabling comparisons of strengths and weaknesses across countries. Researchers will find the Atlas 2005 data useful for health service research. We also hope that mental health professionals and non-governmental organizations will continue to use the Mental Health Atlas in their efforts to advocate for more and better resources for mental health.

Dr Benedetto Saraceno
Director
Department of Mental Health and Substance Abuse

Dr Shekhar Saxena
Co-ordinator
Mental Health: Evidence and Research
Department of Mental Health and Substance Abuse

Section I

Introduction

Methodology

Limitations

Global and Regional Results

Comparison of Data between 2001 and 2004

Introduction

Project Atlas was launched by WHO in 2000 in an attempt to map mental health resources in the world. These data are needed at the country level to assess the current situation and to assist in developing plans and at the regional and global levels to develop an aggregate picture of the available mental health resources and the overall needs. The project thus responds to WHO's objectives as set out in the World Health Report 2001 (WHO, 2001) and in recent resolutions from the governing bodies of WHO on mental health (EB109.R8 on strengthening mental health and its affirmation by WHA55.10).

The analyses of the global and regional data collected in 2001 were compiled and presented in the publication – Atlas: Mental Health Resources in the World (WHO, 2001b); and individual country profiles and some further analyses were presented in Atlas: Country Profiles on Mental Health Resources in the World, 2001. Mental Health Atlas-2005 is the second set of publications from the project, and it presents aggregate results as well as individual country profiles on mental health.

This new edition includes updated and revised information on themes published in Atlas 2001. Atlas 2005 also includes information on new Member States (Timor-Leste) and more Associate Member States, Areas and Territories (e.g. West Bank and Gaza Strip). The general information section has been strengthened considerably, particularly through inclusion of a subsection on epidemiology. And the qualitative information in the country profiles, particularly for low- and middle-income countries is much enriched, as a result of a systematic search on mental health services. This has also led to highlighting issues particularly relevant to these countries, e.g. the issue of migration of trained manpower to high-income countries.

Section I of this publication describes the methodology used, as well as the global and regional analyses. It also explains the limitations of the Atlas data. The global and regional analyses are organized into 16 broad themes. Each theme begins with a definition of the terms used and is followed by a description of the significant findings. The results are presented in tabular form, each followed by a short explanation. The analyses include data received from all 192 WHO Member States. The main limitations of the data are listed after the explanation of the methodology. The specific limitations of each variable are discussed at the end of each theme.

Section II of this publication provides short descriptive profiles for each country. The profiles were generated by computer from the database. This would explain the language for the profile being repetitive in some areas. The countries are arranged in alphabetical order. The profiles of the WHO Associate Members, Territories and Areas include only those which had responded to the questionnaire sent to them as a part of the project. The profiles begin with some general information about each country. The statistics relating to the land areas of each country were obtained from the United Nations (2004) database and other appropriate sources. Only approximate figures are given, as the intention was to provide an estimate of the size of the country – of relevance to a profile on mental health resources – and not accurate figures. The figures for population, gender ratio and ratio of children and elderly in the total population are largely based on United Nations estimates in 2004. The life expectancy, healthy adjusted life expectancy (HALE) and health budget figures were taken from the World Health Report 2004 (WHO, 2004a). Income groupings of countries are based on World Bank 2004 data. However, the GNP/capita for the different countries was obtained from a variety of sources, including the World Bank database. The figures on literacy rate are largely based on UNESCO (2004) data. However, these databases do not always provide information about each country. In such cases, data from different sources, e.g. other international organizations and from countries themselves were included. The final subsection of the general information section in profiles of low- and middle-income countries summarizes epidemiological information available in international databases. The data provided in the general information section should not be read as the official figures for the country but taken as indicative.

The subsequent section on mental health resources includes the broad areas of policy and legislation; finance; mental health facilities, including disability benefits, primary care and training facilities, and community care facilities; distribution of psychiatric beds and professionals; non-governmental organizations; information gathering systems; specific programmes for special sectors of the population; therapeutic drugs and any other information that was made available. Additional sources of information include documents and literature that provided important details about epidemiology and mental health resources in the country. Some qualitative information was obtained from those documents. There is some variation in the quantity of information available for each country depending on the information gathered. Attempts have been made to provide complete references wherever possible, but some citations have remained incomplete due to lack of information.

Methodology

Information for this project was collected in a series of stages or steps.

The initial questionnaire was drafted in 2001 through a process that involved consultations with Regional Offices of WHO and other mental health experts to determine the main subjects about which information was required. Following these consultations, a questionnaire was drafted at WHO Headquarters. A glossary of the terms used in the questionnaire was also prepared to assist the respondents. The definitions used in the glossary are simply working definitions for the purpose of this project and are not official WHO definitions. The draft questionnaire and glossary were discussed with the Regional Offices of WHO and selected mental health experts whose suggestions were then incorporated. The questionnaire was then pilot tested in two countries – one developed, the other developing – and the difficulties presented by both the glossary and questionnaire were once again discussed and amended appropriately. The final questionnaire covered mental health policies, programmes, legislation, mental health budgets, disability benefits, facilities for mental health in primary and community care, number of psychiatric beds and mental health professionals, involvement of non-governmental organizations in mental health, information gathering systems in mental health, special programmes for sub-populations and therapeutic drugs. The aim was to gather basic information from as many countries as possible without going into excessive detail. Once the English version of the questionnaire was finalized, it was translated into four other official languages of WHO: Arabic, French, Russian and Spanish. Responses were obtained through the focal points for mental health in the Ministries of Health in each WHO Member State, Associate Member and Area through WHO Regional Offices. The focal points were requested to complete the questionnaire using all possible sources of information and to follow the definitions provided in the glossary so as to maintain uniformity of the information. They were also requested to provide supporting documents wherever possible.

For Atlas 2005, a comprehensive literature search on mental health services and resources, focussing on low- and middle-income countries was conducted with the help of a librarian specialized in systematic searches. Subject heading based searches on Medline (1996 – February 2004) and Embase Psychiatry (1996 – February 2004) were used. The initial search combining terms 'health services' and 'mental health' yielded 13 726 and 12 438 articles in Medline and Embase, respectively. The resulting searches in each database were then combined with terms for each country in turn. Certain countries were excluded to make the search manageable and to prioritize low- and middle- income countries. WHO member states which are classified as high-income by the World Bank and which are also OECD members were excluded from this search, i.e. Australia, Austria, Belgium, Canada, Denmark, Finland, France, Germany, Greece, Iceland, Ireland, Italy, Japan, Republic of Korea, Luxembourg, Netherlands, New Zealand, Norway, Portugal, Spain, Sweden, Switzerland, Taiwan, United Kingdom, United States of America. For each country the country name was used (e.g. China) in addition to a stem derived from the nationality or language, e.g. Chin$.mp. Terms for nationality and language were obtained from UN Bulletin "Terminology" No.347/Rev.1 and dictionaries. Certain country names were not available as subject headings in one or both databases so over-inclusive search terms were used e.g. Micronesia to search for articles about Tuvalu. The mean number of articles initially obtained for each country was 8.5 (range 0 to 148). Articles were organized using the Windows Reference Manager 10 programme. The abstracts were reviewed separately by two researchers to eliminate unrelated studies, i.e. (1) studies on ethnic populations in developed countries, (2) articles on unrelated populations, e.g. American Indians for a search on India, (3) articles unrelated to services, e.g. efficacy studies on drug, (4) studies examining mental symptoms/disorders as factors affecting services for physical diseases, and (5) services for physical disorders in mentally ill populations. As many articles as possible were retrieved electronically using the WHO online library, the Google search engine and freemedicaljournals.com (including "PubMed"). Additional articles were obtained from the WHO library print holdings. Abstracts of other articles were used.

A comprehensive literature search on epidemiological data of mental health related issues, focussing on low- and middle-income countries was also conducted. Potential terms related to epidemiology, mental health and country (WHO Member States, except all high-income countries) were identified and 4 databases – Medline, Embase Psychiatry, Cinahl and Sociofile – were searched using subject headings (these headings were "exploded" to encompass all subordinate terms) in the first three databases and using keywords derived from its thesaurus for Sociofile. Specificity and sensitivity of the initial search strategy were addressed using abstracts for 4 countries, leading to a step-wise refinement of the search strategy. Specificity was examined by comparing the number of relevant articles to the number of irrelevant ones for each search strategy in each database. To confirm sensitivity, articles derived with the search strategy were compared to the total number of articles for that country. As an additional check on sensitivity, the articles obtained for one country were cross-checked with a researcher who had worked extensively in that country. Income status of WHO member states was examined on basis of current World Bank Classification (in effect until 1st July 2003). A set of criteria similar to the one for mental health services was developed for the elimination of non-mental health/non-epidemiology articles. About two-fifths of the remaining (more than 25 000 abstracts) on epidemiology of mental health in relation to low- and middle income counties were reviewed by two researchers to establish reliability in the elimination process.

In addition to these literature searches, information was obtained from documents received from countries, travel reports submitted by WHO staff, feedback from experts and member associations of the World Psychiatric Association. Additional inputs were also obtained from country data collected by the WHO Offices of the Eastern Mediterranean Region, European Region and American Region.

The updated draft country profiles were then sent to the focal points for mental health in the Ministries of Health in each WHO Member State, Associate Member and Area. The focal points were requested to verify the profile and update it based on all sources of information available with them. They were also requested to provide supporting documents wherever possible. Throughout this process the Project Team was in contact with the Regional Offices and focal points. Clarifications were provided where necessary and regular reminders were sent requesting completion and submission of the verified profiles. The majority of Member States, Associate Members, Areas and Territories have already verified the information in the country profiles. The verification of country profiles of the Democratic People's Republic of Korea, Grenada, the Netherlands, Saint Kitts and Nevis and the United Arab Emirates were still being awaited from the respective Ministries of Health at the time of going to print.

For the purpose of analysis, some continuous variables were grouped into categories based on distribution. Frequency distribution and measures of central tendency (mean, median and standard deviations) were calculated as appropriate. Countries have been grouped by WHO Regions and World Bank income categories based on GNP/capita (World Bank, 2004) for analysis.

Limitations

The data collected in the course of this project have a number of limitations. These should be kept in mind when viewing the results.

While best attempts have been made to obtain information from countries on all variables, some could not provide specific details on a few issues. The most common reason for the missing data is that such data simply do not exist within the countries. It is hoped that these information gaps will be filled in the future. The extent of missing data can be gleaned from the number of countries that have been able to supply details. Each individual chart contains the number (N) of countries, out of a total of 192, whose data could be included in the chart.

The project has used working definitions arrived at through consultations with experts. The aim was to strike a balance between the definitions that are most appropriate and those that the countries currently use. At present, definitions for mental health resources like policy, primary care facilities, community care facilities, health information systems vary from country to country. As a result, countries may have had difficulty in interpreting the definitions provided in the glossary and in reporting accurate information.

Some countries may have had difficulty in providing information about the mental health budget because mental health care in their country is integrated within the primary care system, as recommended by WHO. Most of the questions were framed, so that countries could respond with 'yes' or 'no'. Although this helped in increasing the rate of responses, it failed to take into account differences in coverage and quality. Thus, information related to implementation of policies, programmes or legislation, type of disability benefits, distribution of resources among rural and urban settings, quality of services available at primary or community level, proportion of financing for rural or urban settings, quality of services available for special populations, quality of services provided by non-governmental organizations and quality of information gathering systems cannot be gauged from this data. Attempts have been made to incorporate qualitative data from several sources, but this is still limited. The information collected on the number of psychiatric beds and professionals gives the average figure for the country but does not provide information about distribution across rural or urban settings or distribution across different regions within the country.

Some of the limitations of the Atlas 2001 data, that were due to the fact that they had been collected primarily from Government sources, have been partially removed by incorporating other sources of information. Apart from the verification provided by Governments, the country profiles of the Atlas 2005 are based on information from the literature, epidemiological information, WHO reports on country projects and travel reports of WHO staff. Another rich source of country information has been the pilot trial within 10 countries using a newly developed WHO Assessment Instrument for Mental Health Systems (WHO-AIMS). However, it is still possible that information about the private sector especially that related to availability of psychiatric beds and mental health professionals may be incomplete and may not be representative of the actual figures for the country. Some details may also be missing because the respondents did not have access to the information. This is especially true of the sections on mental health financing and the availability of drugs at primary care level. Some of the data may be old and it is hoped that countries will help WHO to update the information as new data becomes available. While all possible measures have been taken to compile, code and interpret the information given by countries using uniform definitions and criteria, it is possible that some errors may have occurred due to inaccuracies of the data. WHO requests the mental health focal points within the Ministries of Health of Member States to point out any errors for correction in subsequent publications.

Project Atlas is an ongoing activity of WHO and as more accurate and comprehensive information covering all aspects of mental health resources become available and the concepts and definitions of resources become more refined, it is hoped that the database will also become better organized and more reliable.

The information provided in the profiles should be viewed as the best information available with WHO from all sources combined and not as the official viewpoint of the Member States.

Global and Regional Results

The global and regional analyses are organized into 16 broad themes.. These include policies, programmes, legislation, finance, primary care, psychiatric beds, professionals, special programmes in mental health and information gathering systems. The working definitions used for key terms in the questionnaire are given at the beginning of each thematic section. The results of the analyses are presented for the world and for the six WHO Regions. The Member States included in each of the WHO Regions are as follows:

Africa: Algeria, Angola, Benin, Botswana, Burkina Faso, Burundi, Cameroon, Cape Verde, Central African Republic, Chad, Comoros, Congo, Côte d'Ivoire, Democratic Republic of the Congo, Equatorial Guinea, Eritrea, Ethiopia, Gabon, Gambia, Ghana, Guinea, Guinea-Bissau, Kenya, Lesotho, Liberia, Madagascar, Malawi, Mali, Mauritania, Mauritius, Mozambique, Namibia, Niger, Nigeria, Rwanda, Sao Tome and Principe, Senegal, Seychelles, Sierra Leone, South Africa, Swaziland, Togo, Uganda, United Republic of Tanzania, Zambia, Zimbabwe.

Americas: Antigua and Barbuda, Argentina, Bahamas, Barbados, Belize, Bolivia, Brazil, Canada, Chile, Colombia, Costa Rica, Cuba, Dominica, Dominican Republic, Ecuador, El Salvador, Grenada, Guatemala, Guyana, Haiti, Honduras, Jamaica, Mexico, Nicaragua, Panama, Paraguay, Peru, Saint Kitts and Nevis, Saint Lucia, Saint Vincent and the Grenadines, Suriname, Trinidad and Tobago, United States of America, Uruguay, Venezuela.

Eastern Mediterranean: Afghanistan, Bahrain, Djibouti, Egypt, Iran (Islamic Republic of), Iraq, Jordan, Kuwait, Lebanon, Libyan Arab Jamahiriya, Morocco, Oman, Pakistan, Qatar, Saudi Arabia, Somalia, Sudan, Syrian Arab Republic, Tunisia, United Arab Emirates, Yemen.

Europe: Albania, Andorra, Armenia, Austria, Azerbaijan, Belarus, Belgium, Bosnia and Herzegovina, Bulgaria, Croatia, Cyprus, Czech Republic, Denmark, Estonia, Finland, France, Georgia, Germany, Greece, Hungary, Iceland, Ireland, Israel, Italy, Kazakhstan, Kyrgyztan, Latvia, Lithuania, Luxembourg, Malta, Monaco, Netherlands, Norway, Poland, Portugal, Republic of Moldova, Romania, Russian Federation, San Marino, Serbia and Montenegro, Slovakia, Slovenia, Spain, Sweden, Switzerland, Tajikistan, The former Yugoslav Republic of Macedonia, Turkey, Turkmenistan, Ukraine, United Kingdom, Uzbekistan.

South-East Asia: Bangladesh, Bhutan, Democratic People's Republic of Korea, India, Indonesia, Maldives, Myanmar, Nepal, Sri Lanka, Thailand, Timor-Leste.

Western Pacific: Australia, Brunei Darussalam, Cambodia, China, Cook Islands, Fiji, Japan, Kiribati, Lao People's Democratic Republic, Malaysia, Marshall Islands, Micronesia (Federated States of), Mongolia, Nauru, New Zealand, Niue, Palau, Papua New Guinea, Philippines, Republic of Korea, Samoa, Singapore, Solomon Islands, Tonga, Tuvalu, Vanuatu, Viet Nam.

In addition to the Member States, information on mental health is also available from 11 Associate Members, Areas and Territories; this information is given as profiles in Section III, but is not included in the global and regional analyses.

MENTAL HEALTH POLICY

Definitions

- *Mental health policy:* a specifically written document of the Government or Ministry of Health containing the goals for improving the mental health situation of the country, the priorities among those goals and the main directions for attaining them.

A Mental health policy may include the following components:

- *Advocacy:* a combination of individual and social actions designed to raise awareness and to gain political commitment, policy support, social acceptance and health systems support for mental health goals.
- *Promotion:* a process of enabling people to increase control over the determinants of their mental well-being and to improve it.
- *Prevention:* all organized activities in the community to prevent the occurrence as well as the progression of mental disorders, including the timely application of means to promote the mental well-being of individuals and of the community as a whole, and the provision of information and education.
- *Treatment:* relevant clinical and non-clinical care aimed at reducing the impact of mental disorders and improving the quality of life of patients.
- *Rehabilitation:* care given to persons with mental disorders in the form of knowledge and skills to help them achieve their optimum level of social and psychological functioning.

1. Presence of mental health policies in each WHO Region and the world

WHO Regions	Countries (%)	Population coverage* (%)
Africa	50.0	69.4
Americas	72.7	64.2
Eastern Mediterranean	72.7	93.8
Europe	70.6	89.1
South-East Asia	54.5	23.6
Western Pacific	48.1	93.8
World	62.1	68.3

N = 190 *population according to UNO, 2004.

An analysis of the data gathered by Project Atlas shows that only 62.1% of countries, accounting for 68.3% of the population, have a mental health policy. In the African Region only 50.0% of countries have a policy. About one third of the population in the African Region is not covered by a mental health policy. Some countries, however, do have such a policy in draft form, but it has yet to be approved by the Government.

2. Year of initial formulation of the mental health policy

Years	Countries (%)
Up to 1960	6.1
1961 – 1970	0.9
1971 – 1980	7.9
1981 – 1990	22.8
1991 – 2000	53.5
After 2000	8.8

N = 114

3. Year of initial formulation of the mental health policy since 1990

Years	Countries (%)
1991 – 1992	16.9
1993 – 1994	19.7
1995 – 1996	9.9
1997 – 1998	18.3
1999 – 2000	21.1
2001 – 2002	5.6
2003 – 2004	8.5

N = 71

Some 62.3% of countries have formulated their policies since the 1990s. Of these, about one-tenth have done so since 2001.

Most countries that report having a policy also have all the essential components incorporated into them. Treatment issues are covered by 98.1% of countries, prevention by 95.3% of countries, rehabilitation by 93.4% of countries, promotion by 91.4% of countries and advocacy by 80.4% countries. Intersectoral collaboration, collaboration with NGOs, provision of social assistance, human resource development, improvement of community care facilities especially for the underserved (e.g. Maoris in New Zealand) are some of the other components also included in the policies of some countries.

There was a significant association between the presence of a mental health policy and that of a number of different variables: substance abuse policy (χ^2 41.8, $p<0.01$), a national mental health programme ($\chi^2=31.6$, $p<0.01$), disability benefits ($\chi^2=12.1$), primary care training facilities in mental health ($\chi^2=22.9$, $p<0.01$), community care facilities in mental health ($\chi^2=7.80$, $p<0.01$) and presence of NGO activities in mental health ($\chi^2=11.2$, $p<0.01$).

The data on mental health policies have several limitations. Many countries, e.g. in the European Region, might not have a stated policy, but may have a well-developed action plan for mental health. These have not been taken into account in the present analysis. Also, data are not available about the degree to which policies or plans have been implemented. So, it may be possible that although a country reports having a mental health policy, because of incomplete implementation the benefits of the policy may have failed to reach most of the population. The present data refer only to the year when they were initially formulated.

NATIONAL MENTAL HEALTH PROGRAMME

Definitions

- *National mental health programme:* a national plan of action that includes the broad and specific lines of action required in all sectors involved to give effect to the policy. It describes and organizes actions aimed at the achievement of the objectives. It indicates what has to be done, who has to do it, during what time frame and with what resources.
- *Community-based care:* any type of care, supervision and rehabilitation of mental patients outside the hospital by health and social workers based in the community.

4. Presence of national mental health programmes in each WHO Region and the world

WHO Regions	Countries (%)	Population covered*(%)
Africa	76.1	82.9
Americas	76.5	87.9
Eastern Mediterranean	90.9	97.6
Europe	52.9	64.5
South-East Asia	72.7	98.1
Western Pacific	63.0	98.9
World	69.6	90.9

N = 191 *population according to UNO, 2004.

In the world 69.6% of countries, accounting for a population of 90.9%, have a national mental health programme.

5. Year of initial formulation of the national mental health programme

Years	Countries (%)
Up to 1960	2.4
1961 – 1970	2.4
1971 – 1980	7.9
1981 – 1990	26.0
1991 – 2000	51.2
After 2000	10.2

N = 127

6. Year of initial formulation of the national mental health programme since 1990

Years	Countries (%)
1991 – 1992	10.3
1993 – 1994	6.4
1995 – 1996	14.1
1997 – 1998	19.2
1999 – 2000	33.3
2001 – 2002	15.4
2003 – 2004	1.3

N = 78

Some 61.4% of the programmes were formulated since the 1990s. Of these, one-sixth were formulated since 2001.

7. Countries in each WHO Region where the national mental health programme was formulated after 1990*

WHO Regions	1991-2004 (%)
Africa (N = 34)	73.6
Americas (N = 24)	58.5
Eastern Mediterranean (N = 20)	30.0
Europe (N = 25)	76.0
South-East Asia (N = 7)	42.9
Western Pacific (N = 17)	64.7

*from all countries with a national mental health programme

Although in the European Region only 52.9% of countries have a programme, most of these programmes (76.0%) have been formulated since the 1990s. On the other hand, although 90.9% of countries in the Eastern Mediterranean Region have a programme, 70% of those were formulated before 1990.

8. Presence of community care for mental health in each WHO Region and the world

WHO Regions	Countries (%)
Africa	56.5
Americas	75.0
Eastern Mediterranean	68.2
Europe	79.2
South-East Asia	50.0
Western Pacific	66.7
World	68.1

N = 185

Community care facilities exist in only 68.1% of countries, covering 83.3% of the world's population. In the African, Eastern Mediterranean and South-East Asia Regions, such facilities are present in about half the countries. The population coverage is not uniform and is often restricted to a few areas within the country. This is the case in China, India, Paraguay and Zambia.

9. Presence of community care in each income group of countries

Income Group of Countries*	Countries (%)
Low	51.7
Lower Middle	51.9
Higher Middle	90.9
High	97.4

N = 181 * groups are based on GNP/capita of the countries: low (<$755), lower middle ($756-$2995), higher middle ($2996-$9265), high (>$9266).
Source: World Bank, 2004

Across different income groups, community care facilities in mental health are present in 51.7% of the low income countries and in 97.4% of the high income countries.

There were also significant differences between income group and the presence of community care facilities within countries.

Examples of available community care facilities include day-care centres, therapeutic and supervised residential services, crisis residential services, sheltered homes, clubhouses, community mental health services for children and adolescents or the elderly, agricultural psychiatric rehabilitation villages, etc. Comprehensive community care facilities, including the majority of those mentioned above, are found only in the high income countries. The majority of the low income countries and countries belonging to the African, South-East Asia and Western Pacific Regions have limited resources and can afford only a few of these facilities and then only in limited areas.

Some of the European countries that have reported not having a national programme, do have well-developed action plans at state or provincial levels. These are not accounted for in the overall figures. It is possible that some countries that do not appear to have a national mental health programme may have individual programmes directed at specific areas of need. The data presented here refer only to the initial formulation of the programme and not to revisions or updates. The information given here pertains only to the existence of the programmes and not to their implementation. In some countries, community care facilities may only be available in a few areas. Or, they are available as pilot projects and not throughout the whole country as reported, e.g. in India. Further information is required about the quality of care provided through community facilities and the type of personnel involved in providing mental health care at the community level.

MENTAL HEALTH LEGISLATION

Definitions

- *Mental health legislation:* legal provisions for the protection of the basic human and civil rights of people with mental disorders and deals with treatment facilities, personnel, professional training and service structure. Mental health legislation includes provisions concerned with the restraint and protection of individual patients, regulation of compulsory admission, discharge procedures, appeals, protection of property, etc.
- *Disability benefits:* benefits that are payable, as part of a legal right, from public funds in cases of mental disorders that reduce a person's capacity to function.

10. Presence of law in the field of mental health in each WHO Region and the world

WHO Regions	Countries (%)	*Population coverage (%)
Africa	79.5	94.4
Americas	75.0	89.1
Eastern Mediterranean	57.1	70.8
Europe	91.8	90.1
South-East Asia	63.6	95.9
Western Pacific	76.0	13.9
World	78.0	69.1

N = 173 *population according to UNO, 2004

In the world, 78.0% of countries accounting for 69.1% of the population have laws in the field of mental health. In the Eastern Mediterranean Region only 57.1% of countries have laws in the field of mental health compared with 91.8% of countries in the European Region.

11. Year of initiation of the latest law in the field of mental health

Years	Countries (%)
Up to 1960	15.9
1961 – 1970	8.7
1971 – 1980	10.1
1981 – 1990	12.3
1991 – 2000	40.6
After 2000	12.3

N = 138

12. Year of initiation of the latest law in the field of mental health since 1990

Years	Countries (%)
1991 – 1992	6.8
1993 – 1994	5.5
1995 – 1996	8.2
1997 – 1998	28.8
1999 – 2000	27.4
2001 – 2002	17.8
2003 – 2004	5.5

N = 73

13. Countries in each WHO Region with initiation of the latest law in the field of mental health after 1990*

WHO Regions	1991 – 2004 (%)
Africa (N = 30)	30.0
Americas (N = 34)	58.4
Eastern Mediterranean (N = 13)	46.2
Europe (N = 47)	76.6
South-East Asia (N = 6)	16.7
Western Pacific (N = 18)	38.9

*from all countries with laws in mental health

More than half of the existing legislation is recent and has been enacted since 1990. Of this, one-fourth were enacted after 2000. Whereas in the European Region 76.6% of the legislation was enacted since the 1990s, in the South-East Asia Region the figure is only 16.7%. What is striking is that about 16% of the legislation dates from before 1960, when the majority of the current effective methods for treating mental disorders were not available.

14. Presence of disability benefits in each WHO Region and the world

WHO Regions	Countries (%)
Africa	45.5
Americas	90.9
Eastern Mediterranean	85.7
Europe	100
South-East Asia	81.8
Western Pacific	65.4
World	77.8

N = 185

Disability benefits are reported to exist in 77.8% of countries covering a population of 93.0%. They exist in only 45.5% of countries in the African Region compared with 100% of countries in the European Region.

15. Presence of disability benefits in each income group of countries

Income Group of Countries*	Countries (%)
Low	55.2
Lower Middle	88.7
Higher Middle	78.8
High	100

*World Bank, 2004

Only 55.2% of countries in the low income group provide disability benefits for mental health, compared with all countries in the high income group. There were also significant differences for this comparison.

The data on legislation and disability benefits have certain limitations. Some countries do not have separate mental health legislation, although some issues may be covered as a part of wider health legislation. Information on the degree of implementation of the legislation or the extent and effectiveness of it is not available. Some countries have a number of laws on mental health but only the most recent law and its year of enactment were mentioned. Although many countries report about having disability benefits for people with mental disorders, information on the exact kind of disability benefits and their coverage is not available from all countries surveyed. Thus, information about the type of benefits provided or about the sector of the population that benefits is lacking.

SUBSTANCE ABUSE POLICY

Definition

- *Substance abuse policy:* a specifically written document of the Government or Ministry of Health containing goals of prevention and treatment activities related to the use, abuse and dependence of alcohol, prescription and non-prescription including illicit drugs.

  A substance abuse policy is vital to facilitate the planning and improvement of services for the management of people suffering from substance use disorders. The existence of a policy helps to prioritize issues related to substance use and provides direction to governmental or non-governmental organizations to work towards a common goal – the improvement of the services and resources directed towards helping patients affected by substance use disorders. The policy should be comprehensive enough to address the existing problems of the country and should cover both alcohol and illicit drugs.

16. Presence of a substance abuse policy in each WHO Region and the world

WHO Regions	Countries (%)
Africa	50.0
Americas	72.7
Eastern Mediterranean	77.3
Europe	86.3
South-East Asia	72.7
Western Pacific	53.8
World	68.8

N = 189

A substance abuse policy exists in 68.8% of countries of the world, covering a population of 77.1%. However, fewer countries in the African Region (50.0%) and Western Pacific Region (53.8%) have a policy. Almost 30% of countries in the Region of the Americas do not have a substance abuse policy though they have the highest prevalence of both alcohol and drug related disorders, as was found in the GBD, 2000 analysis.

17. Year of initial formulation of the substance abuse policy

Years	Countries (%)
Up to 1960	1.7
1961 – 1970	4.2
1971 – 1980	6.7
1981 – 1990	24.2
1991 – 2000	59.2
After 2000	4.2

N = 120

18. Year of initial formulation of the substance abuse policy since 1990

Years	Countries (%)
1991 – 1992	5.3
1993 – 1994	9.2
1995 – 1996	25.0
1997 – 1998	27.6
1999 – 2000	26.3
2001 – 2002	3.9
2003 – 2004	2.6

N = 76

19. Countries in each WHO Region that formulated a substance abuse policy after 1990*

WHO Regions	1991-2004(%)
Africa (N = 21)	71.5
Americas (N = 21)	66.7
Eastern Mediterranean (N = 16)	37.5
Europe (N = 43)	74.5
South-East Asia (N = 7)	57.1
Western Pacific (N = 12)	41.6

*from all countries with a substance abuse policy

The years since the 1990s saw the formulation of 63.4% of the policies. Of these, 6.5% were formulated since 2001. In the European Region, 74.5% of the policies were formulated since the 1990s compared to only 41.6% and 37.5% of the policies in the Western Pacific and Eastern Mediterranean Regions, respectively.

While some countries may have reported no policy, they may actually have individual plans or programmes for dealing with drug abuse or dependence. In spite of our efforts, it is possible that some countries may have reported the existence of substance abuse policies because they have legislation on substance abuse. This could be because a number of countries do have narcotics related legislation. However, specific details about the substances covered by substance abuse policy, the dates on which the policies were revised and the extent of their implementation are not available.

THERAPEUTIC DRUGS

Definitions

- *Therapeutic drug policy:* a written commitment, endorsed by the Minister of Health or the Cabinet, to ensure accessibility and availability of essential therapeutic drugs. It contains measures for regulating the selection, purchase, procurement, distribution and use of essential and appropriate drugs, including those for mental and neurological disorders. It can also specify the number and types of drugs to be made available to health workers at each level of the health service according to the functions of the workers and the conditions they are required to treat. Under the national policy, drugs may be supplied free of charge to all or selected groups.
- *Essential list of drugs:* the officially approved list of essential drugs that the country has adopted. It is usually adapted from the WHO Model List of Essential Drugs.

20. Presence of a therapeutic drug policy/essential list of drugs in each WHO Region and the world

WHO Regions	Therapeutic Drug Policy/ Essential List of Drugs (%)
Africa	93.5
Americas	90.9
Eastern Mediterranean	95.2
Europe	81.6
South-East Asia	100
Western Pacific	85.2
World	89.3

N = 187

Some 89.3% of countries in the world, covering a population of 91.1%, reported the existence of a therapeutic drug policy or essential list of drugs. In the European Region 81.6% of countries have either one or other of them. All countries in the South-East Asia Region have either a policy or an essential list of drugs.

21. Year of initial formulation of the therapeutic drug policy/essential list of drugs

Years	Countries (%)
Up to 1960	1.5
1961 – 1970	2.2
1971 – 1980	10.3
1981 – 1990	19.1
1991 – 2000	61.0
After 2000	5.9

N = 136

22. Year of initial formulation of the therapeutic drug policy/essential list of drugs since 1990

Years	Countries (%)
1991 – 1992	9.9
1993 – 1994	14.3
1995 – 1996	19.8
1997 – 1998	26.4
1999 – 2000	20.9
2001 – 2002	5.5
2003 – 2004	3.3

N = 91

Two-thirds of the policies or essential lists of drugs were formulated since the 1990s. Of these, one-tenth were formulated since 2001.

Information about availability, most common basic strength and cost of a specific list of drugs was sought.

23. Availability of therapeutic psychotropic drugs in primary care

Drug	Countries (%)
Carbamazepine (N = 185)	91.4
Ethosuximide (N = 183)	37.2
Phenobarbital (N = 185)	93.0
Phenytoin (N = 183)	77.0
Sodium Valproate (N = 184)	67.4
Amitriptyline (N = 184)	86.4
Chlorpromazine (N = 186)	91.4
Diazepam (N = 186)	96.8
Fluphenazine (N = 183)	70.5
Haloperidol (N = 184)	91.8
Lithium (N = 185)	65.4
Biperiden (N = 184)	43.5
Carbidopa (N = 180)	51.1
Levodopa (N = 181)	61.9

N = 180-186.

Among anti-epileptics, phenobarbital is available in 93.0% of countries and phenytoin in 77.0% of countries. Amitriptyline, an anti-depressant, is available in 86.4% of countries. Among anti-psychotics, chlorpromazine is available in 91.4% of countries but fluphenazine in only 70.5% of countries. Lithium, a mood stabilizer, is available in 65.4% of countries. Carbamazepine and sodium valproate which although are anti-epileptics can also act as mood stabilizers and are available in 91.4% and 67.4% of countries, respectively. Anti-Parkinson drugs are available in a lesser number of countries, with biperiden available in only 43.5% of countries.

Although the availability reported by countries is high, it should be kept in mind that these drugs are neither available in all primary care centres of a country nor are they easily available at all times. Thus, effectively, the availability of these drugs would be much lower than that reported.

24. Availability of three* essential therapeutic psychotropic drugs at primary care level in each WHO Region and the world

WHO Regions	Countries (%)
Africa	67.4
Americas	62.9
Eastern Mediterranean	50.0
Europe	62.7
South-East Asia	63.6
Western Pacific	81.5
World	65.1

N = 192 *phenytoin, amitriptyline and chlorpromazine

In the world, 65.1% of countries report having each of the three drugs: amitriptyline (an anti-depressant), chlorpromazine (an anti-psychotic) and phenytoin (an anti-epileptic). In the African Region all three of these drugs are available in 67.4% of countries.

The cost of the aforementioned three drugs varies widely within different WHO Regions and income groups. In order to make a simple comparison, the cost of drugs for treating mental disorders for one year using an average maintenance dose was calculated for all countries.

25. Comparison of median per year expenditure for treating depression with amitriptyline (150mg/day) within different WHO Regions

WHO Regions	Median cost (USD)
Africa	34.38
Americas	21.90
Eastern Mediterranean	60.12
Europe	78.40
South-East Asia	36.14
Western Pacific	54.09

26. Comparison of median per year expenditure for treating psychotic disorders with chlorpromazine (400mg/day) within different WHO Regions

WHO Regions	Median cost (USD)
Africa	49.06
Americas	100.30
Eastern Mediterranean	48.98
Europe	100.45
South-East Asia	28.47
Western Pacific	47.23

27. Comparison of median per year expenditure for treating epilepsy with phenytoin (300mg/day) within different WHO Regions

WHO Regions	Median cost (USD)
Africa	20.59
Americas	42.38
Eastern Mediterranean	34.11
Europe	33.95
South-East Asia	22.34
Western Pacific	44.13

Across different WHO Regions, the cost of treatment for one year using amitriptyline (150 mg/day) varies from $21.90 in the Eastern Mediterranean Region to $78.40 in the European Region; for chlorpromazine (400 mg/day), the cost varies from $28.47 in the South-East Asia Region to $100.45 in the European Region; and for phenytoin (300 mg/day), the cost varies from $20.59 in the African Region to $44.13 in the Western Pacific Region.

28. Comparison of median per year expenditure for treating depression with amitriptyline (150mg/day) in different income groups of countries

Income Group of Countries*	Median cost (USD)
Low	50.37
Lower Middle	49.60
Higher Middle	35.48
High	89.13

*World Bank, 2004

29. Comparison of median per year expenditure for treating psychotic disorders with Chlorpromazine (400mg/day) in different income groups of countries.

Income Group of Countries*	Median cost (USD)
Low	47.89
Lower Middle	35.84
Higher Middle	108.62
High	155.20

*World Bank, 2004

30. Comparison of median per year expenditure for treating epilepsy with phenytoin (300mg/day) in different income groups of countries

Income Group of countries*	Median cost (USD)
Low	16.43
Lower Middle	27.65
Higher Middle	35.04
High	44.35

*World Bank, 2004

Across different income groups the median cost for one year of treatment with amitriptyline (150 mg/day) varies from $35.48 in the higher middle income group to $89.13 in the high income group; for chlorpromazine (400mg/day), the cost varies from $35.84 in the lower middle income group to $155.20 in the high income group; and for phenytoin (300mg/day), the cost varies from $16.43 in the low income group to $44.35 in the high income group. From the analysis of cost it is apparent that low income countries which have a GNP/capita that is at least one-twelfth that of high income countries pay only half the cost for treatment of depression (with amitriptyline) and epilepsy (with phenytoin) and one-fourth of the cost for the treatment of psychosis (with chlorpromazine).

BUDGET FOR MENTAL HEALTH CARE

Definition

- *Specified budget for mental health:* the regular source of money, available in a country's budget, allocated for actions directed towards the achievement of mental health objectives.

31. Presence of a specified budget for mental health care in each WHO Region and the world.

WHO Regions	Countries (%)
Africa	62.2
Americas	78.1
Eastern Mediterranean	71.4
Europe	70.0
South-East Asia	90.0
Western Pacific	59.3
World	69.2

N = 185

In spite of the importance of a separate mental health budget within the total health budget, 30.8% of countries reported not having a specified budget for mental health care. In the Regions of Africa, Eastern Mediterranean and Western Pacific, such a budget is present in 62.2%, 71.4% and 59.3% of countries. On the other hand, 78.1% of countries in the Americas Region have a specified budget for mental health care.

32. Specified budget for mental health as a proportion of total health budget in each WHO Region (N = 101)

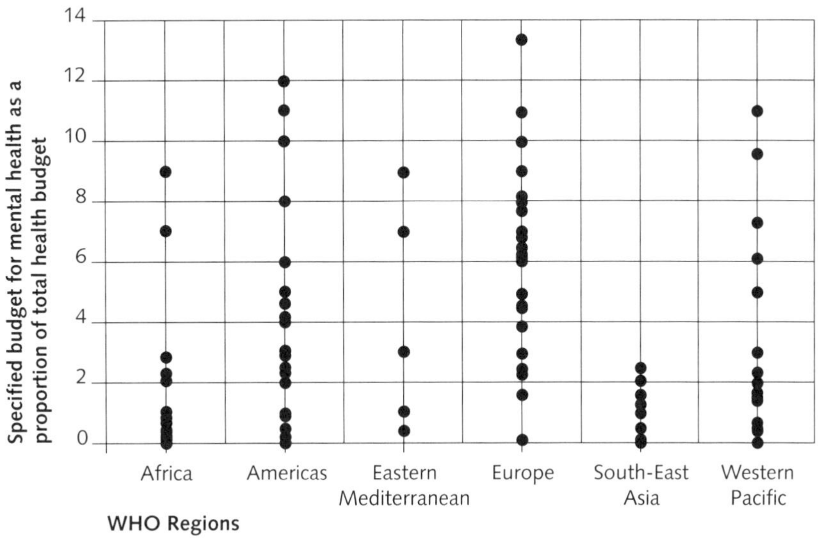

Although only 101 countries have provided information on the actual budget for mental health, this nevertheless covers about 4.8 billion people. Of the 101 countries 20.9%, covering a population of more than 1 billion, spend less than 1% of the total health budget on mental health. In the Regions of Africa and South-East Asia, 70.0% and 50.0% of countries, respectively, spend less than 1% of their health budget on mental health care. More than 61.5% of countries in the European Region spend more than 5% of their health budget on mental health care.

33 a. Specified budget for Mental Health as a proportion of total health budget by GDP/capita (I$) (N = 86)

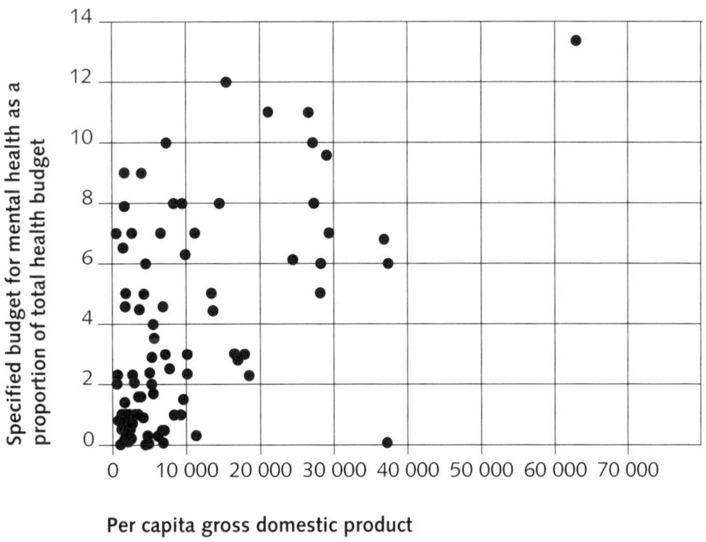

33 b. **Specified budget for Mental Health as a proportion of total health budget by Per Capita Government Expenditure on Health (I$) (N = 101)**

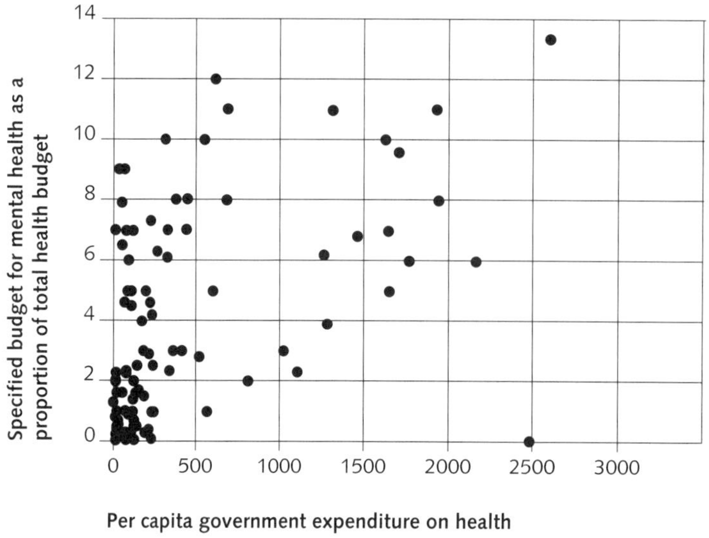

Among low income countries, 29.2% accounting for a population in excess of 0.5 billion spend less than 1% of their budget on mental health care. While, among high income countries, only 0.7% accounting for a population of about 5 million people, spend less than 1% of their health budget on mental health care.

Many European Region countries report that while they do not have a national budget specifically for mental health care, they do allocate budgets to each province or state under their mental health programmes. In many countries mental health is a part of the primary health care system making it difficult to ascertain the budget for mental health care.

The number of countries that reported a specified budget for mental health as a proportion of their total health budget is relatively small. Many countries, especially in the European Region, do not have a separate mental health budget. However, they make financial allocations for mental health within the overall health budget at federal or state level. Some countries have a federal system where individual states are responsible for health expenditure. These countries were not able to provide aggregate figures. It is also possible that some countries have provided the budget allocations for their national mental health programmes. Again, some countries like Austria were unable to provide specific information about the mental health budget as mental health care is fully integrated within the primary care system, as advocated by WHO, and no separate budget exists for mental health. Information is also lacking about budget allocations to Government or non-governmental sectors, for rural or urban sectors and for distribution of budgets for different services and resources. In view of all these limitations the data on mental health budgets should be viewed as preliminary and indicative, even at the country level.

METHODS OF FINANCING MENTAL HEATH CARE

Definitions

- *Out-of-pocket payment:* money spent by the consumer or the consumer's family as the need arises.
- *Tax based funding:* money for mental health services raised through taxation: either through general taxation or through taxes earmarked specifically for mental health services.
- *Social insurance:* everyone above a certain income level is required to pay a fixed percentage of their income to a government-administered health insurance fund. In return, the Government pays for part or all of the consumer's mental health services, should they be needed.
- *Private insurance:* the health care consumer voluntarily pays a premium to a private insurance company. In return, the insurance company pays for part or all of the consumer's mental health services, should they be needed.
- *External grants:* money provided to countries by other countries or international organizations.

The most important source of financing mental health has been reported by 180 countries.

34. Methods of financing* mental health care in each WHO Region and the world

WHO Regions	Mode of finance	Most common method of financing Countries (%) a)	Second most common method of financing Countries (%) b)
Africa	Out-of-pocket payment	38.6	40.0
	Tax Based	54.5	16.0
	Social insurance	0	16.0
	Private insurance	4.5	16.0
	External Grants	2.3	12.0
Americas	Out-of-pocket payment	12.9	25.0
	Tax Based	74.2	25.0
	Social insurance	6.5	40.0
	Private insurance	3.2	10.0
	External Grants	3.2	0
Eastern Mediterranean	Out-of-pocket payment	15.8	57.1
	Tax Based	68.4	21.4
	Social insurance	5.3	7.1
	Private insurance	0	14.3
	External Grants	10.5	0
Europe	Out-of-pocket	0	28.9
	Tax Based	55.1	23.7
	Social insurance	44.9	26.3
	Private insurance	0	21.1
	External Grants	0	0
South-East Asia	Out-of-pocket payment	30.0	50.0
	Tax Based	70.0	25.0
	Social insurance	0	0
	Private insurance	0	0
	External Grants	0	25.0
Western Pacific	Out-of-pocket payment	18.5	37.5
	Tax Based	70.4	18.8
	Social insurance	3.7	25.0
	Private insurance	0	12.5
	External Grants	7.4	6.3
World	Out-of-pocket payment	17.8	36.4
	Tax Based	62.8	21.5
	Social insurance	14.4	22.3
	Private insurance	1.7	14.9
	External Grants	3.3	5.0

a) N = 180 b) N = 121 *based on information provided by countries

World-wide, out-of-pocket payment is the most important method for financing mental health care in 17.8% of countries. In 62.8% of countries the most important method is tax based; in 14.4% of countries: social insurance; in 1.7% of countries: private insurance; and in 3.3% of countries external grants from international organizations and other countries. Across all Regions, tax based financing is the most important financing method in half to almost three-quarters of the countries. Out-of-pocket payment is the most important method of financing in 38.6% of countries in the African Region, in 30% of countries in the South-East Asia Region and in 18.5% of countries in the Western Pacific Region. Out-of-pocket payment is not the primary method of financing mental health in any country in the European Region. In the European Region social insurance is the primary method of financing in 44.9% of countries and in the Americas Region in 6.5% of countries, compared to none in the African and South-East Asia Regions and only 3.7% and 5.3% of countries in the Regions of the Western Pacific and Eastern Mediterranean, respectively. Private insurance and external grants are primary sources of financing in very few countries across the world.

Of the 121 countries that provided details on the second most important method of financing mental health care, 36.4% of countries use out-of-pocket payment, 21.5% tax based, 22.3% social insurance, 14.9% private insurance and 5.0% external grants. Out-of-pocket payment is the second most used method of financing mental health care in 40.0% of countries in the African Region, 25.0% of countries in the Region of the Americas, 57.1% of countries in the Eastern Mediterranean Region, 28.9% of countries in the European Region, 50.0% of countries in the South-East Asia Region and 37.5% of countries in the Western Pacific Region. Social insurance, as the second most important method of financing is used by 40.0% of countries in the Region of the Americas and more than 25.0% of countries in the European and Western Pacific Regions. Importantly, 16.0% of countries in the African Region report using social insurance as the second most common method of financing mental health. In the South-East Asia Region, no country uses social insurance to finance mental health care, not even as the second most common method of financing.

The methods of financing across different income groups also vary.

35. Primary method of financing* mental health care in each income group of countries

Income Group of Countries**	Mode of finance	Most common method of financing Countries (%) a)	Second most common method of financing Countries (%) b)
Low	Out-of-pocket payment	42.9	35.5
	Tax Based	50.0	32.3
	Social insurance	0	16.1
	Private insurance	3.6	3.2
	External Grants	3.6	12.9
Lower Middle	Out-of-pocket payment	16.0	37.1
	Tax Based	72.0	8.6
	Social insurance	8.0	31.4
	Private insurance	0	17.1
	External Grants	4.0	5.7
Higher Middle	Out-of-pocket payment	0	39.1
	Tax Based	63.6	26.1
	Social insurance	30.3	17.4
	Private insurance	0	17.4
	External Grants	6.1	0
High	Out-of-pocket payment	0	32.3
	Tax Based	64.9	22.6
	Social insurance	32.4	22.6
	Private insurance	2.7	22.6
	External Grants	0	0

a) N = 176 b) N = 120 *based on information provided by countries **World Bank, 2004

Across different income groups, tax based care is the primary method of financing mental health in all countries irrespective of their income. Out-of-pocket payment is the primary method in 42.9% of low income countries compared to none in the higher middle income and high income countries. Social insurance is the primary method in 32.4% of high income countries, 30.3% of higher middle income countries and 8% of lower middle income countries. No low income country uses social insurance as its primary method of financing mental health care. Private insurance and external grants are used by a limited number of countries.

Across different income groups, out-of-pocket payment is the second most important financing method in 35.5% of low income countries, 37.1% of lower middle income countries, 39.1% of higher middle income countries and 32.3% of high income countries. Taxes are an important secondary method of financing in 32.3% of low income countries, 8.6% of lower middle income countries, 26.1% of higher middle income countries and 22.6% of high income countries. Social insurance is an important secondary financing method in only 16.1% of low income countries. Private insurance is the second most important method in 22.6% of countries belonging to the high income group and more than 17% of countries belonging to the middle income groups.

The most relevant point to emerge is that although tax based financing is the most important method of financing in the mental health sector, out-of-pocket payment is also a major method of financing. The latter is considered to be an unsatisfactory method for financing mental health care. Unfortunately, it is a common method in low income countries and in some of the poorest Regions of the world – the African, Eastern Mediterranean and South-East Asia Regions. Social insurance and private insurance is more important in the European Region and high income countries. Insurance plays almost no part in financing mental health care in the South-East Asia Region and a minimal part in the Regions of Africa and Western-Pacific. In the Region of the Americas, although tax based financing is the most important, out-of-pocket payment and both social and private insurance are also important methods of financing mental health care.

The information on the sources of financing for mental health care as presented here has several limitations and should be considered both preliminary and indicative. It is derived only from governmental sources, pertains only to the 'most important' method of financing and is not supported at present by actual numbers. Although working definitions of the terms used were provided, it is possible that some countries may not have used them accurately when providing information. Since mental health financing is a relatively new area of investigation most countries do not have the information required to accurately provide data on this. The ratings provided are the estimates of the respondents and are at best approximations. They are not based on available statistics. There is also a lack of information about the proportion of each category of financing for mental health care. This is because this project only sought information ranked by order of importance on each source of financing. It is hoped that in future as countries become more aware of this issue, more accurate and definitive information on mental health financing sources will be available.

MENTAL HEALTH IN PRIMARY CARE AND TRAINING

Definitions

- *Mental health in primary care:* the provision of basic preventive and curative mental health at the first level of the health care system. Usually this means that care is provided by a non-specialist who can refer complex cases to a more specialized mental health professional.
- *Training of primary care personnel:* the provision of essential knowledge and skills in identification, prevention and care of mental disorders to primary health care personnel.

36. Presence of mental health care facilities and treatment facilities for severe mental disorders in primary care in each WHO Region and the world

WHO Regions	Presence of Mental Health Care in Primary Care (%)*	Presence of Treatment Facilities for Severe Mental Disorders in Primary Care (%)**
Africa	82.6	60.9
Americas	93.9	62.5
Eastern Mediterranean	81.8	63.6
Europe	96.1	68.6
South-East Asia	80.0	44.4
Western Pacific	77.8	51.9
World	87.3	61.5

*N = 189 **N = 187

37. Presence of mental health care facilities and treatment facilities for severe mental disorders in each income group of countries

Income Group of Countries*	Presence of Mental Health Care in Primary Care (%)*	Presence of Treatment Facilities for Severe Mental Disorders in Primary Care (%)**
Low	76.3	55.2
Lower Middle	87.0	44.4
Higher Middle	100	72.7
High	97.4	86.8

*World Bank, 2004 **N = 185 ***N = 183

Mental health facilities at primary level are reported to be present in 87.3% of countries and to cover 96.5% of the world's population. However, in actual fact, the population coverage is lower, as primary care services are not distributed evenly across all countries. They are available in more than 77% of countries in the Eastern Mediterranean and Western Pacific Regions and in around 95% of countries in the Americas and European Region. Across income groups they are present in 76.3% of low income countries and 97.4% of high income countries.

In a separate question, respondents were asked about the availability of treatment facilities for severe mental disorders in primary care settings. These were reported to be available in only 61.5% of countries in the world covering 52.8% of the population. The actual population coverage is in fact lower since it is not uniform. Such facilities are available in only 44.4% of countries in the South-East Asia Region. Even in the Regions of Europe and Americas, they are available in only 68.8% and 62.5% of countries. Across different income groups they are available in 55.2% of low income countries, 44.4% of lower middle income countries and 86.8% of high income countries.

38. Presence of training facilities for primary care personnel in mental health in each WHO Region and the world

WHO Regions	Countries (%)
Africa	58.7
Americas	27.3
Eastern Mediterranean	81.8
Europe	68.8
South-East Asia	90.0
Western Pacific	55.6
World	59.7

N = 186

It is not sufficient to have an infrastructure for mental health care at the primary level without having adequately trained staff to detect mental health problems and manage them effectively. In the world, 59.7% of countries have some training facilities for primary care personnel in the field of mental health. Whereas 90.0% of countries of the South-East Asia Region have some training facilities, the same are available in only 27.3% of countries in the Region of the Americas.

39. Presence of training facilities for primary care personnel in mental health in each income group of countries

Income Group of Countries*	Countries (%)
Low	60.3
Lower Middle	61.1
Higher Middle	55.9
High	66.7

N = 182 *World Bank, 2004

Training facilities are available in 60.3% of low income countries and 66.7% of high income countries.

A Kruskal-Wallis one way ANOVA revealed that there was a significant relationship between the presence of primary care activities in mental health and the number of psychiatrists (χ^2= 22.8, p<0.01) and the number of psychiatric nurses (χ^2= 19.7, p<0.01). Primary care treatment facilities for mental disorders also showed a significant relationship with the number health professionals, psychiatric nurses (χ^2= 7.3, p<0.05), psychologists (χ^2= 10.7, p<0.01) and social workers (χ^2= 4.1, p<0.01). In all cases there were a greater number of professionals when primary health care and treatment facilities were available.

Although a large number of countries have reported mental health as an integral part of primary care level, the actual implementation of this at ground level is highly uneven. Often the facilities are restricted to particular areas where specific projects are in place and do not extend to the whole country. Treatment facilities for severe mental disorders in primary care settings across different countries also vary greatly. The quality of care provided was not ascertained through this exercise. More information is required about the different personnel involved in the primary care of psychiatric patients. Whereas in some countries primary care is essentially provided by medical assistants, nurses or other primary care workers, in other countries it is provided by primary care doctors. Training also varies across countries. While some have regular and more comprehensive programmes for different types of personnel, others do not. The data, however, do not reflect these differences in quality and coverage of training activities. Some countries might not have reported having regular training facilities for primary care workers because the latter may have been trained in mental health before their job placements or there may be local facilities for training.

PSYCHIATRIC BEDS

Definition

- *Psychiatric bed:* bed maintained for continuous use by patients with mental disorders. These beds are located in public and private psychiatric hospitals, general hospitals and hospitals for the elderly and children.

The mean number of psychiatric beds in the world per 10 000 population is 4.36 (standard deviation (S.D.) 5.47, median 1.6).

40. Median number of psychiatric beds per 10 000 population in each WHO Region and the world

WHO Regions	Median per 10 000 population
Africa	0.34
Americas	2.60
Eastern Mediterranean	1.07
Europe	8.00
South-East Asia	0.33
Western Pacific	1.06
World	1.69

N = 185

The median figures per 10 000 population vary from 0.33 in the South-East Asia Region to 8.00 in the European Region.

41. Median number of psychiatric beds per 10 000 population in each income group of countries

Income Group of Countries*	Median per 10 000 population
Low	0.24
Lower Middle	1.59
Higher Middle	7.70
High	7.50

N = 181 *World Bank, 2004

The distribution of psychiatric beds across different income countries also varies. The mean and median figures per 10 000 population in low income countries are 0.68 and 0.24, respectively, compared with 8.94 and 7.50, respectively, in high income countries.

There are approximately 1.84 million psychiatric beds in the world and 68.6% of them are in mental hospitals.

42. Approximate proportion of psychiatric beds in different settings in each WHO Region and the world*

WHO Regions	Mental Hospitals (%)	General Hospitals (%)
Africa	73.0	21.4
Americas	80.6	10.3
Eastern Mediterranean	83.0	8.8
Europe	63.5	21.8
South-East Asia	82.7	11.2
Western Pacific	60.1	34.5
World	68.6	19.8

* Other beds may be located in private and military hospitals, hospitals for special groups of population, long-term rehabilitation centres, etc.

Across different Regions, South-East Asia has 82.7% of its psychiatric beds in mental hospitals compared with 63.5% in the European Region. In the Region of the Americas 80.6% of the psychiatric beds are in mental hospitals. The Western Pacific Region has the highest proportion of psychiatric beds in general hospitals (34.5%), followed by Europe with 21.8% of their total psychiatric beds in general hospitals. The Americas have 10.3% of their total psychiatric beds in settings other than mental or general hospitals. These include military hospitals, private set-ups, long-term rehabilitation centres, among others.

43. Approximate proportion of psychiatric beds in mental hospitals in each income group of countries

Income Group of Countries*	Mental Hospitals (%)
Low	74.4
Lower Middle	82.7
Higher Middle	78.8
High	55.0

N = 173 *World Bank, 2004

In low income countries 74.4% of the beds are in mental hospitals. Even, in high income countries the figure is 55.0%.

44. Distribution of psychiatric beds per 10 000 population in each WHO Region and the world.

WHO Regions	Psychiatric Beds per 10 000 population in each category – countries % (Population covered %)			
	0-1	1.01 – 5	5.01 – 10	>10
Africa	78.3 (83.0)	17.4 (17.0)	4.3 (0.0)	–
Americas	29.0 (22.9)	29.0 (29.8)	16.1 (42.7)	25.8 (3.8)
Eastern Mediterranean	50.0 (58.8)	40.9 (40.0)	9.1 (1.2)	–
Europe	–	25.5 (25.7)	49.0 (45.0)	25.5 (29.3)
South-East Asia	75.0 (94.9)	25.0 (5.1)	–	–
Western Pacific	48.1 (10.8)	37.0 (78.3)	7.4 (0.4)	7.4 (10.1)
World	40.5 (44.7)	27.6 (35.8)	19.5 (12.0)	12.4 (7.5)

N = 185

In 40.5% of countries covering 44.7% of the population there is less than one psychiatric bed per 10 000 of the population. In the South-East Asia Region 94.9% of the population has access to less than one bed per 10 000 population. In the Regions of Africa and the Western Pacific, 83.0% and 10.8% of the population, respectively, have access to less than one bed per 10 000 population. In the European Region 25.7% of the population has access to less than 5 psychiatric beds per 10 000 population.

45. Distribution of psychiatric beds per 10 000 population in each income group of countries

Income Group of Countries*	Psychiatric beds per 10 000 population in each category – countries % (Population covered %)			
	0-1	1.01 – 5	5.01 – 10	>10
Low	84.5 (96.0)	12.1 (3.8)	3.4 (0.5)	–
Lower Middle	34.6 (17.3)	44.2 (72.7)	19.2 (4.7)	1.9 (5.5)
Higher middle	12.1 (32.1)	27.3 (28.6)	30.3 (32.1)	30.3 (5.4)
High	2.6 (0)	28.9 (14.0)	36.8 (53.3)	31.6 (33.7)

N = 181 *World Bank, 2004

In 84.5% of low income countries covering a population 96.0%, there is less than one psychiatric bed per 10 000 population. In high income countries more than 10.0% of the population has access to less than 5 psychiatric beds per 10 000 population.

A Kruskal-Wallis one way ANOVA revealed that there was a significant relationship between income groups and the number of psychiatric beds (χ^2=79.1, p<0.01). Countries in the high income group also had the highest number of available beds.

There are some limitations in the data for psychiatric beds. The number of beds reported in general hospital settings, private hospital settings or other settings may be incomplete for some countries due to the absence of definite data. The category of 'other beds', includes beds in private hospitals, military hospitals, hospitals for special populations and long-term rehabilitation centres. No information was available on beds in chronic care versus acute care. Some countries may also have reported beds allocated for neurology within the category of psychiatric beds. Information on the distribution of beds in rural and urban settings or for the number of beds for adult, geriatric and child psychiatry is also not available.

PROFESSIONALS

46. Mental health and related professionals per 100 000 population in the world

Professionals	Mean	Median	Standard Deviation (SD)
Psychiatrists	4.15	1.2	6.07
Psychiatric Nurses	12.97	2.0	26.17
Neurologists	2.13	0.3	3.74
Neurosurgeons	0.58	0.2	1.26
Psychologists working in mental health	7.35	0.6	18.1
Social Workers working in mental health	11.58	0.4	44.96

From the table above it is obvious that not only is there a shortage in the number of professionals in the world as a whole, but there is also a wide variation in the number of professionals among different WHO Regions with the Regions of Africa, South-East Asia and Eastern Mediterranean, especially, lacking adequate numbers of different mental health professionals.

PSYCHIATRISTS

Definition

- *Psychiatrist:* a medical doctor who has had at least two years of post-graduate training in psychiatry at a recognized teaching institution. This period may include training in any sub-speciality of psychiatry.

47. Median number of psychiatrists per 100 000 population in each WHO Region and the world

WHO Regions	Median per 100 000 population
Africa	0.04
Americas	2.00
Eastern Mediterranean	0.95
Europe	9.80
South-East Asia	0.20
Western Pacific	0.32
World	1.20

N = 187

The median number of psychiatrists per 100 000 population varies from 0.04 in the African Region to 9.80 in the European Region.

48. Median number of psychiatrists per 100 000 population in each income group of countries

Income Group of Countries*	Median per 100 000 population
Low	0.05
Lower Middle	1.05
Higher Middle	2.70
High	10.50

N = 183 *World Bank 2004

The median figure for low income countries is 0.05 per 100 000 population and that in the high income countries is 10.50 per 100 000 population.

There are approximately 1 800 psychiatrists for 702 million people in the African Region compared to more than 89 000 psychiatrists for 879 million people in the European Region.

49. Distribution of psychiatrists per 100 000 population in each WHO Region and the world

WHO Regions	Psychiatrists per 100 000 population in each category – countries % (Population covered %)			
	0-1	1.01 – 5	5.01 – 10	>10
Africa	89.1 (83.8)	10.9 (16.2)	–	–
Americas	28.1 (5.1)	53.1 (47.5)	3.1 (1.5)	15.6 (46.0)
Eastern Mediterranean	54.5 (78.3)	45.5 (22.9)	–	–
Europe	2.0 (7.9)	23.5 (15.1)	31.4 (25.2)	43.1 (51.1)
South-East Asia	100 (100)	–	–	–
Western Pacific	66.7 (12.4)	22.2 (78.5)	7.4 (7.6)	3.7 (1.1)
World	47.6 (46.5)	27.3 (34.0)	10.2 (5.8)	15.0 (13.7)

N = 187

In 47.6% of countries covering 46.5% of the world's population there is less than one psychiatrist per 100 000 population. All countries in the South-East Asia Region and 89.1% of countries (covering 83.8% of the population) in the African region have less than one psychiatrist per 100 000 population.

50. Distribution of psychiatrists per 100 000 population in each income group of countries

Income Groups	Psychiatrists per 100 000 population in each category – countries % (Population covered %)			
	0-1	1.01 – 5	5.01 – 10	>10
Low	87.9 (96.5)	10.3 (3.3)	1.7 (0.3)	–
Lower Middle	50.0 (23.4)	35.2 (66.7)	11.1 (3.3)	3.7 (5.6)
Higher middle	24.2 (10.7)	39.4 (44.6)	15.2 (17.9)	21.2 (26.8)
High	–	31.6 (12.1)	18.4 (22.1)	50.0 (65.8)

N = 183

In low income countries, 87.9% of the countries covering 96.5% of the population, have less than one psychiatrist per 100 000 population. Even when available, most psychiatrists are based in large cities and large populations living in rural areas have no access to them.

The data on the number of psychiatrists have certain limitations. Some countries were unable to provide an accurate number of psychiatrists, especially those working in the private sector. Since the source of information in some countries was the national association of psychiatrists, it is possible that psychiatrists who are not members of these associations have not been included. The distribution of psychiatrists within countries is also very uneven with the majority concentrated in urban areas. This distribution creates even greater disparity in their availability than is apparent from the average figures. There are also regional differences in the availability of psychiatrists within a country and this is not reflected in the data.

PSYCHIATRIC NURSES

Definition

- *Psychiatric nurse:* a graduate of a recognized, university-level nursing school with a specialization in mental health. Psychiatric nurses are registered with the local nursing board (or equivalent) and work in a mental health care setting.

51. Median number of psychiatric nurses per 100 000 population in each WHO Region and the world

WHO Regions	Median per 100 000 population
Africa	0.20
Americas	2.60
Eastern Mediterranean	1.25
Europe	24.8
South-East Asia	0.10
Western Pacific	0.50
World	2.00

N = 176

The median number of psychiatric nurses per 100 000 population varies from 0.10 in the South-East Asia Region to 24.8 in the European Region.

52. Median number of psychiatric nurses per 100 000 population in each income group of countries

Income Group of Countries*	Median per 100 000 population
Low	0.16
Lower Middle	1.05
Higher Middle	5.35
High	32.95

N = 172 *World Bank, 2004

Low income countries have a median of 0.16 per 100 000 population, whereas in high income countries the value is 32.95 per 100 000 population.

The Eastern Mediterranean Region has about 6 500 psychiatric nurses for 527 million people, compared with the European Region which has approximately 353 000 psychiatric nurses for 879 million people.

53. Distribution of psychiatric nurses per 100 000 population in each WHO Region and the world

WHO Regions	Psychiatric nurses per 100 000 population in each category – countries % (Population covered %)			
	0-1	1.01 – 10	10.01 – 50	>50
Africa	68.9 (48.7)	31.1 (52.1)	–	–
Americas	40.7 (29.8)	37.0 (63.8)	18.5 (6.4)	3.7 (0.1)
Eastern Mediterranean	50.0 (71.6)	31.8 (27.3)	18.2 (1.1)	–
Europe	6.5 (0.7)	23.9 (23.4)	52.2 (48.2)	17.4 (27.7)
South-East Asia	77.8 (94.8)	22.2 (5.2)	–	–
Western Pacific	63.0 (12.1)	18.5 (76.2)	7.4 (3.1)	11.1 (8.6)
World	45.5 (44.0)	27.8 (41.2)	19.9 (8.4)	6.8 (6.4)

N = 176

In the South-East Asia and Eastern Mediterranean Regions 77.8% and 50.0% of the population, respectively, have access to less than one psychiatric nurse per 100 000 population.

54. Distribution of psychiatric nurses per 100 000 population in each income group of countries

Income Group of Countries*	Psychiatric nurses per 100 000 population in each category – countries % (Population covered %)			
	0-1	1.01 – 10	10.01 – 50	>50
Low	75.9 (85.9)	20.7 (13.9)	3.4 (0.5)	–
Lower Middle	50.0 (20.1)	35.4 (71.1)	14.6 (8.8)	–
Higher middle	23.3 (51.1)	43.3 (21.3)	30.0 (29.8)	3.3 (0.1)
High	5.6 (0.1)	16.7 (37.8)	47.2 (21.2)	30.6 (41.0)

N = 172 *World Bank, 2004

In 75.9% of low income countries (covering 85.9% of population) there is less than one psychiatric nurse per 100 000 population. Almost 25% of the population in high middle income countries has less than 10 psychiatric nurses per 100 000 population.

55. Comparison of mean number of psychiatrists to psychiatric nurses per 100 000 population in each WHO Region and the world

WHO Regions	Mean number of Psychiatrists per 100 000 population	Mean number of Psychiatric Nurses per 100 000 population
Africa	0.26	1.54
Americas	4.54	9.27
Eastern Mediterranean	1.41	6.22
Europe	10.49	34.49
South-East Asia	0.25	0.71
Western Pacific	1.89	8.65
World	4.15	12.97

The ratio of psychiatrists to psychiatric nurses in the Americas is 1:2, compared with a ratio of 1:5 in the Regions of Africa and Western Pacific.

Many of the limitations of the data on psychiatric nurses are similar to those for psychiatrists. However, there are some more specific limitations for this data. The total number of psychiatric nurses in some countries may actually be less as some countries may have reported general nurses, who work in psychiatric facilities, as psychiatric nurses, even though they may not have psychiatric nursing training. Some countries were unable to provide data on psychiatric nurses as they do not have a separate register for different categories of nurses. To expand the information base on the role of nurses in mental health care, WHO is at present collecting information from all countries under a new project- Atlas-Nursing.

NEUROLOGISTS & NEUROSURGEONS

Definitions

- *Neurologist:* a medical doctor who has at least two years of post-graduate training in neurology at a recognized teaching institution.
- *Neurosurgeon:* a medical doctor who has at least two years of post-graduate training in neurosurgery at a recognized teaching institution.

56. Median number of neurologists and neurosurgeons per 100 000 population in each WHO Region and the world

WHO Regions	Median number of neurologists* per 100 000 population	Median number of neurosurgeons** per 100 000 population
Africa	0.02	0.01
Americas	0.70	0.40
Eastern Mediterranean	0.30	0.20
Europe	4.00	1.00
South-East Asia	0.05	0.03
Western Pacific***	0.00	0.00
World	0.30	0.20

*N = 168 **N = 167 ***the median numbers for the Western Pacific Region are 0 as a number of the smaller countries do not have these professionals

In the Western Pacific Region the median number of neurologists or neurosurgeons per 100 000 population are both zero, because many Pacific islands in this Region do not have any neurologists or neurosurgeons. The mean figures for this Region are 0.67 per 100 000 population (neurologists) and 0.43 per 100 000 population (neurosurgeons). The median figures are also low in the African Region (0.02 neurologists and 0.01 neurosurgeons per 100 000 population) and in the South-East Asia Region (0.05 neurologists and 0.3 neurosurgeons per 100 000 population for both groups of professionals). Even in the European Region which has the highest number of these professionals, the median figures per 100 000 population for neurologists and neurosurgeons are 4.00 and 1.00, respectively.

57. Median number of neurologists and neurosurgeons per 100 000 population in each income group of countries

Income Group of Countries*	Median number of neurologists**per 100 000 population	Median number of neurosurgeons*** per 100 000 population
Low	0.02	0.01
Lower Middle	0.35	0.25
Higher Middle	0.95	0.60
High	3.00	0.90

*World Bank, 2000 **N = 164 ***N = 163

The median figures per 100 000 population in low income countries are 0.02 (neurologists) and 0.01 (neurosurgeons). The corresponding figures for high income countries are 3.00(neurologists) and 0.90 (neurosurgeons).

58. Distribution of neurologists per 100 000 population in each WHO Region and the world

WHO Regions	Neurologists per 100 000 population in each category – countries % (Population covered %)			
	0-0.1	0.11 – 1	1.01 – 5	>5
Africa	88.9 (88.3)	11.1 (11.7)	–	–
Americas	15.8 (2.3)	57.9 (11.4)	21.1 (86.4)	5.3 (0.1)
Eastern Mediterranean	31.6 (26.1)	57.9 (72.7)	10.5 (1.1)	–
Europe	–	16.3 (20.8)	38.8 (50.0)	44.9 (29.2)
South-East Asia	88.9 (96.4)	11.1 (4.0)	–	–
Western Pacific	63.0 (3.0)	14.8 (85.8)	18.5 (11.8)	3.7 (0.1)
World	44.0 (40.5)	23.8 (37.8)	17.9 (17.7)	14.3 (3.9)

N = 168

All countries in the African and South-East Asia Regions have less than one neurologist per 100 000 population.

59. Distribution of neurosurgeons per 100 000 population in each WHO Region and the world

WHO Regions	Neurosurgeons per 100 000 population in each category – countries % (Population covered %)			
	0-0.1	0.11 – 0.5	0.51 – 1	>1
Africa	88.9 (88.4)	8.9 (11.6)	2.2 (0.1)	–
Americas	14.3 (0.1)	38.1 (7.9)	23.8 (3.4)	23.8 (87.6)
Eastern Mediterranean	26.3 (20.5)	52.6 (75.0)	15.8 (4.6)	5.3 (0.1)
Europe	10.9 (0.8)	6.5 (2.5)	47.8 (45.9)	34.8 (50.8)
South-East Asia	77.8 (96.1)	22.2 (3.9)	–	–
Western Pacific	70.4 (12.3)	11.1 (0.7)	11.1 (76.7)	7.4.0 (10)
World	47.3 (43.3)	18.0 (10.3)	20.4 (29.3)	14.4 (17.1)

N = 167

All countries in the Regions of Africa and South-East Asia have less than one neurosurgeon per 100 000 population. More than 90% of countries in the Western Pacific and Eastern Mediterranean Regions also have less than one neurosurgeon.

Some of the limitations of the data on these professionals are similar to those for other professions as highlighted earlier, especially those related to urban and rural variations. Information on neurologists and neurosurgeons in the private sector may not have been reported accurately by some countries. Some countries may have reported information on neurologists and neurosurgeons based on membership figures from professional associations, thereby excluding some neurologists and neurosurgeons who are not members of those associations. More comprehensive data on neurologists and neurosurgeons is available in the WHO Atlas – Country Resources for Neurological Disorders (WHO, 2004b).

PSYCHOLOGISTS WORKING IN MENTAL HEALTH

Definition

- *Psychologist working in mental health:* a graduate from a recognized, university-level school of psychology with a specialization in clinical psychology. These psychologists are registered with the local board of psychologists (or equivalent) and work in a mental health setting.

60. Median number of psychologists working in mental health per 100 000 population in each WHO Region and the world

WHO Regions	Median per 100 000 population
Africa	0.05
Americas	2.80
Eastern Mediterranean	0.60
Europe	3.10
South-East Asia	0.03
Western Pacific	0.03
World	0.60

N = 177

The median number of psychologists per 100 000 population varies from 0.03 in the South-East Asia and Western Pacific Region to 3.10 in the European Region and 2.80 in the Region of the Americas.

61. Median number of psychologists working in mental health per 100 000 population in each income group of countries

Income Group of Countries*	Median per 100 000 population
Low	0.04
Lower Middle	0.60
Higher Middle	1.80
High	14.0

N = 173 *World Bank, 2004

The median distribution per 100 000 population in low income countries is 0.04 compared to 14.0 in high income countries.

62. Distribution of psychologists working in mental health per 100 000 population in each WHO Region and the world

WHO Regions	Psychologists working in mental health per 100 000 population in each category – countries % (Population covered %)			
	0-1	1.01 – 10	10.01 – 50	>50
Africa	91.3 (89.7)	8.7 (10.3)	–	–
Americas	32.1 (3.5)	39.3 (10.6)	25.0 (80.3)	3.6 (5.6)
Eastern Mediterranean	72.7 (80.9)	22.7 (19.1)	4.5 (0.1)	–
Europe	26.1 (24.2)	39.1 (56.7)	19.6 (6.2)	15.2 (12.4)
South-East Asia	88.9 (99.9)	11.1 (0.1)	–	–
Western Pacific	84.6 (63.6)	11.5 (35.2)	3.8 (1.1)	–
World	61.6 (66.0)	23.7 (18.4)	10.2 (12.6)	4.5 (3.0)

N = 187

In the world there is less than one psychologist per 100 000 population in 61.6% of countries, accounting for 66.0% of the world's population. Almost the entire population of the South-East Asia Region and 89.7% of the population of the African Region have access to less than one psychologist per 100 000 population.

63. Distribution of psychologists per 100 000 population in each income group of countries

Income Group of Countries*	Psychologists per 100 000 population in each category – countries % (Population covered %)			
	0-1	1.01 – 10	10.01 – 50	>50
Low	91.4 (97.5)	8.6 (2.5)	–	–
Lower Middle	69.4 (58.3)	24.5 (26.5)	6.1 (15.2)	–
Higher Middle	44.8 (28.9)	44.8 (44.4)	6.9 (8.9)	3.4 (17.8)
High	13.5 (6.2)	32.4 (41.2)	35.1 (41.8)	18.9 (11.3)

N = 183 *World Bank, 2004

Among low income countries almost all the population has access to less than one psychologist per 100 000. The number of psychologists actually working in the field of mental health may be less than that reported by countries as some may have included in their figures psychologists working in all health and related sectors.

As with psychiatrists, some of the limitations of the data on psychologists are similar. However, there are some additional limitations. Although the definition of 'psychologist' was provided to countries, some countries may have used a wider definition that includes all psychologists in the country and not simply those working in mental health settings. Information from some countries could not be analysed as they were unable to provide the specific number of psychologists working in mental health out of the total number of psychologists in the country. No information is available on the number of psychologists working in psycho-diagnostics or in therapeutics or rehabilitation settings.

SOCIAL WORKERS WORKING IN MENTAL HEALTH

Definition

- *Social workers working in mental health:* a graduate from a recognized, university-level school of social work, registered with the local board of social workers (or equivalent) and working in a mental health setting.

64. Median number of social workers working in mental health per 100 000 population in each WHO Region and the world

WHO Regions	Median per 100 000 population
Africa	0.05
Americas	1.00
Eastern Mediterranean	0.40
Europe	1.50
South-East Asia	0.04
Western Pacific	0.05
World	0.40

N = 161

The median number of social workers working in mental health per 100 000 population varies from 0.04 in the South-East Asian Region to 1.50 in the European Region.

65. Median number of social workers working in mental health per 100 000 population in each income group of countries

Income Group of Countries*	Median per 100 000 population
Low	0.04
Lower Middle	0.28
Higher Middle	1.50
High	15.70

N = 157 *World Bank, 2004

The median figures per 100 000 population are 0.04 in low income countries and 15.70 in high income countries.

66. Distribution of social workers working in mental health per 100 000 population in each WHO Region and the world

WHO Regions	Social workers working in mental health per 100 000 population in each category – countries % (Population covered %)			
	0-1	1.01 – 10	10.01 – 50	>50
Africa	82.2 (87.6)	13.3 (5.8)	4.4 (6.6)	–
Americas	52.2 (32.6)	30.4 (3.2)	13.0 (63.2)	4.3 (1.0)
Eastern Mediterranean	61.9 (91.0)	33.3 (9.0)	4.8 (0.1)	–
Europe	45.9 (38.5)	18.9 (33.3)	8.1 (0.8)	27.0 (28.2)
South-East Asia	88.9 (86.0)	11.1 (13.6)	–	–
Western Pacific	61.5 (83.6)	30.8 (4.4)	7.7 (12.0)	–
World	64.0 (75.4)	22.4 (10.8)	6.8 (10.5)	6.8 (3.3)

N = 168

In about 64.0% of countries, accounting for about 75.4% of the world's population, there is less than one social worker per 100 000 population. In the African and Eastern Mediterranean Regions more than 85% of the population has access to less than one social worker per 100 000 population, compared to 52.2% of the population in the Americas. Even in Europe, 45.9% of the population has less than one social worker per 100 000 population.

67. Distribution of social workers per 100 000 population in each income group of countries

Income Group of Countries*	Social workers per 100 000 population in each category – countries % (Population covered %)			
	0-1	1.01 – 10	10.01 – 50	>50
Low	92.7 (98.2)	7.3 (1.8)	–	–
Lower Middle	75.0 (78.6)	18.2 (15.8)	6.8 (5.8)	–
Higher Middle	44.4 (67.9)	44.4 (18.9)	7.4 (13.2)	3.7 (1.9)
High	9.7 (0.7)	38.7 (20.0)	19.4 (54.8)	32.3 (24.4)

N = 164 *World Bank, 2004

In low income countries 92.7% of the population has less than one social worker per 100 000 population. In high income countries 38.7% of the population has less than 10 social workers per 100 000.

One of the primary limitations of this data was the interpretation of the definition by different countries. Some countries may have reported social workers working in any health department, although the glossary definition specified that they should be working in a mental health setting. This may have led to over-reporting of social workers in the mental health sector. Information from some countries could not be analysed as they were unable to provide the specific number of social workers working in mental health as a proportion of the total number of social workers in the country. No information is available on the number of social workers in the different mental health settings, e.g. inpatient, outpatient and community services or rural-urban settings.

PROGRAMMES FOR SPECIAL POPULATIONS AND NGOS

Definitions

- *Programmes for special populations:* programmes that address the mental health concerns, including social integration, of the most vulnerable and disorder-prone groups of population such as refugees, people affected by natural and man-made disasters, indigenous people and minorities. Special populations also include people who need special care such as the elderly and children.
- *Non-governmental organizations (NGOs):* voluntary organizations, charitable groups, service-user or advocacy groups, or professional associations.

68. Presence of mental health programmes for special populations in the world

Mental Health Programmes for Special Populations	Countries (%)
Minority Groups	16.5
Refugees	26.2
Disaster Affected Populations	37.7
Indigenous People	14.8
Elderly Persons	50.5
Children	62.4

N = 182–186

Programmes for indigenous people are to be found in 14.8% of countries, programmes for minority groups in 16.5%, programmes for refugees in 26.2%, programmes for disaster-affected populations in 37.7%, programmes for elderly persons in 50.5% and programmes for children in 62.4% of countries.

69. Regional distribution of mental health programmes for children in comparison to the percentage of child population in each WHO Region and the world.

WHO Regions	Countries* (%)	0-14 years population (%)
Africa	37.0	42.6
Americas	81.3	30.4
Eastern Mediterranean	72.7	34.6
Europe	77.6	19.1
South-East Asia	54.5	32.8
Western Pacific	50.0	32.9
World	62.4	31.3

*N = 186

With 42.6% of its population made up of children below 14 years, the African Region only has programmes for children in 37.0% countries, compared to the European Region where 77.6% of countries have a programme. In the European Region, children below the age of 14 years account for 19.1% of the total population. Programmes for children are also limited in the Western Pacific Region where only 50.0% of countries have such programmes.

70. Availability of mental health programmes for children in each income group of countries.

Income Group of Countries*	Countries (%)
Low	34.5
Lower Middle	73.6
Higher Middle	72.7
High	86.8

N = 182 *World Bank, 2004

Whereas 86.8% of high income countries have a programme, only 34.5% of low income countries have one. Additional information on mental health services for children and adolescents will be available in the Atlas-Child and Adolescents being developed by WHO.

71. Regional distribution of mental health programmes for the elderly in comparison with the percentage of elderly population in each WHO Region and the world.

WHO Regions	Countries* (%)	60+ years population (%)
Africa	15.6	5.0
Americas	77.4	9.0
Eastern Mediterranean	54.5	5.6
Europe	63.3	17.8
South-East Asia	54.5	7.3
Western Pacific	50.0	8.1
World	50.5	9.8

*N = 184

Programmes for the elderly are found in even fewer countries. They range from being present in 15.6% of countries in the African Region and 50.0% of countries in the Western Pacific Region, to being present in 77.4% of countries in the Region of the Americas.

72. Availability of mental health programmes for the elderly in each income group of countries.

Income Group of Countries*	Countries (%)
Low	17.9
Lower Middle	50.9
Higher Middle	66.7
High	89.5

N = 180 *World Bank, 2004

Programmes for the elderly are present in 89.5% of high income countries and in only 17.9% of low income countries.

73. Presence of NGO activity in mental health in each WHO Region and the world

WHO Regions	Countries (%)
Africa	89.1
Americas	90.9
Eastern Mediterranean	85.0
Europe	92.0
South-East Asia	90.9
Western Pacific	77.8
World	88.2

N = 187

NGOs are involved in the mental health sector in 88.2% of countries across the world. Across the Regions, availability varies from 77.8% in countries in the Western Pacific Region to 92.0% in the European Region.

74. Presence of NGO activity in mental health in each income group of countries.

Income Group of Countries*	Countries (%)
Low	84.7
Lower Middle	87.0
Higher Middle	93.9
High	91.9

N = 183 *World Bank, 2004

Across the different income groups the figure varies from 84.7% in the low-income countries to 93.9% in the high-income countries.

Among the various activities carried out by NGOs in different countries, advocacy is carried out in 80.5% of countries, promotion in 79.9% of countries, prevention in 74.2% of countries, treatment in 52.2% of countries and rehabilitation in 82.4% of countries.

Although many countries reported the existence of specific programmes, information on the type and quality of the programmes is not available. Some countries may not have specific programmes, but do have psychiatric facilities catering for special groups. Some countries may have had problems in interpreting the definition of special programmes for sub-populations as they differed from those in their own country. Some countries also had difficulty identifying sub-populations present within their country. Information is also lacking about the degree of implementation of the different programmes when available. Although many countries have reported NGO activities in mental health, it is not clear to what extent they cover the population. Information on the quality and coverage of services of NGOs is lacking. Some of the NGOs mentioned are actually international NGOs working in countries and not necessarily local NGOs.

MENTAL HEALTH INFORMATION GATHERING SYSTEMS

Definitions

- *Annual reporting system:* the preparation of information covering health and health services functions and the use of allocated funds for each year by the Government.
- *Information/data collection system:* an organized information gathering activity for service data. It usually incorporates patient admission or discharge rates, outpatient contacts, community contacts and patients subject to mental health legislation.
- *Epidemiological studies:* research studies focusing on extent and nature of mental disorders.

75. Presence of mental health reporting systems in each WHO Region and the world

WHO Regions	Countries (%)
Africa	57.8
Americas	75.8
Eastern Mediterranean	70.0
Europe	87.8
South-East Asia	100
Western Pacific	77.8
World	75.7

N = 185

Across the world, annual mental health reporting systems exist in 75.7% of countries. In the Regions of South-East Asia and Europe, 100% and 87.8% of countries, respectively have some form of annual mental health reporting system, compared with only 57.8% of countries in the African Region.

76. Presence of mental health reporting systems in each income group of countries

Income Group of Countries*	Countries (%)
Low	62.1
Lower Middle	81.5
Higher Middle	81.8
High	86.1

N = 181 *World Bank, 2004

Across income groups, 62.1% of low income countries have an annual mental health reporting system compared with 86.1% of high income countries.

77. Presence of an epidemiological study or data collection system in mental health in each WHO Region and the world

WHO Regions	Countries (%)
Africa	46.7
Americas	71.9
Eastern Mediterranean	52.4
Europe	73.5
South-East Asia	63.6
Western Pacific	51.9
World	60.5

N = 185

A data collection system or an epidemiological study exists in only 60.5% of countries world-wide. Across the different Regions, they are present in 73.5% of the European Region but only in 46.7% of the African Region. All the other Regions have figures varying between 50-70%.

78. Presence of an epidemiological study or data collection system in mental health in each income group of countries

Income Group of Countries*	Countries (%)
Low	48.3
Lower Middle	59.3
Higher Middle	75.0
High	75.7

N = 181 *World Bank, 2004

Across income groups, a data collection system or an epidemiological study is found in 48.3% of low income countries and in 75.7% of high income countries.

More specific information on epidemiology of mental disorders within low and middle income countries can be found within the individual country profiles of this volume.

Comparison of data between 2001 and 2004

A comparison of data collected in the year 2001 with that updated in 2004 would seem natural. However, this should be done only in the light of certain caveats. First, the data collection exercise on many parameters of mental health resources had not been conducted in many countries before, thus some changes in data occurred because the method of data collection improved and due to efforts into triangulation of data sources, i.e. these changes would reflect improvement in reliability of data rather than change in the actual resource base. Second, the denominator for comparisons in the two data sets (years 2001 and 2004) are different as many countries responded to queries in 2004 that they had been unable to previously and a new member state was added. On the other hand, some countries withdrew pieces of information that they felt were unreliable.

Overall, there was a slight increase in countries with a mental health policy, with a 15.5% decrease (66.7% in terms of population covered) noted in the South-East Asia Region (Table 1-3). This counterintuitive finding is related to the fact that India's National Mental Health Programme serves as a policy document at the level of the Health Ministry. India doesn't have a separate policy document with parliamentary approval. The change was due to availability of more reliable information. No major changes were noted in the figures for national mental health programme (Table 4-7). A heartening feature was that more countries were providing community mental health services (Table 8 and 9) than before. These changes were most marked in the Eastern Mediterranean Region (13.7%) and for higher middle-income countries (13.8%).

Similarly, a slight increase was noted in the number of countries with mental health legislation. This trend was more marked in the African (8.4%) and American (7.1%) Regions (Table 10-13). The figures on population covered (13.9%) in comparison to the number of countries with mental health legislation (76%) is low in the Western Pacific Region because China does not have a comprehensive mental health law; instead, laws relating to mental health issues are spread over various other laws. More countries were providing disability benefits in some form; the changes in this regard were most marked in the Eastern Mediterranean Region (10.7%) and the lower middle-income (9.5%) countries (Table 14 and 15).

No major changes occurred in the number of countries with a substance abuse policy (Table 16-19). The apparent increase in the number of countries that initiated their substance abuse policies after the 1990s is due to improvement in reliability of information due to triangulation of data.

A slight increase in the number of countries with a therapeutic drug policy or an essential drug list pertaining to psychotropics was noted. Major changes were not expected really due to the ceiling effect. Almost 90% of countries in all subgroups had such lists/ policies (Table 20-22). Paradoxically a slight decrease (up to 3.6%) seemed to have occurred in the number of countries that made psychotropics available in primary care (Table 23). This was largely due to the fact that some countries had mistakenly mentioned that these drugs were available in primary care setting in 2001, but later they reported that these psychotropics were available only in secondary/tertiary care settings. A 15.5% reduction was noted in the number of countries that made the three essential psychotropics (amitryptiline, chlorpromazine and phenytoin) available in primary care (Table 24). This composite index, suffered as a negative response to any of the three listed drugs, resulted in the overall category being labelled as negative. Some countries, particularly in the European Region mentioned that they have added newer psychotropics to their essential list of drugs to be made available in primary care and are no longer emphasizing the older generation psychotropics. However, this trend was not marked in the African Region. Changes were also noted in the cost of psychotropics (Table 25-30). This was expected because the figure on expenditure on procuring psychotropics is given in dollars and is thus subject to exchange rate fluctuations.

A slight decrease (2.8%) was noted in terms of the number of countries stating that they had a specific budget line for mental health in their health budgets (Table 31). This trend was most prominent in the American (14.5%) and Eastern Mediterranean (8.6%) Regions. On the other hand, 90% (an increase of 23.3%) South-East Asia Region countries reported that they had a specific budget for mental health. Mild alteration in ordering was observed in terms of methods of financing mental health care (for this comparison the most common and second most common methods of financing countries were combined) (Table 34 and 35). There was a decrease (5.4%) in emphasis on out-of-pocket payment and an increase (7.5%) on emphasis on tax based system in the American Region. A few countries in this region also reported that external grants were important means of financing mental health care. In the Eastern Mediterranean Region, a decrease (10.8%) in emphasis on out-of-pocket payment and an increase in emphasis on a tax based system (8.2%) was noted. In the European Region, a slight shift in emphasis from social insurance (5.2%) to private insurance (5.3%) occurred, while in the Western Pacific Region there was an increase in emphasis on out-of-pocket payment (11.2%) and social insurance (5.7%). In terms of income groups of countries, an increase in emphasis on external grants (5.8%) was noted in low-income countries; a decrease in emphasis on social insurance (8.9%) and an increase in emphasis on private insurance (8.0%) were observed in lower middle-income countries; and a decrease in emphasis on social insurance (8.3%) occurred in high-income countries.

No major changes were observed in terms of availability of mental health services in primary care in WHO regions, but an increase (5.7%) was noted in higher middle-income group of countries. More countries (13.6%) in the Eastern Mediterranean Region had made treatment for severe mental disorders available in their primary care. A similar change was observed for higher middle-income (6%) countries (Table 36-37). A 14.6% decrease in the number of countries providing regular training in mental health care to primary health care workers was noted in the American Region, largely because clarifications revealed that some countries had provided ad-hoc training in mental health to primary care workers but were not doing so on a regular basis (Table 38-39).

There was a decrease in median number of beds in regions that had high bed-to-population ratios, i.e. American (0.7 per 10 000 population) and European (0.7 per 10 000 population) Regions and an increase in regions with intermediate bed-to-population ratio, i.e. in the Eastern Mediterranean (0.28 per 10 000 population) and Western Pacific (0.08 per 10 000 population) Regions. No change was observed in regions with low bed-to-population ratio, i.e. in the African and South-East Asia Regions. In congruence with the above findings, a decrease in number of beds was noted in high-income countries (1.20 per 10 000 population), an increase in middle-income (both, higher 2.30 per 10 000 population and lower 0.19 per 10 000 population) groups of countries and no change was observed for low-income countries (Table 42-43). The availability of more reliable figures indicated that the proportion of beds in mental hospital setting had been underestimated in the 2001 data, particularly for American (33%) and Eastern Mediterranean (8.3%) Regions and the higher middle-income group of countries (12%). On the other hand, there was a decrease in proportion of mental health beds in the African (5%), European (7%) and Western Pacific (9.2%) Regions and low-income (11.7%) countries. Despite, the upward change in figures for mental hospital beds, a general trend towards an increase (3.9%) in proportion of general hospital beds to total beds was observed; this was relatively more marked for the African (8.6%), European (11.7%) and Western Pacific (11.8%) Regions. It appears that in reports submitted in 2001, some mental health beds were misclassified in the 'other' category; on the other hand, the figures for general hospital beds were more accurate. A comparison of bed-population ratios at the two time points showed that in general, there was a decrease (3.4%) in the number of countries with more than 10 beds per 10 000 population and a corresponding increase (2.6%) in the number of countries with 5 to 10 beds per 10 000 population. This largely reflected changes in European (a decrease of 13.3% in the former category and an increase of 10.2% in the latter category) and high-income (a decrease of 11.3% in the former category and an increase of 8.2% in the latter category) countries. Many countries in the American Region reported alterations in their bed-to-population ratios as a result of our efforts at triangulation of data sources. This led to an increase (6.4%) being noted in number of countries with less than one bed per 10 000 population and a corresponding decrease (6.5%) in number of countries with 1-5 beds per 10 000 population. A greater member of countries in the Western Pacific Region reported that they had 1-5 beds per 10 000 population (an increase of 7.4%). This trend was also noted for lower middle-income countries (6.5%). Low-income countries reported a decrease in bed-to-population ratios (the number of countries in the less than one bed per 10 000 population category increased by 6.2%). Higher middle-income countries reported a decrease (5%) in the number of countries with less than one bed per 10 000 population (Table 44-45).

Overall, there was an increase in the number of mental health professionals in the world (Table 46). The greatest increase was noted in the number of psychologists (increase in mean: 0.92 per 100 000 population, increase in median: 0.2 per 100 000 population) (especially in the American and to some extent in the European Regions) and social workers (increase in mean: 2.94 per 100 000 population, increase in median: 0.1 per 100 000 population) (especially in the European Region) engaged in mental health care. But, a number of countries noted that it was difficult to give accurate figures for these two groups of professionals as many psychologists and social workers were dealing with mental health issues along with many other responsibilities. Thus, the figures for these groups of mental health professionals are likely an overestimate. The South-East Asia Region showed a decrease in the number of psychiatrists (by about 40%) and psychiatric nurses (by about 60%). Availability of more accurate figures as well as migration of professionals from these to other regions could be reasons for this trend.

When the median number of psychiatrists per 100 000 population was compared it was seen that an increase had occurred on the European Regions (0.8) and in high-income countries (1.5). Overall, there was a decrease (5.1%) in the number of countries with less than one psychiatrist per 100 000 population and a corresponding increase (5.9%) in number of countries with 1-5 psychiatrists per 100 000 population. This was reflected in the situation in the African (where there was a 6.6% decrease in the former category and a 6.6% increase in the latter category) and American (where there was a 5.2% decrease in the former category and a 6.4% increase in the latter category) Regions. More European countries reported having 1-5 (5.1%), and more than 10 (6.4%) psychiatrists per 100 000 population and fewer European countries reported having 5-10 (9.4%) psychiatrists per 100 000 population. Few changes were noted for low-income countries, but a smaller proportion (12.3%) of lower middle-income countries reported having less than one psychiatrist per 100 000 population and a greater number (14.4%) reported having 1-5 psychiatrists per 100 000 population. Similarly, a lower proportion (8.2%) of higher middle-income countries reported that they had less than one psychiatrist per 100 000 population and a greater number (6.5%) reported that they had more than 10 psychiatrists per 100 000 population. Among high-income countries, more countries stated that they had 1-5 (5.9%) and fewer stated that they had 5-10 (10.2%) psychiatrists per 100 000 population (Table 47-50).

A comparison of median number of psychiatric nurses per 100 000 population revealed an increase (0.75) in the Eastern Mediterranean and a decrease in the European (2.7) and Western Pacific (0.6) Regions. A decrease was also noted for high-income countries (0.55), likely due to more accurate definitions used (Table 51-52). A greater number (13%) of Western Pacific Region countries reported that they had less than one psychiatric nurse per 100 000 population and a correspondingly fewer (16.1%) countries reported that they had 1-10 psychiatric nurses per 100 000 population. A greater number of countries in the American (5%),

Eastern Mediterranean (8%) and European (5.5%) Regions had between l and 10 psychiatric nurses per 100 000 population and fewer (5.6%) Eastern Mediterranean countries reported that they had 10-50 psychiatric nurses per 100 000 population. In South East Asia Region, Thailand moved from the category of 1-10 psychiatric nurses per 100 000 population to 10-50 psychiatric nurses per 100 000 population. More (8.7%) lower middle-income group countries reported that they had 1-10 psychiatric nurses per 100 000 population and fewer (5.4%) reported that they had 10-50 psychiatric nurses per 100 000 population. The opposite trend was noted for high-income countries, where 6.6% fewer countries reported having 1-10 and 7.2% more countries reported having 10-50 psychiatric nurses per 100 000 population (table 53-54). The ratio of mean number of psychiatric nurses to mean number of psychiatrists worsened in the South-East Asia Region from 9:1 to 3:1 due to a reduction in the mean number of psychiatric nurses (Table 55).

There was no major change in the median number of neurologists and neurosurgeons in WHO regions, but an increase was observed in the higher middle-income group of countries, where the median number of neurologists increased by 0.45 per 100 000 population (Table 56-57). In the Eastern Mediterranean Region, a greater number (7.9%) of countries reported having 0.1-1 neurologist per 100 000 population and a fewer (7.3%) countries reported having 0-0.1 neurologists per 100 000 population. Fewer (9.7%) countries in the American Region reported having 1-5 neurologists per 100 000 population and more countries (5.3%) in this region reported that they had more than 5 neurologists per 100 000 population. On the other hand, a greater number of countries in the Western Pacific Region reported that they had 1-5 neurologists per 100 000 population (Table 58). More (7.2%) countries in American Region reported having 0-0.1 neurosurgeon per 100 000 population and fewer (9.6%) countries reported that they had more than 0.5 neurosurgeon per 100 000 population (Table 59).

A comparison of median number of psychologists per 100 000 population showed an increase in the Eastern Mediterranean Region (0.4) and in higher middle-income group of countries (1.10) and a decrease in high-income (12.7) countries. The latter result probably reflects the use of tighter definition (Table 60-61). Overall, there was an increase (5.4%) in the number of countries with 1-10 psychologists per 100 000 population and a decrease (6.7%) in the number of countries with less than 1 psychologists per 100 000 population. This trend was supported by figures for the American (6% increase in the former category and a 9.6% decrease in the latter category), European (a 5% increase in the former category and a 5.6% decrease in the latter category) and Eastern Mediterranean (a 18.2% increase in the former category and a decrease of 18.2% in the latter category) Regions and the figures for low-income (a 6.9% increase in the former category and a 6.9% decrease in the latter category) and higher middle-income countries (a 13.8% increase in the former category and a 20.7% decrease in the latter category) and negated to some extent by figures for the Western Pacific Region (a 6.7% decrease in the former category and a 7.3% increase in the latter category) (Table 62-63).

The median number of social workers had decreased in the American (0.9) and European (0.85) Regions and in high-income (9.8) countries (Table 64-65). A greater number of countries in the American Region (14.1%) and in the high-income group (5.5%) reported having 0-1 social workers per 100 000 population and fewer countries in these groups reported that they had 10-50 social workers per 100 000 population (a 10.8% decrease in the American Region and a 9.8% decrease in the high-income group of countries). Similarly, more (7%) countries in the Western Pacific Region reported having 0-1 social workers per 100 000 population and fewer (5.6%) such countries stated that they had 1-10 social workers per 100 000 population. The opposite trend was seen for countries in the Eastern Mediterranean Region (a decrease of 9.5% in the former category and a 9.5% increase in the latter category). In the European Region, also fewer (5.2%) countries reported that they had 10-50 social workers per 100 000 population. Finally, more (5.2%) higher middle-income countries reported having 1-10 social workers per 100 000 population (Table 66-67).

There were no major changes in the overall pattern of services for special populations (Table 68), but there was an increase in services for children and adolescents in the countries of the American (7.1%) and Western Pacific (7.7%) Regions, while a decrease (5.5%) was noted in the South-East Asia Region. Similarly, services for children and adolescents increased in the lower middle-income (13.2%) and higher middle-income (7%) countries (Table 69-70). A similar pattern also emerged for services targeted at the elderly, where more countries in the American (9.7%) and the Western Pacific (11.5%) Regions reported that they had services for the elderly population and fewer (5.5%) countries in the South-East Asia Region reported the presence of such services. Also, a greater number of lower middle-income countries (5.6%) and higher middle-income countries (9.6%) reported the presence of such services (Table 71-72).

Few changes were also noted in the presence of non-governmental organizations (NGOs) in WHO regions. An increase occurred in the number of countries reporting the presence of NGOs in the Eastern Mediterranean (5%) and South-East Asia (10.9%) Regions (Table 73-74).

Regarding mental health reporting systems, a greater number of countries in the African (5.5%), American (8.1%) and South-East Asia (10%) Regions reported their presence, while fewer Eastern Mediterranean (5%) countries reported that they had such systems in place. An increase (9.3%) in the number of countries with such systems was noted in lower middle-income countries, but a decrease (5.1%) occurred in high-income countries (Table 75-76). Similar trends were noted for data collection system/epidemiological studies, where in a greater number of countries in the American (13.8%) and South-East Asia (13.6%) Regions and in the low- (5%), lower middle- (9.3%) and the higher middle-income (6.4%) categories reported the presence of data collection system/epidemiological study (Table 77-78).

In summary:

- Improvements in the availability of mental health resources within different countries are very small, i.e. no substantial changes can be seen between the data collected in 2001 with that updated in 2004.
- Regional imbalances have also remained largely similar. There are marked differences in the availability of mental health resources, particularly between high and low income countries.
- A modest increase can be noted with regard to the overall availability of certain mental health resources. There was an increase in countries with a mental health policy, mental health legislation and a therapeutic drug policy or essential drug list. Also, more countries are providing community mental health services and disability benefits in some form. Finally, there was an increase in the number of mental health professional in the world, with the greatest increase noted in the number of psychologists and social workers.

References

UNESCO (2004) http://www.uis.unesco.org. Accessed in December 2004. UNESCO Institute for Statistics. Montreal.

United Nations (2004) http://unstats.un.org. Accessed in December 2004. United Nations Statistics Divison. New York.

World Bank (2004) http://www.worldbank.org. Accessed in December 2004. World Bank Group. Washington D.C.

World Health Organization (2004a) The World Health Report 2004: Changing History. WHO. Geneva.

World Health Organization (2004b) Atlas: Country Resources for Neurological Disorders 2004. WHO. Geneva.

World Health Organization (2001a) The World Health Report 2001: Mental Health: New Understanding, New Hope. WHO. Geneva.

World Health Organization (2001b) Atlas: Mental Health Resources in the World 2001. WHO. Geneva. WHO/NMH/MSD/MDP/01.1.

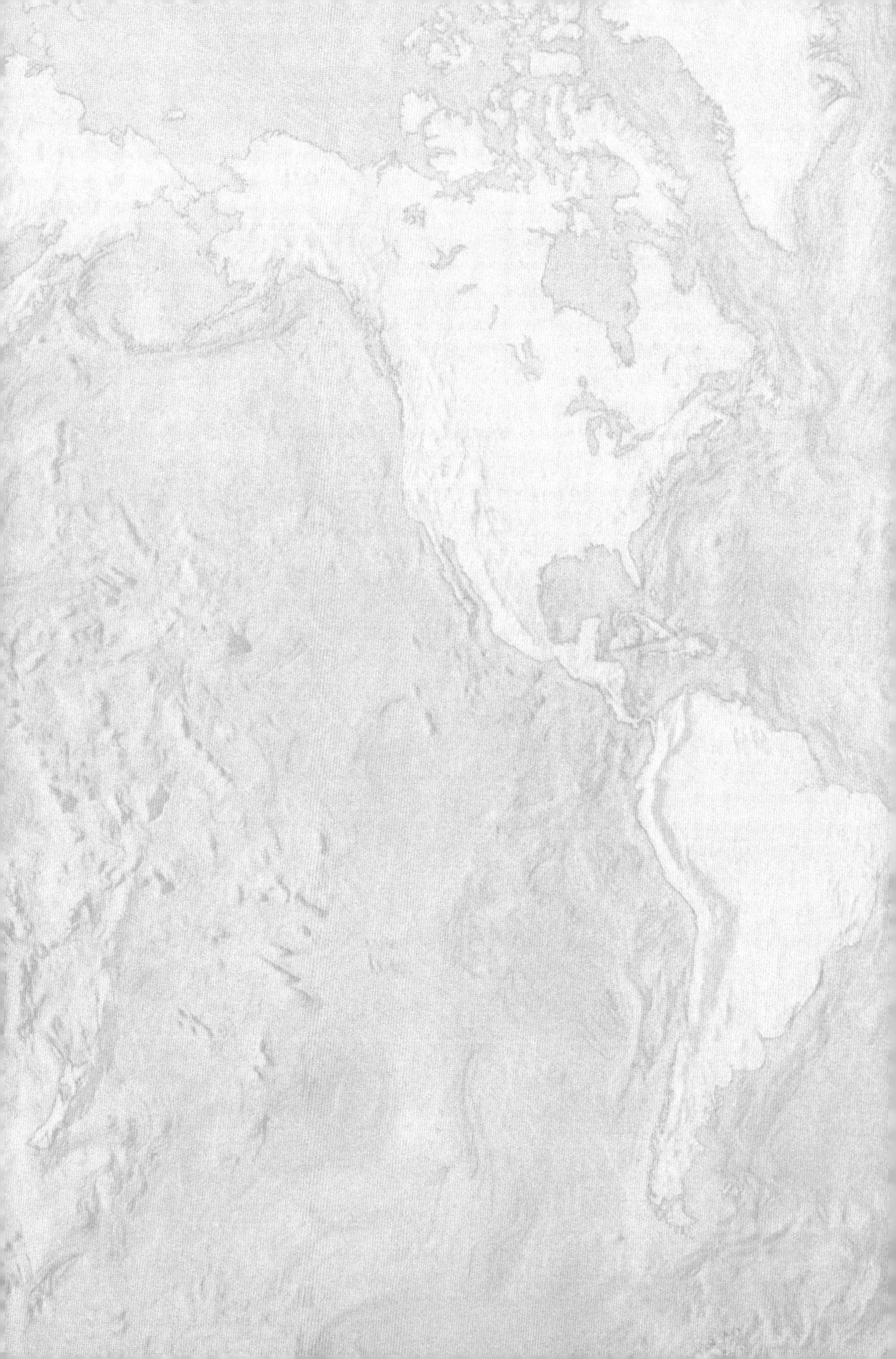

Section II

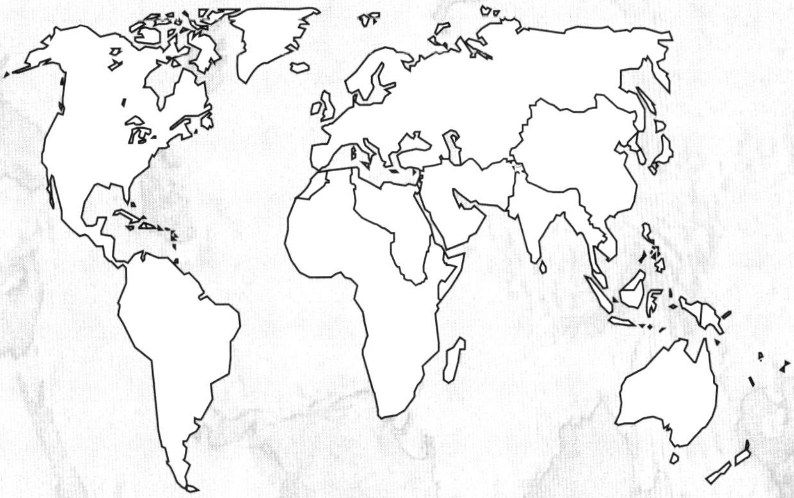

WHO Member States

Afghanistan

A–B

GENERAL INFORMATION

Afghanistan is a country with an approximate area of 652 thousand sq. km. (UNO, 2001). Its population is 24.926 million, and the sex ratio (men per hundred women) is 107 (UNO, 2004). The proportion of population under the age of 15 years is 43% (UNO, 2004), and the proportion of population above the age of 60 years is 5% (WHO, 2004). The literacy rate is 47% for men and 15% for women (UNESCO/MoH, 2004).

The country is a low income group country (based on World Bank 2004 criteria). The proportion of health budget to GDP is 5.2%. The per capita total expenditure on health is 34 international $, and the per capita government expenditure on health is 18 international $ (WHO, 2004).

The main language(s) used in the country is (are) Pashtu, Dari Persian and Turkic. The largest ethnic group(s) is (are) Pashtun (nearly half), and the other ethnic group(s) are (is) Tajik, Hazara and Uzbek. The largest religious group(s) is (are) Sunni Muslim (five sixths).

The life expectancy at birth is 41.9 years for males and 43.4 years for females (WHO, 2004). The healthy life expectancy at birth is 35 years for males and 36 years for females (WHO, 2004).

EPIDEMIOLOGY

Some studies on refugees are available. Mukhamadiev (2003) studied the prevalence of depression in 908 Tadjik refugee women in Afghanistan and found a high prevalence of endogenous depression (28.6%). A 1.5 year follow-up showed good prognosis in subjects who had subsyndromal depression, but not in those with endogenous depression. Rasekh et al (1999) found that symptoms that met the diagnostic criteria for anxiety, depression and PTSD were common in 160 Afghan women (including 80 women currently living in Kabul and 80 Afghan women who had recently migrated to Pakistan) during the Taliban regime. Mghir et al (1995) used the Structured Clinical Interview for DSM-III-R to detect mental illness among 38 children and young adults and identified depression and PTSD in more than one-third of the subjects.

MENTAL HEALTH RESOURCES

Mental Health Policy A mental health policy is present. The policy was initially formulated in 1986.

The components of the policy are advocacy, promotion, prevention, treatment and rehabilitation. The new Afghan Government has identified mental health as one of five health priorities. Since 1986, there has been no new Government policy regarding mental health and the old mental health policy is still followed. The policy outlines prevention, treatment and rehabilitative facilities for mentally ill patients.

Substance Abuse Policy A substance abuse policy is present. The policy was initially formulated in 1988. A new policy on Drug Demand Reduction was formulated in 2002.

National Mental Health Programme A national mental health programme is present. The programme was formulated in 1988. The national mental health programme has the following objectives: provision of mental health care to all, integration of mental health with primary care and community care, services for special population, especially the war-affected. It also outlines services, training, administrative strategies and approaches for promotion of mental health and provision of services for the war-affected. It advocates the development of a nucleus of trained mental health professionals to act as 'master trainers' for primary health care physicians and health workers in their respective provinces in order to ensure at least a minimum provision of mental health services.

National Therapeutic Drug Policy/Essential List of Drugs A national therapeutic drug policy/essential list of drugs is present. It was formulated in 1996.

Mental Health Legislation There is a mental health legislation.

The latest legislation was enacted in 1997.

Mental Health Financing There are budget allocations for mental health.

Details about expenditure on mental health are not available.

The primary source of mental health financing is out of pocket expenditure by the patient or family.

The country has disability benefits for persons with mental disorders. Disability support services are provided for persons with physical, psychiatric, intellectual, sensory or age-related disabilities (or a combination of these) which are likely to continue for a minimum of six months and reduces independent functioning to the extent that ongoing support is required.

Mental Health Facilities Mental health is not a part of primary health care system. Actual treatment of severe mental disorders is not available at the primary level. Community level workers from the local population (villages) have been involved in providing integrated health care for the last 8 years.

Regular training of primary care professionals is not carried out in the field of mental health. Two mental health manuals were prepared in Dari for primary health care doctors and other staff in 1998. WHO has organized mental health training for primary health care physicians. NGOs are running training courses for primary health care doctors, nurses and midwifes, village health volunteers and traditional birth attendants.

There are community care facilities for patients with mental disorders. Mental Health is included in Basic Package for Health Services (BPHS) which covers health service delivery up to district level. New treatment guidelines for common mental health disorder are being formulated (draft is ready). Four Community Mental Health Centers have been established in the capital, but further expansion is required. There are 2 general psychiatric rehabilitation centres with 160 beds.

Psychiatric Beds and Professionals

Total psychiatric beds per 10 000 population	0.055
Psychiatric beds in mental hospitals per 10 000 population	0.031
Psychiatric beds in general hospitals per 10 000 population	0.024
Psychiatric beds in other settings per 10 000 population	0
Number of psychiatrists per 100 000 population	0.036
Number of neurosurgeons per 100 000 population	0.034
Number of psychiatric nurses per 100 000 population	0.07
Number of neurologists per 100 000 population	0.07
Number of psychologists per 100 000 population	0.09
Number of social workers per 100 000 population	0

Currently, there are no social workers, and there are only very few trained psychiatrists. Most doctors working as psychiatrists have either had in-service training or have attended short courses abroad. A three month diploma course was held in 1996 to train some doctors in psychiatry. Postgraduate training in psychiatry is not present. Psychologists get their training from Kabul University. Much of qualified manpower and technical expertise has left the country.

Non-Governmental Organizations NGOs are involved with mental health in the country. They are mainly involved in treatment. The Afghan Government collaborates with non-governmental organizations to rapidly expand basic (mental) health services to underserved populations.

Information Gathering System There is no mental health reporting system in the country. Each hospital maintains registry books on their inpatient and outpatient information. Quarterly reports are submitted by the mental hospital to the Ministry of Public Health.
The country has no data collection system or epidemiological study on mental health.

Programmes for Special Population The country has specific programmes for mental health for disaster affected population. There is a regular programme for traumatized children (trauma and grief programme) which is supported by UNICEF.

Therapeutic Drugs The following therapeutic drugs are generally available at the primary health care level of the country: carbamazepine, phenobarbital, amitriptyline, chlorpromazine, diazepam, haloperidol.
The cost of medicines keeps fluctuating as the local currency is unstable due to the war. Over-the-counter sales of psychotropics occur.

Other Information There is a shortage of staff due to the war and more international support is needed.
A new Mental Health Unit under Primary Care Directorate was established in 2003 (it is not functional as yet). Since mental health is a component of the Basic Package for Health Services, guidelines and treatment protocol for common mental disorders in primary health care have been developed. Treatment guidelines for substance use have also been almost finalized. A strategy for integration of mental health services into primary care was finalized in 2004.

Additional Sources of Information

Mghir, R., Freed, W., Raskin, A., et al (1995) Depression and posttraumatic stress disorder among a community sample of adolescent and young adult Afghan refugees. Journal of Nervous & Mental Disease, 183, 24-30.

Mohit, A., Saeed, K., Mubbashar, M., et al. (1999) Mental health manpower development in Afghanistan: a report on a training course for primary health care physicians. Eastern Mediterranean Health Journal, 5, 373-377.

Mukhamadiev, D. M. (2003) Aspects of depressive states in repatriated female refugees. Zhurnal Nevrologii i Psikhiatrii Imeni S.S. Korsakova, 103, 21-23.

Rasekh, Z., Bauer, H. M., Manos, M. M., et al (1999) Women's health and human rights in Afghanistan. JAMA, 280, 249-255.

van de Put, W. (2002) Addressing mental health in Afghanistan. Lancet, 360, 41-42.

Ventevogel, P., Azimi, S., Jalal, S., et al (2002) Mental health care reform in Afghanistan. Journal of Ayub Medical College, 14, 1-3.

Albania

GENERAL INFORMATION

Albania is a country with an approximate area of 29 thousand sq. km. (UNO, 2001). Its population is 3.193 million, and the sex ratio (men per hundred women) is 104 (UNO, 2004). The proportion of population under the age of 15 years is 27% (UNO, 2004), and the proportion of population above the age of 60 years is 10% (WHO, 2004). The literacy rate is 99.2% for men and 98.3% for women (UNESCO/MoH, 2004).

The country is a lower middle income group country (based on World Bank 2004 criteria). The proportion of health budget to GDP is 3.7%. The per capita total expenditure on health is 150 international $, and the per capita government expenditure on health is 97 international $ (WHO, 2004).

The main language(s) used in the country is (are) Albanian and Greek. The largest ethnic group(s) is (are) Albanian (98.6%), and the other ethnic group(s) are (is) Greek (1.17%). The largest religious group(s) is (are) Muslim (almost 70%), and the other religious group(s) are (is) Orthodox Christian and Roman Catholic.

The life expectancy at birth is 67.3 years for males and 74.1 years for females (WHO, 2004). The healthy life expectancy at birth is 60 years for males and 63 years for females (WHO, 2004).

EPIDEMIOLOGY

There is a paucity of epidemiological data on mental illnesses in Albania in internationally accessible literature. Bilanakis et al (2001) conducted a community survey using Langner and CES-D scales to identify psychiatric morbidity among 217 randomly selected subjects. The results showed that about 26.2% had some psychiatric morbidity and 18.2% had depressive features.

MENTAL HEALTH RESOURCES

Mental Health Policy A mental health policy is present. The policy was initially formulated in 2003.

The focus is given to the following priorities: fighting segregation and social exclusion in the respect of human rights; establishing a Mental Health Department within the Ministry of Health; ensuring the de-institutionalization process; establishing a non-admission policy (partial and gradual) for long term purposes; innovative and flexible use of resources; defining and instituting a separate mental health budget; integrating the mental health services with primary care; providing continuous training and extension of experiences; reviewing the legal frame; involving as many actors on both national and international level as possible; including of the Mental Health Policy into the National Health Strategy.

Substance Abuse Policy A substance abuse policy is absent.

National Mental Health Programme A national mental health programme is present. Details about the year of formulation of the programme are not available.

The national mental health programme in Albania has been actively supported and furthered by the WHO Country Office. WHO supported the establishment by the Minister of Health of the National Steering Committee for Mental Health (NSC) and provided numerous inputs regarding mental health policy and planning. The Policy for Mental Health Services Development in Albania was finalized by the NSC and approved by the Minister of Health in March 2003, and the strategy for its implementation was drafted in September 2004 (awaiting approval). Albanian Mental Health Reform supported by the WHO Country Office in Albania has received the assistance of a wide net of Collaborative Centers and other partners (Birmingham Northern Trust, University of Central England, UK Health Department, Verona University, Asturias Mental Health Services) and also other organizations (UNOPS, Geneva Initiative on Psychiatry).

National Therapeutic Drug Policy/Essential List of Drugs A national therapeutic drug policy/essential list of drugs is present. It was formulated in 1993.

The essential drug list is updated periodically.

Mental Health Legislation During the year 2003-2004 there were efforts, by governmental, intergovernmental and non-governmental partners to review and improve the whole legislative frame with regard to mental health. Laws on social care are also being reconsidered to provide comprehensive answers to the complex needs of the mentally ill.

The latest legislation was enacted in 1996.

Mental Health Financing There are budget allocations for mental health.

The country spends 6% of the total health budget on mental health.

The primary sources of mental health financing in descending order are tax based, private insurances, out of pocket expenditure by the patient or family and grants.

Autonomous budget is allocated only to two psychiatric hospitals; the rest of the mental health services of the country (in- and out-patient units) receive undiscriminated budget within larger health care institutions.

The country has disability benefits for persons with mental disorders. Disability benefits are called invalidity benefits and are based on certain criteria.

Mental Health Facilities Mental health is not a part of primary health care system. Actual treatment of severe mental disorders is not available at the primary level.

Regular training of primary care professionals is not carried out in the field of mental health.

There are community care facilities for patients with mental disorders. Parallel to the elaboration and promotion of the Mental Health Policy, WHO has supported the Ministry of Health in implementing demonstration good practice mental health services in 4 areas and has promoted the implementation of similar services in 2 other areas by UNOPS/PASARP. The community centres provide multidisciplinary care, day care, rehabilitation and outreach services, including assertive outreach in a few cases. They vary in functions, roles and service provision types, depending on the specific conditions of each district. The services provided by the public system through community mental health centres include consultation and treatment, home visits, psychosocial interventions and in few cases assertive outreach. The services provided by the non-governmental non-profit sector are mainly in the form of day centres with focus on rehabilitation. In general, the community services cover urban populations, with exception of two Community Mental Health Centers that do reach rural populations as well, through linkages with respective primary care workers. The catchment areas of the Community Mental Health Centers tend to be around 100 000 inhabitants, which is in line with the proposed catchment area of the drafted Strategy for the Implementation of the Mental Health Policy.

Psychiatric Beds and Professionals

Total psychiatric beds per 10 000 population	2.5
Psychiatric beds in mental hospitals per 10 000 population	2
Psychiatric beds in general hospitals per 10 000 population	0.5
Psychiatric beds in other settings per 10 000 population	0
Number of psychiatrists per 100 000 population	2.2
Number of neurosurgeons per 100 000 population	
Number of psychiatric nurses per 100 000 population	4.2
Number of neurologists per 100 000 population	1
Number of psychologists per 100 000 population	0.2
Number of social workers per 100 000 population	0.4

There are 96 neuropsychiatrists and psychiatrists, with the latter forming 54% of the total. The resources for health care in Albania are low compared to other European countries. The uneven resource distribution leaves entire remote areas out of real health care coverage. The staff consists of only psychiatrists and nurses. There is no special training for nurses working in mental health. There are few outpatient units. The first psychologists to graduate out of the university were in 2000. The involvement of psychologists and social workers in the official mental health structures has started. A curriculum for a 4-year residency training in child and adolescent psychiatry has recently been approved.

Non-Governmental Organizations NGOs are involved with mental health in the country. They are mainly involved in advocacy, promotion and rehabilitation.

Information Gathering System There is no mental health reporting system in the country. The Information gathering system in the country in general is composed of fragmented data blocks reported independently on a vertical line from field services to central institutions. The main institutions that collect data about health care are Ministry of Health and INSTAT. Hospital data are reported as well as primary care data, but they are not aggregated into a unique mental health database either at the Ministry of Health or at INSTAT. The country has no data collection system or epidemiological study on mental health.
Albania was one of the countries selected for WHO's Mental Health System and Service Monitoring exercise, which involved systematic assessment of over 300 indicators related to 10 key components of mental health systems.

Programmes for Special Population The country has specific programmes for mental health for refugees and children. Programmes for special populations are mainly provided by NGOs.

Therapeutic Drugs The following therapeutic drugs are generally available at the primary health care level of the country: carbamazepine, phenobarbital, sodium valproate, amitriptyline, chlorpromazine, fluphenazine, haloperidol, lithium.
Other drugs are included in the essential drug list include clozapine, risperidone, cloimipamine and fluoxetine.

Other Information

Additional Sources of Information

Bilanakis, N., Kaci, M., Malamas, M., et al (2001) Psychiatric morbidity in an urban area of Albania. A community survey. European Journal of Psychiatry, 15, 69-81.

Doornkate, G. (2001) Mental health care reform and development in Albania. Mental Health Reforms, 6, 7-10.

Ministry of Health (2003) Policy for Mental Health Services Development in Albania (supported by WHO).

People' Assembly of the Republic of Albania (1996) Act no. 8092: On Mental Health.

Shehu, T. (1993) Lista E Barnave Thelbesore.

Suli, A., Lazeri, L., Nano, L. (2004) Mental health services in Albania. International Psychiatry, 4, 14-16.

UN Albania (2004) Common Country Assessment.

World Health Organization. (2004) Albania reform. In: Country Projects on Mental Health: Selected Cases. Geneva, World Health Organization, 1-10.

Algeria

GENERAL INFORMATION

Algeria is a country with an approximate area of 2382 thousand sq. km. (UNO, 2001). Its population is 32.339 million, and the sex ratio (men per hundred women) is 102 (UNO, 2004). The proportion of population under the age of 15 years is 32% (UNO, 2004), and the proportion of population above the age of 60 years is 6% (WHO, 2004). The literacy rate is 78% for men and 59.6% for women (UNESCO/MoH, 2004).

The country is a lower middle income group country (based on World Bank 2004 criteria). The proportion of health budget to GDP is 4.1%. The per capita total expenditure on health is 169 international $, and the per capita government expenditure on health is 127 international $ (WHO, 2004).

The main language(s) used in the country is (are) Arabic and French. The largest ethnic group(s) is (are) Arab. The largest religious group(s) is (are) Muslim.

The life expectancy at birth is 67.5 years for males and 71.2 years for females (WHO, 2004). The healthy life expectancy at birth is 60 years for males and 62 years for females (WHO, 2004).

EPIDEMIOLOGY

An epidemiological study done by the Ministry of Health (2004) showed that chronic mental disorders were diagnosed in 0.7% to 1.9% of subjects of different age groups and epilepsy in 0.2% to 0.8% of subjects in different age groups. Chronic mental disorders and epilepsy were more common in those below 40 years of age and in women. There was no rural-urban difference in prevalence of these conditions. The prevalence of posttraumatic stress disorder (PTSD) assessed using the PTSD module of the Composite International Diagnostic Interview Version 2.1 was found to be 37.4% in a community survey conducted on a sample of 653 subjects (de Jong et al, 2001). Conflict-related trauma after age 12 years, torture, poor quality of camp and daily hassles were associated with the occurrence of PTSD. Brunetti et al (1982) compared depression between French (n=125) and Algerian (n=45) women. The one-year prevalence of depressive syndrome (structurally similar in both cultures) for the two samples combined (n=170) was 15% for the mildly impaired and 3% for the more markedly impaired, but the severity of depression was greater in Algerian women. Touari et al (1993) reviewed 3984 clinical interviews of criminals over a period of 23 years. In case histories concerning 1007 criminals, who had committed or attempted homicide, psychosis was identified in 19.9%. Psychotic subjects were older, more likely to have a previous psychiatric history, less likely to come from very large families and less likely to have been raised by both parents. A prevalence survey on psychotrauma on 12 000 school children between the ages of 12 to18 years conducted in 10 regions showed that 9.2% to 29.2% of children in different regions had mental health problems related to trauma (MoH, 2002).

MENTAL HEALTH RESOURCES

Mental Health Policy A mental health policy is present. Details about the year of formulation are not available.
The components of the policy are promotion, prevention, treatment and rehabilitation. The components of the current mental health policy were defined more clearly in the 4 axes of the national mental health programme established since 10 October 2001.

Substance Abuse Policy A substance abuse policy is present. The policy was initially formulated in 1990. A National Bureau for Fighting against Substance Abuse has been set up since 2003.

National Mental Health Programme A national mental health programme is present. The programme was formulated in 2001.
The national mental health programme prioritizes decentralization, primary health care, community approach, availability of psychotropics, adaptation of the mental health legislation, prevention of mental and neurological disorders, psychosocial rehabilitation of people with psychological problems related to violence, education of the public, formation of community and family associations, human resource development, and mental health research.

National Therapeutic Drug Policy/Essential List of Drugs A national therapeutic drug policy/essential list of drugs is present. It was formulated in 1997.
A national list (nomenclature) exists, in which psychotropic drugs are included and are defined based on their medical use. Also, a ministerial circulation letter in 1997 defines the drugs to be distributed at no cost for mentally ill whose care is prioritized in the national mental health programme.

Mental Health Legislation The mental health law is included in the Law on Health Protection and Promotion of 1985. The Law no. 98.09 is the most recent legislation related to mental health. Presently, the mental health legislation is being revised.
The latest legislation was enacted in 1998.

Mental Health Financing There are no budget allocations for mental health.
Details about expenditure on mental health are not available.
The primary source of mental health financing is tax based.
The country has disability benefits for persons with mental disorders. The mentally ill are assessed for disability and benefits are provided accordingly.

Mental Health Facilities Mental health is a part of primary health care system. Actual treatment of severe mental disorders is available at the primary level. There is availability of treatment in primary health care following the integration of mental health care within primary health care as a part of the national mental health programme. There is an organization of intermediary mental heath centres in the structures of primary health care.
Regular training of primary care professionals is carried out in the field of mental health. Training in mental health is provided to doctors and nurses and to the psychologists who provide primary health care.
There are no community care facilities for patients with mental disorders.

Psychiatric Beds and Professionals

Total psychiatric beds per 10 000 population	1.4
Psychiatric beds in mental hospitals per 10 000 population	0.86
Psychiatric beds in general hospitals per 10 000 population	0.2
Psychiatric beds in other settings per 10 000 population	0.36
Number of psychiatrists per 100 000 population	1.1
Number of neurosurgeons per 100 000 population	0.32
Number of psychiatric nurses per 100 000 population	1.1
Number of neurologists per 100 000 population	0.42
Number of psychologists per 100 000 population	0.8
Number of social workers per 100 000 population	0

Some beds have been earmarked for mentally challenged individuals and for children.

Non-Governmental Organizations NGOs are involved with mental health in the country. They are mainly involved in promotion. The APAMM (Association des parents et amis des malades mentaux – Association of parents and friends of the mentally ill) and the AAMMB (Association d'aide aux malades mentaux de Blida – Relief Association for the mentally ill of Bilda) help in the care of the mentally ill. Other associations work in the area of research, such as the Algerian Society of Psychiatry, the Algerian Society for Research in Psychology, the Algerian Society of Psychiatric Epidemiology etc.

Information Gathering System There is mental health reporting system in the country. Presently, several epidemiology studies on different topics related to mental health, such as the psychological consequences of violence, are under development. Furthermore, the Algerian Society of Psychiatric Epidemiology works in the area of epidemiology.
The country has no data collection system or epidemiological study on mental health. There are no national level epidemiological studies, but psychiatric institutions have their own epidemiological data collected through local surveys.
A system exists on mental health data collection since 2002 on various activities such as: care of the victims of violence, mental health activities (till mental health intermediary centre level), hospitalization, distribution of drugs, establishments meant to provide intersectoral care to mentally ill persons with social problems.

Programmes for Special Population The country has specific programmes for mental health for disaster affected population, elderly and children.
An information service which deals with psychiatric emergencies has been operating since September 1997.

Therapeutic Drugs The following therapeutic drugs are generally available at the primary health care level of the country: carbamazepine, ethosuximide, phenobarbital, phenytoin sodium, sodium valproate, amitriptyline, chlorpromazine, diazepam, fluphenazine, haloperidol, carbidopa, levodopa.

Other Information

Additional Sources of Information

Brunetti, P. M., Vincent, P., Neves, J., et al (1982) Epidemiological study of psychological discomfort in French and Algerian samples. Encephale, 8, 615-636.

Chakali, M., Ait, M. A. (1999) A medico-psychological assistance mechanism to adult victims of major traumatism in Blida. Médecine de Catastrophe Urgences Collectives, 2, 188-191.

de Jong, J. T., Komproe, I. H., Van Ommeren, M., et al (2001) Lifetime events and posttraumatic stress disorder in 4 postconflict settings. JAMA, 286, 555-562.

Desrouelles, M., Bersot, H. (1996) Care of the insane in Algeria since the nineteenth century. History of Psychiatry, 7, 549-561.

Enquête Algérienne sur la santé de la famille – 2002 – inscrite dans le cadre du projet pan arabe sur la santé de la famille (Rapport principal – juillet 2004).

Ministère de la Santé de la Population et de la Réforme Hospitalière en Collaboration avec l'UNICEF. Enquête sur la prévalence du psychotraumatisme chez l'enfant d'âge scolaire, Alger, 2002.

Ministère de la Santé de la Population et de la Réforme Hospitalière Programme National de Santé Mentale, Alger, Octobre 2001.

Touari, M., Mesbah, M., Dellatolas, G., et al (1993) Association between criminality and psychosis: a retrospective study of 3984 expert psychiatric evaluations. Revue d'Epidémiologie et de Santé Publique, 41, 218-227.

Andorra

GENERAL INFORMATION

Andorra is a country with an approximate area of 0.45 thousand sq. km. (UNO, 2001). Its population is 0.067 million, and the sex ratio (men per hundred women) is 108 (UNO, 2004). The proportion of population under the age of 15 years is 16% (UNO, 2004), and the proportion of population above the age of 60 years is 22% (WHO, 2004).

The country is a high income group country (based on World Bank 2004 criteria). The proportion of health budget to GDP is 5.7%. The per capita total expenditure on health is 1821 international $, and the per capita government expenditure on health is 1292 international $ (WHO, 2004).

The main language(s) used in the country is (are) Catalán (official) and Spanish. The largest ethnic group(s) is (are) Spanish and Andorran, and the other ethnic group(s) are (is) Portuguese, French and others (70% of the population has a migratory background). The largest religious group(s) is (are) Roman Catholic.

The life expectancy at birth is 76.8 years for males and 83.7 years for females (WHO, 2004). The healthy life expectancy at birth is 70 years for males and 75 years for females (WHO, 2004).

EPIDEMIOLOGY

There is substantial epidemiological data on mental illnesses in Andorra in internationally accessible literature. No attempt was made to include this information here.

MENTAL HEALTH RESOURCES

Mental Health Policy A mental health policy is absent.

Substance Abuse Policy A substance abuse policy is absent. A substance abuse policy is under the active consideration of the Parliament.

National Mental Health Programme A national mental health programme is absent.
So far, Andorra does not have a national mental health plan. However, in 1996, a document from the Regional Office for Europe of WHO described the relevant needs, services and organizational strategies.

National Therapeutic Drug Policy/Essential List of Drugs A national therapeutic drug policy/essential list of drugs is absent.

Mental Health Legislation There is a Law on Guarantee of Rights of People with Discapacity.
Details about the year of enactment of the mental health legislation are not available.

Mental Health Financing There are budget allocations for mental health.
The country spends 3.9% of the total health budget on mental health.
The primary sources of mental health financing in descending order are social insurance, private insurances, out of pocket expenditure by the patient or family and tax based.
The primary care and social services budget are not included in the total health budget. Most doctors in the country have an agreement with the Government such that the patient pays 25% of the cost of consultation and the rest is covered by the national insurance system. If hospitalization is required, the patient pays only 10%.
The country has disability benefits for persons with mental disorders.

Mental Health Facilities Mental health is a part of primary health care system. Actual treatment of severe mental disorders is available at the primary level.
Regular training of primary care professionals is carried out in the field of mental health. In the last two years, about 42 personnel were provided training.
There are community care facilities for patients with mental disorders. The Mental Health Services that have been developed since 1998 are based on the general principles of 'community psychiatry'. The services, including child psychiatry and geriatric psychiatry, are available to everyone covered by the National Insurance System (the great majority of the population). These services are concentrated in the general hospital, which is located in an area of the main urban zone of the country and has good communications. The Mental Health Centre offers an outpatient unit with psychiatric and psychological services together with a day care centre where psycho-social rehabilitation programmes are offered to patients with chronic severe mental disorders. There is a Day-Hospital for less chronic or severe patients. Two apartments with support have been opened in 2004.

Psychiatric Beds and Professionals

Total psychiatric beds per 10 000 population	1.6
Psychiatric beds in mental hospitals per 10 000 population	0
Psychiatric beds in general hospitals per 10 000 population	1.6
Psychiatric beds in other settings per 10 000 population	0
Number of psychiatrists per 100 000 population	10
Number of neurosurgeons per 100 000 population	0
Number of psychiatric nurses per 100 000 population	9
Number of neurologists per 100 000 population	3
Number of psychologists per 100 000 population	30
Number of social workers per 100 000 population	26

There are two occupational therapists and one music therapist. The process of deinstitutionalization has not been necessary in Andorra, since there were no psychiatric institutions till the present time. Several Andorran patients are still resident in private psychiatric institutions, either in France or Spain, as this had been the method of management for chronic psychotic disorders in the past. The mental health team co-operates at different levels with other sectors of health care. It has regular meetings with the Association of General Practitioners, the Social Work Services and the Nursing Centres Network.

Non-Governmental Organizations NGOs are involved with mental health in the country. They are mainly involved in advocacy and rehabilitation. An association of families of mental patients has been formed.

Information Gathering System There is mental health reporting system in the country.
The country has data collection system or epidemiological study on mental health. The information gathering system has been implemented only recently.
There have not been any specific epidemiological studies on mental health, but a National Inquiry on Health has been done.

Programmes for Special Population The country has specific programmes for mental health for elderly and children.
An Addictive Behavior Unit has opened and specific programmes also exist for eating disorders.

Therapeutic Drugs The following therapeutic drugs are generally available at the primary health care level of the country: carbamazepine, ethosuximide, phenobarbital, phenytoin sodium, sodium valproate, amitriptyline, chlorpromazine, diazepam, fluphenazine, haloperidol, lithium, biperiden, carbidopa, levodopa.

Other Information The three greatest matters of concern are: developing the structures and programmes which are still lacking, e.g. a long-stay centre for highly dependent chronic patients; promoting a sensitivity towards cultural and social factors which are liable to affect the mental health of the population among mental health professionals and health professionals in general; and developing a mental health legislation.

Additional Sources of Information

Angola

GENERAL INFORMATION

Angola is a country with an approximate area of 1247 thousand sq. km. (UNO, 2001). Its population is 14.078 million, and the sex ratio (men per hundred women) is 97 (UNO, 2004). The proportion of population under the age of 15 years is 48% (UNO, 2004), and the proportion of population above the age of 60 years is 4% (WHO, 2004). The literacy rate is 57% for men and 29% for women (UNESCO/MoH, 2004).

The country is a low income group country (based on World Bank 2004 criteria). The proportion of health budget to GDP is 4.4%. The per capita total expenditure on health is 70 international $, and the per capita government expenditure on health is 44 international $ (WHO, 2004).

The main language(s) used in the country is (are) Portuguese, Bantu, Ovimbundu, Kimbundu and Kikongo. The largest ethnic group(s) is (are) Ovimbundu, and the other ethnic group(s) are (is) Mbundu, Bakongo, Fiote, Nganguela, Kuanhama and Tchokwe. The largest religious group(s) is (are) Christian (two-thirds of the population).

The life expectancy at birth is 37.9 years for males and 42 years for females (WHO, 2004). The healthy life expectancy at birth is 32 years for males and 35 years for females (WHO, 2004).

EPIDEMIOLOGY

There is a paucity of epidemiological data on mental illnesses in Angola in internationally accessible literature.

MENTAL HEALTH RESOURCES

Mental Health Policy A mental health policy is absent.

Substance Abuse Policy A substance abuse policy is present. The policy was initially formulated in 1989.

National Mental Health Programme A national mental health programme is present. The programme was formulated in 1989.

National Therapeutic Drug Policy/Essential List of Drugs A national therapeutic drug policy/essential list of drugs is present. Details about the year of formulation are not available.

Mental Health Legislation Details about the mental health legislation are not available.

Mental Health Financing There are no budget allocations for mental health.
Details about expenditure on mental health are not available.
The primary source of mental health financing is out of pocket expenditure by the patient or family.
The country has disability benefits for persons with mental disorders.

Mental Health Facilities Mental health is not a part of primary health care system. Actual treatment of severe mental disorders is not available at the primary level. There is no facility in the primary level due to the lack of a mental health policy.
Regular training of primary care professionals is not carried out in the field of mental health.
There are no community care facilities for patients with mental disorders. This inadequacy of community facility is due to lack of training of personnel.

Psychiatric Beds and Professionals

Total psychiatric beds per 10 000 population	0.13
Psychiatric beds in mental hospitals per 10 000 population	0.07
Psychiatric beds in general hospitals per 10 000 population	0.06
Psychiatric beds in other settings per 10 000 population	
Number of psychiatrists per 100 000 population	0
Number of neurosurgeons per 100 000 population	0.032
Number of psychiatric nurses per 100 000 population	0
Number of neurologists per 100 000 population	0.032
Number of psychologists per 100 000 population	0
Number of social workers per 100 000 population	0

Non-Governmental Organizations NGOs are involved with mental health in the country. They are mainly involved in advocacy and rehabilitation.

Information Gathering System There is no mental health reporting system in the country.
The country has data collection system or epidemiological study on mental health. Data from the psychiatric hospital in Luanda is collected.

Programmes for Special Population The country has specific programmes for mental health for disaster affected population and children. There are some NGOs who work for people displaced by war, street children and victims of violence.

Therapeutic Drugs The following therapeutic drugs are generally available at the primary health care level of the country: carbamazepine, phenobarbital, phenytoin sodium, amitriptyline, chlorpromazine, diazepam, fluphenazine, haloperidol, lithium. Prices keep on fluctuating depending on the availability of drugs.

Other Information

Additional Sources of Information

Ministerio da Saude (1989). Programa Nacional de Saude Mental.

Antigua and Barbuda

GENERAL INFORMATION

Antigua and Barbuda is a country with an approximate area of 0.44 thousand sq. km. (UNO, 2001). Its population is 0.077 million, and the sex ratio (men per hundred women) is 92 (UNO, 2004). The proportion of population under the age of 15 years is 28% (UNO, 2004), and the proportion of population above the age of 60 years is 10% (WHO, 2004). The literacy rate is 90% for men and 88% for women (UNESCO/MoH, 2004).

The country is a higher middle income group country (based on World Bank 2004 criteria). The proportion of health budget to GDP is 5.6%. The per capita total expenditure on health is 614 international $, and the per capita government expenditure on health is 374 international $ (WHO, 2004).

The main language(s) used in the country is (are) English. The largest ethnic group(s) is (are) African, and the other ethnic group(s) are (is) British, Portuguese, Lebanese and Syrian. The largest religious group(s) is (are) Anglican, and the other religious group(s) are (is) Roman Catholic.

The life expectancy at birth is 69 years for males and 73.9 years for females (WHO, 2004). The healthy life expectancy at birth is 60 years for males and 64 years for females (WHO, 2004).

EPIDEMIOLOGY

There is a paucity of epidemiological data on mental illnesses in Antigua and Barbuda in internationally accessible literature.

MENTAL HEALTH RESOURCES

Mental Health Policy A mental health policy is absent.

Substance Abuse Policy A substance abuse policy is absent.

National Mental Health Programme A national mental health programme is present. The programme was formulated in 1978.

National Therapeutic Drug Policy/Essential List of Drugs A national therapeutic drug policy/essential list of drugs is present. It was formulated in 2003.

Mental Health Legislation The latest legislation was enacted in 1951.

Mental Health Financing There are budget allocations for mental health.
The country spends 3% of the total health budget on mental health.
The primary sources of mental health financing in descending order are tax based and social insurance.
The Medical Benefit Scheme for chronic mental illness is the source of financing for medication.
The country does not have disability benefits for persons with mental disorders.

Mental Health Facilities Mental health is a part of primary health care system. Actual treatment of severe mental disorders is available at the primary level. Treatment is administered by the 6 mental health clinics in the country.
Regular training of primary care professionals is not carried out in the field of mental health.
There are community care facilities for patients with mental disorders. Community care is also administered from the 6 clinics.

Psychiatric Beds and Professionals

Total psychiatric beds per 10 000 population	17.9
Psychiatric beds in mental hospitals per 10 000 population	17
Psychiatric beds in general hospitals per 10 000 population	0.7
Psychiatric beds in other settings per 10 000 population	0.2
Number of psychiatrists per 100 000 population	2
Number of neurosurgeons per 100 000 population	0
Number of psychiatric nurses per 100 000 population	4.5
Number of neurologists per 100 000 population	0
Number of psychologists per 100 000 population	3
Number of social workers per 100 000 population	

There are 5 social workers, but none work in mental health. Antigua and Barbuda provided long-term care services for Leeward Island for a long time in exchange for a nominal fee. There is an old style mental hospital with psychiatric care at the general hospital.

Non-Governmental Organizations NGOs are involved with mental health in the country. They are mainly involved in advocacy, promotion and rehabilitation.

Information Gathering System There is no mental health reporting system in the country.
The country has no data collection system or epidemiological study on mental health.

Programmes for Special Population The country has specific programmes for mental health for children. The child and family guidance centre at the general hospital is run by an NGO (Collaborative Committee for the Promotion of Emotional Health in Children).

Therapeutic Drugs The following therapeutic drugs are generally available at the primary health care level of the country: carbamazepine, ethosuximide, phenobarbital, phenytoin sodium, sodium valproate, amitriptyline, chlorpromazine, diazepam, fluphenazine, haloperidol, lithium, carbidopa, levodopa.
Benztropine is available.

Other Information

Additional Sources of Information

Argentina

A–B

GENERAL INFORMATION

Argentina is a country with an approximate area of 2780 thousand sq. km. (UNO, 2001). Its population is 38.871 million, and the sex ratio (men per hundred women) is 96 (UNO, 2004). The proportion of population under the age of 15 years is 27% (UNO, 2004), and the proportion of population above the age of 60 years is 14% (WHO, 2004). The literacy rate is 97% for men and 97% for women (UNESCO/MoH, 2004).

The country is a higher middle income group country (based on World Bank 2004 criteria). The proportion of health budget to GDP is 9.5%. The per capita total expenditure on health is 1130 international $, and the per capita government expenditure on health is 604 international $ (WHO, 2004).

The main language(s) used in the country is (are) Spanish. The largest ethnic group(s) is (are) European. The largest religious group(s) is (are) Roman Catholic.

The life expectancy at birth is 70.8 years for males and 78.1 years for females (WHO, 2004). The healthy life expectancy at birth is 62 years for males and 68 years for females (WHO, 2004).

EPIDEMIOLOGY

Di Marco (1982) carried out a representative general population survey (n=3411) in the Greater Buenos Aires area using the Present State Examination (PSE) and found a prevalence of mental disorders to be 26% (30.8% in females and 20.3% in males). About 13% of the population had neurotic disorders, especially of depressive type, 6% had affective psychosis, 4% schizophrenic psychosis and 1.3% paranoid states. The prevalence rate of psychiatric disorder was associated with gender and socioeconomic level. The National Study on Consumption of Addictive Substances showed that almost 91.4% of the adult population reported a lifetime use of alcohol and 66.2% reported using it in the last thirty days. Almost 6.6% of the subjects (11.9% men and 1.6% women), mostly young people from low socioeconomic background had consumed alcohol in large amounts in the previous month (>70 grams/day) and 4.3% (6.7% men and 1.7% women) were dependent on it. The prevalence of lifetime use of any illegal substance, was 10.09% (SEDRONAR, 1999). However, alcohol consumption represented the main cause for diagnosis of mental disorders (Ministry of Health, 2004a). In a household survey in a middle- and lower-class section of Greater Buenos Aires, Tarnopolsky et al (1975) reported that disorders related to alcohol use were present in one-sixth of adults. They were present almost exclusively among males and were more prevalent among those with lower levels of education, occupation and residential status and among migrants. A survey of three Buenos Aires hospitals revealed that 5% of all the cases attended during a single week were related to the consumption of alcohol and drugs. Lack of formal education, unemployment and marital separation were associated with substance abuse by males (especially in the case of alcohol abuse among older men and the abuse of psychoactive and illegal drugs among the young), while women tended to take overdoses of psychoactive drugs in times of personal crisis (Miguez & Grimson, 1989). In a study conducted on more than 1200 school going adolescents of both sexes and 51 male adolescents in a drug treatment programme, Moss et al (1998) found that older age, deviant behaviour, deviant peer behaviour, school related problems and familial drug abuse were associated with drug abuse in study subjects. Alvarez (1996) showed a strong association between drug use and drug consumption by friends or sibs and consumption of tobacco or alcohol. Serfaty et al (1991) found severe depression in 4.5% of the sample of adolescents (n=553) who had applied for military service. Sadness in childhood, drug abuse by sibs, family conflict and suicidal ideations were associated with the occurrence of depression. Chemerinski et al (1998) assessed a consecutive series of 398 patients with probable Alzheimer's Disease (AD) for the presence of generalized anxiety disorder (GAD) using a standardized neuropsychiatric evaluation. 5% of patients showed GAD during the 4 weeks preceding the psychiatric evaluation. Vasquez et al (2000) studied 149 hospital patients for delirium and found that 20.5% suffered from delirium with severity of illness, chronicity and fever being the main factors associated with it. Official mortality statistics showed that crude rate of suicides increased from 6.3 per 100 000 in 1997 to 8.4 per 100 000 in 2002. Suicides were more common in those in the age range of 15 to 24 years and to a smaller degree in the age range of 50 to 54 and 65 to 69 years (Ministry of Health, 2004b). Rizzi et al (1998) reviewed reports of autopsies of all violent deaths in women aged 12-44 years over a 5-year period (n=272) and found that suicide accounted for 17.6% of all violent deaths.

MENTAL HEALTH RESOURCES

Mental Health Policy A mental health policy is present. The policy was initially formulated in 1957.
The components of the policy are advocacy, promotion, prevention, treatment and rehabilitation. It was revised in 2001 through a process that involved multiple stakeholders (politicians, mental health professionals, NGOs and public servants). Regular funds for its implementation were allocated.

Substance Abuse Policy A substance abuse policy is present. The policy was initially formulated in 1987. The substance abuse policies are established by the National Secretariat of Prevention and Action against Narcotraffic that reports to the President. It has a specific budget for its implementation and is supported by a legislation on substance abuse that was formulated in 1990.

National Mental Health Programme A national mental health programme is present. The programme was formulated in 1998. Its main focus is on strategy for services reform, promotion and prevention, integration of mental health services with primary care and consolidation of specialized services. As Argentina is a federal country, different regional mental health programmes are currently in place in different provinces. Consultations for updating the national mental health programme have been initiated in 2004.

National Therapeutic Drug Policy/Essential List of Drugs A national therapeutic drug policy/essential list of drugs is absent.

Mental Health Legislation The most recent legislation in this area is one on mental health in primary care. It also covers promotion/prevention, users' rights and advocacy and it conforms to International Human Rights Laws. However, it does not contain regulations on involuntary treatment, mental health services, admission and discharge procedures and housing/employment facilities for the patients. A specific budget has not been assigned to it. Data on percentage of involuntary admissions is not available. The National Law regarding admissions (Law 229/4) was passed in 1982.
The latest legislation was enacted in 2001.

Mental Health Financing There are budget allocations for mental health.
Details about expenditure on mental health are not available.
The primary sources of mental health financing in descending order are tax based, social insurance, private insurances and out of pocket expenditure by the patient or family.
At national level, the budget for a health area (e.g. mental health) depends on the ministerial office to which it belongs. Various regions make their own budget allocations for mental health; for example Buenos Aires assigns 2% of health budget to mental health. At the national level, approximately 10% of mental health expenses are allocated to public psychiatric hospitals. Data regarding other expenses such as public and private general hospitals, ambulatory clinics, community care, etc. are not available.
The country has disability benefits for persons with mental disorders.

Mental Health Facilities Mental health is a part of primary health care system. Actual treatment of severe mental disorders is available at the primary level. Facilities are not uniform across the country (less than 25 % of the population is covered by mental health services through primary care. Usually patients reach the specialist system directly or through referral from other sources. Regular training of primary care professionals is not carried out in the field of mental health.
There are community care facilities for patients with mental disorders. Facilities are not uniform across the country. A budget for community services is available in some provinces.

Psychiatric Beds and Professionals

Total psychiatric beds per 10 000 population	6
Psychiatric beds in mental hospitals per 10 000 population	5.4
Psychiatric beds in general hospitals per 10 000 population	0
Psychiatric beds in other settings per 10 000 population	
Number of psychiatrists per 100 000 population	13.25
Number of neurosurgeons per 100 000 population	1.1
Number of psychiatric nurses per 100 000 population	
Number of neurologists per 100 000 population	1.6
Number of psychologists per 100 000 population	106
Number of social workers per 100 000 population	11

The number of psychiatric nurses, occupational therapists is not known. There are 43 000 psychologists but the specific number working for mental health is not available. There are 225 facilities in Argentina with psychiatric beds. Psychiatric beds are almost equally divided between public and private psychiatric institutions. 80% of these beds are occupied by long stay patients (>1 year); 15.0% medium stay (3 months to 1 year) and 5.0% short stay (<3 months). There are no psychiatric beds in prison for offenders with mental disorders. Hospitals for forensic purposes and general hospitals receive patients sent by the judge. Private hospitals also assist forensic services if the patient can afford the expenses. Mental health professionals are concentrated in the urban centres.

Non-Governmental Organizations NGOs are involved with mental health in the country. These organizations participate in mental health issues related to women, children, domestic violence and consumers. NGOs are often registered with the ministry.

Information Gathering System There is no mental health reporting system in the country.
The country has no data collection system or epidemiological study on mental health. There are no general studies, only isolated ones like the one for Buenos Aires.

Programmes for Special Population The country has specific programmes for mental health for minorities, disaster affected population, indigenous population, elderly and children.
Some special programmes carried out in collaboration with national and international organizations. The Forensic Psychiatric System involves civil and penal areas, each with its own legislation. The Constitution of Argentina provides the ethical and juridical framework for the purpose and operation of prisons and other safety psychiatric institutes from the penitentiary services. Unimputability and the implementation of safety measures according to danger are ruled by the Penal Code from 1921 (last modified in 1997). In the civil area, the Civil Code (1997) in force at the national level looks into the issue of involuntary care. The objective of care of forensic patients is to avoid prolonged hospital stay and to integrate the patient into the community through a self-managed sys-

tem. While admitted, some forensic patients are allowed to attend day care centres for occupational therapy. After discharge from the hospital, supervision is maintained for 4 years. Though a number of programmes cover forensic psychiatry, a specific course leading to recognition as a forensic psychiatrist has not been organized.

Therapeutic Drugs The following therapeutic drugs are generally available at the primary health care level of the country: carbamazepine, phenobarbital, sodium valproate, amitriptyline, chlorpromazine, diazepam, haloperidol, lithium.

Other Information Methods to assess quality of care at primary care level are unavailable, however, tools for quality assurance are available at secondary and tertiary levels.

Additional Sources of Information

Alvarez, A. (1996) Risk factors for the consumption of illegal drugs. Study in 1904 18-year-old boys in the city of Buenos Aires Medicina., 56, 23-28.

Chemerinski, E., Petracca, G., Manes, F., et al (1998) Prevalence and correlates of anxiety in Alzheimer's disease. Depression & Anxiety, 7,166-170.

Di Marco, G. (1982) Prevalence of mental disorders in the metropolitan area of the Republic of Argentina (Prevalencia de desordenes mentales en el area metropolitana de la Republica Argentina). Acta Psiquiatrica y Psicologica de America Latina, 28, 93-102.

Folino, J. O., Vasquez, J. M., Sarmiento, D. (2000) Forensic psychiatry in the province of Buenos Aires. International Journal of Law and Psychiatry, 23, 567-577.

Miguez, H. A., Grimson, R. W. (1989) Emergency consultations for abuse of psychoactive substances in Buenos Aires hospitals. Boletin de la Oficina Sanitaria Panamericana, 107, 296-306.

Ministry of Health (2004a).

Ministry of Health (2004b) Mortality Statistics of the National Programme of Statistics of Health (PNES).

Moss, H. B., Bonicatto, S., Kirisci, L., et al (1998) Substance abuse and associated psychosocial problems among Argentina adolescents: sex heterogeneity and familial transmission. Drug & Alcohol Dependence, 52, 221-230.

Rizzi, R. G., Cordoba, R. R., Maguna, J. J., et al (1998) Maternal mortality due to violence. International Journal of Gynaecology & Obstetrics, 63 (Supp.l) 1, 19-24.

SEDRONAR (1999) National Study on Consumption of Addictive Substances.

Serfaty, E., Andrade, J., D'Aquila, H., et al (1995) Severe depression and risk factors in Buenos Aires. Acta Psiquiatrica y Psicologica de America Latina, 41, 35-39.

Tarnopolsky, A., Olmo, G. D., Levav (Lubchansky), I., et al (1975) Survey of alcoholism and excessive drinking in a suburb of Buenos Aires. Psychological Medicine, 5, 193-205.

Vazquez, F., O'Flaherty, M., Michelangelo, H., et al (2000) Epidemiology of delirium in elderly inpatients. Medicina, 60, 555-560.

Armenia

GENERAL INFORMATION

Armenia is a country with an approximate area of 30 thousand sq. km. (UNO, 2001). Its population is 3.052 million, and the sex ratio (men per hundred women) is 94 (UNO, 2004). The proportion of population under the age of 15 years is 19% (UNO, 2004), and the proportion of population above the age of 60 years is 13% (WHO, 2004). The literacy rate is 99.7% for men and 99.2% for women (UNESCO/MoH, 2004).

The country is a lower middle income group country (based on World Bank 2004 criteria). The proportion of health budget to GDP is 7.8%. The per capita total expenditure on health is 273 international $, and the per capita government expenditure on health is 112 international $ (WHO, 2004).

The main language(s) used in the country is (are) Armenian and Russian. The largest ethnic group(s) is (are) Armenian. The largest religious group(s) is (are) Armenian Apostolic Christian.

The life expectancy at birth is 67 years for males and 73 years for females (WHO, 2004). The healthy life expectancy at birth is 59 years for males and 63 years for females (WHO, 2004).

EPIDEMIOLOGY

Recent data (2000-2002) obtained on a representative sample (n=395) by means of a specially elaborated unified questionnaire and properly adapted and standardized Symptom Checklist (SCL-90R), Beck Depression Inventory (BDI) and Hospital Anxiety and Depression Scale (HADS) suggested high levels of emotional disorders in comparison to that reported in Western Europe and Russia. Anxiety and depression were significantly higher in those areas reporting an inability to access medical aid due to financial reasons. Surprisingly, no substantial differences were seen in the level of anxiety and depression as well as on the majority of SCL-90R scores between respondents from disaster and non-disaster areas (Khachaturyan, 2002; Khachaturyan & Nersesyan, 2004). Armenian et al (2000) interviewed 1785 adult victims, identified through stratified population sampling 2 years after the 1988 earthquake, with the National Institute of Mental Health (NIMH) Disaster Interview Schedule/Disaster Supplement. A comparison of pure PTSD (without comorbidity, n=154 cases) and controls (without psychiatric diagnoses, n=583) showed that PTSD was positively associated with geographic location (level of destruction) and loss to the family, and negatively associated with level of education, being accompanied at the moment of the earthquake and making new friends after the earthquake. Armenian et al (2002) also reported a rate of 52% for depression. A comparison of cases of pure depression (no comorbidity) with controls revealed that depression was positively associated with female gender, geographic location (level of destruction) and loss to the family, and negatively associated with receiving disaster related assistance and social support after the earthquake and alcohol use. Goenjian et al (1994a) evaluated 179 adults 1 1/2 years after the 1988 earthquake with the Posttraumatic Stress Disorder (PTSD) Reaction Index. PTSD reaction index score was associated with nearness to the epicentre (higher exposure) and loss of family members. Although there was no difference in total mean score on the PTSD Reaction Index, the elderly had higher scores on arousal symptoms and lower scores on intrusive symptoms in comparison to young adults. In another study, Goenjian et al (1994b) assessed 202 adults exposed in 1988 to political violence in Azerbaijan and/or the earthquake in Armenia. High rates of severe posttraumatic stress reactions were found among the most highly exposed individuals, irrespective of the type of trauma. The same group of workers (Goenjian et al, 2000) evaluated 78 non-treatment-seeking subjects with self-report instruments approximately 1.5 and 4.5 years after the 1988 earthquake in Armenia and the 1988 pogroms against Armenians in Azerbaijan. No significant differences in PTSD severity, profile or course were seen between the two groups. Those exposed to severe trauma (earthquake or violence) had high initial and follow-up PTSD scores that did not remit over the 3-year interval, though the depressive symptoms subsided. Posttraumatic stress, anxiety and depressive reactions were highly intercorrelated within and across both time intervals. Goenjian (1993) found high rates of psychiatric morbidity (post-traumatic stress disorder: 74%, major depressive disorder: 22%) in a sample of 582 school children. In a sample of 231 children, Pynoos et al (1993) found that the Children's Post-traumatic Stress Disorder Reaction Index (CPTSD-RI) score was strongly correlated with a clinical diagnosis of PTSD and that there was a strong positive correlation between proximity to the epicentre and overall severity of post-traumatic stress reaction. Analyses controlling for exposure revealed that girls reported more persistent fears than boys. Goenjian et al (1995) evaluated 218 school-age children using the Child Posttraumatic Stress Disorder Reaction Index, the Depression Self-Rating Scale and the section on separation anxiety disorder from the Diagnostic Interview for Children and Adolescents. They found high rates of current PTSD, depressive disorder (and the co-occurrence of PTSD and depression) among victims residing in the two heavily impacted cities. Separation anxiety disorder was comparatively less frequent, Severity of post-traumatic stress and depressive reactions were highly correlated and each with the extent of loss of family members. Najarian (1996) found that two groups of children with high exposure to the earthquake (those remaining in the earthquake city and those relocated to another place) demonstrated significantly higher rates of PTSD, depression and behavioural difficulties in comparison to a control group. There were no differences between the relocated children and those who remained in the earthquake zone. An article comparing suicide patterns across different countries that were a part of the erstwhile USSR reports that during 1984-1990 the rate of suicide was 3.5 cases per 100 000 inhabitants in the Caucasus (Georgia, Azerbaijan and Armenia) (Wasserman et al, 1998).

MENTAL HEALTH RESOURCES

Mental Health Policy A mental health policy is present. The policy was initially formulated in 1994.

The components of the policy are advocacy, promotion and prevention.

Substance Abuse Policy A substance abuse policy is present. The policy was initially formulated in 1992.

National Mental Health Programme A national mental health programme is absent.

National Therapeutic Drug Policy/Essential List of Drugs A national therapeutic drug policy/essential list of drugs is present. Details about the year of formulation are not available.

Mental Health Legislation The law regulates the rights of mentally disturbed individuals (excluding any discrimination for psychiatric patients), provision of professional medical aid and social insurance, as well as issues of compulsory and non-compulsory treatment.
The latest legislation was enacted in 2004.

Mental Health Financing There are budget allocations for mental health.
The country spends 4.5% of the total health budget on mental health.
The primary source of mental health financing is tax based.
The treatment of psychiatric patients is financed by the state. However, in the situation of slender budgets for public health care, the funding of the psychiatric service is obviously inadequate.
The country has disability benefits for persons with mental disorders. Chronically mentally ill patients receive monthly payments.

Mental Health Facilities Mental health is a part of primary health care system. Actual treatment of severe mental disorders is not available at the primary level. Treatment of severe mental disorders is carried out by specialized centres and psychiatric dispensaries (specialized outpatient departments).
Regular training of primary care professionals is carried out in the field of mental health. In the last two years, about 175 personnel were provided training. Treatment of patients is organized in close cooperation with the local primary care service. Regulations for continuous training of family doctors in the field of mental health are in the stage of development. Since 1999, mental health issues are considered in postgraduate training and respecialization (concerning experienced general practice physicians) programmes for family doctors. Special emphasis is placed on identification and management of neurotic and somatoform disorders, affective (especially mild and masked depressive) disorders, drug use disorders, behavioural syndromes connected with physiological disturbances and other physical factors, personality disorders and developmental disorders. Approximately 250 family doctors have been trained in the field of mental health since 1999.
There are community care facilities for patients with mental disorders. Each community and locality has its mental health providers.

Psychiatric Beds and Professionals

Total psychiatric beds per 10 000 population	4.8
Psychiatric beds in mental hospitals per 10 000 population	4.78
Psychiatric beds in general hospitals per 10 000 population	0.02
Psychiatric beds in other settings per 10 000 population	0
Number of psychiatrists per 100 000 population	4
Number of neurosurgeons per 100 000 population	1.2
Number of psychiatric nurses per 100 000 population	0
Number of neurologists per 100 000 population	9.8
Number of psychologists per 100 000 population	0.4
Number of social workers per 100 000 population	0.08

Psychiatric provision in Armenia is carried out by two kinds of medical service: outpatient and inpatient. It is represented through the network of dispensaries, hospitals and health centres within the various communities. In recent years, the policy of reducing hospital beds has been implemented and new day hospitals have been opened; the development of night hostels is proposed. The psychiatric hospitals have been broken up into smaller units; whereas they formerly had 500-1000 beds, at present the greatest number of beds in any one is 400.

Non-Governmental Organizations NGOs are involved with mental health in the country. They are mainly involved in advocacy and promotion. In 1999, with the assistance of the international organization Médecins Sans Frontières, it became possible to open a rehabilitation workshop at one of the biggest psychiatric hospitals.

Information Gathering System There is mental health reporting system in the country.
The country has data collection system or epidemiological study on mental health.

Programmes for Special Population The country has specific programmes for mental health for refugees, disaster affected population and children.
In 2000, the Association of Child Psychiatrists and Psychologists (ACPP) and the Geneva Initiative on Psychiatry (GIP) successfully implemented a project entitled 'Public Education and Training of Professionals Working with Children in Primary Health Care

System of Armenia.' One of the outcomes of this project was the creation of the Child and Adolescent Mental Health Care Project (CAMHCP). This programme attempts to respond to the mental health needs of children and adolescents in Armenia by a quick response to requests and referrals, involving parents and teachers in the early detection of behavioural problems in a multidisciplinary, supportive and therapeutic environment.

Therapeutic Drugs The following therapeutic drugs are generally available at the primary health care level of the country: carbamazepine, ethosuximide, phenobarbital, phenytoin sodium, sodium valproate, amitriptyline, chlorpromazine, diazepam, fluphenazine, haloperidol, lithium, levodopa.

Other Information

Additional Sources of Information

Anonymous (2000) Making mental health law reform in Armenia. www.mentalhealth.am

Armenian, H. K., Morikawa, M., Melkonian, A. K., et al (2000) Loss as a determinant of PTSD in a cohort of adult survivors of the 1988 earthquake in Armenia: implications for policy. Acta Psychiatrica Scandinavica, 102, 58-64.

Armenian, H. K., Morikawa, M., Melkonian, A. K., et al (2002) Risk factors for depression in the survivors of the 1988 earthquake in Armenia. Journal of Urban Health, 79, 373-382.

Goenjian, A. (1993) A mental health relief programme in Armenia after the 1988 earthquake. Implementation and clinical observations. British Journal of Psychiatry, 163, 230-239.

Goenjian, A. K., Najarian, L. M., Pynoos, R. S., et al (1994a) Posttraumatic stress disorder in elderly and younger adults after the 1988 earthquake in Armenia. American Journal of Psychiatry, 151, 895-901.

Goenjian, A. K., Najarian, L. M., Pynoos, R. S., et al (1994b) Posttraumatic stress reactions after single and double trauma. Acta Psychiatrica Scandinavica, 90, 214-221.

Goenjian, A. K., Pynoos, R. S., Steinberg, A. M., et al (1995) Psychiatric comorbidity in children after the 1988 earthquake in Armenia. Journal of the American Academy of Child & Adolescent Psychiatry, 34, 1174-1184.

Goenjian, A. K., Steinberg, A. M., Najarian, L. M., et al (2000) Prospective study of posttraumatic stress, anxiety, and depressive reactions after earthquake and political violence. American Journal of Psychiatry, 157, 911-916.

Khachaturyan A. M. (2002) Psychosomatic performance of population in Armenia. European Journal of Public Health (Supplement – Abstracts of the 10th Annual EUPHA Meeting. Dresden, Germany, 28-30 November 2002), 67-68.

Khachaturyan, A. M., Nersesyan, A. K. (2004) Mental performance of population of disaster and non-disaster area in Armenia. Mental health perspectives in public health. Proceedings of the International Psychiatric Conference, 7-10 October 2004, 61-62.

Najarian, L. M., Goenjian, A. K., Pelcovitz, D., et al (1996) Relocation after a disaster: posttraumatic stress disorder in Armenia after the earthquake. Journal of the American Academy of Child & Adolescent Psychiatry, 35, 374-383.

Pynoos, R. S., Goenjian, A., Tashjian, M., et al (1993) Post-traumatic stress reactions in children after the 1988 Armenian earthquake. British Journal of Psychiatry, 163, 239-247.

Wasserman, D., Varnik, A., Dankowicz, M. (1998) Regional differences in the distribution of suicide in the former Soviet Union during perestroika, 1984-1990. Acta Psychiatrica Scandinavica, Supplement 394, 5-12.

Yeghiyan, M., Gasparyan, K., Grigorian, H. (2002) Contemporary child and adolescent mental health in Armenia. Mental Health Reforms, 7, 12-13.

Australia

A–B

GENERAL INFORMATION

Australia is a country with an approximate area of 7741 thousand sq. km. (UNO, 2001). Its population is 19.913 million, and the sex ratio (men per hundred women) is 99 (UNO, 2004). The proportion of population under the age of 15 years is 20% (UNO, 2004), and the proportion of population above the age of 60 years is 17% (WHO, 2004). The literacy rate is 99% for men and 99% for women (UNESCO/MoH, 2004).

The country is a high income group country (based on World Bank 2004 criteria). The proportion of health budget to GDP is 9.2%. The per capita total expenditure on health is 2532 international $, and the per capita government expenditure on health is 1718 international $ (WHO, 2004).

The main language(s) used in the country is (are) English. The largest ethnic group(s) is (are) Caucasian, and the other ethnic group(s) are (is) Asian and indigenous groups. The largest religious group(s) is (are) Anglican, and the other religious group(s) are (is) Roman Catholic.

The life expectancy at birth is 77.9 years for males and 83 years for females (WHO, 2004). The healthy life expectancy at birth is 71 years for males and 74 years for females (WHO, 2004).

EPIDEMIOLOGY

There is substantial epidemiological data on mental illnesses in Australia in internationally accessible literature. No attempt was made to include this information here.

MENTAL HEALTH RESOURCES

Mental Health Policy A mental health policy is present. The policy was initially formulated in 1992.

The components of the policy are advocacy, promotion, prevention, treatment and rehabilitation. The national mental health policy together with the Statement of Rights and Responsibilities and the three consecutive National Mental Health Plans is a foundation document of the National Mental Health Strategy, the umbrella for mental health reform in Australia. The aims of the policy are to: promote the mental health of the Australian community and, where possible, prevent the development of mental health problems; reduce the impact of mental disorders on individuals, families and the community; and assure the rights of people with mental disorders. The national mental health policy discusses twelve key policy areas including: consumer rights; promotion and prevention; service mix; mainstreaming of mental health services; mental health workforce; legislation; research and evaluation; and monitoring and accountability. The Policy is implemented through the National Mental Health Strategy and the 5-year National Mental Health Plans (1992-1997; 1998-2003; 2003-2008).

Substance Abuse Policy A substance abuse policy is present. The policy was initially formulated in 1985. The National Drug Strategy 2004-2009 provides a framework for a coordinated, integrated approach to drug issues in the Australian community. It is a national policy framework that is complemented, supported and integrated with a range of national, state, territory, governmental and non-governmental strategies, plans and initiatives. It builds upon the experience and achievements of its policy predecessor, the National Drug Strategic Framework 1998-99 to 2003-04, and is overseen and guided by key advisory and decision making bodies. Its mission is to improve health, social and economic outcomes by preventing the uptake of harmful drug use and reducing the harmful effects of licit and illicit drugs in Australian society.

National Mental Health Programme A national mental health programme is present. The programme was formulated in 1992. The programme progressed through the first and second National Mental Health Plans. Under the National Mental Health Strategy, the Australian Government and all State and Territory Governments are working to achieve reform of mental health care in Australia. The private sector is also engaged in reform activity. The current National Mental Health Plan 2003-2008 has four priority themes: mental health promotion and prevention of mental illness; increasing service responsiveness; strengthening quality; and fostering research, innovation and sustainability. The Plan aims to continue the reform processes previously begun and to engage with other sectors such as housing, education, welfare, justice and employment. Under the Plan there is also an increased focus on issues of recovery and rehabilitation and the need for a broad Government and community response.

National Therapeutic Drug Policy/Essential List of Drugs A national therapeutic drug policy/essential list of drugs is present. It was formulated in 1991.

Mental Health Legislation Mental health legislation in Australia is the responsibility of each of the eight State and Territory Governments. In 1996, under the National Mental Health Strategy, a Rights Analysis Instrument was developed by the Federal Attorney-General's Department for assessing compliance of state and territory legislation with national and international standards. All jurisdictions have undertaken such assessment and suitable amendments to legislation have been incorporated based on assessment findings. The assessments looked for conformity with the United Nations Principles for the Protection of Persons with Mental Illness and for the Improvement of Mental Health Care and the National Mental Health Statement of Rights and Responsibilities. Details about the year of enactment of the mental health legislation are not available.

Mental Health Financing There are budget allocations for mental health.

The country spends 9.6% of the total health budget on mental health.

The primary sources of mental health financing in descending order are tax based, private insurances and out of pocket expenditure by the patient or family.
The figure 6.4% refers to the proportion of the total health budget spent on specialized mental health services (excluding alcohol and drug services). When all health services are taken into account, an estimated 9.6% of total recurrent health expenditure is spent on mental disorders. The Federal Government share is about one-third and the remaining is provided by the State and Territory Government with some contribution from the private sector. Between 1993 and 2002, federal spending grew by 128% and state and territory funding by about 40%. In this period, the state and territory spending on community care increased by 145%; NGOs increased their share of the mental health budget from 2% to 5%. In 2000, only 20% of mental health resources were accounted for by stand-alone psychiatric institutions, down from 49% in 1993. Financing arrangements differ across states and territories. State funded specialized mental health services are largely funded through block grants. Victoria funds specialized mental health services on the basis of unit costs – number of beds available and staff employed. Some other states use a case-mix system for their acute hospitals where providers are funded according to the number and type of patients treated (the classification system used for this is the Australian National Diagnosis Related Groups). In cases where the case-mix system is restricted to acute care, community care is funded on block grants. Under the Australian system all citizens are eligible to free medical care in the public sector and the national health insurance system covers some portion of the expenses incurred under the private sector. Private mental health care is also funded by private insurance (almost one-third of the population has private health insurance) and workers' compensation insurance. The country has disability benefits for persons with mental disorders.

Mental Health Facilities Mental health is a part of primary health care system. Actual treatment of severe mental disorders is available at the primary level. Primary care is now acknowledged as part of the mental health workforce. The majority of Divisions of General Practice have developed and implemented mental health projects that focus on partnership development. In 2001-2002, the 'Better Outcomes in Mental Health Care' initiative was launched to advance primary mental health care. It provides incentive payments for general practitioners to provide mental health care and in particular to deliver focused psychological strategies. It supports ongoing general practitioner education and access to allied health specialists to provide non-pharmacological treatments and multi-disciplinary care. Changes were also made to the Medicare Benefits Schedule to fund psychiatrists for case conferencing with general practitioners. Regular training of primary care professionals is carried out in the field of mental health.
There are community care facilities for patients with mental disorders. Detailed information can be obtained from the Government website and also other published literature.

Psychiatric Beds and Professionals

Total psychiatric beds per 10 000 population	3.9
Psychiatric beds in mental hospitals per 10 000 population	1.2
Psychiatric beds in general hospitals per 10 000 population	2.7
Psychiatric beds in other settings per 10 000 population	1
Number of psychiatrists per 100 000 population	14
Number of neurosurgeons per 100 000 population	0.6
Number of psychiatric nurses per 100 000 population	53
Number of neurologists per 100 000 population	3
Number of psychologists per 100 000 population	5
Number of social workers per 100 000 population	5

All state and territories have transferred the management of public mental health services to the mainstream health system. Psychiatric beds in stand alone psychiatric hospitals have been reduced. In 2002, 83% of acute psychiatric beds were in general hospitals (up from 55% in 1993). The proportion of clinical staff providing ambulatory mental health care has grown from 24% in 1993 to 40% in 2002. Australia has supply side control on the number of medical practitioners by limiting the number of places in Australian medical schools, all of which are in public universities.

Non-Governmental Organizations NGOs are involved with mental health in the country. They are mainly involved in advocacy, promotion, prevention, treatment and rehabilitation. NGOs are often funded by the Government and provide support services like a wide range of accommodation, rehabilitation, recreational and social support and advocacy programmes.

Information Gathering System There is mental health reporting system in the country. The information collected through the annual National Mental Health Survey of mental health services is collated and analysed nationally and reported through the National Mental Health Report. There is a mental health information development strategy developed under the Second National Mental Health Plan. Priorities include the development of a mental health information infrastructure and implementation of nationally agreed clinical mental health outcome measures. Information development priorities are being updated under the National Mental Health Plan 2003-2008. The country has data collection system or epidemiological study on mental health. The data collection systems covers all public specialist mental health services. A national epidemiological study on the mental health of the Australian population was conducted in 1996. Populations included in the study were adults aged between 18 and 24 years, children and adolescents and people living with a psychotic illness. Results are available in a number of reports on the National Survey of Mental Health and Wellbeing.

Australia has a mental health reporting system. National information on mental health in Australia is published annually in the National Mental Health Report.

Programmes for Special Population The country has specific programmes for mental health for minorities, refugees, disaster affected population, indigenous population, elderly and children.
A Community Awareness Programme was launched in the mid 1990s aimed at destigmatizing mental illness. School, community and media based activities are also under way. 'MindMatters' resources containing material related to mental health promotion and prevention and early intervention have been provided to all secondary schools in Australia and 73% have participated in professional development. Similarly 'Mindmatters Plus' and 'Families Matter' have been launched to assist children with high support needs and families. A National Action Plan for Depression was released in November 2000. An innovative alliance, 'Beyondblue: the national depression initiative' was formed between a number of sectors to progress the activities of the Action Plan. Telepsychiatry is now considered an important component of mental health service delivery to rural and remote areas. Kids Help Line, a national telephone counselling service, has introduced internet and web-based counselling for children. Special programmes are being developed for specific population groups including Aboriginal people and Torres Strait Islanders. However, there is still a shortage of indigenous health workers and an ongoing need to improve the links between indigenous specific services and mainstream services. The report 'Towards a National Approach to Forensic Mental Health' was released in 2000 as a guide for discussion and planning of good practice. The forensic mental health services are the responsibility of the states and territories with the Federal Government advocating strategies and standards. Key issues include – availability of appropriately secure forensic hospitals; shifting care out from institutions to the community; on-site mental health liaison/assessment services in the courts; systematic mental health assessment of all new receptions into prisons; multidisciplinary services; easily accessible consultation/ liaison services to the general mental health programmes.

Therapeutic Drugs The following therapeutic drugs are generally available at the primary health care level of the country: carbamazepine, ethosuximide, phenobarbital, phenytoin sodium, sodium valproate, amitriptyline, chlorpromazine, diazepam, fluphenazine, haloperidol, lithium, biperiden, carbidopa, levodopa.

Other Information Consumer rights and consumer and carer participation at all stages in the planning and delivery of mental health services is an impetus for the reform within the mental health system. Consumers and carers have been included in all national planning groups since the advent of the National Mental Health Strategy, and mental health leads the health industry in this area. A number of advisory groups have been established to increase consumer and carer input at the national, state and territory levels. The Mental Health Council of Australia (MHCA) includes consumers and carers as 25% of its membership. It was established as the peak national NGO to represent and promote the interests of the mental health sector. At the service delivery level, by 2002, 89% of organizations had established a specific, formal mechanism for consumer participation in local service issues as against 33% in 1994. The participation, however, is variable across jurisdictions and services. National Standards for Mental Health Services were developed in 1997 for use in assessing service quality and act as a guide to continuous quality improvement. All public mental health services in Australia, and many private services, are undergoing review against the National Standards as part of a quality assurance and accreditation cycle. National Practice Standards for the Mental Health Workforce were endorsed in 2002. These workforce standards target the professions of psychiatry, nursing, social work, psychology and occupational therapy and address the shared knowledge and skills required when working in a multi-disciplinary mental health environment. The National Practice Standards are designed to be used in conjunction with the National Standards for Mental Health Services. In a major mental health industry development initiative all public mental health services are participating in the routine collection of consumer outcome measures together with the bulk of the private sector.

Additional Sources of Information

Australian Health Ministers, National Mental Health Plan 2003-2008, Canberra: Australian Government, 2003.

Casey, D. (2000) Mental Health Rights Analysis. Mental Health and Special Programs Branch.

Commonwealth Department of Health and Aged Care (2000) National Mental Health Report 2000: Sixth Annual Report: Changes in Australia's Mental Health Services under the First National Mental Health Plan of the National Mental Health Strategy 1993-98. Canberra: Commonwealth of Australia.

Henderson, S. (2000) Focus on psychiatry in Australia. British Journal of Psychiatry, 176, 97-101.

Hickie, I., Groom, G. (2002) Primary care-led mental health service reform: an outline of the Better Outcomes in Mental Health care initiative. Australasian Psychiatry, 10, 376-382.

http://www.mentalhealth.gov.au

Laugharne, J. (1999) Poverty and mental health in Aboriginal Australia. Psychiatric Bulletin, 23, 364-66.

Leitch, E., Macleod, B., Whiteford, H. (1993) The National Mental Health Policy: implications for public psychiatric services in Australia. Australian and New Zealand Journal of Psychiatry, 27, 186-191.

Mullen, P. E., Briggs, S., Dalton, T., et al (2000) Forensic mental health services in Australia. International Journal of Law and Psychiatry, 23, 433-452.

Singh, B. S., McGorry, P. D. (1998) The second National Mental Health Plan: an opportunity to take stock and move forward. Medical Journal of Australia, 169, 435-437.

Watchirs H. (2000) Application of Rights Analysis Instrument to Australian Mental Health Legislation. Canberra: Commonwealth of Australia.

Whiteford, H. (1993) Australia's National Mental Health Policy. Hospital and Community Psychiatry, 44, 963-66.

Whiteford, H. (2000) Introduction: the Australian mental health survey. Australian and New Zealand Journal of Psychiatry, 34, 193-96.

Whiteford, W., Buckingham, B., Manderscheid, R. (2002) Australia's National Mental Health Strategy. British Journal of Psychiatry, 180, 210-215.

Whiteford, H., Thompson, I., Casey, D. (2000) The Australian mental health system. International Journal of Law and Psychiatry, 23, 403-417.

Austria

GENERAL INFORMATION

Austria is a country with an approximate area of 84 thousand sq. km. (UNO, 2001). Its population is 8.12 million, and the sex ratio (men per hundred women) is 96 (UNO, 2004). The proportion of population under the age of 15 years is 16% (UNO, 2004), and the proportion of population above the age of 60 years is 21% (WHO, 2004). The literacy rate is 99% for men and 99% for women (UNESCO/MoH, 2004).
The country is a high income group country (based on World Bank 2004 criteria). The proportion of health budget to GDP is 8%. The per capita total expenditure on health is 2259 international $, and the per capita government expenditure on health is 1566 international $ (WHO, 2004).
The main language(s) used in the country is (are) German. The largest religious group(s) is (are) Roman Catholic.
The life expectancy at birth is 76.4 years for males and 82.2 years for females (WHO, 2004). The healthy life expectancy at birth is 69 years for males and 74 years for females (WHO, 2004).

EPIDEMIOLOGY

There is substantial epidemiological data on mental illnesses in Austria in internationally accessible literature. No attempt was made to include this information here.

MENTAL HEALTH RESOURCES

Mental Health Policy A mental health policy is present. The policy was initially formulated in 1999.
The Federal Minister responsible for health matters reports every 3 years about activities of the Ministry of Health to the Parliament.

Substance Abuse Policy A substance abuse policy is present. The policy was initially formulated in 1997. Though at the federal level there is no fixed drug strategy, different provinces have adopted their own drug plans based on the traditional Austrian Drug policy (The Narcotic Substances Act, 1997) principles. Details can be obtained from the document 'Report on the Drug Situation-2000'.

National Mental Health Programme A national mental health programme is absent.
There are mental health plans at the level of all nine provinces, however, there are regional differences. For instance, some provinces already follow the principle of sectorization, others do not. Since 1997, there has been a National Hospital Plan, which involves a certain degree of obligation on individual provinces to fulfil its requirements until 2005. These include a few pages on psychiatry, with a subsection on community services (development period also until 2005). This plan is continuously adapted (latest version July 2003) and contains suggestions for the establishment of psychiatric units in general hospitals. Until now, nine of 23 planned psychiatric units in general hospitals have been created, with several others in advanced planning stage for 2005. The country has a plan for national action with regard to prevention of suicides.

National Therapeutic Drug Policy/Essential List of Drugs A national therapeutic drug policy/essential list of drugs is absent.

Mental Health Legislation Though there is a legislation related to confinement of mentally ill persons in hospitals (1990/1997), there is no comprehensive mental health act or any obligation to provide adequate services. Under the scope of forensic psychiatric services, the penal reform in 1975 brought the treatment of mentally ill offenders under the jurisdiction of the Ministry of Justice. The patients were to be committed to designated institutions for an indefinite period of time, but since the institution was still in the planning phase, actual treatment took place in hospitals. With the opening of the institution in 1985, a large number of male forensic patients were transferred out of psychiatric hospitals. The last reform came with the formulation of the inpatient civil commitment in 1991, which intended to improve the situation of mentally ill patients involuntarily admitted in psychiatric hospitals. It provided for patient's lawyers at psychiatric hospitals. The Austrian Penal Code has legislation for assessment of offences committed by individuals with mental disorders and takes relevant measures for involuntary treatment. In 1991, the Psychology Act and Psychotherapy Act established the state certified professions of 'clinical/health psychologists' and 'psychotherapists'. The Health Care and Nursing Act of 1997 redefined the nursing professions and especially psychiatric nursing, including aspects of community psychiatric nursing.
The latest legislation was enacted in 1997.

Mental Health Financing There are no budget allocations for mental health.
Details about expenditure on mental health are not available.
The primary sources of mental health financing in descending order are social insurance, tax based, private insurances and out of pocket expenditure by the patient or family.
There are no special allocations for mental health as mental health is a part of the primary health care system. Psychiatric services are funded by a variety of sources (among others health insurance), which sometimes leads to difficulties in transition between in-, day- and outpatient as well as medical and social services. Clinical/health psychologists can be partly reimbursed by social security, and psychotherapists can be partly reimbursed by health insurance. The Austrian Hospital and Major Equipment Plan limits the rate of psychiatric beds (including day hospital places). The financing arrangements are such that it is more attractive to have day hospitals.

The country has disability benefits for persons with mental disorders. Different laws are present like the Federal Longterm Care Allowance Act, Provincial Longterm Care Allowance Act, Social Maintenance Act and Disabled Persons Employment Act. Patients with mental disorders can receive benefits based on the provisions made by these acts.

Mental Health Facilities Mental health is a part of primary health care system. Actual treatment of severe mental disorders is available at the primary level. General practitioners usually work in solo practices which are accessible also for patients with mental health problems. From there, patients may be referred to psychiatrists who also work in solo practices and in some cases (about 120 out of 540) have a contract with social security.

Regular training of primary care professionals is carried out in the field of mental health.

There are community care facilities for patients with mental disorders. Responsibility for providing community care lies with the federal provinces. Since the mid 1970s – starting with the WHO/EURO project 'Mental health services in pilot study areas' – Austrian psychiatry has gradually moved away from large mental hospitals to community-based services. The number of community psychiatric services has been steadily increasing over the last 15 years. There are now at least 1000 tax funded services/projects (counselling services, residential facilities, day structure services, vocational rehabilitation services) run by more than 250 providers (usually charitable and private organizations). Nearly all are multi-professionally staffed and often non-psychiatric professionals dominate. It has been suggested that the reduction in suicide mortality might be related to the increase in community psychiatric services. Given the federal character of the country, this development has occurred at different speeds in different provinces. Some provinces have quite advanced community-based psychiatric services, while others still lag behind. In community-based services like day hospitals, crisis intervention services and hostels for psychiatric patients, multidisciplinary teamwork prevails. In some parts of the country, there are procedures for the systematic supervision of such teams.

Psychiatric Beds and Professionals

Total psychiatric beds per 10 000 population	6.5
Psychiatric beds in mental hospitals per 10 000 population	4.5
Psychiatric beds in general hospitals per 10 000 population	2
Psychiatric beds in other settings per 10 000 population	
Number of psychiatrists per 100 000 population	11.8
Number of neurosurgeons per 100 000 population	1.7
Number of psychiatric nurses per 100 000 population	37.8
Number of neurologists per 100 000 population	8.2
Number of psychologists per 100 000 population	49
Number of social workers per 100 000 population	103.4

Psychotherapists can be clinical/health psychologists, psychiatrists and also others who have undergone training in psychotherapy. Since there is a large overlap between these professions, their numbers cannot be simply added. Over the last 3 decades, there has been a reduction of almost 60% in bed strength. These beds are distributed over more than 30 psychiatric and general hospitals and only three hospitals have more than 500 beds. This has gone hand in hand with diversification (e.g. Austria has many day hospitals) and specialization (e.g. child and adolescent psychiatry, geriatric psychiatry, substance abuse etc.). However, this process has not been even throughout the country. Almost three-fifths of psychiatrist work in private (mostly ambulatory) practice, but only a fraction of these (one-ninth) had contact with social security (i.e. they were accessible to those who could not afford to pay commercial fees). Almost 5% of neurosurgeons and 20% of neurologists have a contract with social security. There is a state certified profession of psychotherapy (psychologists, psychiatrists, but also person without any other professional background who have undergone training in psychotherapy; 5495 in the year 2002, i.e. 68 per 100 000 population). Most clinical and health psychologists (90% are trained in both disciplines and more than 40% are also trained as psychotherapists) and psychotherapists are in private practice. The majority of psychiatric nurses work in psychiatric or general hospitals.

Non-Governmental Organizations NGOs are involved with mental health in the country. They are mainly involved in advocacy, promotion, prevention, treatment and rehabilitation. There are few initiatives to promote mental health in relation to positive or negative factors in society. However, the Austrian Society of Psychiatrists is carrying out a de-stigmatization project for schizophrenia. Some local anti-stigma initiatives exist (e.g. school projects in the provinces of Lower Austria and of Tyrol).

Information Gathering System There is no mental health reporting system in the country. Mental health details are mentioned only in hospital discharges and mortality figures.

The country has data collection system or epidemiological study on mental health.

The only service use data routinely available on a countrywide basis are data about 'hospitalization, originating in the performance related hospital financing system based on the 'Diagnosis Related Groups' (DRG).

Programmes for Special Population The country has specific programmes for mental health for refugees, disaster affected population, elderly and children.

Patients who are fit to stand trial are detained in special institutions in the prison system. Those who are not fit to stand trials may be detained in these special institutions or in other psychiatric hospitals. There are also three small forensic outpatient clinics run by universities. Many of the discharged mentally ill offenders have to accept, as an additional condition for release, the services of a probational officer.

Therapeutic Drugs The following therapeutic drugs are generally available at the primary health care level of the country: carbamazepine, ethosuximide, phenytoin sodium, sodium valproate, amitriptyline, diazepam, fluphenazine, haloperidol, lithium, biperiden, carbidopa, levodopa.
The drugs are dispensed through pharmacies.

Other Information The fragmentation of responsibilities at national and local level makes the cooperation between different providers of services and the intersectoral cooperation difficult. The federal structure has also restricted the establishment of common definition of services and quality assurance criteria outside hospitals.

Additional Sources of Information

Austrian Parliament (1990) Unterbringungsgesetz (Civil Commitment Law). BGBl 155.

European Monitoring Centre for Drugs and Drug Addiction and the Austrian Federal Ministery of Social Security and Generations(2000). Report on the Drug Situation. Bundesministerium für soziale Sicherheit und Generationen, Wien.

Katschnig, H., Ladinser, E., Scherer, M., et al (2001) Österreichischer Psychiatriebericht 2001, Teil 1: Daten zur psychiatrischen und psychosozialen Versorgung der österreichischen Bevölkerung (Report on Psychiatry in Austria). Bundesministerium für soziale Sicherheit und Generationen, Wien (available for download in German: www.gesundheit.bmsg.gv.at).

Ludwig-Boltzmann-Institut für Suchtforschung (1999) Handbuch Alkohol – Österreich. Zahlen, Daten, Fakten, Trends (Handbook Alcohol – Austria). Bundesministerium für Arbeit, Gesundheit und Soziales, Wien.

Mental Health in Austria. Selected Annotated Statistics from the Austrian Mental Health reports 2001 and 2003. Vienna: The Federal Ministry of Health and Women.

Osterreichischer Krankenanstalten – und Grobgeräteplan OKAP/GGP (2003) Bundesministerium Für Soziale Sicherheit und Generationen.

Österreichisches Bundesinstitut für Gesundheitswesen (1998) Struktureller Bedarf in der psychiatrischen Versorgung, (Structural Needs for organizing Psychiatric Services), Wien.

Österreichisches Bundesinstitut für Gesundheitswesen (2001) Evaluierung der dezentralen Fachabteilungen für Psychiatrie (Evaluation of psychiatric units in general hospitals), Wien.

Schanda,H., Ortwein-Swoboda, G., Knecht, G., et al (2000) The situation of forensic psychiatry in Austria: setback or progress? International Journal of Law and Psychiatry, 23, 481-492.

Sonneck, G (1999) Suizidprävention in Österreich (Suicide prevention in Austria). Bundesministerium für Arbeit, Gesundheit und Soziales, Wien.

Azerbaijan

GENERAL INFORMATION

Azerbaijan is a country with an approximate area of 87 thousand sq. km. (UNO, 2001). Its population is 8.447 million, and the sex ratio (men per hundred women) is 95 (UNO, 2004). The proportion of population under the age of 15 years is 28% (UNO, 2004), and the proportion of population above the age of 60 years is 9% (WHO, 2004). The literacy rate is 99% for men and 96% for women (UNESCO/MoH, 2004).

The country is a lower middle income group country (based on World Bank 2004 criteria). The proportion of health budget to GDP is 1.6%. The per capita total expenditure on health is 48 international $, and the per capita government expenditure on health is 32 international $ (WHO, 2004).

The main language(s) used in the country is (are) Azerbaijanis and Russian. The largest ethnic group(s) is (are) Azerbaijani (four-fifths), and the other ethnic group(s) are (is) Russian and Armenian. The largest religious group(s) is (are) Muslim (five-sixths), and the other religious group(s) are (is) Russian Orthodox and Armenian Apostolic.

The life expectancy at birth is 63 years for males and 68.6 years for females (WHO, 2004). The healthy life expectancy at birth is 56 years for males and 59 years for females (WHO, 2004).

EPIDEMIOLOGY

There are some articles comparing the prevalence of PTSD and other mental disorders and associated factors between two groups of populations – Armenians affected by the 1988 earthquake and Armenians affected by violence in Azerbaijan (Goenjian et al, 1994, 2000). These studies showed that after exposure to severe trauma (earthquake or violence) adults are at high risk of developing severe and chronic posttraumatic stress reactions that are persistent. Gulakmedove et al (2002) found that among 9500 children with psychoneurological illnesses, 2336 suffered from mental deficiency. An article comparing suicide patterns across different countries that were a part of the erstwhile USSR reports that during 1984-1990 the rate of suicide was 3.5 cases per 100 000 inhabitants in the Caucasus (Georgia, Azerbaijan and Armenia) (Wasserman et al, 1998).

MENTAL HEALTH RESOURCES

Mental Health Policy A mental health policy is absent.

With the help of international organizations (including the Geneva Initiative on Psychiatry and the International Consortium for Mental Health Services) a working group has been established to draft the documents on mental health policy and national mental health programme. The main priority is a programme of deinstitutionalization and the simultaneous development of community services.

Substance Abuse Policy A substance abuse policy is present. The policy was initially formulated in 1996.

National Mental Health Programme A national mental health programme is absent.

National Therapeutic Drug Policy/Essential List of Drugs A national therapeutic drug policy/essential list of drugs is present. It was formulated in 1999.

Mental Health Legislation The law focuses on the protection of civil and human rights of mentally ill people and regulates the provision of mental health services. Several acts related to privileged services to refugees have been passed because of their large numbers. Order 145 simplifies the admission of refugees to psychiatric institutions.

The latest legislation was enacted in 2001.

Mental Health Financing There are budget allocations for mental health.

The country spends 1.6% of the total health budget on mental health.

The primary sources of mental health financing in descending order are tax based, out of pocket expenditure by the patient or family, private insurances and grants.

Hospital treatment is expensive by the average standards.

The country has disability benefits for persons with mental disorders. Disability benefits do not correspond to minimum subsistence levels.

Mental Health Facilities Mental health is a part of primary health care system. Actual treatment of severe mental disorders is available at the primary level. Primary health care is provided at regional level by psychiatrist but general physicians do not provide that service at the primary health care level.

Regular training of primary care professionals is not carried out in the field of mental health.

There are community care facilities for patients with mental disorders. Currently a community based programme is being developed with the help of NGOs.

Psychiatric Beds and Professionals

Total psychiatric beds per 10 000 population	7.1
Psychiatric beds in mental hospitals per 10 000 population	6.9
Psychiatric beds in general hospitals per 10 000 population	0.11
Psychiatric beds in other settings per 10 000 population	0.09
Number of psychiatrists per 100 000 population	5
Number of neurosurgeons per 100 000 population	0.4
Number of psychiatric nurses per 100 000 population	3.9
Number of neurologists per 100 000 population	5.2
Number of psychologists per 100 000 population	0.2
Number of social workers per 100 000 population	0.3

Psychologists and social workers are being trained. Most professionals charge fees for their services. Psychiatrists have to undergo refresher training for 4 months after every 5 years. The official involvement of clinical psychologists in the provision of mental health services has not been established.

Non-Governmental Organizations NGOs are involved with mental health in the country. They are mainly involved in advocacy, promotion and rehabilitation.

Information Gathering System There is mental health reporting system in the country.
The country has data collection system or epidemiological study on mental health. Annual data on the mentally ill is forwarded to the Central Statistics Department.

Programmes for Special Population The country has specific programmes for mental health for refugees. In the state programme of health of refugees there is a section on mental health assistance. Some small projects on psychosocial rehabilitation of refugees, particularly children and invalids have been implemented. However, educational programmes for the refugees need to be established in order to help them to be aware of mental health problems and to reduce the stigma associated with mental health. This information would also benefit them when they return to their own country. Order No. 145 allows a simplified process of acceptance of refugees by psychiatric institutions, irrespective of their country of origin.
Some special pharmacies that supply medicines free of charge to refugees have been established.

Therapeutic Drugs The following therapeutic drugs are generally available at the primary health care level of the country: carbamazepine, phenobarbital, amitriptyline, chlorpromazine, diazepam, haloperidol, lithium.

Other Information

Additional Sources of Information

Goenjian, A. K., Najarian, L. M., Pynoos, R. S., et al (1994) Posttraumatic stress reactions after single and double trauma. Acta Psychiatrica Scandinavica, 90, 214-221.

Goenjian, A.K., Steinberg, A.M., Najarian, L.M., et al (2000) Prospective study of posttraumatic stress, anxiety, and depressive reactions after earthquake and political violence. American Journal of Psychiatry, 157, 911-916.

Gulakhmedove, H., Musabekova, G.N., Aliyeva, N.A. (2002) Retarded children and their families face challenges in Azerbaijan. Mental Health Reforms, 7, 12-13.

Ismayilov, F. (2004) Mental health services in Azerbaijan. International Psychiatry, 3, 16-17.

Ismayilov, N. V., Ismayilov, F. (2002) Mental health of refugees: the case of Azerbaijan. World Psychiatry, 1, 121-122.

Wasserman, D., Varnik, A., Dankowicz, M. (1998) Regional differences in the distribution of suicide in the former Soviet Union during perestroika, 1984-1990. Acta Psychiatrica Scandinavica, Supplement 394, 5-12.

Bahamas

GENERAL INFORMATION

Bahamas is a country with an approximate area of 14 thousand sq. km. (UNO, 2001). The country is an archipelago of about 700 islands and 2 400 cays. Thirty islands are inhabited. Its population is 0.317 million, and the sex ratio (men per hundred women) is 97 (UNO, 2004). The proportion of population under the age of 15 years is 29% (UNO, 2004), and the proportion of population above the age of 60 years is 8% (WHO, 2004). The literacy rate is 94.5% for men and 96.3% for women (UNESCO/MoH, 2004). The country is a high income group country (based on World Bank 2004 criteria). The proportion of health budget to GDP is 5.7%. The per capita total expenditure on health is 1220 international $, and the per capita government expenditure on health is 695 international $ (WHO, 2004).

The main language(s) used in the country is (are) English. The largest ethnic group(s) is (are) African (descent). The largest religious group(s) is (are) Anglican, and the other religious group(s) are (is) Baptist and Roman Catholic.

The life expectancy at birth is 69.4 years for males and 75.7 years for females (WHO, 2004). The healthy life expectancy at birth is 61 years for males and 66 years for females (WHO, 2004).

EPIDEMIOLOGY

There is substantial epidemiological data on mental illnesses in the Bahamas in internationally accessible literature. No attempt was made to include this information here.

MENTAL HEALTH RESOURCES

Mental Health Policy A mental health policy is absent.
The policy is being developed.

Substance Abuse Policy A substance abuse policy is absent. A policy is currently before the Cabinet.

National Mental Health Programme A national mental health programme is absent.
The programme is being developed.

National Therapeutic Drug Policy/Essential List of Drugs A national therapeutic drug policy/essential list of drugs is present. It was formulated in 1997.

Mental Health Legislation The mental health legislation is under review.
Details about the year of enactment of the mental health legislation are not available.

Mental Health Financing There are budget allocations for mental health.
The country spends 11% of the total health budget on mental health.
The primary source of mental health financing is tax based.
The country has disability benefits for persons with mental disorders.

Mental Health Facilities Mental health is a part of primary health care system. Actual treatment of severe mental disorders is available at the primary level. Cases are only assessed and then referred to specialized centres.
Regular training of primary care professionals is not carried out in the field of mental health.
There are community care facilities for patients with mental disorders.

Psychiatric Beds and Professionals

Total psychiatric beds per 10 000 population	11.96
Psychiatric beds in mental hospitals per 10 000 population	11.69
Psychiatric beds in general hospitals per 10 000 population	0.27
Psychiatric beds in other settings per 10 000 population	0
Number of psychiatrists per 100 000 population	4.7
Number of neurosurgeons per 100 000 population	0.3
Number of psychiatric nurses per 100 000 population	21.6
Number of neurologists per 100 000 population	1
Number of psychologists per 100 000 population	3
Number of social workers per 100 000 population	3.7

Besides trained psychiatrist there are other trained doctors who deliver psychiatric care.

Non-Governmental Organizations NGOs are involved with mental health in the country. They are mainly involved in prevention and treatment. The majority of the NGOs work in the field of substance abuse.

Information Gathering System There is mental health reporting system in the country.
The country has no data collection system or epidemiological study on mental health. A data collection system is being developed.

Programmes for Special Population The country has specific programmes for mental health for disaster affected population, elderly and children.

Therapeutic Drugs The following therapeutic drugs are generally available at the primary health care level of the country: carbamazepine, phenobarbital, phenytoin sodium, sodium valproate, amitriptyline, chlorpromazine, diazepam, fluphenazine, haloperidol, lithium, carbidopa, levodopa.

Other Information More emphasis needs to be placed on developing psychiatry in a general hospital set-up.

Additional Sources of Information

Bahrain

GENERAL INFORMATION

Bahrain is a country with an approximate area of 0.71 thousand sq. km. (UNO, 2001). The country is an archipelago of low desert islands, of which the largest is Manama. Its population is 0.739 million, and the sex ratio (men per hundred women) is 135 (UNO, 2004). The proportion of population under the age of 15 years is 29% (UNO, 2004), and the proportion of population above the age of 60 years is 4% (WHO, 2004). The literacy rate is 91.5% for men and 84.2% for women (UNESCO/MoH, 2004).
The country is a high income group country (based on World Bank 2004 criteria). The proportion of health budget to GDP is 4.1%. The per capita total expenditure on health is 664 international $, and the per capita government expenditure on health is 458 international $ (WHO, 2004).
The main language(s) used in the country is (are) Arabic and English. The largest ethnic group(s) is (are) Arab. The largest religious group(s) is (are) Muslim.
The life expectancy at birth is 72.1 years for males and 74.5 years for females (WHO, 2004). The healthy life expectancy at birth is 64 years for males and 64 years for females (WHO, 2004).

EPIDEMIOLOGY

There is substantial epidemiological data on mental illnesses in Bahrain in internationally accessible literature. No attempt was made to include this information here.

MENTAL HEALTH RESOURCES

Mental Health Policy A mental health policy is present. The policy was initially formulated in 1993.
The components of the policy are advocacy, promotion, prevention, treatment and rehabilitation.

Substance Abuse Policy A substance abuse policy is present. The policy was initially formulated in 1983.

National Mental Health Programme A national mental health programme is present. The programme was formulated in 1989.

National Therapeutic Drug Policy/Essential List of Drugs A national therapeutic drug policy/essential list of drugs is present. It was formulated in 1975.

Mental Health Legislation The latest mental health legislation is Decree 3.
The latest legislation was enacted in 1975.

Mental Health Financing There are budget allocations for mental health.
Details about expenditure on mental health are not available.
The primary sources of mental health financing in descending order are tax based and out of pocket expenditure by the patient or family.
The country has disability benefits for persons with mental disorders.

Mental Health Facilities Mental health is a part of primary health care system. Actual treatment of severe mental disorders is available at the primary level. Primary care is provided only after stabilization of the case. There are 23 primary care centres, each within 5 km of the catchment area, and have all psychiatric drugs. Any new drugs can be procured within a day.
Regular training of primary care professionals is carried out in the field of mental health. The psychiatry department is involved in the training of family physicians. Child care workers have been trained on issues related to mental health and behavioural disorders.
There are community care facilities for patients with mental disorders. There are regular home visits through outreach programmes of the hospital. The psychiatric community care was started in 1979 and forms an important aspect of mental health delivery system along with primary care. During community visits, family members are encouraged to participate in the treatment. Patients are given information on treatment, management and other educational items related to their illness. A day care centre that can provide services for 40 clients exists.

Psychiatric Beds and Professionals

Total psychiatric beds per 10 000 population	3.3
Psychiatric beds in mental hospitals per 10 000 population	3.3
Psychiatric beds in general hospitals per 10 000 population	0
Psychiatric beds in other settings per 10 000 population	0
Number of psychiatrists per 100 000 population	5
Number of neurosurgeons per 100 000 population	0.3
Number of psychiatric nurses per 100 000 population	23
Number of neurologists per 100 000 population	1
Number of psychologists per 100 000 population	0.8
Number of social workers per 100 000 population	1.5

Psychiatric training is undertaken in the country with licensing from the Arab Board of Psychiatry. Beds have been earmarked for treatment of drug abusers and management of mentally challenged individuals.

Non-Governmental Organizations NGOs are involved with mental health in the country. They are mainly involved in advocacy, promotion, prevention and rehabilitation.

Information Gathering System There is mental health reporting system in the country. Data are available from the Bahrain Health Statistics, 1999.
The country has data collection system or epidemiological study on mental health. Data collection is hospital-based.

Programmes for Special Population The country has specific programmes for mental health for elderly and children.

Therapeutic Drugs The following therapeutic drugs are generally available at the primary health care level of the country: carbamazepine, phenytoin sodium, sodium valproate, amitriptyline, chlorpromazine, diazepam, fluphenazine, haloperidol, lithium, biperiden.
All drugs available at the psychiatric hospital can be made available to health centres on request and according to needs of known patients.

Other Information

Additional Sources of Information

Al-Haddad, M. K. (1989) Community psychiatry in Bahrain. World Health Forum, 10, 432.

Bangladesh

GENERAL INFORMATION

Bangladesh is a country with an approximate area of 144 thousand sq. km. (UNO, 2001). Its population is 149.665 million, and the sex ratio (men per hundred women) is 105 (UNO, 2004). The proportion of population under the age of 15 years is 37% (UNO, 2004), and the proportion of population above the age of 60 years is 5% (WHO, 2004). The literacy rate is 50.3% for men and 31.4% for women (UNESCO/MoH, 2004).

The country is a low income group country (based on World Bank 2004 criteria). The proportion of health budget to GDP is 3.5%. The per capita total expenditure on health is 58 international $, and the per capita government expenditure on health is 26 international $ (WHO, 2004).

The main language(s) used in the country is (are) Bangla. The largest ethnic group(s) is (are) Bangla (nine-tenths). The largest religious group(s) is (are) Muslim (four-fifths).

The life expectancy at birth is 62.6 years for males and 62.6 years for females (WHO, 2004). The healthy life expectancy at birth is 55 years for males and 53 years for females (WHO, 2004).

EPIDEMIOLOGY

In a study on 1288 primary school children screened with the Rutter B2 Scale, 13.4% had behaviour disorders (males 20.4%, females 9.9%). Emotional, conduct and undifferentiated disorders were detected in 3.2, 8.9 and 1.2% of cases. Psychiatric morbidity was greater in higher school grades (Rabbani & Hossain, 1999). A two-phase survey on over 10 000 children aged 2-9 revealed that the prevalence rates of severe and mild mental retardation were 0.6% and 1.4%, respectively. Mild mental retardation was strongly and significantly associated with low socioeconomic status (Islam et al, 1993). Further analyses showed that significant risk factors of serious mental retardation in rural and urban areas were maternal goiter and postnatal brain infections, and in rural areas consanguinity and landless agriculture. Risk factors for mild cognitive disabilities included maternal illiteracy, landlessness, maternal history of pregnancy loss and small for gestational age at birth. Durkin et al (1993, 2000) used a structured measure for assessment of 162 children affected by a flood, who had been evaluated earlier, and found that an additional 10% had aggressive behaviours and 34% had enuresis. A survey for physical and psychiatric disorders of the entire population (n=1181) of a village revealed a point-prevalence rate of 6.5% (3.6% of subjects had psychiatric disorders alone and 2.9% had both psychiatric and physical disorders). Depressive and anxiety states were common and psychiatric disorders occurred more frequently in women (Choudhury et al, 1981). A study that covered 4751 health facilities throughout Bangladesh evaluated deaths among women aged 10-50 years by examining medical records and interview. Among 28 998 deaths in women aged 10-50 years 11.4% were attributable to suicide. Regional variations were noted (Appleby, 2000). Neurotic disorders were reported to be common in general practice (Alam, 1978) and medical outpatients (31%) (Chowdhury et al, 1975). Schizophrenia, affective disorders and anxiety neurosis were common among adult psychiatric outpatients (77%) (Ahmed, 1978), and dissociative disorder (Hysteria) (21.65%) and epilepsy (19.59%) among child psychiatry outpatients (Rahim et al, 1997).

MENTAL HEALTH RESOURCES

Mental Health Policy A mental health policy is absent.

Substance Abuse Policy A substance abuse policy is present. The policy was initially formulated in 1990.

National Mental Health Programme A national mental health programme is present. The programme was formulated in 1984.

National Therapeutic Drug Policy/Essential List of Drugs A national therapeutic drug policy/essential list of drugs is present. It was formulated in 1983.

Mental Health Legislation There is the Lunacy Act. A national workshop on the draft of the Mental Health Act was held in 1999 to formulate the final version of the act and for its enactment.

The latest legislation was enacted in 1912.

Mental Health Financing There are budget allocations for mental health.

The country spends 0.5% of the total health budget on mental health.

The primary sources of mental health financing in descending order are tax based, out of pocket expenditure by the patient or family and grants.

The country has disability benefits for persons with mental disorders. Lifetime pension is provided for mentally handicapped children after the death of the father or mother who was receiving some pension.

Mental Health Facilities Mental health is a part of primary health care system. Actual treatment of severe mental disorders is available at the primary level. Efforts are being made to provide cheaper drugs at primary level.

Regular training of primary care professionals is carried out in the field of mental health. In the last two years, about 6000 personnel were provided training. Training on mental health for primary care physicians and health workers is being conducted by the Ministry of Health and Family Welfare. They are trained to develop diagnostic skills, to participate in activities to collect data, to develop biological, psychological and social orientation towards all health problems and to develop training abilities to further train other mental health staff. Medical administrators have also been trained on mental health issues.

There are community care facilities for patients with mental disorders. Periodic mental health extension services are being provided at the primary care level by the Institute of Mental Health Research, Dhaka. Public education and family counselling with the supervision of specialists are done. Though specific rehabilitation programmes are not available in an organized form, efforts are being made to implement day care facilities, sheltered workshops and rehabilitation programmes for chronic schizophrenics.

Psychiatric Beds and Professionals

Total psychiatric beds per 10 000 population	0.065
Psychiatric beds in mental hospitals per 10 000 population	0.03
Psychiatric beds in general hospitals per 10 000 population	0.009
Psychiatric beds in other settings per 10 000 population	0.024
Number of psychiatrists per 100 000 population	0.05
Number of neurosurgeons per 100 000 population	0.01
Number of psychiatric nurses per 100 000 population	0.06
Number of neurologists per 100 000 population	0.02
Number of psychologists per 100 000 population	0.002
Number of social workers per 100 000 population	0.001

There is one occupational therapist and 4011 medical assistants. The number of mental health professionals is inadequate. Prior to 1957, there were no psychiatric services in Bangladesh. One mental hospital was established at Pabna in 1957, and in 1969 the first outdoor clinic started functioning in Dhaka Medical College. Since the 1970s, more institutes were opened. In 1981, the OTMH institute was opened with the help of WHO to cater to mental health exclusively; it was later renamed as the National Institute of Mental Health. Mental health care is provided at the primary level by primary care physicians and health workers, at the secondary level by the district hospital, though unfortunately, only one such hospital is equipped to provide the services, and at tertiary level by teaching hospitals.

Non-Governmental Organizations NGOs are involved with mental health in the country. They are mainly involved in treatment and rehabilitation.

Information Gathering System There is mental health reporting system in the country. There are some figures related to incidence and prevalence of mental disorders.
The country has data collection system or epidemiological study on mental health. Only hospital based service data collection is present.
A WHO supported country wide population-based survey on mental disorders has been undertaken recently.

Programmes for Special Population The country has specific programmes for mental health for elderly and children. The National Institute has special units for child and adolescent and elderly population. All other groups are cared for by the general adult psychiatry units.

Therapeutic Drugs The following therapeutic drugs are generally available at the primary health care level of the country: carbamazepine, phenobarbital, phenytoin sodium, sodium valproate, amitriptyline, chlorpromazine, diazepam, fluphenazine, haloperidol, lithium, levodopa.

Other Information

Additional Sources of Information

Ahmed, S. U. (1978) Analysis of the epidemiological data of 600 psychiatric patients. Bangladesh Medical Research Council Bulletin, 4, 43-48.

Ahsan, N. (2001) Mental Health & Substance Abuse: A Country Report from Bangladesh. Institute of Mental Health & Research.

Alam, M. N. (1978) Psychiatric morbidity in general practice. Bangladesh Medical Research Council Bulletin, 4, 38-42.

Appleby, L. (2000) Suicide in women. Lancet, 355, 1203-1204.

Chowdhury, A. K., Alam, M. N., Ali, S. M., et al (1981) Dasherkandi project studies. Demography, morbidity and mortality in a rural community of Bangladesh. Bangladesh Medical Research Council Bulletin, 7, 22-39.

Chowdhury, A. K., Salim, M., Sakeb, N., et al (1975) Some aspects of psychiatric morbidity in the out-patient population of a general hospital. Bangladesh Medical Research Council Bulletin, 1, 51-59.

Durkin, M. S., Khan, N., Davidson, L. L., et al (1993) The effects of a natural disaster on child behavior: evidence for posttraumatic stress. American Journal of Public Health, 83, 1549-1553.

Durkin, M., Khan, N. Z., Davidson, L. L., et al (2000) Prenatal and postnatal risk factors for mental retardation among children in Bangladesh. American Journal of Epidemiology, 152, 1024-1033.

Islam, S., Durkin, M. S., Zaman, S. S. (1993) Socioeconomic status and the prevalence of mental retardation in Bangladesh. Mental Retardation, 31, 412-417.

Rabbani, M. G., Hossain, M. M. (1999) Behaviour disorders in urban primary school children in Dhaka. Bangladesh. Public Health, 113, 233-236.

Rahim, D. A., Ali, S. M., Rabbani, M. G., et al (1997) Analysis of psychiatric morbidity of outpatient children in Mitford Hospital, Dhaka. Bangladesh Medical Research Council Bulletin, 23, 60-62.

Barbados

A–B

GENERAL INFORMATION

Barbados is a country with an approximate area of 0.43 thousand sq. km. (UNO, 2001). Its population is 0.271 million, and the sex ratio (men per hundred women) is 95 (UNO, 2004). The proportion of population under the age of 15 years is 19% (UNO, 2004), and the proportion of population above the age of 60 years is 13% (WHO, 2004). The literacy rate is 99.7% for men and 99.7% for women (UNESCO/MoH, 2004).
The country is a higher middle income group country (based on World Bank 2004 criteria). The proportion of health budget to GDP is 6.5%. The per capita total expenditure on health is 940 international $, and the per capita government expenditure on health is 623 international $ (WHO, 2004).
The main language(s) used in the country is (are) English. The largest ethnic group(s) is (are) African (descent), and the other ethnic group(s) are (is) Caucasian, East Indian and Chinese. The largest religious group(s) is (are) Christian, and the other religious group(s) are (is) Hindu, Muslim, Jew and Rastafarian.
The life expectancy at birth is 70.5 years for males and 77.9 years for females (WHO, 2004). The healthy life expectancy at birth is 63 years for males and 68 years for females (WHO, 2004).

EPIDEMIOLOGY

A 12-month study of all persons in the 18-54-year age group presenting with a psychosis for the first time was carried out on the population of Barbados. Information was collected using World Health Organization screening and measurement instruments. On an island of just over a quarter of a million, 40 out of the 53 patients that met the inclusion criteria were categorized as S+ (narrow) schizophrenia, giving an incidence rate of 2.8/10 000. The incidence rate for broad schizophrenia was calculated at 3.2/10 000, which is significantly lower than the comparable rate for London's African-Caribbeans of 6.6/10 000. The very high rate for broad schizophrenia among African-Caribbean people in the UK is probably due to environmental factors like migration and psychosocial stressors (Mahy et al, 1999). Mansoor and Edwards (1991) used the Michigan Alcohol Screening Test (MAST) and found that 18% were problem drinkers among 203 emergency admissions. Problem drinking was found in 31% of males and 5% of females.70% of all problem drinkers had a first degree family relative who drank compared to 28% of non-drinkers. A high prevalence of alcoholism (48%) was found among smokers. Comorbid medical complications were high. House staff detected just over half of male (56%) and female (60%) alcoholics who were MAST-positive. Studies on attempted suicide/parasuicide are also available (Mahy, 1987a, b).

MENTAL HEALTH RESOURCES

Mental Health Policy A mental health policy is present. The policy was initially formulated in 2004.

Substance Abuse Policy A substance abuse policy is present. The policy was initially formulated in 1995. A National Council on Substance Abuse (NCSA) Act sets the roles and functions of the NCSA. It was promulgated in March 1996.

National Mental Health Programme A national mental health programme is present. The programme was formulated in 2001.
A National Mental Health Framework Plan is present. It was formulated with an active collaboration between the Ministry of Health and PAHO. A draft of a revised plan was ready in September 2004.

National Therapeutic Drug Policy/Essential List of Drugs A national therapeutic drug policy/essential list of drugs is present. It was formulated in 1989.

Mental Health Legislation The Mental Health Act is of 1980. The Mental Health Act- Laws of Barbados (Chapter 45) is the most recent legislation.
The latest legislation was enacted in 1985.

Mental Health Financing There are budget allocations for mental health.
The country spends 12% of the total health budget on mental health.
The primary sources of mental health financing in descending order are tax based, out of pocket expenditure by the patient or family, private insurances and social insurance.
The country has disability benefits for persons with mental disorders.

Mental Health Facilities Mental health is a part of primary health care system. Actual treatment of severe mental disorders is available at the primary level. Primary care is provided through a mental health team providing services in each polyclinic.
Regular training of primary care professionals is not carried out in the field of mental health. A training programme for primary care personnel was carried out by PAHO in May 1999. Another training programme for core clinical mental health professionals was conducted by PAHO in February 2004.
There are community care facilities for patients with mental disorders. It is provided through mental health personnel and mental health officers working out of the psychiatric hospital. There are District Psychiatric Nursing Services across the country which provide the bulk of community care. They collectively make up to 6000 domiciliary visits per year.

Psychiatric Beds and Professionals

Total psychiatric beds per 10 000 population	26
Psychiatric beds in mental hospitals per 10 000 population	22
Psychiatric beds in general hospitals per 10 000 population	0.3
Psychiatric beds in other settings per 10 000 population	4
Number of psychiatrists per 100 000 population	3
Number of neurosurgeons per 100 000 population	1
Number of psychiatric nurses per 100 000 population	97
Number of neurologists per 100 000 population	0.7
Number of psychologists per 100 000 population	9
Number of social workers per 100 000 population	2

Two social workers are trained in psychiatry social work till the masters level. Barbados has one large mental hospital. The private set-ups have no fixed number of psychiatric beds. Mental health officers play an important role in psychiatric care. A training programme for core clinical mental health professionals was conducted by PAHO in February 2004.

Non-Governmental Organizations NGOs are involved with mental health in the country. They are mainly involved in advocacy, promotion and prevention.

Information Gathering System There is mental health reporting system in the country.
The country has data collection system or epidemiological study on mental health. The annual health reporting system and data collection system are being upgraded.

Programmes for Special Population The country has specific programmes for mental health for elderly and children.
The child guidance clinic is a weekly outpatient affair. The liaison service is in its infancy. There are also substance abuse related programmes. Services in forensic psychiatry are also present.

Therapeutic Drugs The following therapeutic drugs are generally available at the primary health care level of the country: carbamazepine, ethosuximide, phenobarbital, phenytoin sodium, sodium valproate, amitriptyline, chlorpromazine, diazepam, fluphenazine, haloperidol, lithium, carbidopa, levodopa.

Other Information

Additional Sources of Information

Evans, C. (1999) Psychiatry in Barbados: a personal experience. Psychiatric Bulletin, 23, 49-51.

Fisher, L. E. (1981) Social organization and stigmatization of mental patients in Barbados. Illinois Sociological Association.

Mahy, G. (1987a) Attempted suicide in Barbados. West Indian Medical Journal, 36, 31-34.

Mahy, G. (1987b) Completed suicide in Barbados. West Indian Medical Journal, 36, 91-94.

Mahy, G. E., Mallett, R., Leff, J., et al (1999) First-contact incidence rate of schizophrenia on Barbados. British Journal of Psychiatry, 175, 28-33.

Mansoor, G. A., Edwards, C. N. (1991) Questionnaire detection of problem drinkers among acute medical admissions. West Indian Medical Journal, 40, 65-68.

Belarus

GENERAL INFORMATION

Belarus is a country with an approximate area of 208 thousand sq. km. (UNO, 2001). Its population is 9.851 million, and the sex ratio (men per hundred women) is 88 (UNO, 2004). The proportion of population under the age of 15 years is 16% (UNO, 2004), and the proportion of population above the age of 60 years is 19% (WHO, 2004). The literacy rate is 99.8% for men and 99.6% for women (UNESCO/MoH, 2004).

The country is a lower middle income group country (based on World Bank 2004 criteria). The proportion of health budget to GDP is 5.6%. The per capita total expenditure on health is 464 international $, and the per capita government expenditure on health is 402 international $ (WHO, 2004).

The main language(s) used in the country is (are) Belarusian and Russian. The largest ethnic group(s) is (are) Belarusian (five-sixths), and the other ethnic group(s) are (is) Russian. The largest religious group(s) is (are) Orthodox Christian (four-fifths) among those who rank themselves as religious (about half of the population).

The life expectancy at birth is 62.6 years for males and 74.3 years for females (WHO, 2004). The healthy life expectancy at birth is 57 years for males and 65 years for females (WHO, 2004).

EPIDEMIOLOGY

Aleksandrovskii (1991) found a 38% rate of psychiatric morbidity in a sample of 300 persons living in a polluted area of Byelorussia after the Chernobyl nuclear disaster in 1986. Havenaar et al (1996) used the General Health Questionnaire (12-item version) and the Munich Diagnostic Checklist for DSM-III-R in a two-stage survey of a broad based population sample affected by the disaster (n=1617). Psychiatric disorders were present in 35.8% (affective: 16.5%, anxiety: 12.6%). Dysthymia, general anxiety disorder, adjustment disorders and 'not otherwise specified syndromes' made up almost two-thirds of the observed morbidity (22.9%). A higher prevalence of mental health problems was observed among people who have been evacuated and in mothers with children under 18 years of age. In a later study, Havenaar et al (1997) studied two population samples 6 1/2 years after the event (n=3044), one from the region close to the accident site and one from a region 500 miles away, with a variety of self-report questionnaires and a standardized psychiatric interview. The prevalence of psychological distress and DSM-III-R psychiatric disorders was exceptionally high in both regions. Scores on the self-report scales were consistently higher in the exposed region; however, a higher risk of DSM-III-R psychiatric disorders could be demonstrated only among women with children less than 18 years of age. Kolominsky et al (1999) compared children who had suffered prenatal radiation exposure (n=138) and a control group (n=122) at the age of 6-7 and 10-11 years. The exposed group manifested a relative increase in the prevalence of specific developmental speech-language disorders (18.1% vs. 8.2% at 6-7 years; 10.1% vs. 3.3% at 10-11 years) and emotional disorders (20.3% vs. 7.4% at 6-7 years; 18.1 vs. 7.4% at 10-11 years). The mean IQ of the exposed group was lower than that of the control group, and there were more cases of borderline IQ (IQ=70-79) (15.9% vs. 5.7% at 6-7 years; and 10.1% vs. 3.3% at 10-11 years). In utero thyroid exposure was not related to IQ, but educational level of parents was moderately associated with IQ. In an extension of this study (Igumnov & Drozdovitch, 2000) compared 250 children at the age of 6-7 and 10-12 years who had been exposed in utero with a control group of 250 children. No statistically significant distinctions in average IQ were found between the different subgroups of children in relation to the gestational age at the time of the Chernobyl accident. Exposed children had a higher relative risk of emotional disorders (OR=2.67, P<0.001) but not for mental retardation, hyperkinetic disorders and other mental and behavioural disorders. In both studies, there was a moderate correlation between high personal anxiety in parents and emotional disorders in children. In a study using multivariate analysis, Little (1993) suggested that there was no increase in the rate of congenital abnormalities like Trisomy 21 following the nuclear disaster. Similar conclusions were reached by Laziuk et al (2002) who analysed the annual and monthly prevalence of Down syndrome (n=2786) in Belarus for a 19-year period (1981 to 1999). Based on data obtained from national registers, Razvodovskii (2002) showed a strong positive correlation between the incidence of alcoholic psychoses and alcohol use disorders and the level of alcoholic beverage consumption per capita in Belarus from 1970 to 1999. Wasserman et al (1998) reported that suicide rates were high (25.6 per 100 000) in the Slavic region (Russia, the Ukraine and Belarus) of the former USSR. Declines in suicide rates from 1984 to 1986-1988 occurred in all republics, with the largest decreases in Russia and Belarus, at 42% for men and 20% for women (Varnik et al, 1998). Suicide rates have risen in Belarus since 1990 and are higher in rural than in urban areas. The regional distribution of suicide rates suggests a north-south variation that may be a result of ethnic and cultural differences between the regions (Kondrichin & Lester, 1998).

MENTAL HEALTH RESOURCES

Mental Health Policy A mental health policy is absent.

Prevention of mental ill-health is a part of the National Policy, even though there is no national mental health programme for the country.

Substance Abuse Policy A substance abuse policy is present. The policy was initially formulated in 2000. The following have been developed, adopted and implemented: Outline for state alcohol-control policy, (decree No. 23, 2000), Outline for state policy for controlling abuse of narcotics and psychotropic substances in the Republic of Belarus (decree No. 583, 1996), the state programme for comprehensive measures to combat abuse of and illegal trade in narcotics and psychotropic substances for the period 2001-2005 (decree No. 25, 2001), the state programme of national activities to prohibit and eliminate drunkenness and alcoholism (decree No. 1332, 2000). The coordination of intersectoral activities at a state level is governed by the Interministerial Commission on Drug Abuse and Crime, under the Council of Security, and the Interministerial Commission on Control of Drugs and Psychotropic Substances, under the Council of Ministers.

National Mental Health Programme A national mental health programme is absent.
There is no national mental health plan in Belarus. Mental health plans are included within the framework of the annually developed Health Ministry Plans. Currently, the Health Ministry is trying to establish the legislative basis for mental health programmes by amendments to the Law 'On Health Care' and is involved in the development of standards for psychiatric care. Some measures have been planned for a transition to the use of ICD-10.

National Therapeutic Drug Policy/Essential List of Drugs A national therapeutic drug policy/essential list of drugs is present. It was formulated in 2003.
The supply of medication for maintenance treatment sometimes gets interrupted due to shortages.

Mental Health Legislation There is legislation on psychiatric care that guarantees the rights of the citizens. Provision of health care to the population is regulated by the following laws: 'On Health' drafted in 2002; 'On psychiatric care and guarantees for the rights of citizens receiving care', 1999; 'On veterans', 1992; 'On social protection for victims of the Chernobyl nuclear accident', 1991; 'On social protection for the disabled', 1991; and the Regulatory Legislation of the Ministry of Health (directive No. 24 Protocol [standards] applicable to diagnosis and treatment in the sphere of mental health and behavioural disorders' 2002).
The latest legislation was enacted in 1999.

Mental Health Financing There are no budget allocations for mental health.
Details about expenditure on mental health are not available.
The primary sources of mental health financing in descending order are tax based, social insurance and out of pocket expenditure by the patient or family.
The Ministry of Health plans expenditure on a per capita expenditure basis using budgetary allocations. For this purpose, planning and funding of expenditure on health, including that on mental health services, is determined by the volume and type of medical care.
The country has disability benefits for persons with mental disorders. Public disability benefits are given to mental health invalids. Mental health patients including working ones are treated free of charge at polyclinics.

Mental Health Facilities Mental health is a part of primary health care system. Actual treatment of severe mental disorders is available at the primary level. Specialized primary health care is rendered at the polyclinic by therapists and neuropathologists; at the psychiatric and narcologic clinics by psychiatrists and narcologists; at the hospital in cases of psychosis by psychiatrists and narcologists. The national system of psychiatric care has been developed based on the needs of society, as stipulated by the community as a whole and by the consumers of these services in particular. In the past, such care was mainly provided at large psychiatric institutions. At present, it is provided as near as possible to the patient's home, aiming to shift the provision of care from the inpatient to the outpatient level. Establishing a network of outpatient clinics, psychotherapeutic facilities and socio-psychological care at each area polyclinic, integration of psychiatric care into GP practice, developing cooperation with social services and NGOs are also being planned.
Regular training of primary care professionals is carried out in the field of mental health. In the last two years, about 720 personnel were provided training.
There are no community care facilities for patients with mental disorders. Community care services have not fully developed. There are psychiatric wards in general hospitals and specialized psychiatric teams in polyclinics even in rural areas, but there are few day care centres or psychosocial programmes. Day-patient psychiatric care for adults is provided by day clinics located within and outside psychiatric institutions. In order to prevent suicide, telephone mental health helpline services have been set up and are still being set up throughout Belarus.

Psychiatric Beds and Professionals

Total psychiatric beds per 10 000 population	8
Psychiatric beds in mental hospitals per 10 000 population	7.5
Psychiatric beds in general hospitals per 10 000 population	0.5
Psychiatric beds in other settings per 10 000 population	0
Number of psychiatrists per 100 000 population	10.1
Number of neurosurgeons per 100 000 population	1.5
Number of psychiatric nurses per 100 000 population	25.6
Number of neurologists per 100 000 population	15.4
Number of psychologists per 100 000 population	1.14
Number of social workers per 100 000 population	0

The current focus continues to be on an inpatient (in mental and general hospitals) rather than an outpatient care. Staffing norms are being developed, along with norms for ratios of psychiatrists, psychotherapists, drug-abuse specialists and psychologists which will make it possible to provide mental health care through multidisciplinary teams with intensive use of technology and minimum isolation of patients. Outpatient psychiatric care for adults is provided by psychiatrists, psychotherapists and psychologists at surgeries located in specialized mental-health institutions. Positions for psychotherapists and psychologists also exist in surgeries in municipal general hospitals. Psychiatric beds are organized on the basis of age (adults, children, adolescents and geriatric), by sex (male, female, mixed) and by category of disorder (treatment of depression, anxiety disorders, post-suicide, psychoses and somatic disorders). There are in-patient facilities for mandatory treatment of psychiatric patients who have committed offences contemplated by the Criminal Code. The number of psychiatric beds fell from 11 370 (11.1 per 10 000 population) to 7868 (8.0 per 10 000 population) between 1999 and 2004, i.e. by 30.8%.During the same period, the number of beds for drug-abuse patients fell from 4490 (4.4 per 10 000 population) to 1347 (1.4 per 10 thousand population), i.e. by more than two thirds. There are no specialized drug-abuse clinics in Belarus; beds for drug-abuse patients are provided in psychiatric hospitals. Psychiatric care is provided in part outside the Ministry of Health system, e.g. in Ministry of Labour and Social Protection establishments – at homes for chronic mental health patients without any family or social ties and in Ministry of internal affairs establishments – at penal establishments of the prison service. There is a move towards deinstitutionalization, replacing long- term hospitalization with various forms of outpatient treatment, medico-social and socio-legal care. In the 1990s itself, a reduction of nearly 12% in mental health beds and 30% in substance abuse beds was achieved. Treatment by psychotherapy is being introduced at outpatient clinics. Limited services are available in the private sphere, mostly for drug abuse and psychotherapy. However, no effective mechanisms presently exist for the quality control of private services and for ensuring the right balance between governmental services and developing private practices within the mental health field. Separate wards are available for the treatment of children and elderly. Demented patients are usually referred to institutions for chronic psychiatric patients that are under the jurisdiction of Ministry of Social Welfare. Multidisciplinary teams with the participation of doctors, nurses, psychologists, and social workers usually provide care in mental health facilities, but the number of psychologists and social workers is still insufficient. Preparations for the assignment of social workers to the staff of psychiatric institutions are under way.

Non-Governmental Organizations NGOs are not involved with mental health in the country. The current legislation authorizes the establishment of social organizations. Professional non-governmental organizations exist in Belarus (the Belarusian Psychiatric Association, the Belarusian Association of Psychotherapists) and issue their own publications. There are associations of users of psychiatric services and their relatives, although they are non-operational and their registration has lapsed. There are also a number of social organizations that deal with rehabilitation for drug users.

Information Gathering System There is mental health reporting system in the country.
The country has no data collection system or epidemiological study on mental health.
Since 1998, the suicidal behaviour of the population of Minsk city has been studied as an indicator of mental health. It is also planned to collect information on suicides and parasuicides throughout the country.

Programmes for Special Population The country has specific programmes for mental health for disaster affected population and children. The disaster affected population are those affected by the Chernobyl accident.
Outpatient paediatric psychiatric care is provided by child psychiatrists, psychotherapists and psychologists at clinics in children's hospitals. Day-patient paediatric mental health care is provided at situated within and outside mental health institutions. Inpatient psychiatric care for children is provided in children's mental health clinics, located in psychiatric hospitals and general children's hospitals. Psychiatric care is also provided by Ministry of Education Establishments at preschool establishments and schools for children with psychiatric disorders.

Therapeutic Drugs The following therapeutic drugs are generally available at the primary health care level of the country: carbamazepine, ethosuximide, phenobarbital, phenytoin sodium, sodium valproate, amitriptyline, chlorpromazine, diazepam, fluphenazine, haloperidol, lithium, carbidopa, levodopa.
The essential list of drugs (decree N° 43, 2003) which must be available at mental health hospitals is renewed every two years. In 2004, the Ministry of Health drew up a formulary of drugs whose use is authorized in Belarus. Supplies of drugs to treat mental and behavioural disorders are sufficient to meet demand.

Other Information

Additional Sources of Information

Aleksandrovskii, I. A., Rumiantseva, G. M., Iurov, V. V., et al (1991) Dynamics of mental adaptation disorders in chronic stress among the population after the accident at the Chernobyl nuclear power plant. Zhurnal Nevropatologii i Psikhiatrii Imeni S-S-Korsakova, 91, 3-6.

Havenaar, J. M., Rumyantzeva, G. M., Van den Brink, et al (1997) Long-term mental health effects of the Chernobyl disaster: an epidemiologic survey in two former Soviet regions. American Journal of Psychiatry, 154, 1605-1607.

Havenaar, J. M., Van den Brink, W., Van den Bout, J., et al (1996) Mental health problems in the Gomel region (Belarus): an analysis of risk factors in an area affected by the Chernobyl disaster. Psychological Medicine, 26, 845-855.

Igumnov, S., Drozdovitch, V. (2000) The intellectual development, mental and behavioural disorders in children from Belarus exposed in utero following the Chernobyl accident. European Psychiatry: the Journal of the Association of European Psychiatrists, 15, 244-253.

Karpenko, E. (1998) Nursing development in Belarussian psychiatry. Mental Health Reforms, 3, 11-12.

Kolominsky, Y., Igumnov, S., Drozdovitch, V. (1999) The psychological development of children from Belarus exposed in the prenatal period to radiation from the Chernobyl atomic power plant. Journal of Child Psychology & Psychiatry & Allied Disciplines, 40, 299-305.

Kondrichin, S. V., Lester, D. (1998) Suicide in Belarus. Crisis: Journal of Crisis Intervention & Suicide, 19, 167-171.

Laziuk, G. I., Zatsepin, I. O., Verger, P., et al (2002) Down syndrome and ionizing radiation: causal effect or coincidence. Radiatsionnaia Biologiia, Radioecologiia, 42, 678-683.

Little, J. (1993) The Chernobyl accident, congenital anomalies and other reproductive outcomes. Paediatric and Perinatal Epidemiology, 7, 121-151.

Poznyak, V., Solodkaya, T. (1999) Mental health care in Belarrus Today. Mental Health Reforms, 1, 12-16.

Razvodovskii, I. E. (2002) Alcoholism and alcoholic psychosis in Belarus in 1970-1999. Zhurnal Nevrologii i Psikhiatrii Imeni S.S. Korsakova, 102, 58-63.

Varnik, A., Wasserman, D., Dankowicz, M., et al (1998) Marked decrease in suicide among men and women in the former USSR during perestroika. Acta Psychiatrica Scandinavica, 98, 13-19.

Wasserman, D., Varnik, A., Dankowicz, M. (1998) Regional differences in the distribution of suicide in the former Soviet Union during perestroika, 1984-1990. Psychiatrica Scandinavica, 98, 5-12.

Belgium

GENERAL INFORMATION

Belgium is a country with an approximate area of 33 thousand sq. km. (UNO, 2001). Its population is 10.339 million, and the sex ratio (men per hundred women) is 96 (UNO, 2004). The proportion of population under the age of 15 years is 17% (UNO, 2004), and the proportion of population above the age of 60 years is 22% (WHO, 2004). The literacy rate is 99% for men and 99% for women (UNESCO/MoH, 2004).

The country is a high income group country (based on World Bank 2004 criteria). The proportion of health budget to GDP is 8.9%. The per capita total expenditure on health is 2481 international $, and the per capita government expenditure on health is 1778 international $ (WHO, 2004).

The main language(s) used in the country is (are) Dutch, French and German. The largest ethnic group(s) is (are) Fleming (half), and the other ethnic group(s) are (is) Walloon. The largest religious group(s) is (are) Roman Catholic.

The life expectancy at birth is 75.2 years for males and 81.5 years for females (WHO, 2004). The healthy life expectancy at birth is 69 years for males and 73 years for females (WHO, 2004).

EPIDEMIOLOGY

There is substantial epidemiological data on mental illnesses in Belgium in internationally accessible literature. No attempt was made to include this information here.

MENTAL HEALTH RESOURCES

Mental Health Policy A mental health policy is present. The policy was initially formulated in 1988.

It was amended in 1990. Now, since both Federal Government and communities are in charge of different parts of mental health, there is a national and a community mental health policy.

Substance Abuse Policy A substance abuse policy is present. The policy was initially formulated in 1921. It has been amended several times and is now in the process of being renewed.

National Mental Health Programme A national mental health programme is present. The programme was formulated in 1990. Various adaptations have been made over time. Belgium has suicide prevention programmes but not at a national level.

National Therapeutic Drug Policy/Essential List of Drugs A national therapeutic drug policy/essential list of drugs is present. Details about the year of formulation are not available.

There is no list of essential drugs since all officially registered drugs are available.

Mental Health Legislation There is a Royal decision of May 2000 changing the previous one of 1976 concerning the fixation of maximum number of beds in psychiatric services. The communities are in charge of all non-hospital mental health care such as sheltered housing, centres for mental health, etc. The Federal Government is in charge of hospitals, location of psychiatric care and quality of hospital care.

The latest legislation was enacted in 2000.

Mental Health Financing There are budget allocations for mental health.

The country spends 6% of the total health budget on mental health.

The primary sources of mental health financing in descending order are social insurance, private insurances, out of pocket expenditure by the patient or family and tax based.

The country has disability benefits for persons with mental disorders. Different parameters like ability to work and measurement of handicap are assessed.

Mental Health Facilities Mental health is a part of primary health care system. Actual treatment of severe mental disorders is available at the primary level.

Regular training of primary care professionals is carried out in the field of mental health.

There are community care facilities for patients with mental disorders. The forensic psychiatry services are limited to some experimental areas.

Psychiatric Beds and Professionals

Total psychiatric beds per 10 000 population	22.1
Psychiatric beds in mental hospitals per 10 000 population	12.9
Psychiatric beds in general hospitals per 10 000 population	2.6
Psychiatric beds in other settings per 10 000 population	6.6
Number of psychiatrists per 100 000 population	18
Number of neurosurgeons per 100 000 population	1.5
Number of psychiatric nurses per 100 000 population	
Number of neurologists per 100 000 population	1

Number of psychologists per 100 000 population
Number of social workers per 100 000 population

Psychiatrists include adult psychiatrists, child psychiatrics and neuropsychiatrists; some of the latter exclusively work in the area of neurology. Hence, the figure for psychiatrists is an overestimate, while that for neurologists is an underestimate. Figures for psychiatric nurses, psychologists and social workers are not available because these professional titles are not recognized by the federal authority, therefore they are not registered.

Non-Governmental Organizations NGOs are involved with mental health in the country. They are mainly involved in promotion, prevention and rehabilitation.

Information Gathering System There is mental health reporting system in the country.
The country has data collection system or epidemiological study on mental health. The document containing psychiatric information is known as the Minimal Psychiatric Dataset.

Programmes for Special Population The country has specific programmes for mental health for minorities, refugees, disaster affected population, indigenous population, elderly and children. There are services for prisoners too.

Therapeutic Drugs The following therapeutic drugs are generally available at the primary health care level of the country: carbamazepine, ethosuximide, phenobarbital, phenytoin sodium, sodium valproate, amitriptyline, diazepam, haloperidol, lithium, biperiden, carbidopa, levodopa.
Drugs are partially or wholly reimbursed. Carbidopa and levodopa are always prescribed in association with others.

Other Information

Additional Sources of Information

Baro F., Prims A., de Schouwer, P. (1984). Belgium: psychiatric care in a pluralist system. In: Mental Health Care in the European Community, S. P. Mangen (Ed.). Croom Helm. pp 42-54.

Centraal Ziekenhuisbestand, Public Federal Service of Health, Food Chain Safety and Environment, October 6th, 2004.

Der Minister van Consumentenzaken, Volksgezondheid en Leefmilieu and Aelvoet, M. (2000). Legislation Concerning Mental Health.

Federale databank van de beoefenaars van de gezondheidszorgberoepen, Public Federal Service of Health, Food Chain Safety and Environment, January, 2004.

Simoens-Desmet, A. (1998) Rapport National 1998 du Resume Psychiatrique Minimum. Ministere des Affaires Sociale. Se la Santè, Publique et de l'Environment.

Belize

GENERAL INFORMATION

Belize is a country with an approximate area of 23 thousand sq. km. (UNO, 2001). Its population is 0.261 million, and the sex ratio (men per hundred women) is 102 (UNO, 2004). The proportion of population under the age of 15 years is 37% (UNO, 2004), and the proportion of population above the age of 60 years is 6% (WHO, 2004). The literacy rate is 76.7% for men and 77.1% for women (UNESCO/MoH, 2004).

The country is a higher middle income group country (based on World Bank 2004 criteria). The proportion of health budget to GDP is 5.2%. The per capita total expenditure on health is 278 international $, and the per capita government expenditure on health is 125 international $ (WHO, 2004).

The main language(s) used in the country is (are) English and Spanish. The largest ethnic group(s) is (are) Mestizo (almost half of the population) and Creole (one-fourth), and the other ethnic group(s) are (is) indigenous groups (Mopan, Yucatec and Ketch) and Garifuna. The largest religious group(s) is (are) Roman Catholic.

The life expectancy at birth is 67.4 years for males and 72.4 years for females (WHO, 2004). The healthy life expectancy at birth is 58 years for males and 62 years for females (WHO, 2004).

EPIDEMIOLOGY

There is a paucity of epidemiological data on mental illnesses in Belize in internationally accessible literature. McClusky (1999) conducted an ethnographic study on domestic violence against rural Belizean women of Mayan origin.

MENTAL HEALTH RESOURCES

Mental Health Policy A mental health policy is absent.

There is a written document that gives policy directions that need to be adopted by the country in order to become the official mental health policy.

Substance Abuse Policy A substance abuse policy is absent.

National Mental Health Programme A national mental health programme is absent.

National Therapeutic Drug Policy/Essential List of Drugs A national therapeutic drug policy/essential list of drugs is present. Details about the year of formulation are not available.

Mental Health Legislation The country has a mental health legislation dated 1965 and based on the British model, which is currently being reviewed and updated to ensure that it adheres to international human rights standards. Multiple stakeholder groups are involved in this process. The latest addition to the legislation was enacted in 1998 after the Mental Health Association extensively lobbied for the decriminalization of suicide, as well as ensuring that survivors of suicide attempts received professional help rather than face criminal charges.

The latest legislation was enacted in 1998.

Mental Health Financing There are budget allocations for mental health.

The country spends 1% of the total health budget on mental health.

The primary sources of mental health financing in descending order are tax based, out of pocket expenditure by the patient or family, private insurances.

The country has disability benefits for persons with mental disorders. If patients have worked they are entitled to social security benefits.

Mental Health Facilities Mental health is a part of primary health care system. Actual treatment of severe mental disorders is not available at the primary level. It is available mainly at secondary level.

Regular training of primary care professionals is not carried out in the field of mental health.

There are community care facilities for patients with mental disorders. For over ten years, Belize has followed a community-based approach to addressing mental health issues. Psychiatric nurse practitioners (PNP) who are trained in field work, function under the supervision of the psychiatrist to provide services to patients in their respective communities. Every district hospital has PNPs working out of the Mental Health Clinic. This helps in the integration of community psychiatric services with general health services. An acute psychiatric unit exists within a general hospital. No day hospital service is currently in place. Most patients have to travel only short distances to their clinics.

Psychiatric Beds and Professionals

Total psychiatric beds per 10 000 population	2.3
Psychiatric beds in mental hospitals per 10 000 population	2.1
Psychiatric beds in general hospitals per 10 000 population	0.2
Psychiatric beds in other settings per 10 000 population	0
Number of psychiatrists per 100 000 population	1.3
Number of neurosurgeons per 100 000 population	0.9
Number of psychiatric nurses per 100 000 population	0.5
Number of neurologists per 100 000 population	0.9
Number of psychologists per 100 000 population	0
Number of social workers per 100 000 population	4.3

The social workers were not trained as psychiatric social workers. There are no occupational therapist currently working in the programme. The country has one psychiatric institution; and in 2001, a General Hospital Psychiatric Unit was opened that can accommodate approximately four patients. It is anticipated that an additional psychiatric unit will be constructed at the referral hospital in Belize City. In addition, there are 3 private hospitals which admit psychiatric patients occasionally. The country has one psychiatric institution, the Rockview Hospital, one psychiatrist and two clinical psychologist (who are working in the private sector) working in country. Currently, there are 10 Psychiatric Nurse Practitioners working at district clinics and the outpatient clinic in Belize City, and 13 additional PNPs are being trained at the University of Belize. This is the second training of Psychiatric Nurse Practitioners as mental health is not included in the regular training of primary health care providers. The psychiatrist is based in the capital but visit district clinics every six weeks. They also visit the mental hospital and other health facilities. Psychiatric Nurse Practitioners can prescribe medication and admit patients to the hospital, though there is no legal provision for prescription by nurses. Time for Continuing Medical Education was limited.

Non-Governmental Organizations NGOs are involved with mental health in the country. They are mainly involved in advocacy, promotion, prevention and rehabilitation. The Mental Health Association helps in raising awareness about issues related to mental well-being and advocates on behalf of those with mental illness and their families. Dedicated work by psychiatric nurses led to the formation of Mental Health Consumer Associations in almost each district. Two of these groups are very active, and since their formation were instrumental in lobbying for the availability of new drugs.

Information Gathering System There is no mental health reporting system in the country. The Psychiatric Unit has recently developed key indicators which will be included in the update of the Belize Health Information System.
The country has data collection system or epidemiological study on mental health. Data collection is currently done through psychiatric units in each of the six districts. An anthropological and epidemiological overview of the mental health situation in Belize was conducted in 1993 (Bonander et al, 2000). Preliminary results are available. The high use of drugs among young people was revealed in two studies: the National Secondary School Prevalence Survey conducted in 2002 and the Global Youth Tobacco Survey conducted in 2003.

Programmes for Special Population There is no specific programme, but patients belonging to any special group of population can go for consultation as outpatients, depending on their needs.
The National Drug Advisory Council, which is a part of the Ministry of Health, has a well organized drug prevention programme.

Therapeutic Drugs The following therapeutic drugs are generally available at the primary health care level of the country: carbamazepine, ethosuximide, phenobarbital, sodium valproate, amitriptyline, chlorpromazine, diazepam, fluphenazine, haloperidol, lithium.
A selected list of the newer psychotropic drugs were added to the National Drug Formulary recently.

Other Information Issues of stigma and discrimination continue to be a major problem and are often a hindrance for mental health consumers advocating for better services. With limited human resources for mental health, the Psychiatric Nurses have played an instrumental role in meeting the direct needs of the communities in which they serve. Beside their main duties, they have provided ongoing counselling for survivors of domestic violence, including rape and child abuse, HIV/AIDS Counselling etc.

Additional Sources of Information

Bonander J, Kohn R, Arana B, Levav I: An anthropological and epidemiological overview of mental health in Belize. Transcultural Psychiatry 37:1; 57-72, 2000.

Cayetano, C. (April 2004) The need to prioritize the mental health services.

Central Statistical Office, Population Census (2000) Major Findings. Ministry of Budget Management. 2000.

Sharma, D. (1998). Recommendations for the development of a National Mental Health Program, PAHO.

Herzberg, J. L., O Neill-Byrne, J., O Neill-Byrne, K., et al (1996) Belize: a new psychiatric service revisited. Psychiatric Bulletin, 20, 237-38.

McClusky, L. J. (1999) Domestic violence among Belizean Maya. Humanity & Society, 23, 319-338.

National Health Information Surveillance Unit, Ministry of Health Belmopan. 2003.

Benin

GENERAL INFORMATION

Benin is a country with an approximate area of 113 thousand sq. km. (UNO, 2001). Its population is 6.918 million, and the sex ratio (men per hundred women) is 97 (UNO, 2004). The proportion of population under the age of 15 years is 45% (UNO, 2004), and the proportion of population above the age of 60 years is 4% (WHO, 2004). The literacy rate is 54.8% for men and 25.5% for women (UNESCO/MoH, 2004).

The country is a low income group country (based on World Bank 2004 criteria). The proportion of health budget to GDP is 4.4%. The per capita total expenditure on health is 39 international $, and the per capita government expenditure on health is 18 international $ (WHO, 2004).

The main language(s) used in the country is (are) French. The largest ethnic group(s) is (are) African. The largest religious group(s) is (are) indigenous groups (four-fifths), and the other religious group(s) are (is) Christian.

The life expectancy at birth is 50.1 years for males and 52.4 years for females (WHO, 2004). The healthy life expectancy at birth is 43 years for males and 44 years for females (WHO, 2004).

EPIDEMIOLOGY

There is a paucity of epidemiological data on mental illnesses in Benin in internationally accessible literature. Some studies on common conditions like depression and panic disorder in clinical samples are available (Bertschy, 1992; Bertschy et al, 1992).

MENTAL HEALTH RESOURCES

Mental Health Policy A mental health policy is absent.

Substance Abuse Policy A substance abuse policy is present. The policy was initially formulated in 1999.

National Mental Health Programme A national mental health programme is present. The programme was formulated in 1997.

National Therapeutic Drug Policy/Essential List of Drugs A national therapeutic drug policy/essential list of drugs is present. It was formulated in 1998.

Mental Health Legislation Details about the mental health legislation are not available.

Mental Health Financing Details about disability benefits for mental health are not available.

Details about expenditure on mental health are not available.

The primary sources of mental health financing in descending order are out of pocket expenditure by the patient or family and tax based.

Mental health care for the chronically sick persons with very low or no resources is financed from the state budget. Private insurance companies do not provide for the care of mentally ill people.

The country does not have disability benefits for persons with mental disorders. Treatment is provided free.

Mental Health Facilities Mental health is a part of primary health care system. Actual treatment of severe mental disorders is not available at the primary level. This will be possible only when decentralization is done.

Regular training of primary care professionals is not carried out in the field of mental health.

There are no community care facilities for patients with mental disorders. It is available only where pilot projects are going on.

Psychiatric Beds and Professionals

Total psychiatric beds per 10 000 population	0.08
Psychiatric beds in mental hospitals per 10 000 population	
Psychiatric beds in general hospitals per 10 000 population	0.03
Psychiatric beds in other settings per 10 000 population	0.05
Number of psychiatrists per 100 000 population	1.2
Number of neurosurgeons per 100 000 population	0.05
Number of psychiatric nurses per 100 000 population	0
Number of neurologists per 100 000 population	0.05
Number of psychologists per 100 000 population	0.05
Number of social workers per 100 000 population	0.02

Ten psychologists are in training. Four-fifths of the psychiatrists practice in the southern side of the country where the population mainly consists of the majority ethnic community, i.e. the Fon.

Non-Governmental Organizations NGOs are involved with mental health in the country. They are mainly involved in advocacy, promotion, prevention and treatment.

Information Gathering System Details about mental health reporting systems are not available.

The country has no data collection system or epidemiological study on mental health. Only thesis works related to epidemiological studies exist.

Programmes for Special Population The country has specific programmes for mental health for elderly and children. SMRR cares for children with psychiatric problems and the university for the elderly with psychiatric problems.

Therapeutic Drugs The following therapeutic drugs are generally available at the primary health care level of the country: carbamazepine, phenobarbital, phenytoin sodium, sodium valproate, amitriptyline, chlorpromazine, diazepam, fluphenazine, haloperidol, levodopa.

Other Information

Additional Sources of Information

Bertschy, G. (1992) Panic disorder in Benin, West Africa. American Journal of Psychiatry, 149, 1410.

Bertschy, G., Viel, J. F., Ahyi, R. G., et al (1992) Depression in Benin: an assessment using the Comprehensive Psychopathological Rating Scale and the principal component analysis. Journal of Affective Disorders, 25, 173-180.

Bhutan

GENERAL INFORMATION

Bhutan is a country with an approximate area of 47 thousand sq. km. (UNO, 2001). Its population is 2.325 million, and the sex ratio (men per hundred women) is 102 (UNO, 2004). The proportion of population under the age of 15 years is 41% (UNO, 2004), and the proportion of population above the age of 60 years is 6% (WHO, 2004). The literacy rate is 56% for men and 28% for women (UNESCO/MoH, 2004).

The country is a low income group country (based on World Bank 2004 criteria). The proportion of health budget to GDP is 3.9%. The per capita total expenditure on health is 64 international $, and the per capita government expenditure on health is 58 international $ (WHO, 2004).

The main language(s) used in the country is (are) Chhokey, Ngalopkha (in the west), Sharchopkha (in the east) and Nepali (in the south). The largest ethnic group(s) is (are) Tibetan, Indo-Mongoloid and indigenous (three-fourths), and the other ethnic group(s) are (is) Nepalese. The largest religious group(s) is (are) Mahayana Buddhist (seven-tenths), and the other religious group(s) are (is) Hindu.

The life expectancy at birth is 60.2 years for males and 62.4 years for females (WHO, 2004). The healthy life expectancy at birth is 53 years for males and 53 years for females (WHO, 2004).

EPIDEMIOLOGY

There is a paucity of epidemiological data on mental illnesses in Bhutan in internationally accessible literature. Some data are available on Bhutanese refugees living in Nepal. These are described under the relevant section in Nepal.

MENTAL HEALTH RESOURCES

Mental Health Policy A mental health policy is present. The policy was initially formulated in 1997.
The components of the policy are advocacy, promotion, prevention and treatment.

Substance Abuse Policy A substance abuse policy is present. The policy was initially formulated in 1988. The Narcotic Drugs and Psychotropic Substances Notification deals with definitions, offences and penalties and prohibition, control and regulation.

National Mental Health Programme A national mental health programme is present. The programme was formulated in 1997. The primary objectives of the programme are to integrate mental health into primary care and to help in improvement of general health care, undertake public education and to reduce problems related to neuropsychiatric conditions and training of personnel.

National Therapeutic Drug Policy/Essential List of Drugs A national therapeutic drug policy/essential list of drugs is present. It was formulated in 1987.

Mental Health Legislation There is no mental health legislation.

Mental Health Financing There are budget allocations for mental health.
The country spends 0.17% of the total health budget on mental health.
The primary sources of mental health financing in descending order are tax based, grants and social insurance.
The country has disability benefits for persons with mental disorders. Mentally ill patients are exempted from paying labour tax. Some are given cash benefits.

Mental Health Facilities Mental health is a part of primary health care system. Actual treatment of severe mental disorders is available at the primary level. Some drugs like chlorpromazine and diazepam are available at the basic health unit.
Regular training of primary care professionals is carried out in the field of mental health. In the last two years, about 100 personnel were provided training.
There are community care facilities for patients with mental disorders. Basic emergency and follow-up services are done by health workers in the community but more training is required.

Psychiatric Beds and Professionals

Total psychiatric beds per 10 000 population	0
Psychiatric beds in mental hospitals per 10 000 population	0
Psychiatric beds in general hospitals per 10 000 population	0
Psychiatric beds in other settings per 10 000 population	0
Number of psychiatrists per 100 000 population	0.3
Number of neurosurgeons per 100 000 population	0
Number of psychiatric nurses per 100 000 population	0.16
Number of neurologists per 100 000 population	0
Number of psychologists per 100 000 population	0
Number of social workers per 100 000 population	0

There is one occupational therapist. There is a shortage of trained mental health staff.

Non-Governmental Organizations NGOs are not involved with mental health in the country.

Information Gathering System There is mental health reporting system in the country. All mental illnesses are lumped under the heading of mental disorders; moreover, reporting may not be correct.
The country has data collection system or epidemiological study on mental health. JDWNR hospital in Thimpu has started maintaining patient treatment data since July 1999.

Programmes for Special Population The mental health programme, being in an early stage, is not able to provide special care.

Therapeutic Drugs The following therapeutic drugs are generally available at the primary health care level of the country: phenobarbital, diazepam.
Most of the listed drugs are available at the referral hospitals and district hospitals and some of the drugs in basic health units. Those marked out above are only those drugs available at basic health units.

Other Information

Additional Sources of Information

Health Services Administration (1997) Project HSD 05: Mental Health Programme.
Ministry of Home Affairs (1988) The Narcotic Drugs and Psychotropic Substances Notification.
Report on Community-Based Mental Health Programme (as part of National Mental Health Programme).
Royal Government of Bhutan (1987) National Drug Policy.

Bolivia

GENERAL INFORMATION

Bolivia is a country with an approximate area of 1099 thousand sq. km. (UNO, 2001). Its population is 8.973 million, and the sex ratio (men per hundred women) is 99 (UNO, 2004). The proportion of population under the age of 15 years is 38% (UNO, 2004), and the proportion of population above the age of 60 years is 7% (WHO, 2004). The literacy rate is 93.1% for men and 80.7% for women (UNESCO/MoH, 2004).

The country is a lower middle income group country (based on World Bank 2004 criteria). The proportion of health budget to GDP is 5.3%. The per capita total expenditure on health is 125 international $, and the per capita government expenditure on health is 83 international $ (WHO, 2004).

The main language(s) used in the country is (are) Spanish, Quechua and Aymara. The largest ethnic group(s) is (are) Quechua, and the other ethnic group(s) are (is) Aymara. The largest religious group(s) is (are) Roman Catholic (almost 95%), and the other religious group(s) are (is) indigenous groups.

The life expectancy at birth is 61.8 years for males and 64.7 years for females (WHO, 2004). The healthy life expectancy at birth is 54 years for males and 55 years for females (WHO, 2004).

EPIDEMIOLOGY

There is a paucity of epidemiological data on Bolivia. But some studies suggest that articles in relation to drug use and abuse may be available in other languages. An interesting study that employed ethnographic methods suggested that migration changed the rates of mental pathology in a special ethnographic population group (Chiriguanos) (Pages et al, 1981).

MENTAL HEALTH RESOURCES

Mental Health Policy A mental health policy is present. The policy was initially formulated in 1985.

The components of the policy are advocacy, promotion, prevention, treatment and rehabilitation. It was revised in 2001 through a process that included consultations with stakeholder groups that included politicians, mental health professionals and civil servants. Between 10 to 25% of its original content was put into practice.

Substance Abuse Policy A substance abuse policy is present. The policy was initially formulated in 1977. It was revised in 2001, and a regular budget was set aside for its implementation. Currently, about 10-25% of the policy goals have been implemented. There is also a specific legislation for substance abuse from 1988.

National Mental Health Programme A national mental health programme is present. The programme was formulated in 1972. It was revised in 2001, and a regular budget was set aside for its implementation. Currently, about 10-25% of the programme has been implemented by national authorities. Its main components are strategy of services reform, promotion and prevention, integration of mental health services in primary care and development of specialized services.

National Therapeutic Drug Policy/Essential List of Drugs A national therapeutic drug policy/essential list of drugs is present. It was formulated in 1992.

The national programme of essential drugs has grown steadily from 1991 onwards.

Mental Health Legislation The mental health legislation was revised in 2001. There are regular funds for its implementation. It focuses on promotion and prevention, human rights, regulation of mental health services, etc., but there is no reference to regulation of involuntary treatment.

The latest legislation was enacted in 1978.

Mental Health Financing There are budget allocations for mental health.

The country spends 0.2% of the total health budget on mental health.

The primary sources of mental health financing in descending order are out of pocket expenditure by the patient or family, tax based, social insurance and private insurances.

The country has disability benefits for persons with mental disorders.

Mental Health Facilities Mental health is a part of primary health care system. Actual treatment of severe mental disorders is not available at the primary level. Less than 25 % of the population is covered by this kind of service. Mental health care is provided by primary health care psychiatrists. A referral system is in place.

Regular training of primary care professionals is not carried out in the field of mental health.

There are community care facilities for patients with mental disorders. The community care system for the mentally ill includes outpatient clinics, preventive/promotion interventions, home interventions, residential facilities and vocational training, however, these are available for less than 25% of the population. Primary health care doctors and nurses are responsible for taking care of patients with mental disorders in the community.

Psychiatric Beds and Professionals

Total psychiatric beds per 10 000 population	0.791
Psychiatric beds in mental hospitals per 10 000 population	0.51
Psychiatric beds in general hospitals per 10 000 population	0.04
Psychiatric beds in other settings per 10 000 population	
Number of psychiatrists per 100 000 population	0.9
Number of neurosurgeons per 100 000 population	0.8
Number of psychiatric nurses per 100 000 population	
Number of neurologists per 100 000 population	0.5
Number of psychologists per 100 000 population	5
Number of social workers per 100 000 population	

About half of mental health professionals of various disciplines are employed in the public sector.

Non-Governmental Organizations NGOs are involved with mental health in the country. They are mainly involved in advocacy, promotion, prevention and rehabilitation. These organizations participate in mental health activities related to women, children, domestic violence and substance abuse.

Information Gathering System There is mental health reporting system in the country. Both ICD-10 and DSM-IV are used for recording purposes.
The country has no data collection system or epidemiological study on mental health.

Programmes for Special Population The country has specific programmes for mental health for elderly and children.

Therapeutic Drugs The following therapeutic drugs are generally available at the primary health care level of the country: carbamazepine, phenobarbital, phenytoin sodium, sodium valproate, amitriptyline, chlorpromazine, diazepam, haloperidol, lithium, biperiden, carbidopa, levodopa.
The essential list of drugs was revised in 2003.

Other Information

Additional Sources of Information

Darras, C. (1997) Local health services: some lessons from their evolution in Bolivia. Blackwell Science Ltd., 2, 356-62.

Pages, L. F., Servy, E., Marangunich, L., et al (1981) Migration and mental disorders in the Chiraguano civilization. Acta Psiquiatrica y Psicologica de America Latina, 27, 15-27.

Bosnia and Herzegovina

A–B

GENERAL INFORMATION

Bosnia and Herzegovina is a country with an approximate area of 51 thousand sq. km. (UNO, 2001). Its population is 4.186 million, and the sex ratio (men per hundred women) is 98 (UNO, 2004). The proportion of population under the age of 15 years is 16% (UNO, 2004), and the proportion of population above the age of 60 years is 15% (WHO, 2004). The literacy rate is 98.4% for men and 91.1% for women (UNESCO/MoH, 2004).

The country is a lower middle income group country (based on World Bank 2004 criteria). The proportion of health budget to GDP is 7.5%. The per capita total expenditure on health is 268 international $, and the per capita government expenditure on health is 99 international $ (WHO, 2004).

The main language(s) used in the country is (are) Bosnian, Serbian and Croatian. The largest ethnic group(s) is (are) Bosniac, and the other ethnic group(s) are (is) Croat, Serb, Roma and Slovenian. The largest religious group(s) is (are) Muslim, and the other religious group(s) are (is) Catholic and Orthodox Christian.

The life expectancy at birth is 69.3 years for males and 76.4 years for females (WHO, 2004). The healthy life expectancy at birth is 62 years for males and 66 years for females (WHO, 2004).

EPIDEMIOLOGY

Community studies in war torn areas showed enormous increase of mental disorders (total: over 60%, neurotic disorder: over 40%, psychotic disorders: about 20%). Dahl et al (1998) assessed 209 displaced women in a war zone in 1994 using a 10-item Posttraumatic Symptom Scale (PTSS-10). The proportion of caseness (defined by a score of six or more symptoms) was highest (71%) among women who had survived the most severe trauma (concentration camps or other kinds of detention) in comparison to others (47%) with less severe trauma. Caseness was also associated with severity of trauma and marital support (absent husband) in a multivariate analysis. Goldstein et al (1997) found that the majority of children in their sample had faced multiple stresses (separations from family, bereavement, close contact with war and combat and extreme deprivation) and that the prevalence and severity of experiences were not significantly related to a child's gender, wealth or age, but were related to their region of residence. Almost 94% of the children met DSM-IV criteria for posttraumatic stress disorder. High levels of other symptoms were also found. Children with greater symptoms had witnessed the death, injury or torture of a member of their nuclear family, were older and came from a large city. Allwood et al (2002) assessed 791 children aged 6 to 16 years during the 1994 siege in Sarajevo with the help of the Impact of Event Scale, PTSD Reaction Index, the Children's Depression Inventory, the Child Behavior Checklist, and the War Experience Questionnaire (completed by children and their teachers). Nearly 41% had clinically significant PTSD symptoms. Children were adversely affected by exposure to both violent and non-violent war-traumas. An additive effect of trauma exposure on trauma reactions was also found. As part of a UNICEF-sponsored Psychosocial Programme in Bosnia, Smith et al (2001) collected data from a representative sample of 339 children aged 9-14 years, their mothers and their teachers in order to investigate risk and moderating factors in children's psychological reactions to war. Self-report data from children revealed high levels of post-traumatic stress symptoms and grief reactions, but normal levels of depression and anxiety. Mothers' self-reports also indicated high levels of post-traumatic stress reactions, but normal levels of depression and anxiety. Structural equation modelling showed that child distress was related to both their level of exposure and to maternal reactions. Among the children and adolescents there was an increase of neurotic and psychotic disorders in the very beginning of the first year of the war, and a decrease of the same diagnoses during the second year. Stein et al (1999) who examined 147 displaced children residing in refugee centres in Bosnia reported that symptoms of posttraumatic stress, anxiety and depression showed a greater decrease in boys relative to girls over time. A study on soldiers showed that alcohol abuse was 3.7 times more frequent in participants of combat actions compared to those who did not have such assignment (Plavljanic & Mijic, 1997). Loga et al (1999) reported that stress/reactive psychoses increased and alcoholic psychoses decreased in clinical samples during the war. Studies on Bosnian refugees in Croatia are detailed under the relevant section of Croatia.

MENTAL HEALTH RESOURCES

Mental Health Policy A mental health policy is present. The policy was initially formulated in 1996.
The components of the policy are advocacy, promotion, prevention, treatment and rehabilitation. Basic elements of the mental health policy are: decentralization and sectorization of mental health services; intersectoral activity; comprehensiveness of services; equality in access and utilization of psychiatric service resources; nationwide accessibility of mental health services; continuity of services and care, together with the active participation of the community.

Substance Abuse Policy A substance abuse policy is absent. A substance abuse policy is in the implementation phase. Government and Parliament of Federation of Bosnia and Herzegovina have approved the Action Plan for Prevention and Treatment of Addictions, while a similar Plan still needs to be approved by the Parliament of Republic of Srpska. The best achievements in prevention and treatment of addictions are in two Cantons – Sarajevo and Tuzla.

National Mental Health Programme A national mental health programme is present. The programme was formulated in 1996.
The national plan needs are: postdoctoral study seminars on stress, PTSD, trauma psychology, treatment of war trauma; training programmes for staff including doctors, psychologists, psychiatric nurses, social workers, teachers and students of medicine and psychology; psychiatric and psychological services for individual and group counselling, psychotherapy for psychiatric patients, supervision of staff; mobile professional emergency teams for psychological trauma, with screening for PTSD, depression, suicidal states and

other kinds of psychiatric emergencies; institutions for forensic psychiatry; telepsychiatry service for assessment of callers and their reported problems; national plan for mental health care.

National Therapeutic Drug Policy/Essential List of Drugs A national therapeutic drug policy/essential list of drugs is present. It was formulated in 1996.

Mental Health Legislation The mental health legislation is in the form of a general law, 'Law on protection of persons with mental health'. A similar law in the Republic of Srpska is awaiting the approval of the Parliament.
The latest legislation was enacted in 2000.

Mental Health Financing There are no budget allocations for mental health.
Details about expenditure on mental health are not available.
The primary sources of mental health financing in descending order are social insurance and out of pocket expenditure by the patient or family.
Local authorities also contribute a small proportion of financing of mental health care.
The country has disability benefits for persons with mental disorders. The Complete Health Care Insurance takes care of any disability benefits.

Mental Health Facilities Mental health is a part of primary health care system. Actual treatment of severe mental disorders is available at the primary level. Primary care services are available for some cases.
Regular training of primary care professionals is carried out in the field of mental health. In the last two years, about 200 personnel were provided training. A network of community mental health centres is operational. An efficient and useful training of the staff in these centres has been carried out. Training programmes for family doctors and general practitioners are also available.
There are community care facilities for patients with mental disorders. Community care services are partially developed and are in the process of development. After the war, 38 community mental health centres (with catchment areas of 25 000-50 000 inhabitants) were proposed in Bosnia and Herzegovina and 7 in Republic of Sprska with funding by World Bank. These were to be established within or appended to the existing health centres and serve a catchment area of 50 000 to 100 000 inhabitants. Their aims were to provide clinical services for the mentally ill people and psychosocial rehabilitation to those traumatised by war. They offer a variety of services. Most personnel have changed their attitudes to mental health and relevant service provision and devoted to implement mental health reforms. Studies show that mental health personnel would like to have more influence on decision making for future service and policy improvements and that service users are satisfied with the service provided.

Psychiatric Beds and Professionals

Total psychiatric beds per 10 000 population	3.6
Psychiatric beds in mental hospitals per 10 000 population	2.4
Psychiatric beds in general hospitals per 10 000 population	1
Psychiatric beds in other settings per 10 000 population	0.2
Number of psychiatrists per 100 000 population	1.8
Number of neurosurgeons per 100 000 population	0.08
Number of psychiatric nurses per 100 000 population	10
Number of neurologists per 100 000 population	0.4
Number of psychologists per 100 000 population	0.5
Number of social workers per 100 000 population	0.03

Even during the war (1992-1995), WHO and the Universities in Sarajevo and Tuzla conducted a one year post-graduate course on 'Psychological Trauma and Healing' for psychiatrists, psychologists and social workers. There is continuous education in the field of mental health since 1999. Sarajevo University in cooperation with Centro di Studi in Trieste, Italy and within the TEMPUS Project organized postgraduate study 'Community psychiatry' for young psychiatrists, psychologists and social workers. Sarajevo University, in cooperation with Umea University, Sweden, is organizing a full postgraduate study in Child and Adolescent Psychiatriy and Psychology.

Non-Governmental Organizations NGOs are involved with mental health in the country. They are mainly involved in advocacy, promotion, prevention, treatment and rehabilitation. Many NGOs and international organizations, e.g. UNICEF, Médicins sans Frontières, Save the Children and Oxfam, have mental health programmes in the country with a focus on crisis counselling but a long term perspective. They have established accessible counselling centres and trained local counsellors and supervisors. Others like SweBiH (Swedish-Bosnian Association for Psychological and Social assistance to Bosnia & Herzegovina, founded by Swedish East Europe Committee and financed by SIDA), and HNI Bosnia-Hercegovina have focused on training of personnel from different professions. Users are a key element in the operation of mental health services. Five associations of former psychiatric patients, have organized under the umbrella Alliance at the state level.

Information Gathering System There is mental health reporting system in the country. But the system is not fully functional. The lacks of the system now represent a danger to the implementation and the future of the system itself.
The country has no data collection system or epidemiological study on mental health. There is a need for development at the national level of a data set on mental health.

Programmes for Special Population The country has specific programmes for mental health for refugees, disaster affected population and children. It is estimated that in the Srpska Republic, there are more than 500,000 refugees (from ex-Yugoslavia, Croatia, etc.) and about 20,000 internal displaced persons (from Kosovo and the Federal Republic of Yugoslavia). These refugees are living in collective shelters, in private accommodation, or with relatives and friends all over the country. The more vulnerable subjects have developed serious psychiatric disorders. In the country, there are only 5 centres for community-based rehabilitation. The main clinical problems which most urgently require attention are: enduring personality change, post-traumatic stress disorder and suicide. Special centres or special programmes within psychiatric clinics are urgently needed to treat existing problems of these kinds. The main goals of projects concerned with psycho-social support and rehabilitation of persons with PTSD are: education and training for nurses, doctors, psychologists, social workers, teachers, and students of medicine and psychology, as well as volunteers; detection of traumatised persons, as a consequence of stressful experiences; development of a programme for the treatment and evaluation of each high-risk group; psychological and psychiatric help, as well as psycho-social support and rehabilitation for psychologically traumatised persons with symptoms of PTSD or anxious-depressive and psychosomatic reactions; prevention of suicide.
The reorganization of services for the mentally ill is aimed at both war victims and others; and this is organized at community mental health centres. Similarly, a public mental health approach was used to develop and implement a school-based postwar trauma/grief intervention programme for adolescents. This approach included the development of multilateral partnerships with various stakeholders, systematic assessment that yields a detailed understanding of the specific range and severity of trauma and loss experiences, current adversities and trauma reminders among the affected population, and a training programme aimed at developing the capacities of local service providers and an indigenous support infrastructure so that the intervention programme could be directed and sustained by people within the communities served.

Therapeutic Drugs The following therapeutic drugs are generally available at the primary health care level of the country: carbamazepine, phenobarbital, phenytoin sodium, sodium valproate, amitriptyline, chlorpromazine, diazepam, fluphenazine, haloperidol, lithium, biperiden, carbidopa, levodopa.

Other Information The country comprises of two separate entities – Bosnia and Herzegovina and Srpsca Republic. The information is a combination of information available from both parts.
The country comprises of two entities Federation of Bosnia and Herzegovina and Republic of Srpska, as well as District Brcko. The first neuropsychiatry unit was set up in Sarajevo University in 1947, and since then the psychiatric services have gradually expanded (Ceric et al, 1995).

Additional Sources of Information

Allwood, M. A., Bell-Dolan, D., Husain, S. A. (2002) Children's trauma and adjustment reactions to violent and nonviolent war experiences. Journal of the American Academy of Child & Adolescent Psychiatry, 41, 450-457.

Beganovic, M., Lagerkvist, B., Masic, I., et al (1999) Rehabilitation of war victims in the Federation of Bosnia and Hercegovina with special reference to physical injuries. Medicinski Arhiv, 53, 179-180.

Ceric, I., Gavranovic, M., Oruc, L. (1995) History of the neuropsychiatric health service in Bosnia-Herzegovina. Medicinski Arhiv, 49, 117-119.

Ceric, I., Loga, S., Sinanovic, O., et al (1999) Reconstruction of mental health services in the Federation of Bosnia-Herzegovina. Medicinski Arhiv, 53, 127-130.

Dahl, S., Mutapcic, A., Schei, B. (1998) Traumatic events and predictive factors for posttraumatic symptoms in displaced Bosnian women in a war zone. Journal of Traumatic Stress, 11, 137-145.

De Clercq, L., Lagerkvist, B., Kapetanovic, T., et al (2000) Assessment of community mental health care in The Federation of Bosnia-Hercegovinia (FBH) after the 1992-95 war. Medicinski Arhiv, 55, 105-112.

de Jong, K., Ford, N., Kleber, R. (1999) Mental health care for refugees from Kosovo: the experience of Medicins sans Frontieres. Lancet, 353, 1616-1617.

Goldstein, R. D., Wampler, N. S., Wise, P. H. (1997) War experiences and distress symptoms of Bosnian children. Pediatrics, 100, 873-878.

Lagerkvist, B., Jacobsson, L. (2001) Development of community psychiatry in Bosnia-Herzegovina with focus on support from Sweden. Medicinski Arhiv, 55, 33-35.

Lagerkvist, B., Maglajlic, R. A., Puratic, V., et al (2003) Assessment of community mental health centres in Bosnia and Herzegovina as part of the ongoing mental health reform. Medicinski Arhiv, 57, 31-38.

Loga, S., Ceric, I., Stojak, R., et al (1999) Psychosocial research during the war in Sarajevo. Medicinski Arhiv, 53, 139-144.

Plavljanic, R., Mijic, R. (1997) Alcohol abuse in soldiers of the Herzegovina Corps of the Republic of Serbia Army during the 1992-1994 war. Vojnosanitetski Pregled, 54, 469-472.

Saltzman, W. R., Layne, C. M., Steinberg, A. M., et al (2003) Developing a culturally and ecologically sound intervention program for youth exposed to war and terrorism. Child & Adolescent Psychiatric Clinics of North America, 12, 319-342.

Smith, P., Perrin, S., Yule, W., et al. (2002) War exposure among children from Bosnia-Hercegovina: psychological adjustment in a community sample. Journal of Traumatic Stress, 15, 147-56.

Stein, B., Comer, D., Gardner, W., et al (1999) Prospective study of displaced children's symptoms in wartime Bosnia. Social Psychiatry & Psychiatric Epidemiology, 34, 464-469.

Botswana

A–B

GENERAL INFORMATION

Botswana is a country with an approximate area of 582 thousand sq. km. (UNO, 2001). Its population is 1.795 million, and the sex ratio (men per hundred women) is 97 (UNO, 2004). The proportion of population under the age of 15 years is 39% (UNO, 2004), and the proportion of population above the age of 60 years is 4% (WHO, 2004). The literacy rate is 76.1% for men and 81.5% for women (UNESCO/MoH, 2004).

The country is a higher middle income group country (based on World Bank 2004 criteria). The proportion of health budget to GDP is 6.6%. The per capita total expenditure on health is 381 international $, and the per capita government expenditure on health is 252 international $ (WHO, 2004).

The main language(s) used in the country is (are) English and Setswana (official). The largest ethnic group(s) is (are) Setswana speaking tribes. The largest religious group(s) is (are) Christian.

The life expectancy at birth is 40.2 years for males and 40.6 years for females (WHO, 2004). The healthy life expectancy at birth is 36 years for males and 35 years for females (WHO, 2004).

EPIDEMIOLOGY

Ben-Tovim and Cushnie (1986) ascertained the one-year prevalence of schizophrenia among individuals aged 15 years or older living in six villages in a remote area of Botswana. All cases were diagnosed independently by two experienced psychiatrists, following ICD-9 rubrics. DSM-III criteria were also applied, separately. Accurate contemporary population estimates of the villages were available. The age-adjusted prevalence of schizophrenia was 5.3 per 1000 in terms of ICD-9, or 4.3 per 1000 by DSM-III, which has an upper age limit for onset of 45 years. Ben-Tovim (1983, 1985) encountered substantial psychiatric morbidity in primary level psychiatric care facilities in Botswana, but he found that acute psychoses and culture-bound syndromes were rare. Lobatse Mental Hospital reports indicate that acute psychotic conditions are a common cause of admissions. Almost 18% of admissions at the main national referral hospital were HIV positive (Sidandi et al, 2004). Ben-Tovim and Boyce (1988) compared patient profiles in psychiatric hospitals of Botswana and South Australia. The patients in Botswana in comparison to Australia had shorter duration of illness, were likely to suffer from psychotic illnesses rather than personality and neurotic illnesses and were more likely to suffer from violence against property or others rather than self. A few articles on sexual behaviour and HIV and wife abuse were also accessible (Herring, 2001; Mmidi & Delmonico, 2001; Maundeni, 2002).

MENTAL HEALTH RESOURCES

Mental Health Policy A mental health policy is present. Details about the year of formulation are not available.

Substance Abuse Policy A substance abuse policy is present. Details about the year of formulation are not available. The plan to develop a substance abuse policy is in the advanced stage.

National Mental Health Programme A national mental health programme is present. The programme was formulated in 1992. Plans are under way to have the programme evaluated.

National Therapeutic Drug Policy/Essential List of Drugs A national therapeutic drug policy/essential list of drugs is present. It was formulated in 1992.

Revision of the policy is under way.

Mental Health Legislation The mental disorders act is under revision and will be soon replaced by the Mental Health Act of Botswana.

The latest legislation was enacted in 1971.

Mental Health Financing There are budget allocations for mental health.

The country spends 1% of the total health budget on mental health.

The primary source of mental health financing is tax based.

The country does not have disability benefits for persons with mental disorders.

Mental Health Facilities Mental health is a part of primary health care system. Actual treatment of severe mental disorders is available at the primary level.

Regular training of primary care professionals is carried out in the field of mental health. In the last two years, about 343 personnel were provided training. Facilities for training community mental health nurses is present. It is an 18 months post-basic course which teaches nurses to function effectively in the community, district and tertiary psychiatric hospitals. The training is comprehensive.

There are community care facilities for patients with mental disorders. Community care is mainly provided by family welfare educators based in primary care facilities. A community mental health nurse can provide all aspects of mental health and psychiatric nursing as well as render promotional, preventive, therapeutic and rehabilitative mental health services. They also provide consultative services due to the lack of trained psychiatrists and also train other non-specialized colleagues in the field of mental health.

Psychiatric Beds and Professionals

Total psychiatric beds per 10 000 population	1.1
Psychiatric beds in mental hospitals per 10 000 population	0.7
Psychiatric beds in general hospitals per 10 000 population	0.4
Psychiatric beds in other settings per 10 000 population	0
Number of psychiatrists per 100 000 population	0.4
Number of neurosurgeons per 100 000 population	0.1
Number of psychiatric nurses per 100 000 population	9
Number of neurologists per 100 000 population	0
Number of psychologists per 100 000 population	0.3
Number of social workers per 100 000 population	3

One neurologist visits from South Africa. There are 821 family welfare educators, 9 occupational therapists and 6 occupational therapy assistants.

Non-Governmental Organizations NGOs are involved with mental health in the country. They are mainly involved in advocacy, promotion, prevention and rehabilitation. Research is also an activity of NGOs.

Information Gathering System There is mental health reporting system in the country.
The country has data collection system or epidemiological study on mental health.

Programmes for Special Population There are no services for special population groups.

Therapeutic Drugs The following therapeutic drugs are generally available at the primary health care level of the country: carbamazepine, phenobarbital, phenytoin sodium, sodium valproate, amitriptyline, chlorpromazine, diazepam, fluphenazine, haloperidol, lithium, biperiden, carbidopa, levodopa.

Other Information

Additional Sources of Information

Ben-Tovim, D. I. (1983) A psychiatric service to the remote areas of Botswana. British Journal of Psychiatry, 142, 199-203.

Ben-Tovim, D. I. (1985) DSM-III in Botswana: a field trial in a developing country. American Journal of Psychiatry, 142, 342-345.

Ben-Tovim, D. I. (1987) Development psychiatry. Mental health and primary health care in Botswana. Tavistock Publications Ltd., London, UK.

Ben-Tovim, D. I., Boyce, G. P. (1988) A comparison between patients admitted to psychiatric hospitals in Botswana and South Australia. Acta Psychiatrica Scandinavica, 78, 222-226.

Ben-Tovim, D. I., Cushnie, J. M. (1986) The prevalence of schizophrenia in a remote area of Botswana. British Journal of Psychiatry, 148, 576-580.

Central Statistics Office, Government Printer, Gaborone

Herring, B. (2001) HIV and sexual compulsivity. Sexual Addiction & Compulsivity, 8, 81-82.

Kgosidintsi, A. (1996) The Role of the community health nurse in Botswana: the needs and problems of carers of schizophrenic clients in the community. Curations: South African Journal of Nursing, 19, 38-42.

Maundeni, T. (2002) Wife abuse among a sample of divorced women in Botswana: a research note. Violence Against Women, 8, 257-274.

Mmidi, M., Delmonico, D. L. (2001) Compulsive sexual behavior and HIV in Africa: a first look. Sexual Addiction & Compulsivity, 8, 169-183.

Sidandi, P. O., et al (2003) Lobatse Mental Hospital Report 2003.

Wankiiri, V. B. (1994). Training of community health nurses in Botswana. World Health Forum, 15, 260-261.

Brazil

GENERAL INFORMATION

Brazil is a country with an approximate area of 8547 thousand sq. km. (UNO, 2001). Its population is 180.655 million, and the sex ratio (men per hundred women) is 97 (UNO, 2004). The proportion of population under the age of 15 years is 28% (UNO, 2004), and the proportion of population above the age of 60 years is 8% (WHO, 2004). The literacy rate is 88% for men and 88.3% for women (UNESCO/MoH, 2004).

The country is a lower middle income group country (based on World Bank 2004 criteria). The proportion of health budget to GDP is 7.6%. The per capita total expenditure on health is 573 international $, and the per capita government expenditure on health is 238 international $ (WHO, 2004).

The main language(s) used in the country is (are) Portuguese. The largest ethnic group(s) is (are) Portuguese (descent), and the other ethnic group(s) are (is) mixed Caucasian and African (descent). The largest religious group(s) is (are) Roman Catholic (almost 70%), and the other religious group(s) are (is) Protestant.

The life expectancy at birth is 65.7 years for males and 72.3 years for females (WHO, 2004). The healthy life expectancy at birth is 57 years for males and 62 years for females (WHO, 2004).

EPIDEMIOLOGY

Andrade et al (2002) conducted a community survey for mental disorders in adults (n=1464) using Composite International Diagnostic Interview (CIDI-1.1). The life time, 1-year and 1-month prevalence of ICD-10 mental disorders were 45.9%, 26.8% and 22.2%, respectively. The most prevalent disorders (lifetime, 12-month and 1-month, respectively) were: nicotine dependence (25%, 11.4%, 9.3%), any mood disorder (18.5%, 7.6%, 5%) with depressive episode the most common mood disorder (16.8%, 7.1%, 4.5%), any anxiety disorder (12.5%, 7.7%, 6%), somatoform disorder (6%, 4.2%, 3.2%) and alcohol abuse/dependence (5.5%, 4.5%, 4%). No gender differences were found in overall morbidity. However, if substance use disorders were excluded, women had a higher risk for non-psychotic disorders. Kohn et al (2004) examined 1464 subjects utilizing the CIDI 1.1 and the DSM-III-R criteria and found that the lifetime prevalence for major depression was 12.6 %, for alcohol use disorders 14.9%, for non-affective psychosis 2.1% and for bipolar disorder 1.3%. In a multi-site study, Almeido Filho et al (1997), employed a two-stage methodology to assess 6476 subjects. Age-adjusted prevalence of cases ranged from 19% to 34% with anxiety and alcohol use disorders being the commonest (18% and 8% respectively). A number of studies that used only a screening instrument for ascertaining caseness found rates between 22.7% and 37.5% (De Lima et al, 1999; Faria et al, 1999). Higher rates were found among women (24.5%-26.5%) in comparison to men (11.7%-17.9%) (De Jesus et al, 1993; De Lima et al, 1999). An inverse relationship was seen between level of income, schooling and prevalence of minor psychiatric disorders (De Lima et al, 1999). Faria et al (1999) found that pesticide poisoning was strongly associated with minor psychiatric disorders in a population of farm workers. Herrera et al (2002) interviewed 1656 individuals aged over 65 years and found that 7.7% suffered from dementia (55.1% Alzheimer's disease, 9.3% vascular type and 14.4% mixed type). Age, female gender and low educational level were significantly associated with a higher prevalence of dementia. The prevalence of Organic Brain Syndrome in the elderly varied from 5.9% to 29.8% and of depression from 19.7% to 35.1% in a community study done in three cities (Veras & Murphy 1994). Moreira et al (1996), assessed 1091 individuals selected through a population-based multistage random sampling using the CAGE questionnaire and found the rate of dependence to be 9.3%. Chaieb and Castellarin (1998) compared age and sex matched alcoholics (identified by the use of CAGE questionnaire) and non-alcoholics. Alcohol dependence was associated with male gender, smoking (in self and family members) and low educational, employment and income status. De Carvalho (1986) identified drug abuse in 23.8% of college students with cannabis, amphetamines, tranquilizers and cocaine abuse being the most prevalent. Moreira et al (2001) found erectile dysfunction of some degree in 39.5% to 46.2% of respondents in three large population surveys. Age, marital status (never married), educational attainment (low), race/ethnicity (black), homo/bisexuality and a history of physical and mental illnesses were associated with an increased prevalence of erectile dysfunction. Silva et al (1999) reviewed data in files catalogued by the Legal Medical Institution and other indirect sources of information and found that suicide occurred more often among single men between 21 and 30 years of age. They also reported that the rate of suicide was not increasing and that the preferential method for committing suicide was hanging. Baus et al (2002) assessed 478 elementary and high school students during the 4th National Survey on Drug Abuse. Regular use (6 or more times per month) of alcohol, marijuana, solvent drugs and amphetamines was found in 24.2%, 4.9%, 2.5% and 2.3% of students, respectively. Age, gender, social status and living with both parents were significantly associated with drug abuse. Girls were more likely to consume weight loss drugs, stimulants and tranquilizers, and boys were more likely to use solvent drugs. Guardiola et al (2000) found ADHD in 18% of 484 first-graders while applying DSM-IV criteria and 3.5% using neuropsychological criteria.

MENTAL HEALTH RESOURCES

Mental Health Policy A mental health policy is present. The policy was initially formulated in 1991.
The components of the policy are advocacy, promotion, prevention, treatment and rehabilitation. It was revised in 2001. There are regular funds for its implementation. 50-75% of its original content was put into practice.

Substance Abuse Policy A substance abuse policy is present. The policy was initially formulated in 2000. It was revised in 2001, and has a specific budget for its implementation. A specific legislation for substance abuse exists since 1978.

National Mental Health Programme A national mental health programme is present. The programme was formulated in 1991. It was revised in 2001. There is a specific budget for its implementation and 50% to 75% of it is already implemented. Its main components are strategy of services reform, integration of mental health services into primary care and development of specialized services. The various states in the country have different mental health programmes currently in place.

National Therapeutic Drug Policy/Essential List of Drugs A national therapeutic drug policy/essential list of drugs is present. It was formulated in 1978.

Mental Health Legislation There is a mental health legislation. Funding is available for its implementation. It focuses on human rights (conforms to International Human Rights laws), regulation of involuntary treatment, regulation of mental health services, admission and discharge procedures, housing, accommodation and employment facilities for patients. Brazil's Psychiatric Reform Law shifted the emphasis from hospital-based care to community-based care. In Brazil, the national laws are hierarchically superior to state laws. Some subjects like penal laws are exclusively federal while others like laws that regulate penitentiary and health services can be either federal or state. The national laws that are relevant to the field of forensic psychiatry are the Federal Constitution, the Penal Execution Law, the Health Organic Law, the Penal Code and the Penal Procedural Code. Different states have their own laws in addition to the above. There is a provision for recognition of guilty but mentally ill. Under Brazilian law, notwithstanding competence, the defendant is submitted to trial. This is possible because the defendant has a passive role.
The latest legislation was enacted in 2001.

Mental Health Financing There are budget allocations for mental health.
The country spends 2.5% of the total health budget on mental health.
The primary sources of mental health financing in descending order are tax based, social insurance, private insurances and out of pocket expenditure by the patient or family.
Approximately 2.0% is spent on general hospitals, 80.0% in psychiatric hospitals, 15.0% in ambulatory clinics and 3.0% in community care. There is a plan to audit psychiatric hospitals. The new laws permit remuneration for consultations performed by professionals like psychologists, nurses, social workers and for management at centres of psychosocial attention. The slow growth of mental health care in private general hospitals is hypothesized to be related to the low rates paid for psychiatric services by the Government.
The country has disability benefits for persons with mental disorders.

Mental Health Facilities Mental health is a part of primary health care system. Actual treatment of severe mental disorders is not available at the primary level. This kind of service is available for less than 25% of the population. Mental health care is provided by primary health care doctors and nurses. A system of referral is in place.
Regular training of primary care professionals is not carried out in the field of mental health.
There are community care facilities for patients with mental disorders. The community care system for the mentally ill includes outpatient clinics, preventive/promotion interventions, home interventions all of them available for less than 25% of the treated population, and residential facilities available to 50 to 75% of the treated population. Current services involve an active participation of multi-disciplinary teams. Over the last one and a half decade, hundreds of new services including day care centres have been created. However, services are heavily concentrated in the most developed regions and state capitals.

Psychiatric Beds and Professionals

Total psychiatric beds per 10 000 population	2.56
Psychiatric beds in mental hospitals per 10 000 population	2.44
Psychiatric beds in general hospitals per 10 000 population	0.12
Psychiatric beds in other settings per 10 000 population	
Number of psychiatrists per 100 000 population	4.8
Number of neurosurgeons per 100 000 population	
Number of psychiatric nurses per 100 000 population	
Number of neurologists per 100 000 population	
Number of psychologists per 100 000 population	31.8
Number of social workers per 100 000 population	

More data are being collected on human resources in mental health. There was a gradual closing down of hospital beds even before the new law (2001). In the last one and a half decades, the number of beds came down from 85 000 to about 43 000. 30% of these beds are occupied by long stay patients (>1 year). Of the over 6000 general hospitals in Brazil, less than 2% had psychiatric units. There has been a gradual growth of the private sector particularly for care of drug abuse patients. There is a provision of forensic psychiatric hospitals, but all states do not have them. A system of progressive discharge helps in acceptance and integration of forensic psychiatric patients in the community. Mental health professionals are concentrated in the south and south-east of the country. Brazil is the only country in South America where the profession of psychology is regulated. This is important as more than 90% of the causes are conducted by private institutions. Almost two-thirds of psychologists are employed in private institutions. Continuing education is neither required nor regulated. Psychologists cannot prescribe medication, and few can directly admit patients to hospitals. Psychiatric nursing started to develop in Brazil since 1970, when community care began to be emphasized. Due to the creation of new services, the prospects of employment of nurses have risen.

Non-Governmental Organizations NGOs are involved with mental health in the country. They are mainly involved in advocacy, promotion, treatment and rehabilitation. They participate in activities related to women, children, domestic violence and consumers.

Information Gathering System There is mental health reporting system in the country. ICD-10 is used for recording purposes. The mental health components are for inpatients, admission and discharge and for outpatient care consultations.
The country has data collection system or epidemiological study on mental health. The Statistics Department from the Unified Health System (DATASUS) is in charge of the data collection system for mental disorders. Data collection is conducted in parts of the system: hospitals and outpatient clinics.

Programmes for Special Population The country has specific programmes for mental health for elderly and children.

Therapeutic Drugs The following therapeutic drugs are generally available at the primary health care level of the country: carbamazepine, phenobarbital, phenytoin sodium, amitriptyline, chlorpromazine, diazepam, haloperidol, lithium, biperiden.
The National Therapeutic Drugs Policy was revised in 1999.

Other Information

Additional Sources of Information

Almeida-Filho, N., de Jesus, M. J., Coutinho, E., et al (2004) Brazilian multicentric study of psychiatric morbidity. Methodological features and prevalence estimates. British Journal of Psychiatry, 171, 524-529.

Andrade, V. M., Bueno, F.A. (2001) Medical psychology in Brazil. Journal of Clinical Psychology in Medical Settings, 8, 9-13.

Andrade, L., Walters, E. E., Gentil, V., et al (2002) Prevalence of ICD-10 mental disorders in a catchment area in the city of Sao Paulo, Brazil. Social Psychiatry & Psychiatric Epidemiology, 37, 316-325.

Baus, J., Kupek, E., Pires, M. (2002) Prevalence and risk factors associated with drug use among school students, Brazil. Revista de Saude Public, 36, 40-46.

Botega, N. J. (2002) Psychiatric units in Brazilian general hospitals: a growing philanthropic field. International Journal of Social Psychiatry, 48, 97-102.

Chaieb, J. A., Castellarin, C. (1998) Smoking associated with alcoholism: introduction to the major human dependencies. Revista de Saude Publica, 32, 246-254.

Csillag, C. (2001) Psychiatric reform law comes into effect in Brazil. Lancet, 357, 1346.

De Carvalho, F.V. (1986) Drug use among university students in the state of Sao Paulo, Brazil. Bulletin on Narcotics, 38, 37-40.

de Jesus, M. J., Almeida-Filho, N., Coutinho, E., et al (1993) The epidemiology of psychotropic use in the city of Sao Paulo. Psychological Medicine, 23, 467-474.

De Lima, M. S., Hotopf, M., Mari, J. J., et al (1999) Psychiatric disorder and the use of benzodiazepines: an example of the inverse care law from Brazil. Social Psychiatry & Psychiatric Epidemiology, 34, 316-322.

de Toledo Ferraz, M. P., Carlini, E. A. (2003) Brazilian public mental health policy: education and research. International Psychiatry, 1, 15-16.

Faria, N. M., Facchini, L. A., Fassa, A. G., et al (1999) A cross-sectional study about mental health of farm-workers from Serra Gaucha (Brazil). Revista de Saude Publica, 33, 391-400.

Guardiola, A., Fuchs, F. D., Rotta, N. T., et al (2000) Prevalence of attention-deficit hyperactivity disorders in students. Comparison between DSM-IV and neuropsychological criteria. Arquivos de Neuro-Psiquiatria, 58, 401-407.

Herrera, Jr. E., Caramelli, P., Silveira, A. S. B., et al (2002) Epidemiologic survey of dementia in a community-dwelling Brazilian population. Alzheimer Disease & Associated Disorders, 16, 103-108.

Kantorski, L. P. (2002). Mental health care in Brazil. Journal of Psychiatric and Mental Health Nursing, 9, 251-253.

Kohn R., Caldas de Almeida, J. M., Miranda C. T., et al (2004) Mental disorders in Latin America and the Caribbean: a serious public health challenge. (Accepted for publication: Pan American Journal of Public Health).

Moreira, Jr. E. D., Abdo, C. H., Torres, E. B., et al (2001) Prevalence and correlates of erectile dysfunction: results of the Brazilian study of sexual behavior. Urology, 58, 583-588.

Moreira, L. B., Fuchs, F. D., Moraes, R. S., et al (1996) Alcoholic beverage consumption and associated factors in Porto Alegre, a southern Brazilian city: A population-based survey. Journal of Studies on Alcohol, 57, 253-259.

Silva, J. A. S., Silva, C. N., Silva, J. A. S., et al (1999) Epidemiology of suicide in the city of Salvador (BA). Revista Brasileira de Neurologia e Psiquiatria, 3, 19-25.

Taborda, J. G. V., Cardoso, R. G., Morana, H. C. P.(2000). Forensic psychiatry in Brazil. International Journal of Law and Psychiatry, 23, 579-588.

Veras, R. P., Murphy, E. (1994) The mental health of older people in Rio de Janeiro. International Journal of Geriatric Psychiatry, 9, 285-295.

Brunei Darussalam

GENERAL INFORMATION

Brunei Darussalam is a country with an approximate area of 6 thousand sq. km. (UNO, 2001). Its population is 0.366 million, and the sex ratio (men per hundred women) is 108 (UNO, 2004). The proportion of population under the age of 15 years is 30% (UNO, 2004), and the proportion of population above the age of 60 years is 4% (WHO, 2004). The literacy rate is 96.3% for men and 91.4% for women (UNESCO/MoH, 2004).

The country is a high income group country (based on World Bank 2004 criteria). The proportion of health budget to GDP is 3.1%. The per capita total expenditure on health is 638 international $, and the per capita government expenditure on health is 507 international $ (WHO, 2004).

The main language(s) used in the country is (are) Malay, Chinese and English. The largest ethnic group(s) is (are) Malay (two-thirds), and the other ethnic group(s) are (is) Chinese and Iban. The largest religious group(s) is (are) Muslim.

The life expectancy at birth is 74.8 years for males and 77.4 years for females (WHO, 2004). The healthy life expectancy at birth is 65 years for males and 66 years for females (WHO, 2004).

EPIDEMIOLOGY

There is substantial epidemiological data on mental illnesses in Brunei Darussalam in internationally accessible literature. No attempt was made to include this information here.

MENTAL HEALTH RESOURCES

Mental Health Policy A mental health policy is absent.

Though the country has no mental health policy, certain components of the policy like advocacy, prevention, etc. are undertaken from time to time on an ad-hoc basis.

Substance Abuse Policy A substance abuse policy is present. Details about the year of formulation are not available. The substance abuse policy deals with misuse of illicit drugs and prohibition of alcohol.

National Mental Health Programme A national mental health programme is absent.

Though at present the country lacks a national mental health programme, it has been identified as one of the six priority programmes under the National Committee of Health Promotion formed in March 2000.

National Therapeutic Drug Policy/Essential List of Drugs A national therapeutic drug policy/essential list of drugs is present. It was formulated in 1993.

Mental Health Legislation The Lunacy Act is under the process of revision.

The latest legislation was enacted in 1929.

Mental Health Financing There are no budget allocations for mental health.

Details about expenditure on mental health are not available.

The primary source of mental health financing is tax based.

The country has disability benefits for persons with mental disorders. There is a mental illness allowance given from the Ministry of Youth, Culture and Sports.

Mental Health Facilities Mental health is not a part of primary health care system. Actual treatment of severe mental disorders is not available at the primary level. Treatment is undertaken at the psychiatric units of two hospitals and 6 other outpatient psychiatric clinics under the care of psychiatrists.

Regular training of primary care professionals is not carried out in the field of mental health. Training of primary care personnel in mental health is done on an ad-hoc basis and is integrated into the CME for doctors, nurses and other health professionals.

There are community care facilities for patients with mental disorders. There are three day-care centres and one community care team.

Psychiatric Beds and Professionals

Total psychiatric beds per 10 000 population	1.2
Psychiatric beds in mental hospitals per 10 000 population	0
Psychiatric beds in general hospitals per 10 000 population	1.2
Psychiatric beds in other settings per 10 000 population	0
Number of psychiatrists per 100 000 population	1.9
Number of neurosurgeons per 100 000 population	0.6
Number of psychiatric nurses per 100 000 population	0.3
Number of neurologists per 100 000 population	0.9
Number of psychologists per 100 000 population	0.3
Number of social workers per 100 000 population	1

The 6 social workers and 1 clinical psychologist provide some services for the mental health units but are not specifically allocated to mental health. The geographic distribution of mental health facilities is uneven because of their limited number, e.g. inpatient facilities may be relatively inaccessible for the population residing in the rural interior areas to the west.

Non-Governmental Organizations NGOs are involved with mental health in the country. They are mainly involved in rehabilitation.

Information Gathering System There is mental health reporting system in the country.
The country has no data collection system or epidemiological study on mental health.

Programmes for Special Population There are no special facilities at present and support services are provided through mental health services coordinating with other programmes.

Therapeutic Drugs The following therapeutic drugs are generally available at the primary health care level of the country: carbamazepine, phenobarbital, phenytoin sodium, sodium valproate, amitriptyline, chlorpromazine, diazepam, haloperidol, lithium, carbidopa, levodopa.

Other Information The system of primary care clinics as such is well developed and a regular flying doctor service covers most populous areas.

Additional Sources of Information

Government document (1929) Lunacy Enactment, Chapter 48.

Bulgaria

A–B

GENERAL INFORMATION

Bulgaria is a country with an approximate area of 111 thousand sq. km. (UNO, 2001). Its population is 7.829 million, and the sex ratio (men per hundred women) is 94 (UNO, 2004). The proportion of population under the age of 15 years is 14% (UNO, 2004), and the proportion of population above the age of 60 years is 22% (WHO, 2004). The literacy rate is 99.1% for men and 98.1% for women (UNESCO/MoH, 2004).

The country is a lower middle income group country (based on World Bank 2004 criteria). The proportion of health budget to GDP is 4.8%. The per capita total expenditure on health is 303 international $, and the per capita government expenditure on health is 248 international $ (WHO, 2004).

The main language(s) used in the country is (are) Bulgarian and Turkish. The largest ethnic group(s) is (are) Bulgarian (five-sixths), and the other ethnic group(s) are (is) Turks. The largest religious group(s) is (are) Bulgarian Orthodox Christian (five-sixths), and the other religious group(s) are (is) Muslim.

The life expectancy at birth is 68.8 years for males and 75.6 years for females (WHO, 2004). The healthy life expectancy at birth is 63 years for males and 67 years for females (WHO, 2004).

EPIDEMIOLOGY

Dimitrova et al (1997) reviewed registers and reported that projected psychiatric morbidity had increased by 4% over the period 1989-93 to 2.4%. As a part of a WHO collaborative project, Saunders et al (1993) determined the prevalence of hazardous and harmful alcohol use among patients attending primary health care facilities in several countries including Bulgaria. After non-drinkers and known alcoholics had been excluded, 18% of subjects had a hazardous level of alcohol intake and 23% had experienced at least one alcohol-related problem in the previous year. Popova (1996) found that between 1961 and 1991 suicide rates had doubled to 17.2/100 000 population. Suicide was associated with mental illness, gender (male) and age (elderly). Akabaliev and Iliev (2002) conducted a study on all documented completed suicides (n=353) due to poisoning in a region of Bulgaria during the period of socioeconomic transition and crisis (1990-2000). Age, female gender, local and rural residence, pensioner status, intake of drugs, pesticide and corrosive intoxications and receipt of medical aid were significantly associated with lethal suicidal poisoning when compared to lethal accidental poisoning. Men predominated in the working age group and women in the pensioners' age group. Men tended to use poisons and corrosives while women used drug overdoses as means of committing suicide. Iliev et al (2000) found that younger age and female gender were associated with deliberate self-poisoning in a retrospective study on a representative sample (n=311) from a regional toxicological centre. Almost half of the subjects had a psychiatric disorder with adjustment disorder (53.6%) and depressive and schizophrenic disorders (26.8%) being the leading diagnoses. Milev and Mikhov (1992) reviewed hospital data (n=9235) and found that female subjects were four times more likely to attempt suicide. More than half of the patients were below 24 years and were single. Iliev et al (2001) studied the whole caseload (n=571) of acute overdose with psycho-active substances in a regional toxicology center (catchment area served 8.8% of the population of the country) in a 10 year period between 1990 and 2000. Alcohol (62.8%) and opioid (15.3%) intoxications were common especially among severe intoxications. The lethality rate was 1.6%. Serious reading and writing disorders were detected in 14.8% of all pupils in a study done in the setting of a single school. These disorders were encountered in 29.3% of children with low marks and in only 1% of those with good marks (Bircheva, 1979).

MENTAL HEALTH RESOURCES

Mental Health Policy A mental health policy is present. The policy was initially formulated in 2004.
It was adopted by the Council of Ministries along with an Action plan for the period 2005-2012. This policy incorporates all the relevant elements of the National Health Strategy 'Better health for better future' and develops the main principles of the mental health reform formulated since 2001. The main goals are: to substitute for centrally funded, hierarchically administered institutions a network of client-orientated and market regulated autonomous services with a variety of profiles; to substitute for outmoded psychiatric institutions a network of comprehensive community-based mental health services; and to integrate mental health services in the general health system. Suicide, drug and alcohol abuse and learning disabilities are subject to other policy documentation.

Substance Abuse Policy A substance abuse policy is present. The policy was initially formulated in 2001. The policy covers the areas of prevention, treatment and rehabilitation. A specific legislation on psychoactive substances and their precursors also exists. A National Drug Service was created at the Ministry of Health to implement the Act of Drugs and their Precursors.

National Mental Health Programme A national mental health programme is present. The programme was formulated in 2001. The mental health programme includes several demonstration projects related with the basic principles of the reform – a pilot community mental health center, mobile teams for crisis intervention, acute psychiatric wards and protected homes. An important part of the programme is the international epidemiological study on stress related disorders in Bulgaria (EPIBUL) in cooperation with WHO and Michigan University. A comprehensive national suicide prevention programme is present.

National Therapeutic Drug Policy/Essential List of Drugs A national therapeutic drug policy/essential list of drugs is present.
Details about the year of formulation are not available.
Pharmacotherapy is widely applied, and access to new drugs is unimpaired.

Mental Health Legislation Bulgaria does not have a specific mental health act. There are some provisions in two chapters in the actual Public Health Act (enacted 1973) that postulate rules for involuntary treatment of mentally ill persons. During the last few years, partial changes have been made in Bulgaria (i.e. exclusion of sections on compulsory admission for alcohol and drug abusers without psychotic symptoms and compulsory work activity in the course of such treatment; a new option for outpatient and day care treatment under compulsion). In the new Health Act (2004), in a separate chapter for mental health, there are more detailed provisions for compulsory treatment, informed consent, definition of the mental health services and responsible institutions and patients' rights. The Bulgarian Penal Code for offenders with mental illness was formulated in 1968. The Health Services Act (1999) made access to specialist care conditional on referral from primary care.
The latest legislation was enacted in 1973.

Mental Health Financing There are budget allocations for mental health.
The country spends 2.5% of the total health budget on mental health.
The primary sources of mental health financing in descending order are tax based, social insurance, out of pocket expenditure by the patient or family and private insurances.
The Bulgarian Ministry of Health funds 11 large governmental psychiatric hospitals. Some hospitals and dispensaries are financed by the Ministry of Finance and local municipalities. From the 1st of July 2000 with the introduction of the new health insurance system, inpatient services are financed through taxes (state budget) and outpatient services through the National Health Insurance Fund. According to the Health Insurance Law all citizens in the country have a compulsory health insurance. This makes outpatient health services accessible to about 90% of the population in the country. The funding for NGO projects is exclusively from external donors on a grant basis.
The country has disability benefits for persons with mental disorders.

Mental Health Facilities Mental health is a part of primary health care system. Actual treatment of severe mental disorders is not available at the primary level. Severe mental disorders are treated by specialists.
Regular training of primary care professionals is carried out in the field of mental health. In the last two years, about 450 personnel were provided training. The programme for training of the GPs in mental health is in its preliminary stage. A module for mental health training was introduced within the post-graduate training for GPs a few years ago.
There are no community care facilities for patients with mental disorders. There are very few community care facilities such as day centres, sheltered houses, etc. for patients with mental disorders. Pilot projects for such services are run by NGOs, National Mental Health Programme, Stability Pact SEE Mental Health Project and some are planned for the future under the PHARE project (starting 2005). With the process of reform in psychiatry, the existing system of mental health services will be changed and community-based mental health care will be introduced. At present, Bulgarian psychiatrists do not practise the components of modern community-based psychiatry in a way that meets international standards. The implementation of these components would require the development of new training programmes based on experiences derived from these pilot services.

Psychiatric Beds and Professionals

Total psychiatric beds per 10 000 population	8.3
Psychiatric beds in mental hospitals per 10 000 population	4.1
Psychiatric beds in general hospitals per 10 000 population	1.9
Psychiatric beds in other settings per 10 000 population	2.3
Number of psychiatrists per 100 000 population	9
Number of neurosurgeons per 100 000 population	1.6
Number of psychiatric nurses per 100 000 population	15
Number of neurologists per 100 000 population	15
Number of psychologists per 100 000 population	0.9
Number of social workers per 100 000 population	0.3

The other specialists are working in private set-ups. Mental health needs are defined from a medical point of view. This implies that control of symptoms is the most important service and it underestimates the need for other types of intervention programmes – occupational, psychological, etc. Staffs, mainly composed of psychiatrists, dominate the treatment process and reflect a paternalistic treatment model. Some special residential facilities under the social welfare administration provide care for chronically mentally ill patients. The delivery of outpatient services is based on geographical responsibility. There is a lack of coordination between hospitals and outpatient services in terms of procedures for referral and follow-up. About 100, 80 and 20 beds are available for treatment of drug abusers, forensic cases, and children, respectively. Mental health needs are defined from a medical point of view. The introduction of National Health Insurance prompted several psychiatrists to leave their salaried positions within the Government system and establish private specialist services. Postgraduate training in child and adolescent psychiatry is available.

Non-Governmental Organizations NGOs are involved with mental health in the country. They are mainly involved in advocacy, promotion, prevention, treatment and rehabilitation. The Geneva Initiative on Psychiatry is helping in the training of psychiatric nurses and future trainers. Open Society Foundation is also interested in promoting activities in mental health reform.

Information Gathering System There is mental health reporting system in the country. It is based on the national and regional centres for health information.
The country has data collection system or epidemiological study on mental health.

Programmes for Special Population The country has specific programmes for mental health for minorities, refugees, elderly and children. Most of the programmes are run by NGOs and have a limited scope of action. There are programmes for women victims of violence. There are well established psychiatric services for children, for alcohol and drug abusers and for forensic psychiatry. There are also psychiatrists who work predominantly with elderly mentally ill.
WHO in collaboration with the Bulgarian Institute for Human Relations has been involved in a project to improve the mental health and well-being of the community through engaging adolescents in prevention and promotion related activities. Every city has a child psychiatric ambulatory unit; some of these units have a day-treatment centre.

Therapeutic Drugs The following therapeutic drugs are generally available at the primary health care level of the country: carbamazepine, ethosuximide, sodium valproate, amitriptyline, chlorpromazine, fluphenazine, haloperidol, biperiden, carbidopa, levodopa.
Some medicines are reimbursed totally or partially by the health insurance system. Only the tablet form of fluphenazine is reimbursed. A combination of Carbidopa and Levodopa is reimbursed.

Other Information There are no procedures for the cost assessment of psychiatric disability or psychiatric care. The significance of stigmatization and discrimination because of mental illness is not widely recognized. This leads to a poor quality of life for mentally ill patients and their relatives, as well as to a poor quality of services offered. However, the process of recognition of the importance of patients' participation in the decision-making process has started.

Additional Sources of Information

Achkova, M., Polnareva, N. (1999) Child and adolescent psychiatry in Bulgaria. In: H. Remschmidt, H. van Engeland (Eds). Child and Adolescent Psychiatry in Europe. Historical Development, Current Situation and Future Perspectives. Darmstadt, Steinkopff. pp33-40.

Akabaliev, V., Iliev, Y. (2002) Suicides among death cases from acute poisoning in the period of socio-economic transition 1990-2000 in Plovdiv region. Bulgarian Medicine, 10, 22-25.

Bircheva, E. (1979) Reading and writing disorders in elementary school students with varying achievement. Problemi Na Khigienata, 4, 136-142.

Borissov, V., Rathwell, T. (1996) Health care reforms in Bulgaria: an initial appraisal. Social Science & Medicine, 42, 1501-1510.

Delcheva, et al (1998) Cost of schizophrenia. Bulletin of the Bulgarian Psychiatric Association, 3-4, 14-18.

Dimitrova, Z., Dumanov, V. G., Ivanova Petrova, G. (1997) Trends in registered psychiatric morbidity and forecasting psychotropic drug needs in Bulgarian hospitals. Acta Pharmaceutica Hungarica, 67, 73-79.

Dontschev, P., Gordon, H. (1997) Forensic psychiatry in Bulgaria. Criminal Behaviour & Mental Health, 7, 141 – 151.

Iliev, Y. T., Akabaliev, V. H., Avgarska, L. P. (2001) Some characteristics of acute poisoning with psychoactive substances in the period of socioeconomic transition 1990-2000. Folia Medica (Plovdiv), 43, 33-39.

Iliev, Y. T., Mitrev, I. N., Andonova, S. G., et al (2000) Psychopathology and psychosocial causes in adult deliberate self-poisoning in Plovdiv region, Bulgaria. Folia Medica (Plovdiv), 42, 30-33.

Mihova, Z., Fercheva, A. (1999) Training in therapeutic nursing. Mental Health Reforms, 4, 8-10.

Milev, V., Mikhov, D. (1992) Attempted suicide by poisoning in the Sofia region. British Journal of Psychiatry, 160, 560-562.

Popova, S. (1996) Suicide in Bulgaria. Evaluation, risk factors and preventive measures. Romanian Journal of Legal Medicine, 4, 43-46.

Saunders, J. B., Aasland, O. G., Amundsen, A., et al (1993) Alcohol consumption and related problems among primary health care patients: WHO collaborative project on early detection of persons with harmful alcohol consumption--I. Addiction, 88, 349-362.

Tomov, T., Mladenova, M., Lazarova, I. et al (2004) Bulgaria mental health country profile. International Review of Psychiatry, 16, 93-106.

Burkina Faso

GENERAL INFORMATION

Burkina Faso is a country with an approximate area of 274 thousand sq. km. (UNO, 2001). Its population is 13.393 million, and the sex ratio (men per hundred women) is 96 (UNO, 2004). The proportion of population under the age of 15 years is 49% (UNO, 2004), and the proportion of population above the age of 60 years is 4% (WHO, 2004). The literacy rate is 18.5% for men and 8.1% for women (UNESCO/MoH, 2004).

The country is a low income group country (based on World Bank 2004 criteria). The proportion of health budget to GDP is 3%. The per capita total expenditure on health is 27 international $, and the per capita government expenditure on health is 16 international $ (WHO, 2004).

The main language(s) used in the country is (are) French. The largest ethnic group(s) is (are) Mossi, and the other ethnic group(s) are (is) Dioula, Peulh, Gourmantché, Bobo, Gourounsi, Samo. The largest religious group(s) is (are) Muslim, and the other religious group(s) are (is) indigenous groups.

The life expectancy at birth is 40.6 years for males and 42.6 years for females (WHO, 2004). The healthy life expectancy at birth is 35 years for males and 36 years for females (WHO, 2004).

EPIDEMIOLOGY

In a community study, Ouedraogo et al (1997) found enuresis in 12.9% in a sample of 1575 adolescents. Among them, 78.9% had primary enuresis. Ouedraogo et al (1998a) estimated the prevalence of disorders in child and adolescent population in a psychiatric hospital. The most current pathologies were epilepsy (31.5%), psychoses (25.7%) and adjustment disorders (21.5%). Ouedraogo and Ouango (1998) found paranoid schizophrenia to be the predominant subtype of schizophrenia among psychiatric patients. Ouedraogo et al (1998b) found that psychosocial support and parity play an important role in postpartum depression among patients admitted to maternity wards.

MENTAL HEALTH RESOURCES

Mental Health Policy A mental health policy is absent.
Some features of mental health policy are defined in the Public Health Code.

Substance Abuse Policy A substance abuse policy is present. Details about the year of formulation are not available. Substance abuse issues are also discussed in the Public Health Code.

National Mental Health Programme A national mental health programme is present. The programme was formulated in 2002.

National Therapeutic Drug Policy/Essential List of Drugs A national therapeutic drug policy/essential list of drugs is present. It was formulated in 1996.

Mental Health Legislation The Public Health Code has references to mental health.
The latest legislation was enacted in 1994.

Mental Health Financing There are no budget allocations for mental health.
Details about expenditure on mental health are not available.
Details about sources of financing are not available.
Details about disability benefits for mental health are not available.

Mental Health Facilities Mental health is a part of primary health care system. Actual treatment of severe mental disorders is available at the primary level. Psychiatric units are present in national and regional hospitals and one in an isolation hospital. Regular training of primary care professionals is carried out in the field of mental health. In the last two years, about 50 personnel were provided training.
There are community care facilities for patients with mental disorders. Traditional treatment by healers provide community care. Since 1983, the mental health system has been gradually decentralized.

Psychiatric Beds and Professionals

Total psychiatric beds per 10 000 population	0.18
Psychiatric beds in mental hospitals per 10 000 population	0.06
Psychiatric beds in general hospitals per 10 000 population	0.12
Psychiatric beds in other settings per 10 000 population	0
Number of psychiatrists per 100 000 population	0.05
Number of neurosurgeons per 100 000 population	0
Number of psychiatric nurses per 100 000 population	0.4
Number of neurologists per 100 000 population	0.01
Number of psychologists per 100 000 population	0.03
Number of social workers per 100 000 population	0.02

Non-Governmental Organizations NGOs are involved with mental health in the country. They are mainly involved in advocacy, treatment and rehabilitation.

Information Gathering System There is mental health reporting system in the country. Data are only available at the hospital level; abstracts can be obtained from the Health Statistical Report 1996.
The country has data collection system or epidemiological study on mental health.
A National Health Information System consists of data related to epidemiological study and hospital data. They are included in the National Health Statistics Report 1996 and the Mental Health Activities Assessment 2000.

Programmes for Special Population The country has specific programmes for mental health for children. In 2001, new strategies were developed to look into the children with mental conditions.

Therapeutic Drugs The following therapeutic drugs are generally available at the primary health care level of the country: carbamazepine, phenobarbital, chlorpromazine, diazepam, fluphenazine, haloperidol.

Other Information

Additional Sources of Information

Ouedraogo, A., Kere, M., Lankoande, J., et al (1998b) Screening of post-partum depressive states in the Yalgado Ouedraogo National Hospital Center maternity ward in Ouagadougou Burkina Faso. Journal de Gynécologie, Obstétrique et Biologie de la Reproduction, 27, 611-616.

Ouedraogo, A., Kere, M., Ouedraogo, T. L., et al (1997) Epidemiology of enuresis in children and adolescents aged 5-16 years in Ouagadougou (Burkina Faso). Archives de Pédiatrie, 4, 947-951.

Ouedraogo, A., Ouango, J. G. (1998) Clinical aspects of adult schizophrenia in the psychiatric service at the Yalgado Ouedraogo National Hospital Center of Ouagadougou (Burkina Faso). Dakar Medical, 43, 194-197.

Ouedraogo, A., Ouedraogo, T. L., Zallé, M. L. (2000) Problèmes médicopsychologiques en milieu carcéral au Burkina Faso: résultats d'une enquête préliminaire par questionnaire auprès des prisonniers de la Maison d'Arrêt et de Correction de Ouagadougou. Psychopathologie Africaine, 30, 317-328.

Ouedraogo, A., Sanou, Z. (1995) Decentralization of psychiatric care in Burkina Faso. World Health Forum, 16, 276-277.

Ouedraogo, A., Siranyan, S., Ouedraogo, T. L. (1998a) Psychiatric morbidity in children and adolescents: a five-year retrospective study of the hospital data of the YO-HNC Psychiatric Department in Ouagadougou (Burkina-Faso). Neuropsychiatrie de l'Enfance et de l'Adolescence, 46, 135-140.

Burundi

GENERAL INFORMATION

Burundi is a country with an approximate area of 28 thousand sq. km. (UNO, 2001). Its population is 7.068 million, and the sex ratio (men per hundred women) is 96 (UNO, 2004). The proportion of population under the age of 15 years is 45% (UNO, 2004), and the proportion of population above the age of 60 years is 4% (WHO, 2004). The literacy rate is 57.7% for men and 43.6% for women (UNESCO/MoH, 2004).

The country is a low income group country (based on World Bank 2004 criteria). The proportion of health budget to GDP is 3.6%. The per capita total expenditure on health is 19 international $, and the per capita government expenditure on health is 11 international $ (WHO, 2004).

The main language(s) used in the country is (are) French and Swahili. The largest ethnic group(s) is (are) Hutu, and the other ethnic group(s) are (is) Tutsi and Twa. The largest religious group(s) is (are) Roman Catholic, and the other religious group(s) are (is) Protestant and Muslim.

The life expectancy at birth is 38.7 years for males and 43 years for females (WHO, 2004). The healthy life expectancy at birth is 33 years for males and 37 years for females (WHO, 2004).

EPIDEMIOLOGY

There is a paucity of epidemiological data on mental illnesses in Burundi in internationally accessible literature. A study showed that sexual abuse is not as uncommon as thought (Baribwira et al, 1994). Some data are available on Burundese refugees living in Tanzania. These are described under the relevant section in Tanzania.

MENTAL HEALTH RESOURCES

Mental Health Policy A mental health policy is absent.

Substance Abuse Policy A substance abuse policy is absent.

National Mental Health Programme A national mental health programme is present. The programme was formulated in 1998.

National Therapeutic Drug Policy/Essential List of Drugs A national therapeutic drug policy/essential list of drugs is present. It was formulated in 1998.

Mental Health Legislation Details about the mental health legislation are not available.

Mental Health Financing There are no budget allocations for mental health.

Details about expenditure on mental health are not available.

The primary sources of mental health financing in descending order are out of pocket expenditure by the patient or family and tax based.

The country does not have disability benefits for persons with mental disorders.

Mental Health Facilities Mental health is a part of primary health care system. Actual treatment of severe mental disorders is not available at the primary level. Personnel are not trained as yet, and the number of drugs are limited.

Regular training of primary care professionals is not carried out in the field of mental health.

There are community care facilities for patients with mental disorders. Community care is available only in four provinces and is undertaken by an NGO.

Psychiatric Beds and Professionals

Total psychiatric beds per 10 000 population	0.1
Psychiatric beds in mental hospitals per 10 000 population	0.1
Psychiatric beds in general hospitals per 10 000 population	0
Psychiatric beds in other settings per 10 000 population	0
Number of psychiatrists per 100 000 population	0.02
Number of neurosurgeons per 100 000 population	0.02
Number of psychiatric nurses per 100 000 population	0
Number of neurologists per 100 000 population	0.06
Number of psychologists per 100 000 population	0.2
Number of social workers per 100 000 population	1.5

There is a special workers school and the university produces psychologists.

Non-Governmental Organizations NGOs are involved with mental health in the country. They are mainly involved in advocacy, promotion, prevention, treatment and rehabilitation.

Information Gathering System There is no mental health reporting system in the country. The personnel are untrained and the questionnaires do not contain questions on mental disorders.
The country has no data collection system or epidemiological study on mental health. The system is being built.

Programmes for Special Population There are no special programmes for any population group.

Therapeutic Drugs The following therapeutic drugs are generally available at the primary health care level of the country: carbamazepine, phenobarbital, phenytoin sodium, sodium valproate, amitriptyline, chlorpromazine, diazepam, fluphenazine, haloperidol, lithium, biperiden, levodopa.
There is also an essential list of drugs which was initially made in 1980, and the last revision was done in 1994.

Other Information

Additional Sources of Information

Baribwira, C., Muteganya, D., Ndihokubwayo, J. B., et al (1994) Aspects of sexually transmissible diseases in young children in Burundi: gonorrhea caused by sexual abuse. Médecine Tropicale, 54, 231-233.

Cambodia

GENERAL INFORMATION

Cambodia is a country with an approximate area of 181 thousand sq. km. (UNO, 2001). Its population is 14.482 million, and the sex ratio (men per hundred women) is 95 (UNO, 2004). The proportion of population under the age of 15 years is 41% (UNO, 2004), and the proportion of population above the age of 60 years is 5% (WHO, 2004). The literacy rate is 80.8% for men and 59.3% for women (UNESCO/MoH, 2004).
The country is a low income group country (based on World Bank 2004 criteria). The proportion of health budget to GDP is 11.8%. The per capita total expenditure on health is 184 international $, and the per capita government expenditure on health is 27 international $ (WHO, 2004).
The main language(s) used in the country is (are) Khmer. The largest ethnic group(s) is (are) Khmer (nine-tenths). The largest religious group(s) is (are) Buddhism.
The life expectancy at birth is 51.9 years for males and 57.1 years for females (WHO, 2004). The healthy life expectancy at birth is 46 years for males and 50 years for females (WHO, 2004).

C–D

EPIDEMIOLOGY

De Jong et al (2001) conducted epidemiological surveys to establish the rate of PTSD in 4 post-conflict zones, Algeria, Cambodia, Ethiopia and Gaza, using the PTSD module of CIDI. The sample consisted of adults (aged >=16 years) who were randomly selected from community populations (Cambodia, n=610). PTSD was prevalent in 28.4% of the population surveyed in Cambodia compared to 37.4% in Algeria, 15.8% in Ethiopia and 17.8% in Gaza. The following risk factors were associated with PTSD in Cambodia: conflict-related trauma after age 12 years, psychiatric history and current illness, youth domestic stress, death or separation in the family and alcohol abuse in parents. A number of studies have addressed mental health issues of Cambodian refugees in camps in the Thai-Cambodian border. These are presented under the relevant section in Thailand. Some studies which have looked at issues related to substance use disorders were accessible.

MENTAL HEALTH RESOURCES

Mental Health Policy A mental health policy is absent.
A draft was submitted to the Ministry of Health, but it has not been formally recognized yet. The development of the mental health policy is emerging as a national priority as a component of the national health policy.

Substance Abuse Policy A substance abuse policy is present. Details about the year of formulation are not available.

National Mental Health Programme A national mental health programme is absent.
A national mental health plan 2003-2020 has been prepared with inputs from WHO, mental health professionals, NGOs and other stakeholders. It focuses on promotion and prevention, access to care, integration of mental health care with primary and general health care, and development of mental health legislation and community care.

National Therapeutic Drug Policy/Essential List of Drugs A national therapeutic drug policy/essential list of drugs is present. It was formulated in 1997.
The National Sub-committee on Mental Health is trying to improve the distribution and availability of psychotropics. The basic essential drugs are available. Second generation drugs are freely available in private pharmacies but are expensive.

Mental Health Legislation There is no mental health legislation. However, a draft is present which is to be finalized soon.
Details about the year of enactment of the mental health legislation are not available.

Mental Health Financing There are budget allocations for mental health.
Details about expenditure on mental health are not available.
The primary sources of mental health financing in descending order are out of pocket expenditure by the patient or family, grants and tax based.
In the public sector, patients pay small consultation fees in public services, but prescribed medicines are provided free of charge.
The country does not have disability benefits for persons with mental disorders. There is a Disability Action Council composed of personnel from the Government, non-governmental and international organizations and religious organizations. The Government provides support in kind, and the main funding is provided by international donors. The Council is dealing with themes like raising awareness, drafting legislation and community work. Pilot studies are being conducted in villages to ascertain the prevalence of disability, both physical and mental. Further studies would be conducted to ascertain service availability.

Mental Health Facilities Mental health is a part of primary health care system. Actual treatment of severe mental disorders is available at the primary level. It is available in some provincial and referral hospitals and is currently in the six most populous of the twenty-three provinces and municipalities.
Regular training of primary care professionals is carried out in the field of mental health. A two-year training in mental health for general practitioners (102) and nurses in one province was organized by the Harvard Trauma Programme in Cambodia. The Transcultural Psychosocial Organization also trained several general practitioners and nurses. The Cambodian Mental Health

Development Programme offers training for mental health care in primary care to general practitioners, military and police doctors. Besides this, the municipal health department of some areas also offer training. Training has been provided to staff, albeit to a small group (e.g. about 100 out of 3000 doctors), who have then gone on to train community leaders like teachers, monks, village elders in identification of mental health problems. Training of primary care officials has been carried out in the field of mental health since 1997. Several NGOs have included primary health care training in their project design. Outpatient services have been developed as an offshoot of such training programmes.
There are community care facilities for patients with mental disorders. Since there are no existing mental hospitals, it is felt that general hospital facilities for treatment of mental disorders needs to be developed. Some clinics are beginning to operate with the help of the newly trained professionals. Two community-based day care centres have been set up with the help of NGOs. An effort is being made to integrate grass root workers in the care of mentally ill under the broader framework of general health. Traditional healers are also being included in the rehabilitation process in rural settings.

Psychiatric Beds and Professionals

Total psychiatric beds per 10 000 population	0
Psychiatric beds in mental hospitals per 10 000 population	0
Psychiatric beds in general hospitals per 10 000 population	0
Psychiatric beds in other settings per 10 000 population	0
Number of psychiatrists per 100 000 population	0.16
Number of neurosurgeons per 100 000 population	0.009
Number of psychiatric nurses per 100 000 population	0.22
Number of neurologists per 100 000 population	0
Number of psychologists per 100 000 population	0.45
Number of social workers per 100 000 population	0.05

Psychiatric services before 1975 included only one psychiatric hospital. Between 1979 and 1992, there were no mental health services though services and training programmes were available at some of the refugee camps in the Thai-Cambodian border. Currently, mental outpatient services are available in 12 out of 67 referral hospitals in the country. A 4-bedded ward is being developed for treatment of drug users. It may also be used for admission of acutely ill psychiatric patients. Training programmes in the country for psychiatrists and psychiatric nurses were established in 1994 with Norwegian (NORCOMH, NORAD, Norwegian Ministry of Foreign Affairs) financial assistance through the University of Oslo and IOM, the Association of Medical Doctors in Asia (Japan) and the Ministry of Health. 30% of the qualified psychiatrists are not involved in mental health work at a clinical level as they are in other health care positions and two-thirds are in the capital city. Psychiatrists are allowed part-time private practice. In one province, where there is no psychiatrist, a psychiatric nurse has been authorized to prescribe medication if needed on telephonic consultation with psychiatrists in Pnom Penh.

Non-Governmental Organizations NGOs are involved with mental health in the country. They are mainly involved in advocacy, promotion, prevention, treatment and rehabilitation. Six NGOs are active in the mental health area. These NGOs are funded by donations from international NGOs and organizations. There is a proposal to organize all NGOs in a council to utilize their resources more effectively. The Transcultural Psychosocial Organization (TPO) and the Social Service du Combodge (SSC) train village level workers and social workers, develop self-help groups and aid in providing assistance and referral to mentally ill for treatment in 6 out of 21 provinces. In addition, the TPO supports mental health groups for land mine victims and amputees at the WARS (War Amputees rehabilitation Services) centre and has developed a manual entitled Community mental health in Cambodia for training workers. The SSC runs a day care centre with help from the Municipality Government. The Centre for Child Mental Health (CCMH) is a comprehensive child and adolescent assessment and treatment centre in Pnom Penh and it has an outreach project in another city.

Information Gathering System There is mental health reporting system in the country. Very few data are reported.
The country has no data collection system or epidemiological study on mental health. There have been some form of epidemiological research but analysis is awaited.

Programmes for Special Population The country has specific programmes for mental health for children. There is a small clinic for children. A post-conflict family support programme has begun in Battambang under the aegis of the International Organization for Migration.
Programmes of care and rehabilitation for landmine victims have included mental health.

Therapeutic Drugs The following therapeutic drugs are generally available at the primary health care level of the country: phenobarbital, phenytoin sodium, amitriptyline, chlorpromazine, diazepam, haloperidol.
Carbamazepine, fluphenazine and lithium though available are not present in primary care.

Other Information Cambodia is in active transition from a post conflict situation to one of peace and development and that while the challenges are enormous; progress is being made under difficult circumstances. The Khmer Rouge shut the only mental hospital in 1975 and only a few traditional healers were allowed to practice and care for the mentally ill. After the Pol Pot regime was overthrown in 1979, the traditional healers gained more importance, though formal mental health care was not restored. It is only after 1990, when the international community started rebuilding the country that western methods of psychiatric care were introduced. The first western services were introduced in 1995. The Canadian Marcel Roy Foundation for Children of Cambodia started a child mental health clinic at a hospital in 1994. In the same year the International Organization for Migration along with the Norwegian council for Mental Health started the Cambodian Mental Health Training Programme to train 10 local doctors as psychiatrists. Psychiatry was included in the curricula of doctors and nurses in 1995. In 1996, the Harvard Training Programme in Cambodia started an outpatient department in the Siem Riep Provincial Hospital and in the following year provided psychiatric training to 48 doctors and medical assistants. An Office for Mental Health has been established within the Ministry of Health and budget has been provided for procuring essential psychotropic drugs, though no other financial support is currently available. The Ministry of Health feels that there is a huge scope for a close collaboration with WHO in developing programmes and policies in the field of mental health.

Additional Sources of Information

de Jong, J. T. V. M., Komproe, I. H., Van Ommeren, M., et al (2001) Lifetime events and posttraumatic stress disorder in 4 postconflict settings. JAMA, 286, 555-562.

Savin, D. (2000) Developing psychiatric training and services in Cambodia. Psychiatric Services, 51, 935.

Somasundaram, D. J., Van de Put, W. A. C. M., Eisenbruch, M., et al (1999) Starting mental health services in Cambodia. Social Science and Medicine, 48, 1029-1046.

Cameroon

C–D

GENERAL INFORMATION

Cameroon is a country with an approximate area of 475 thousand sq. km. (UNO, 2001). Its population is 16.296 million, and the sex ratio (men per hundred women) is 99 (UNO, 2004). The proportion of population under the age of 15 years is 42% (UNO, 2004), and the proportion of population above the age of 60 years is 6% (WHO, 2004). The literacy rate is 77% for men and 59.8% for women (UNESCO/MoH, 2004).

The country is a low income group country (based on World Bank 2004 criteria). The proportion of health budget to GDP is 3.3%. The per capita total expenditure on health is 42 international $, and the per capita government expenditure on health is 16 international $ (WHO, 2004).

The main language(s) used in the country is (are) French and English (official). The largest ethnic group(s) is (are) Cameroon Highlanders, and the other ethnic group(s) are (is) Equatorial Bantu, Kirdi, Fulani, Baka/Pygmees, Northwest Bantu and other African groups. The largest religious group(s) is (are) indigenous groups and Christian, and the other religious group(s) are (is) Muslim.

The life expectancy at birth is 47.2 years for males and 49 years for females (WHO, 2004). The healthy life expectancy at birth is 41 years for males and 42 years for females (WHO, 2004).

EPIDEMIOLOGY

There is a paucity of epidemiological data on mental illnesses in Cameroon in internationally accessible literature. A rapid assessment study revealed that the use of cannabis, heroin and cocaine was common. Solvents were mainly used by street children (Wansi et al, 1996). Studies suggest that child sexual abuse may require public health attention (Mabassa et al, 1999; Menick, 2002).

MENTAL HEALTH RESOURCES

Mental Health Policy A mental health policy is present. The policy was initially formulated in 1998.

The components of the policy are advocacy, promotion, prevention, treatment and rehabilitation. Formation and legislation are also a component of the policy. The process of drafting began in 1992, but the mechanism for its implementation is still being worked out.

Substance Abuse Policy A substance abuse policy is present. The policy was initially formulated in 1992. The mechanism for its implementation is still being worked out.

National Mental Health Programme A national mental health programme is present. The programme was formulated in 1999. It is included in the National Sectorial Strategy for Health.

National Therapeutic Drug Policy/Essential List of Drugs A national therapeutic drug policy/essential list of drugs is present. It was formulated in 1999.

Mental Health Legislation Activities related to a mental health legislation have been issued in the draft form.

Details about the year of enactment of the mental health legislation are not available.

Mental Health Financing There are budget allocations for mental health.

The country spends 0.1% of the total health budget on mental health.

The primary sources of mental health financing in descending order are tax based, out of pocket expenditure by the patient or family and private insurances.

Mental health has been included as a public health priority since 1989 with a designation of a mental health national coordinator, but greater priority was given to family planning and hospital medicine. In 2003, the mental health sub-directorate was cancelled with a risk of rolling back of financing for mental health. For example, the 2000-2001 budget addressed mental health programme activities with particular regard to the development of community-based mental health and with a plan to implement it over the next three years, but these activities could not be implemented.

The country has disability benefits for persons with mental disorders. It is available only for public servants who have mental illness.

Mental Health Facilities Mental health is not a part of primary health care system. Actual treatment of severe mental disorders is not available at the primary level. Mental health care in the primary health set-up is being developed as a part of the mental health action plan.

Regular training of primary care professionals is carried out in the field of mental health. Training modules exist for training primary care personnel. Training of primary care workers commenced in 2004.

There are no community care facilities for patients with mental disorders.

Psychiatric Beds and Professionals

Total psychiatric beds per 10 000 population	0.08
Psychiatric beds in mental hospitals per 10 000 population	0.07
Psychiatric beds in general hospitals per 10 000 population	0.0007
Psychiatric beds in other settings per 10 000 population	
Number of psychiatrists per 100 000 population	0.03
Number of neurosurgeons per 100 000 population	0.03
Number of psychiatric nurses per 100 000 population	0.2
Number of neurologists per 100 000 population	0.03
Number of psychologists per 100 000 population	0
Number of social workers per 100 000 population	0.1

Psychologists get training in clinical psychology while working (but without structured clinical supervision). Some psychologists in the private sector carry out counselling.

Non-Governmental Organizations NGOs are involved with mental health in the country. They are mainly involved in advocacy, promotion, prevention and rehabilitation.

Information Gathering System There is no mental health reporting system in the country. Data collection is poor because of insufficient staff.
The country has no data collection system or epidemiological study on mental health. Service reorganization (as prescribed in the existing sectorial strategy document) will allow for standardization of the epidemiological collection system.
An information gathering network is not yet developed due to a lack of trained and motivated staff and a lack of infrastructure.

Programmes for Special Population The country has specific programmes for mental health for disaster affected population.

Therapeutic Drugs The following therapeutic drugs are generally available at the primary health care level of the country: carbamazepine, ethosuximide, phenobarbital, phenytoin sodium, sodium valproate, amitriptyline, chlorpromazine, diazepam, fluphenazine, haloperidol, biperiden, carbidopa, levodopa.

Other Information Even if political and budget programmes are present, the plans in mental health are very slow to activate because of low priority, which leads to ineffective use of even existing human resources and capacities.

Additional Sources of Information

Home Office, United Kingdom. Report of fact-finding mission to Cameroon. London: Country Information and Policy Unit, Immigration and National Directorate, Home Office, United Kingdom, 2004.

Mbassa Menick D., Ngoh, F. (1999) Reconciliation and/or mediation settlements in cases of sexual abuse of minors in Cameroon. Médecine Tropicale, 59, 161-164.

Menick, D. M. (2002) Sexual abuse at schools in Cameroon: results of a survey-action program in Yaounde. Médecine Tropicale, 62, 58-62.

Wansi, E., Sam-Abbenyi, A., Befidi-Mengue, R., et al (1996) Rapid assessment of drug abuse in Cameroon. Bulletin on Narcotics, 48, 79-88.

Canada

GENERAL INFORMATION

Canada is a country with an approximate area of 9971 thousand sq. km. (UNO, 2001). Its population is 31.743 million, and the sex ratio (men per hundred women) is 98 (UNO, 2004). The proportion of population under the age of 15 years is 18% (UNO, 2004), and the proportion of population above the age of 60 years is 17% (WHO, 2004). The literacy rate is 99% for men and 99% for women (UNESCO/MoH, 2004).

The country is a high income group country (based on World Bank 2004 criteria). The proportion of health budget to GDP is 9.5%. The per capita total expenditure on health is 2792 international $, and the per capita government expenditure on health is 1978 international $ (WHO, 2004).

The main language(s) used in the country is (are) English and French. The largest ethnic group(s) is (are) British and French (descent), and the other ethnic group(s) are (is) other European. The largest religious group(s) is (are) Roman Catholic, and the other religious group(s) are (is) Anglican and other Christian (United Church).

The life expectancy at birth is 77.2 years for males and 82.3 years for females (WHO, 2004). The healthy life expectancy at birth is 70 years for males and 74 years for females (WHO, 2004).

EPIDEMIOLOGY

There is substantial epidemiological data on mental illnesses in Canada in internationally accessible literature. No attempt was made to include this information here.

MENTAL HEALTH RESOURCES

Mental Health Policy A mental health policy is present. The policy was initially formulated in 1988.

The components of the policy are advocacy, promotion, prevention, treatment and rehabilitation. Each of the provinces and territories in Canada have a mental health policy. The components of these policies can include support for advocacy, promotion, prevention, treatment and rehabilitation. The Federal Government is involved in health care at several broad levels: maintaining Canada's Health Act (the overarching legal framework that sets the minimum standards for health insurance in each province), financing (through taxation), health promotion, provision of services to federal inmates in custody and direct funding of services to aboriginal populations and military personnel. By virtue of having to meet the standards outlined in Canada's Health Act, Canada has thirteen interlocking health insurance plans and thirteen separate service delivery systems. Provided minimum standards are met, each province may adapt services and legislation to meet its own needs. Thus, there can be a significant variation in service access, programme coverage, funding, human resources and legislation across the country. Since the federal involvement in health and therefore mental health is restricted, there are few national policies or programmes relating to mental health treatment or service delivery. One exception to this is the 'Report on the Task Force on Mental Health' (1991) published by the Correctional Services of Canada pertaining to federally incarcerated inmates. The Federal Government regularly releases National Action Plans, strategies and discussion documents relating to health and mental health. Often these are the result of national consensus-building exercises. While these are not policy statements per se, they are meant to stimulate thinking and guide provincial service developments. Perhaps the most important of these policy-type document is the 'Mental Health for Canadians: Striking a Balance' (1988) which provided a set of guiding principles to assist Canadians engaged in developing and reviewing mental health related policies and programmes. The Federal Government does not have jurisdiction over treatment/rehabilitation but is involved in policy coordination, knowledge development, strengthening communities, professional participation, mutual aid, human rights and citizenship and reducing inequalities. Since Canada's drug policy includes many issues related to federal law enforcement, the Federal Government provides leadership and undertakes national co-ordination on issues pertaining to alcohol and drugs by working collaboratively with Provincial Governments. Canada's Health Act limits the powers of the Federal Government in matters of health delivery and programming. Provision is under the provinces or territories. In all provinces but one, the local ministries have divested authorities for direct service delivery to regional authorities and they carry out functions within the geographical areas. At the provincial level, mental health services are provided through a variety of means: primary care, general hospital care, community service, specialized treatment facilities, psychiatric hospitals, community providers, NGOs and consumer-run organizations. The extent to which all of these are organized under a single administration differ from one province to another. Implementation of evidence-based therapies and best practice models of service delivery are explicit aims of the mental health policies in most provinces.

Substance Abuse Policy A substance abuse policy is present. The policy was initially formulated in 1998.

National Mental Health Programme A national mental health programme is absent.

Mental health programming occurs in the provincial level. Most provinces have an elected or appointed regional health board which has the responsibility for the planning and operation of all health, including mental health, services for a defined population.

National Therapeutic Drug Policy/Essential List of Drugs A national therapeutic drug policy/essential list of drugs is absent.

Mental Health Legislation The latest legislation on mental health is Ontario's Brian's Law. Each of Canada's provinces can frame their own laws. While certain themes run throughout with respect to the key criteria for civil commitment (such as dangerousness to others) and underlying principles (such as promotion of the least restrictive alternative), provincial mental health acts may differ

widely on specific issues such as the extent to which they permit grave disability or need for treatment as criteria for involuntary confinement. The most recent legislation in mental health has been the Amendment to Ontario's Mental Health Act (Brian's Law). Across the country, people are debating about including Community Treatment Orders, a legal mechanism for ensuring compliance to treatment outside hospital settings, and three provinces have legislated involuntary community commitment. All people in Canada are entitled to the rights and freedoms enshrined in the Charter of Rights and Freedom. Besides this, there are common laws which are judgements passed by the judges in different trials and which become a precedent for future cases. In Canada, the Federal Government is responsible for enacting legislation governing criminal law. This is embodied in a set of statutes known as the Criminal Code of Canada. The provinces and territories are each responsible for delivery of health and enact their own laws related to services and care of mental health patients. The Criminal Code has undergone two recent amendments. Firstly, an offender with mental disorder can now be found guilty but nonetheless exempt from criminal responsibility. Secondly, well defined circumstances and procedures, including time lines, have been established to conduct psychiatric assessments of offenders. A revision to the mental disorder provisions of the Criminal Code are expected by the spring of 2005.
The latest legislation was enacted in 2000.

Mental Health Financing There are budget allocations for mental health.
Details about expenditure on mental health are not available.
The primary sources of mental health financing in descending order are tax based, out of pocket expenditure by the patient or family, private insurances and social insurance.
There are no federal budgets for mental health, but each province has its own health and mental health budget. Virtually all necessary medical services have a tax based funding source. However, private services are paid for by patients themselves or through private insurances and form just less than one-third of the total health bill. The cornerstone of the Canadian health care system is a national health insurance programme called the Medicare. It is administered by the provinces and territories and regulated and partly financed through block transfer payments by the National Government. The Medicare pays basic medical and hospital bills. The direct and indirect costs related to mental health problems are estimated to be among the costliest of all conditions and represent nearly one-sixth of the national corporate net operating profits. Since 1970, more funds have been allotted to community care programmes, but this forms only about one-twentieth of the provincial mental health budget. Provincial health insurance plans fund general practitioners but do not usually cover services provided by other mental health professionals.
The country has disability benefits for persons with mental disorders.

Mental Health Facilities Mental health is a part of primary health care system. Actual treatment of severe mental disorders is available at the primary level. In a 'shared care' system, primary practitioners provide care while in collaboration with a psychiatrist. However, serious patients are often referred to the psychiatrist and primary practitioners take care of stabilized and less serious patients. About 50% of medical treatment for mental and emotional disorders are provided through the primary care system.
Regular training of primary care professionals is carried out in the field of mental health. Though training is provided regularly, there are no official national figures for the number of persons trained per year.
There are community care facilities for patients with mental disorders. Canada uses a range of assertive community-based treatment strategies in combination with crisis intervention and residential treatment options. Case management is key to the success of community care. There are also community-based crisis response systems and these include phone lines, walk-in clinics, mobile crisis teams, free-standing crisis centres, hospital emergency departments with holding beds and inpatient psychiatric units. The other element in community care is supported housing. In some provinces, innovative arrangements between the Ministry of Health and Social Service Ministries have led to coordinated approaches, but in general, coordination between treatment and essential support services is sub-optimal. There are relatively few home care programmes existing in the country.

Psychiatric Beds and Professionals

Total psychiatric beds per 10 000 population	19.34
Psychiatric beds in mental hospitals per 10 000 population	9.1
Psychiatric beds in general hospitals per 10 000 population	5.06
Psychiatric beds in other settings per 10 000 population	5.18
Number of psychiatrists per 100 000 population	12
Number of neurosurgeons per 100 000 population	
Number of psychiatric nurses per 100 000 population	44
Number of neurologists per 100 000 population	
Number of psychologists per 100 000 population	35
Number of social workers per 100 000 population	

The figures for professionals date back to 1991-93. The figures for social workers, occupational therapists and recreational therapists working for mental health are not known. Psychiatrists are mainly concentrated in the cities and vast remote areas lack psychiatrists. Non-medical professionals usually work within agencies or hospital settings on a salaried basis but may also offer services in a private practice. Secondary level care is provided by general hospital psychiatry units. They form an important part of the crisis response system, consultation and family education and general assessment and treatment. There is an increasing trend to have community-based tertiary care units having well-staffed specialized units. Between 1950 and 2000, almost 80% of beds for mentally ill patients were eliminated from psychiatric hospitals. Only three sub-specialities are recognized in psychiatry: child, geriatric and forensic. Members of other sub-speciality practices such as addiction or administration have sought credentialing from US organizations. About 10% of psychiatrists are child psychiatrists. International medical graduates have accounted for about a quarter of the supply of physicians in Canada, this portion doubling in the province of Newfoundland and the Saskatchewan. The current shortage of physicians and the fact that their average age is 49 years have spurred a renewed effort to streamline the entry of prospective immigrants through the Medical Council of Canada, provincial licensing colleges and medical schools. Psychiatrists are required to accumulate 400 Continuing Medical Education credits over a 5-year period to maintain speciality certification.

Non-Governmental Organizations NGOs are not involved with mental health in the country. Though there are no official NGOs in Canada, there are numerous self-help and advocacy groups. Some like Canadian Mental Health Association – National (CMHA) have been instrumental in altering views across Canada about consumer capacities and necessary elements of a system of care. Provinces are now funding consumer survivor development initiatives. Twelve NGOs (Canadian Alliance on Mental Illness and Health), including the Canadian Psychiatric Association, have urged the Government to identify specific mental health goals, a policy framework embracing both mental illness and mental health promotion, adequate resources to sustain the plan and an annual public reporting mechanism.

Information Gathering System There is mental health reporting system in the country. Hospital morbidity data, mortality data, national surveys, etc. provide sources for annual reporting on mental health.
The country has data collection system or epidemiological study on mental health. There are surveys on selected epidemiological data on mental health (such as stress and depression). Administrative databases describing hospital morbidity and mortality also exist. The 'Population Mental Health in Canada' provides a good summary of the population mental health indicators taken from the most recent National Population Health Survey. Health Survey Cycle 1.2 by Statistics Canada collected national statistics on five mental disorders – bi-polar disorder, panic disorder, social anxiety, agoraphobia and uni-polar depression – as well as information on alcohol and illicit drug dependence. This information is available on the Statistics Canada web site at: http://www.statcan.ca/english/concepts/health/cycle1

Programmes for Special Population The country has specific programmes for mental health for minorities, refugees, disaster affected population, indigenous population, elderly and children. There are services for the mentally disordered offenders and developmentally disabled patients.
Until recently, drug abuse management services were delivered separately from mental health services. Efforts are being made to integrate the two in some provinces. Forensic services have been developed along somewhat different lines in different provinces. Almost all seem to have small-medium secure regional forensic units; there are 3 maximum security forensic hospitals in Canada. Telehealth programmes appear to provide some relief to poorly resourced communities.

Therapeutic Drugs The following therapeutic drugs are generally available at the primary health care level of the country: carbamazepine, ethosuximide, phenobarbital, phenytoin sodium, sodium valproate, amitriptyline, chlorpromazine, diazepam, fluphenazine, haloperidol, lithium, biperiden, carbidopa, levodopa.
Costing and dosing has been taken from the Ontario Drug Benefit Formulary/Comparative Index (1998). These are recommended prices. At times people pay more, e.g. as dispensing fees, or at times they pay less as their insurances cover them. Elderly patients are eligible for special benefits.

Other Information

Additional Sources of Information

Arboleda-Flörez, J. El Sistema de Salud Mental en el Canadà.

Durbin, J., Goering, P., Wasylenki, D. (2000) Canada's mental health system. International Journal of Law and Psychiatry, 23, 345-59.

Eaves, D., Lamb, D., Tien, G. (2000) Forensic psychiatric services in British Columbia. International Journal of Law and Psychiatry, 23, 615-631.

el-Guebaly, N. (2004) Canadian psychiatry: a status report. International Psychiatry, 6, 12-15.

Gourlay, D. (1998) A fiscal and legislative governance map of the Canadian health and mental health systems in Canada. For: Mental Health Promotion Unit, Health Issues Division, Health Programs and Promotions Branch and Health Canada.

Government of Ontario Press Releases (1988) Mental Health for Canadians: Striking a Balance. Authority of the Minister of National Health and Welfare.

Stephens, T. (1998) Population mental health in Canada. Ottawa Mental Health Promotion Unit, Health Canada.

Cape Verde

GENERAL INFORMATION

Cape Verde is a country with an approximate area of 4 thousand sq. km. (UNO, 2001). The country is an archipelago with mostly mountainous islands. Its population is 0.472 million, and the sex ratio (men per hundred women) is 92 (UNO, 2004). The proportion of population under the age of 15 years is 38% (UNO, 2004), and the proportion of population above the age of 60 years is 6% (WHO, 2004). The literacy rate is 85.4% for men and 68% for women (UNESCO/MoH, 2004).

The country is a lower middle income group country (based on World Bank 2004 criteria). The proportion of health budget to GDP is 4.5%. The per capita total expenditure on health is 165 international $, and the per capita government expenditure on health is 138 international $ (WHO, 2004).

The main language(s) used in the country is (are) Portuguese and Criuolo. The largest ethnic group(s) is (are) Creole, and the other ethnic group(s) are (is) African. The largest religious group(s) is (are) Roman Catholic, and the other religious group(s) are (is) indigenous groups.

The life expectancy at birth is 66.6 years for males and 72.9 years for females (WHO, 2004). The healthy life expectancy at birth is 59 years for males and 63 years for females (WHO, 2004).

EPIDEMIOLOGY

There is a paucity of epidemiological data on mental illnesses in Cape Verde in internationally accessible literature. Neto and Barros (2000) assessed loneliness in students from Cape Verde and Portugal using standardized instruments. They found loneliness to be associated with neuroticism and dissatisfaction with life.

MENTAL HEALTH RESOURCES

Mental Health Policy A mental health policy is absent.
The national health policy covers some aspects of mental health.

Substance Abuse Policy A substance abuse policy is present. The policy was initially formulated in 1996.

National Mental Health Programme A national mental health programme is present. The programme was formulated in 1986.

National Therapeutic Drug Policy/Essential List of Drugs A national therapeutic drug policy/essential list of drugs is present. It was formulated in 1979.

Mental Health Legislation Some old laws dating back to the pre-independence period, i.e. prior to 1975 do exist, but there is no legislation after that period except one on restriction on tobacco consumption of 1995.
The latest legislation was enacted in 1975.

Mental Health Financing There are budget allocations for mental health.
Details about expenditure on mental health are not available.
The primary source of mental health financing is tax based.
The country has disability benefits for persons with mental disorders. Disability benefits for Government employees exist in the form that they are allowed to draw their salaries in spite of not working.

Mental Health Facilities Mental health is a part of primary health care system. Actual treatment of severe mental disorders is available at the primary level. Patients are treated by admission to hospital. Rehabilitation is done with the help of family support. Regular training of primary care professionals is carried out in the field of mental health.
There are no community care facilities for patients with mental disorders.

Psychiatric Beds and Professionals

Total psychiatric beds per 10 000 population	0.78
Psychiatric beds in mental hospitals per 10 000 population	0
Psychiatric beds in general hospitals per 10 000 population	0.78
Psychiatric beds in other settings per 10 000 population	0
Number of psychiatrists per 100 000 population	0.9
Number of neurosurgeons per 100 000 population	
Number of psychiatric nurses per 100 000 population	
Number of neurologists per 100 000 population	
Number of psychologists per 100 000 population	0.9
Number of social workers per 100 000 population	0.2

Occupational therapy is present at the Centre for Occupational Therapy. Only one occupational therapist is present.

Non-Governmental Organizations NGOs are involved with mental health in the country. They are mainly involved in advocacy and prevention.

Information Gathering System There is mental health reporting system in the country.
The country has no data collection system or epidemiological study on mental health. The central hospitals have systems of registering admissions/discharges of inpatients.
Hospital data from the central hospital is collected.

Programmes for Special Population There are no special programmes for any specified population.

Therapeutic Drugs The following therapeutic drugs are generally available at the primary health care level of the country: carbamazepine, ethosuximide, phenobarbital, phenytoin sodium, sodium valproate, amitriptyline, chlorpromazine, diazepam, fluphenazine, haloperidol, biperiden, carbidopa, levodopa.

Other Information

Additional Sources of Information

Neto, F., Barros, J. (2000) Psychosocial concomitants of loneliness among students of Cape Verde and Portugal. Journal of Psychology, 134, 503-514.

Central African Republic

GENERAL INFORMATION

Central African Republic is a country with an approximate area of 623 thousand sq. km. (UNO, 2001). Its population is 3.912 million, and the sex ratio (men per hundred women) is 95 (UNO, 2004). The proportion of population under the age of 15 years is 43% (UNO, 2004), and the proportion of population above the age of 60 years is 6% (WHO, 2004). The literacy rate is 64.7% for men and 33.5% for women (UNESCO/MoH, 2004).
The country is a low income group country (based on World Bank 2004 criteria). The proportion of health budget to GDP is 4.5%. The per capita total expenditure on health is 58 international $, and the per capita government expenditure on health is 30 international $ (WHO, 2004).
The main language(s) used in the country is (are) French. The largest ethnic group(s) is (are) Baya and Banda, and the other ethnic group(s) are (is) Mandjia and Sara. The largest religious group(s) is (are) Roman Catholic, and the other religious group(s) are (is) Protestant, indigenous groups and Muslim.
The life expectancy at birth is 42.1 years for males and 43.7 years for females (WHO, 2004). The healthy life expectancy at birth is 37 years for males and 38 years for females (WHO, 2004).

EPIDEMIOLOGY

There is a paucity of epidemiological data on mental illnesses in Central African Republic in internationally accessible literature.

MENTAL HEALTH RESOURCES

Mental Health Policy A mental health policy is absent.
The national mental health policy formulation had to be stopped because of serious military-political events in the country. The situation analysis for this policy formulation is complete and funding is being sought to revive the activities.

Substance Abuse Policy A substance abuse policy is absent.

National Mental Health Programme A national mental health programme is absent.

National Therapeutic Drug Policy/Essential List of Drugs A national therapeutic drug policy/essential list of drugs is present. It was formulated in 2002.

Mental Health Legislation Details about the mental health legislation are not available.

Mental Health Financing There are no budget allocations for mental health.
Details about expenditure on mental health are not available.
The primary source of mental health financing is out of pocket expenditure by the patient or family.
The country does not have disability benefits for persons with mental disorders.

Mental Health Facilities Mental health is a part of primary health care system. Actual treatment of severe mental disorders is available at the primary level. Neuroleptics are very cheap. A campaign against drug abuse has been undertaken by the Ministry of Health.
Regular training of primary care professionals is not carried out in the field of mental health.
There are no community care facilities for patients with mental disorders.

Psychiatric Beds and Professionals

Total psychiatric beds per 10 000 population	0.07
Psychiatric beds in mental hospitals per 10 000 population	0
Psychiatric beds in general hospitals per 10 000 population	0.07
Psychiatric beds in other settings per 10 000 population	0
Number of psychiatrists per 100 000 population	0.03
Number of neurosurgeons per 100 000 population	0
Number of psychiatric nurses per 100 000 population	0.03
Number of neurologists per 100 000 population	0.03
Number of psychologists per 100 000 population	0.08
Number of social workers per 100 000 population	0.03

Non-Governmental Organizations NGOs are involved with mental health in the country. They are mainly involved in prevention and rehabilitation.

Information Gathering System There is no mental health reporting system in the country.
The country has data collection system or epidemiological study on mental health. An annual statistics report in psychiatry and mental health service does exist.

Programmes for Special Population The country has specific programmes for mental health for refugees, indigenous population and children.

Therapeutic Drugs The following therapeutic drugs are generally available at the primary health care level of the country: carbamazepine, phenobarbital, chlorpromazine, diazepam.
The essential drug list was revised in 2004.

Other Information

Additional Sources of Information

Chad

GENERAL INFORMATION

Chad is a country with an approximate area of 1284 thousand sq. km. (UNO, 2001). Its population is 8.854 million, and the sex ratio (men per hundred women) is 98 (UNO, 2004). The proportion of population under the age of 15 years is 47% (UNO, 2004), and the proportion of population above the age of 60 years is 5% (WHO, 2004). The literacy rate is 54.5% for men and 37.5% for women (UNESCO/MoH, 2004).

The country is a low income group country (based on World Bank 2004 criteria). The proportion of health budget to GDP is 2.6%. The per capita total expenditure on health is 17 international $, and the per capita government expenditure on health is 13 international $ (WHO, 2004).

The main language(s) used in the country is (are) French and Arabic. The largest ethnic group(s) is (are) Toubou forming the majority in north, Arab in the Sahelian zone and Sara in the Soudanian zone. The largest religious group(s) is (are) Muslim (half).

The life expectancy at birth is 46.1 years for males and 49.3 years for females (WHO, 2004). The healthy life expectancy at birth is 40 years for males and 42 years for females (WHO, 2004).

EPIDEMIOLOGY

There is a paucity of epidemiological data on mental illnesses in Chad in internationally accessible literature. Katz and Katz (2002) found that social strain accounted for a significant proportion of variance in depressive symptoms and somatic complaints of intellectually disabled people.

MENTAL HEALTH RESOURCES

Mental Health Policy A mental health policy is absent.

Substance Abuse Policy A substance abuse policy is present. The policy was initially formulated in 1996.

National Mental Health Programme A national mental health programme is present. The programme was formulated in 1998.

National Therapeutic Drug Policy/Essential List of Drugs A national therapeutic drug policy/essential list of drugs is present. Details about the year of formulation are not available.

Mental Health Legislation Details about the mental health legislation are not available.

Mental Health Financing There are budget allocations for mental health.
Details about expenditure on mental health are not available.
The primary sources of mental health financing in descending order are out of pocket expenditure by the patient or family, social insurance and private insurances.
The country has disability benefits for persons with mental disorders. Benefits are available only for public servants who get their full salary for the initial 6 months and then half the salary.

Mental Health Facilities Mental health is not a part of primary health care system. Actual treatment of severe mental disorders is not available at the primary level. Very few psychotropics are included in the essential drug list and treatment is difficult.
Regular training of primary care professionals is not carried out in the field of mental health.
There are no community care facilities for patients with mental disorders. Only traditional treatment is available at the community level.

Psychiatric Beds and Professionals

Total psychiatric beds per 10 000 population	0.02
Psychiatric beds in mental hospitals per 10 000 population	0.01
Psychiatric beds in general hospitals per 10 000 population	0.01
Psychiatric beds in other settings per 10 000 population	0
Number of psychiatrists per 100 000 population	0.01
Number of neurosurgeons per 100 000 population	0.01
Number of psychiatric nurses per 100 000 population	0.01
Number of neurologists per 100 000 population	0
Number of psychologists per 100 000 population	0.01
Number of social workers per 100 000 population	0

These resources are not widely used.

Non-Governmental Organizations NGOs are involved with mental health in the country. They are mainly involved in advocacy, promotion, prevention and rehabilitation.

Information Gathering System There is mental health reporting system in the country. Mental disorders are grouped as 'other disorders'.
The country has data collection system or epidemiological study on mental health.

Programmes for Special Population There are no special programmes for any population group.

Therapeutic Drugs The following therapeutic drugs are generally available at the primary health care level of the country: carbamazepine, phenobarbital, chlorpromazine, diazepam, haloperidol, levodopa.

Other Information

Additional Sources of Information

Katz, S., Katz, S. (2002) Assessing the loneliness of workers with learning disabilities. British Journal of Developmental Disabilities, 48, 91-94.

Chile

GENERAL INFORMATION

Chile is a country with an approximate area of 757 thousand sq. km. (UNO, 2001). Its population is 15.997 million, and the sex ratio (men per hundred women) is 98 (UNO, 2004). The proportion of population under the age of 15 years is 27% (UNO, 2004), and the proportion of population above the age of 60 years is 11% (WHO, 2004). The literacy rate is 95.8% for men and 95.6% for women (UNESCO/MoH, 2004).

The country is a higher middle income group country (based on World Bank 2004 criteria). The proportion of health budget to GDP is 7%. The per capita total expenditure on health is 792 international $, and the per capita government expenditure on health is 348 international $ (WHO, 2004).

The main language(s) used in the country is (are) Spanish. The largest ethnic group(s) is (are) Mestizo (two-thirds), and the other ethnic group(s) are (is) European and Native American. The largest religious group(s) is (are) Roman Catholic (70%), and the other religious group(s) are (is) Evangelical and Protestant Christian.

The life expectancy at birth is 73.4 years for males and 80 years for females (WHO, 2004). The healthy life expectancy at birth is 65 years for males and 70 years for females (WHO, 2004).

EPIDEMIOLOGY

Araya et al (2001) interviewed 3870 adults from households selected by a probabilistic sampling design using the Clinical Interview Schedule-Revised (CIS-R). Almost 13% of the respondents met ICD-10 criteria for psychiatric illness. Female gender, low socio-economic status, unemployment, low education, marital separation and single parenthood were associated with increased prevalence of mental disorders. In another study using a probabilistic design, Vincente et al (2002) assessed 2978 individuals from 4 regions of Chile using CIDI. The life time and 6-month prevalence of DSM-III-R defined psychiatric disorder was 36% and 23%, respectively. The most common lifetime diagnoses were agoraphobia (11%), major depressive disorder (9%), dysthymia (8%) and alcohol dependence (6%). The Third National Study of the Consumption of Drugs, conducted on a nationally representative sample of 31,665 individuals in the age group of 12 to 64 years, showed that 17.5% of individuals reported the life time use of one of the three illicit drugs (marijuana: 16.8%, coca paste: 2.3% and cocaine hydrochloride: 4.0%). The one-year and one-month prevalence of use of any of the three drugs were 5.3% and 2.2%, respectively. Lifetime use of anxiolytics, alcohol and tobacco was reported to be 28.4%, 84.4% and 71.9%. Use of drugs was associated with male sex (except anxiolytics) and the youth (19-25 years) (Fuentealba et al, 2000). Florenzano et al (1993) reported the use of alcohol and tobacco by more than 50% and marijuana by more than 10% of the youth. Frequent use of tobacco (smoking), alcohol and marijuana was reported by 32%, 15.5% and 5% of the sample. Substance abuse, except cigarette smoking was more prevalent among males, those older than 15 years and in youth coming from dysfunctional families. Araneda et al (1996) reported the prevalence of problem drinking to be 9% in male and 3% female university students. Fuentealba Herrera et al (1995) who used the locally validated Michigan Alcoholism Screening Test (MAST) reported the prevalence for abnormal drinking to be 40.3% in the major care givers of families living in extreme poverty (46.2% in males and 3.3% in females). In a community sample, Busto et al (1996) reported that the 1-year prevalence of benzodiazepine dependence (DSM-III-R) was 3.3%. Wolf et al (2002) assessed three groups of women with young children (n=1256) from Chile and Costa Rica using Center for Epidemiological Studies – Depression scale and found prominent depressive symptoms in 35-50% of the mothers. Durkin (1993) compared survey data from households affected by earthquakes in USA (n=288) and Chile (n=116) and an unexposed reference population in USA. Prevalence rates of major depression in the Chile sample were the same as in the exposed US sample, and 2.7 times the background US rate. While the exposed US posttraumatic stress disorder (PTSD) rate was only slightly higher than the US background rate, the Chile PTSD rate was 7 times the US rates. Jardesic and Araya (1995) found the prevalence of postpartum depression as assessed by the Edinburgh Postnatal Depression Scale to be 36.7% in 542 women attending primary health care clinics. Women from lower socioeconomic status and those not currently married were more likely to be depressed. In a WHO study on psychiatric comorbidity in primary health care patients with chronic medical illnesses, Fullerton et al (2000) used GHQ and CIDI and found that two-thirds of the Chilean group had a coexisting psychiatric diagnosis compared to 31% of the global study group. The most frequent diagnoses in the Chilean sample were somatization disorders (25%), harmful alcohol use (14%), depression (35%) and hypochondriasis (6%). Women tended to have higher prevalence of mental disorders. Mendez et al (1997) reviewed death certificates of deceased in a region and found that suicide rates had increased in the early nineties, particularly in males that led to the male:female ratio of 4.8:1. They did not find an age effect but noted a seasonal pattern with increase in suicide rates both in summer and winter months. Bralio et al (1987) used the Achenbach's Child Behavior Checklist that was standardized in Chile for assessing a representative sample of primary school going children (n=517) and reported a prevalence of approximately 15% for behavioural and emotional problems. Toledo et al (1997) found that 24.2% of first-grade children had a syndromal psychiatric diagnosis and 17.2% had significant disability. ADHD and enuresis were the commonest diagnosis and 10% had a family history of psychiatric illness.

MENTAL HEALTH RESOURCES

Mental Health Policy A mental health policy is present. The policy was initially formulated in 1993.

The components of the policy are advocacy, promotion, prevention, treatment and rehabilitation. There is a National Plan on Mental Health and Psychiatry (2000). The policy addresses primary and specialist care, bed reduction and community based secondary services. Other important components include activities with sectors other than health, support to consumers and family organizations and social inclusion. It was developed through the participation of multiple stakeholders: politicians, mental health professionals, NGOs, public servants and consumers. Between 20 to 25 % of its original content has been put into practice.

Substance Abuse Policy A substance abuse policy is present. The policy was initially formulated in 1993. It was formulated by the Ministry of Interior with the participation of different sectors (Justice, Health, Education, Labour, Police, etc). It was revised in 2003. It has a specific budget for its implementation, and between 20 to 25% of its content has already been implemented.

National Mental Health Programme A national mental health programme is present. The programme was formulated in 1999. The National Mental Health and Psychiatry Programme has only been implemented for those covered by the public health insurance programme (FONASA), i.e. almost two-thirds of the Chilean population (those on lower income). The priorities of the programme are: depression, alcohol and drug abuse and dependence, victims of domestic violence, schizophrenia, dementia and ADHD. Between 20 to 25 % of the programme has been implemented by local, regional and national authorities.

National Therapeutic Drug Policy/Essential List of Drugs A national therapeutic drug policy/essential list of drugs is present. It was formulated in 1990.
The policy is meant both for primary and specialized level. It allows for psychotropic medications for specialized treatment.

Mental Health Legislation The most recent legislation in the area was in the form of a chapter about mental health in the general health legislation. Less than 20% has been implemented because funds for its implementation were inadequate. Its components include rights of users of mental health services (it conforms to international human rights laws), regulation of involuntary treatment, regulation of mental health services and admission and discharge procedures. A legislation on domestic violence and alcohol and drug abuse also exists.
The latest legislation was enacted in 2001.

Mental Health Financing There are budget allocations for mental health.
The country spends 2.33% of the total health budget on mental health.
The primary sources of mental health financing in descending order are social insurance, tax based, out of pocket expenditure by the patient or family and private insurances.
Mental health services receive funding from the public social health insurance system (FONASA), which covers two-thirds of the population. Until 1990, most of this funding for mental health went to mental hospitals, but over the last one and a half decade about one-third has been spent on implementation of community programmes and incorporation of mental health in primary care. Currently, approximately 12.0% of the amount spent on mental health is spent on general hospitals; 36.0% in psychiatric hospitals; 33.0% in ambulatory clinics and 19.0% in community care. The National Council for Drug Control (CONACE) under the Ministry of the Interior has allocated funds to the health sector for the management of drug abuse. Private insurance (ISAPRES) covers almost one-fifth of the population. Private health insurance pays for only a very limited number of psychiatry and psychology sessions. Those covered under FONASA can get services from private sector if they make higher co-payment (out of pocket).
The country has disability benefits for persons with mental disorders. Mental health is considered a disability for getting public and private disability benefits for those covered by insurance (the working population). There are also social security benefits for people with no working insurance and low family income. Between 70 and 80% of all the eligible persons actually receive the benefits. Schizophrenia, major depression, mental retardation, Alzheimer and organic psychosis are considered eligible for state/public and private disability benefits.

Mental Health Facilities Mental health is a part of primary health care system. Actual treatment of severe mental disorders is available at the primary level. Treatment of severe mental disorders is available at specialized centres in all regions, mainly on an ambulatory basis. Primary care is available for depression, victims of domestic violence and alcohol abuse in most areas of the country. Overall, about 35% of the population receives treatment for mental health disorders through primary care. Nurses, social workers, psychologists and primary care physicians are responsible for treating mental disorders in primary health care. Psychiatrists meet primary care teams once a month to see and discuss the most difficult cases in about 25% of primary care facilities. All urban primary health care clinics (and approximately 50% overall) have incorporated psychologists to their health teams. The programme for treatment of depression has led to the treatment of over 100 000 people in the last 4 years (three-fifths of the people in need of treatment). Only 7% of these were referred for specialized treatment.
Regular training of primary care professionals is not carried out in the field of mental health. Training in family medicine has included some mental health components. The Psychiatric Society conducts periodic courses for general practitioners.
There are community care facilities for patients with mental disorders. Each of the 28 health districts have at least one mental health and psychiatric community team of psychiatrist, psychologist and at least one other mental health professional. A community care network has been developed with different programmes (protected homes [more than 700 places], day care units [more than 1300], admittance service, outpatient care, psychosocial rehabilitation programmes, social clubs, protected workshops, etc.) which are at different levels of development within the country, but which are far from meeting the people's needs. Ten districts still don't have

inpatient psychiatric beds and a few do not have day care facilities, sheltered homes and psychosocial facilities. Almost 50% of clients receive preventive interventions, home interventions, family interventions, have access to residential facilities, vocational training and employment programmes. Nurses, psychologists, occupational therapists, social workers and psychiatrists are responsible for taking care of patients with severe mental disorders in the community.

Psychiatric Beds and Professionals

Total psychiatric beds per 10 000 population	1.27
Psychiatric beds in mental hospitals per 10 000 population	1.04
Psychiatric beds in general hospitals per 10 000 population	0.24
Psychiatric beds in other settings per 10 000 population	0.13
Number of psychiatrists per 100 000 population	4
Number of neurosurgeons per 100 000 population	0.4
Number of psychiatric nurses per 100 000 population	1.1
Number of neurologists per 100 000 population	0.8
Number of psychologists per 100 000 population	15.7
Number of social workers per 100 000 population	1.5

There are 16.4 general nurses per 100 000 population with partial time for mental health. Among the 8021 social workers only a small number work in mental health. There are 200 occupational therapists. There are at present more than 800 acute and 800 long stay beds in the public sector and 240 long stay beds in private nursing homes. Just over one-third of admitted individuals are long-stay patients. Beds have also been specified for child, forensic (20 high security and 80 medium security) and drug abuse management services. Admissions to long stay wards was stopped in 2000. The private sector provides for some beds for acute care, child and adolescent and drug abuse services. Residential facilities are also available for patients with drug abuse. The Ministry of Health provides technical support for these small private hospitals and programmes and also for a few services in the non-health setting. About one-third of psychiatrists and half of clinical psychologists work in the private sector, which makes community-based human resource scarce. There are just over 50 child psychiatrists and only about half of the health districts have one. Clinical psychologists have to become accredited by the National Commission for the Accreditation of Clinical Psychologists. An 'addiction rehabilitation technician' certificate was recently created by the Ministry of Health, requiring two years of training.

Non-Governmental Organizations NGOs are involved with mental health in the country. They are mainly involved in advocacy, promotion, prevention, treatment and rehabilitation. There are two main types of mental health NGOs: those formed by professionals, which act as service providers (e.g. therapeutic communities for alcohol and drug abuse, psychosocial rehabilitation programmes, treatment for survivors of torture), and those formed by consumers and families (e.g. self-help groups for alcohol and drug abuse, relatives and friends of people with mental disabilities). They are active in sensitizing the community, defending the rights of patients, advocacy and provision of services particularly rehabilitative services.

Information Gathering System There is mental health reporting system in the country. ICD-10 is used for recording purposes. The country has data collection system or epidemiological study on mental health. Data collection is conducted both on inpatient and outpatient care. Mental health components include, besides diagnosis, length of stay, primary health care mental health consultations, drug intoxication and death rates caused by suicide. The Departamento de Estatistica e Informacion en Salud (Health Statistics Department) is in charge of data collection performed on part of the mental health system for the population covered by the public health system.

The National Plan for Mental Health and Psychiatry Information System covers the activities of primary and specialist care and evaluation and research of outcomes of specific programmes with specific funding. Further information will be obtained through general household surveys.

Programmes for Special Population The country has specific programmes for mental health for elderly and children. There is a programme called PRAIS which is involved in compensation and total health care programme for victims of political violence. There are also programmes for victims of domestic violence and depression.

Specific programmes, namely depression in primary care (oriented particularly towards women), treatment of drug addiction, forensic psychiatry, provision of atypical anti-psychotics to treatment-resistant patients and sheltered homes, have been assigned specific funding. Combined work with the Ministry of Education has led to project on training teachers on the prevention of alcohol and drug abuse and mental health programmes for grade 1 and 2 children. Intellectually disabled children are now integrated into regular school classes. Special services are also available for victims of human rights violation during the military dictatorship. The Ministry of Justice and the Women's National Service have established a few centres for children and women who have suffered physical violence.

Therapeutic Drugs The following therapeutic drugs are generally available at the primary health care level of the country: carbamazepine, ethosuximide, phenobarbital, phenytoin sodium, amitriptyline, chlorpromazine, diazepam, haloperidol. Fluphenazine is available in some places.

Other Information Development is under way for a national forensic psychiatry system with medium complexity units (2 working, 1 in the stage of designing) and one unit of high complexity (under construction) as well as ambulatory care and sheltered homes. In 2001, the following new programmes started: primary health care programme on depression, implementation of 20 new day hospitals and development of new treatment and rehabilitation plans for people with drug dependence or abuse problems.
Though the efficient social health insurance system covers a significant proportion of the population for mental as well as other health interventions and public sector services are open to all, there are large waiting lists and long waiting times. A study on consumer satisfaction with care in psychiatric outpatient department has begun. The Mental Health Unit in the Ministry of Health has also recently developed several guidelines with the collaboration of health professionals, consumers and families. It is introducing an accreditation system for mental health facilities using PAHO/WHO standards. A National Commission for the Protection of People with Mental Illness and Civil Rights has been formed to go into complaints of clients.

Additional Sources of Information

Araneda, J. M., Repossi, A., Puente, C. (1996) What, how much and when the university student drinks. Revista Medica de Chile, 124, 377-388.

Araya, R., Rojas, G., Fritsch, R., et al (2001) Common mental disorders in Santiago, Chile: prevalence and socio-demographic correlates. British Journal of Psychiatry, 178, 228-233.

Bralio, S., Seguel, X., Montenegro, H. (1987) Prevalence of mental disorders in the schoolchild population of Santiago de Chile. Acta Psiquiatrica y Psicologica de America Latina, 33, 316-325.

Busto, U. E., Ruiz, I., Busto, M., et al (1996) Benzodiazepine use in Chile: impact of availability on use, abuse, and dependence. Journal of Clinical Psychopharmacology, 16, 363-372.

Diario Official de la Republica de Chile (1995) Sanciona el trafico ilicito de estupefacientes y sustancias sicotropicas, 11.

Division of Health Program (1993) Politicas y plan nacional de salud mental.

Durkin, M. E. (1993) Major depression and post-traumatic stress disorder following the Coalinga and Chile earthquakes: a cross-cultural comparison. Journal of Social Behavior & Personality, 8, 5.

Executive Secretary (1993) Political and National Plan of the Prevention and Control of Drugs. Republic of Chile.

Florenzano, R., Pino, P., Marchandon, A. (1993) Risk behavior in adolescent students in Santiago de Chile. Revista Medica de Chile, 121, 462-469.

Fuentealba, R., Cumsille, F., Araneda, J. C., et al (2000) Consumption of licit and illicit drugs in Chile: results of the 1998 study and comparison with the 1994 and 1996 studies. Pan American Journal of Public Health, 7, 79-87.

Fuentealba, H. R., Flores, G. M., Fernandez, C. A. (1995) Application of the Michigan Alcoholism Screening Test in heads of the family. Acta Psiquiatrica y Psicologica de America Latina, 41, 206-213.

Fullerton, C., Florenzano, R., Acuna, J., et al (2000) Comorbidity of chronic diseases and psychiatric disorders among patients attending public primary care. Revista Medica de Chile, 128, 729-734.

Jadresic, E., Araya, R. (1995) Prevalence of postpartum depression and associated factors in Santiago, Chile. Revista Medica de Chile, 123, 694-699.

Mendez, J. C. V., Opgaard, A. J., Escalier, S., et al (1997) Epidemiology of suicide at the second region of Chile. Revista Chilena de Neuro-Psiquiatria, 35, 465-472.

Ministerio de Salud (2000) Plan Nacional de Salud Mental y Psiquiatria.

Ministerio de Salud (2000) Plan Nacional de Salud Mental y Psiquiatria, Resumen Ejecutivo.

Ministerio de Salud (1999) Las Enfermedades Mentales en Chile, Magnitud y Consecuencias.

Pemjean, A. (2003) Psychiatric country profile: Chile. International Psychiatry, 1, 13-15.

Stewart, C. L. (2004) Chile mental health country profile. International Review of Psychiatry, 16, 73-82.

Toledo, V. de la, Barra F., Lopez, C., et al (1997) Psychiatric diagnosis in a cohort of first grade basic course children from the Western area of Santiago de Chile.

Vicente, B., Rioseco, P., Saldivia, S., et al (2002) Chilean study on the prevalence of psychiatric disorders (DSM-III-R/CIDI) (ECPP). Revista Medica de Chile, 130, 527-536.

Wolf, A. W., De, Andraca, I., Lozoff, B. (2002) Maternal depression in three Latin American samples. Social Psychiatry & Psychiatric Epidemiology, 37, 169-176.

China

GENERAL INFORMATION

China is a country with an approximate area of 9597 thousand sq. km. (UNO, 2001). Its population is 1.313 billion, and the sex ratio (men per hundred women) is 105 (UNO, 2004). The proportion of population under the age of 15 years is 22% (UNO, 2004), and the proportion of population above the age of 60 years is 10% (WHO, 2004). The literacy rate is 92.1% for men and 77.9% for women (UNESCO/MoH, 2004).

The country is a lower middle income group country (based on World Bank 2004 criteria). The proportion of health budget to GDP is 5.5%. The per capita total expenditure on health is 224 international $, and the per capita government expenditure on health is 83 international $ (WHO, 2004).

The main language(s) used in the country is (are) Mandarin. The largest ethnic group(s) is (are) Han, and the other ethnic group(s) are (is) Zhuang and Man.

The life expectancy at birth is 69.6 years for males and 72.7 years for females (WHO, 2004). The healthy life expectancy at birth is 63 years for males and 65 years for females (WHO, 2004).

EPIDEMIOLOGY

Zhang et al (1998) used the Chinese Scale of Mental Disability and Intellectual Impairment and found the point prevalence and life-time prevalence of all disorders (except neurosis) to be 1.12% and 1.35%, respectively. An increase in the prevalence of all mental disorders, particularly alcohol use disorders, Alzheimer's disease and affective disorders was noted. A number of studies (e.g. Wang et al, 2000) have examined the prevalence of dementia in different regions in large samples (>1000) using a two-stage procedure in which the initial screening was done with the MMSE and diagnosis was confirmed by clinical interviews. The prevalence rates were in the range of 1.0% to 4.2%. Dementia was more common in women and the prevalence rate increased with age. Zhang et al (2001) assessed 5913 subjects over the age of 55 years from urban and rural communities, selected through a stratified multiple stage cluster sampling method, using a three-phase strategy in which the final evaluation was done by neurologists or psychiatrists using the DSM-IV, NINCDS-ADRDA and NINCDS-AIREN criteria. The age-standardized prevalence was 4.2% for dementia (all causes), 2.0% for Alzheimer's disease and 1.5% for vascular dementia. The rate of Alzheimer disease (AD) doubled every 5 years with age, though that of vascular dementia (VD) increased little with age. Liu et al (2003) analysed 17 studies published in Chinese from 1990-1999, and found the prevalence rates for the population aged 60 years and over were 1.26% for AD and 0.74% for VD. The prevalence of AD was 2.10% in women and 0.76% in men, while the prevalence of VD was 0.71 and 0.69%, respectively. The prevalence of AD increased with age, but there was no association between VD and gender. Yan et al (2002) reported that the annual incidence rate of senile dementia was 0.9% in those above 60 years of age. The rate increased in almost each 5-year age groups to reach 5.1% in the 90 years (and above) age group. Niu et al (2000) assessed 991 current smokers from 488 randomly selected nuclear families by using the Fagerstrom Test of Nicotine Dependence (FTND) questionnaire and the Revised Tolerance Questionnaire (RTQ). The prevalence of nicotine dependence as defined by FTND (cut off - 7/8) and RTQ (cut off - 27/28) were 12.7% and 11.1%, respectively. Wei et al (1999) assessed 23 513 adults and found that the point prevalence of alcohol dependence (DSM-III-R) was 3.4% (males 6.6%, females 0.1%). Jiang et al (1995) assessed 6567 subjects with a screening questionnaire and the Present State Examination. The 1-year prevalence rate of benzodiazepine dependence rate was reported to be 1.63%. Chen et al (1999) conducted a meta-analysis on 10 cross-sectional studies (n=13 565) of depression in elderly subjects. The pooled prevalence of depression was 3.9% (rural 5.1%, urban 2.6%). Chen et al (2004) interviewed 1736 urban subjects aged 65 and over using the GMS -AGECAT. Age-standardized prevalence was 2.2%. Yan et al (2002) reported that the annual incidence rate of senile depression was 1.3% in those above 60 years of age. Zhang et al (1999) assessed women at an antenatal clinic (n=1052) with the Edinburgh Postpartum Depression Scale 7 days after delivery and found a rate of 15% for postpartum depression. Shen et al (1998) used the GHQ-12 and the Present State Examination in an urban elderly sample. The prevalence of neurosis was 2.1% (3.5% in women and 4.0% in men). The prevalence declined with age. Neurasthenia, depressive and anxiety neurosis were common. Wang et al (2000) assessed 181 and 157 randomly selected subjects from two earthquake affected villages. Counter-intuitively, subjects from the village that faced greater damage (but received more support) had lower rates of PTSD. The incidence of DSM-IV PTSD within 9 months was 19.8% and 30.3% for the two villages. Zhang et al (1992) studied 509 college freshmen. Bulimia, as per Chinese and DSM-III-R criteria, was diagnosed in 1.1% of subjects. Review of data from different sources (e.g. National Disease Surveillance Point system, Chinese Public Health Annuals) have given varying rates of suicide (4.8 to 19.6 per 100 000), but there is unanimity that the rates are greater in women, in rural areas and in the elderly (e.g. Ji et al, 2001). Jenkins (2002) collated mortality data from the Ministry of Health for the period 1995-99 with an estimated rate of unreported deaths. The annual suicide rate was estimated at 23/100 000, accounting for 3.6% of all deaths. The rate in women was 25% higher than in men, primarily due to large number of suicides in young rural women. Rural suicide rates were three times higher than urban rates across both sexes, for all age-groups and over time. Phillips et al (2002) interviewed close associates of people who died due to suicide (n=519) or other injuries (n=536). After adjustment for different socio-demographic variables, the predictors for suicide were: depression score, previous suicide attempt, acute stress at time of death, low quality of life, high chronic stress, severe interpersonal conflict in the 2 days before death and a blood relative or friend with previous suicidal behaviour. Suicide risk increased substantially with exposure to multiple risk factors from 30% for those with 2 or 3 risks to 96% for those with 6 or more risks. Hesketh et al (2002) administered a self-administered questionnaire to 1576 middle school students and found that the frequency of severe depressive symptoms, suicidal ideation and suicide attempts was 33%, 16% and 9%, respectively. A number of large (sample size >1000) community studies have been conducted on behavioural problems in school age children and adolescents using a variety of reliable tools (e.g. Liu et al, 2001). The prevalence rate of behavioral problems had been reported to be in the range of 7% to 23%. Boys have more behavioral problems, particularly externalizing problems and girls have more internalizing problems. Leung et al (1996) conducted a two-stage study on 3069 schoolboys and found the prevalence rates for hyperkinetic disorder (ICD-10), ADDH (DSM-III) and ADHD (DSM- III-R) respectively, were 0.8%, 6.1% and 8.9%. Liu et al (2000) assessed 3344 children in the 6-16 years age group and found the overall prevalence of nocturnal enuresis was 4.3%, with a significantly higher prevalence in boys. Zou et al (1994) assessed 85170 children (<14 years) using the WHO description of mental retardation and standard psychological tests. The prevalence of mental retardation was 1.2%, with the proportion of mild, moderate, severe and profound MR being 60.6%, 22.7%, 9.6%, and 7.1%, respectively.

MENTAL HEALTH RESOURCES

Mental Health Policy A mental health policy is present. The policy was initially formulated in 1987.
The components of the policy are prevention, treatment and rehabilitation.
In September 2004, the Proposal on Further Strengthening Mental Health Work had been agreed by the Ministries of Health, Education, Security, Civil Affairs, Justice, Finance and the China Disabled Person's Federation, and it was transmitted in the name of the General Office of the State Council to all departments of and to all institutions directly under the State Council (including the People's Congress, the National Committee of the Chinese People's Political Consultative Conference, the Supreme Court and the military) and to provincial Governments. In the proposals, principles, aims, organization and leadership, intervention for key populations, treatment and rehabilitation for mental disorders, mental health team building, research and surveillance and legal rights protection are indicated; especially the community-based mental health service model is stressed.

Substance Abuse Policy A substance abuse policy is present. The policy was initially formulated in 1987.

National Mental Health Programme A national mental health programme is present. The programme was formulated in 1992. The Ministries of Health, Civil Affairs, Security and the China Disabled Person's Federation jointly enacted the National Mental Health Project of China (2002-10) in April 2002. The three main areas of focus are: integrated care and multisectoral links, equity, community care, training of mental health professionals, increasing research, development of a mental health legislation. Specific targets have been set. A national disaster mental health response plan is being developed.

National Therapeutic Drug Policy/Essential List of Drugs A national therapeutic drug policy/essential list of drugs is present. It was formulated in 1995.

Mental Health Legislation There is no existing mental health legislation. At the national level, although there is no existing mental health law, the Criminal Law (1980), the Criminal Procedure Law (1980), the Civil Law (1987), the Civil Procedure Law (1982), the Law on the Protection of Disabled Persons (1990), the Law on Maternal and Infant Health Care (1994), and the Marriage Law (2001) deal with some mental health issues. The national mental health law is in the process of being drafted since 1986; the 15th draft was finished and is being reviewed by relevant departments. The Ministry of Health is hoping it will be enacted before 2007. Provincial laws are also in different stages of development. The Shanghai Mental Health Regulations came into effect in 2002. It requires that all medium-size general hospitals and community medical centres should set up outpatient mental health services.

Mental Health Financing There are budget allocations for mental health.
The country spends 2.35% of the total health budget on mental health.
The primary source of mental health financing in decending order are out of pocket expenditure by the patient or family, social insurance and tax based.
Insurance coverage of mental health issues is variable. Some like those covering Government employees are generous (so unemployment is doubly hard on ill people); others like those for people in the country side (funded from pooled resources of the community) are very basic. Less than 15% of the population are entitled to comprehensive health insurance that covers psychiatric disorders. Economic Reforms have partially diminished many insurance systems and pushed up health care costs. Inpatient care is expensive (a one month fee, approximately $100, is equivalent of average wage of 4 months in urban areas and 8 months in rural areas). For long-stay patients, two-thirds of the expenses are borne by the persons/family and the remaining by the state.
The country has disability benefits for persons with mental disorders. The law for disabled persons was formulated in 1990 and offers some benefits in getting jobs and public welfare. Other benefits are covered under the National Health Care Insurance. The family, work units and community organizations are also supposed to help the disabled.

Mental Health Facilities Mental health is a part of primary health care system. Actual treatment of severe mental disorders is available at the primary level. In some bigger cities like Beijing or Shanghai treatment at primary care level is available.
Regular training of primary care professionals is carried out in the field of mental health. In the last two years, about 600 personnel were provided training. In 1999, a programme for training physicians from general hospitals in mental health was initiated by the WHO/ Beijing Collaborating Centre for Research and Training in Mental Health. About 600 physicians were trained. Since then, short training

programmes have been conducted by WHO consultants for doctors, nurses and other participants from hospitals, schools, media etc. on mental disorders, communication skills, psychosocial management of stress and trauma. WHO and the German Academic Exchange Service (DAAD) are collaborating with Chinese academic institutions and conduct short training programmes for doctors, paediatricians and health care workers in psychosocial management of children and adolescents. Trainers training courses have also been set up. There are community care facilities for patients with mental disorders. The community-based care for mentally ill individuals has developed under the initiative of the China Disabled Federation since 1991. Until now, 243 counties are covered under the cooperation with local health bureau, security department, civil administrative bureau, etc. The plan relies on collective industrial therapy in the community, guardianship networks (doctors, local officials, family members and possibly volunteers) and less restrictive treatments in hospitals. The national government has allocated some money for this project; however, most of the funding is supposed to be generated locally. Some provinces like Shanghai have relatively more community facilities like nursing homes, counseling centres and hotlines. A few locations have community-based suicide prevention programmes.

Psychiatric Beds and Professionals

Total psychiatric beds per 10 000 population	1.06
Psychiatric beds in mental hospitals per 10 000 population	0.87
Psychiatric beds in general hospitals per 10 000 population	0.1
Psychiatric beds in other settings per 10 000 population	0.09
Number of psychiatrists per 100 000 population	1.29
Number of neurosurgeons per 100 000 population	0.63-0.79
Number of psychiatric nurses per 100 000 population	1.99
Number of neurologists per 100 000 population	0.79-0.95
Number of psychologists per 100 000 population	
Number of social workers per 100 000 population	0

Three Ministries, Health, Civil Affairs (i.e. Welfare) and Security (i.e. police) provide inpatient services. Some mental health units also exist under the Ministry of Industry and Mining and the People's Liberation Army. The Ministry of Health provides services to mentally ill patients who are not mentally ill offenders, drug abusers or people without work ability, money and carers; the Ministry of Civil Affairs to the patients without work ability, money and carers but not mentally ill offenders or drug abusers; the Ministry of Security to mentally ill offenders and drug abusers. Through a meeting system, the three main Ministries and the China Disabled Person's Federation coordinate; however, formal horizontal linkages are not very strong. Setting-up of private hospitals has been permitted since 1985. There are a few (around 150) child psychiatry beds. About 150 qualified child psychiatrists are practicing in cities. Two national examination systems exist, one for psychological counsellors, another for psychotherapists. There is a national training programme for physicians from general hospitals. There is no formal system of psychiatric social workers and occupational therapists. Some mental health staff is leaving the sector because financial crisis at psychiatric hospitals (due to low occupancy rates) results in much lower incomes than for staff in other medical disciplines.

Non-Governmental Organizations A few NGOs are involved with mental health in the country. They are mainly involved in advocacy, promotion and rehabilitation. The most important one is the China Disabled Person's Federation, a semi-NGO. NGOs have been consulted in the process of developing the national mental health programme and the mental health legislation. Telephone hotlines are being set up in many cities by NGOs.

Information Gathering System There is no mental health reporting system in the country. In the annual report of the Ministry of Health, there is a mention of the number of mental hospitals, beds and psychiatrists.
The country has data collection system or epidemiological study on mental health. There were epidemiological studies for mental disorders in the country, and systematic studies were carried out by the WHO Collaborating Centre since 1982. Many local areas have done or planned to do their own epidemiological surveys.

Programmes for Special Population The country has specific programmes for mental health for disaster affected population, elderly and children. A five-year project on mental health promotion for children and adolescents has been launched by the Ministry of Health. To facilitate this, national workshops on mental health knowledge have been held for school teachers, school physicians and paediatricians. A PsychoSunlight Project has been designed for college students to promote their ability to cope with college life and prepare to go into society. Two large projects have targeted the elderly; these will help in the development of treatment guidelines for dementia, and screening scales for differentiation between normal aging and early dementia. An emergency psychosocial response plan for disaster affected population is being drafted. A set of four mental health education books were compiled for adolescents, women, working staff and the elderly. On the World Mental Health Day 2004, 3000 sets of these books were presented to the Chinese Central Youth League, the All-China Women's Federation, the All-China Federation of Trade Unions and the Chinese National Committee on Ageing, respectively. Many cities conducted different activities to promote mental health for the public on this day. Telephone hotlines are being set up in many cities and some are focussed on specific population groups (e.g. women or adolescents) and issues (e.g. AIDS). The research group from the Institute of Mental Health, Beijing, carried out the post-earthquake and post-flood studies.

Therapeutic Drugs The following therapeutic drugs are generally available at the primary health care level of the country: carbamazepine, phenobarbital, phenytoin sodium, sodium valproate, amitriptyline, chlorpromazine, diazepam, fluphenazine, haloperidol, lithium.
Artane 6-8 mg is used to treat side-effects of anti-psychotics.

Other Information Among all the cities of China, Shanghai has the most developed psychiatric set-up. It includes community follow-up programmes, guardianship networks, work therapy stations, mental health services in factories, day hospitals, night hospitals and family support groups. Services at each of the three levels-municipal, district and grass-root level are available. Non-psychiatric medical and paramedical staff helps in care-giving. Services for special population like for children, elderly and AIDS patients are also available. Different hotline services can be accessed. Further details can be obtained from Zhang et al (1994, 1997).

Additional Sources of Information

Chen, R., Copeland, J. R. M., Wei, L. (1999) A meta-analysis of epidemiological studies in depression of older people in The People's Republic of China. International Journal of Geriatric Psychiatry, 14, 821-830.

Chen, R., Hu, Z., Qin, X., et al (2004) A community-based study of depression in older people in Hefei, China--the GMS-AGECAT prevalence, case validation and socio-economic correlates. International Journal of Geriatric Psychiatry, 19, 407-13.

Hao, W., Yang, D., Xiao, S. Y., et al (1999) Alcohol consumption and alcohol-related problems: Chinese experience from six area samples, 1994. Addiction, 94, 1467-1476.

Hesketh, T., Ding, Q. J., Jenkins, R. (2002) Suicide ideation in Chinese adolescents. Social Psychiatry & Psychiatric Epidemiology, 37, 230-235.

Jenkins, R. (2002) Addressing suicide as a public-health problem. Lancet, 359, 813-814.

Ji J.L., Kleinman A., Becker, A.E. (2001) Suicide in contemporary China: a review of China's distinctive suicide demographics in their sociocultural context. Harvard Review of Psychiatry, 9, 1-12.

Jiang, Z., Guo, H., Zhu, Z. (1995)An epidemiological survey on use and abuse of antianxiety drugs among Beijing residents. Chinese Journal of Neurology & Psychiatry, 28, 12-15.

Leung, P. W. L., Luk, S. L., Ho, T. P., et al (1996) The diagnosis and prevalence of hyperactivity in Chinese schoolboys. British Journal of Psychiatry, 168, 486-496.

Liu, L., Guo, X., Zhou, Y. et al (2003) Prevalence of dementia in China. Dementia and Geriatric Cognitive Disorders, 15, 226-30.

Liu, X., Sun, Z., Neiderhiser, J. M., et al (2001) Behavioral and emotional problems in Chinese adolescents: parent and teacher reports. Journal of the American Academy of Child & Adolescent Psychiatry, 4, 828-836.

Liu, X., Sun, Z., Uchiyama, M., et al (2000) Attaining nocturnal urinary control, nocturnal enuresis, and behavioral problems in Chinese children aged 6 through 16 years. Journal of the American Academy of Child & Adolescent Psychiatry, 39, 1557-1564.

Ministry of Health, PRC (2004) Infant mortality rates and life expectancy at birth. China Health Statistical Yearbook. 175.

Ministry of Health, PRC (2004) Total Expenditure of Health. China Health Statistical Yearbook. 79.

Niu, T., Chen, C., Ni, J., et al (2000) Nicotine dependence and its familial aggregation in Chinese. International Journal of Epidemiology, 29, 248-252.

Pearson, V. (1995) Mental health care in China. The Royal College of Psychiatrists and Gaskell. United Kingdom.

Pearson, V. (1996) The Chinese equation in mental health policy and practice: order plus control equal stability. International Journal of Law and Psychiatry, 19, 437-458.

Pearson, V., Phillips, M. R. (1994) The social context of psychiatric rehabilitation in China. British Journal of Psychiatry, 165 (suppl. 24), 11-18.

Phillips, M. R. (2000) Mental health services in China. Epidemiologia e Psychiatria Sociale, 9, 84-88.

Phillips, M. R., Yang, G., Zhang, Y., et al (2002) Risk factors for suicide in China: a national case-control psychological autopsy study. Lancet, 360, 1728-1736.

Shen, Y. C., Li, S. R., Chen, C. H., et al (1998) An epidemiological survey on neuroses of urban elderly in Beijing. Psychiatry & Clinical Neurosciences, 52, 288-290.

Wang, W., Wu, S., Cheng, X., et al (2000) Prevalence of Alzheimer's disease and other dementing disorders in an urban community of Beijing, China. Neuroepidemiology, 19, 194-200.

Wang, X. D., Gao, L., Shinfuku, N., et al (2000) Longitudinal study of earthquake-related PTSD in a randomly selected community sample in north China. American Journal of Psychiatry, 157, 1260-1266.

WHO (2002) Working with countries: mental health policy and service development projects.

WHO. Geneva. WHO/MSD/MPS/02.1.

Yan, F., Li, S., Liu, J., et al. (2002) Incidence of senile dementia and depression in elderly population in Xicheng District, Beijing, an epidemiologic study. Chung-Hua i Hsueh Tsa Chih [Chinese Medical Journal], 82,1025-1028.

Zhang, F. C., Mitchell, J. E., Li, K., et al (1992) The prevalence of anorexia nervosa and bulimia nervosa among freshman medical college students in China. International Journal of Eating Disorders, 12, 209-214.

Zhang, M. Y., Ji, J. L., Yan, H. Q. (1997) New perspectives in mental health services in Shanghai. American Journal of Psychiatry, 154, 55 - 58.

Zhang, M. Y., Yan, H. Q., Phillips, M. R. (1994) Community-based psychiatric tehabilitation in Shanghai. British Journal of Psychiatry, 165, 70-79.

Zhang, R., Chen, Q., Li, Y. (1999) Study for the factors related to postpartum depression. Chung-Hua Fu Chan Ko Tsa Chih [Chinese Journal of Obstetrics & Gynecology], 34, 231-233.

Zhang, W. X., Shen, Y. C., Li, S. R. (1998) Epidemiological investigation on mental disorders in 7 areas of China. Chinese Journal of Psychiatry, 31, 69-72.

Zhang, Z., Wei, J., Hong, X. (2001) Prevalence of dementia and major subtypes in urban and rural communities of Beijing. Chinese Journal of Neurology, 34, 199-203.

Zou, Q. H., Lei, Z. W., Zhang, Z. X. (1994) An epidemiological study on etiology of mental retardation. Chung-Hua i Hsueh Tsa Chih [Chinese Medical Journal], 74, 134-137.

Colombia

GENERAL INFORMATION

Colombia is a country with an approximate area of 1139 thousand sq. km. (UNO, 2001). Its population is 44.914 million, and the sex ratio (men per hundred women) is 98 (UNO, 2004). The proportion of population under the age of 15 years is 31% (UNO, 2004), and the proportion of population above the age of 60 years is 7% (WHO, 2004). The literacy rate is 92.1% for men and 92.2% for women (UNESCO/MoH, 2004).

The country is a lower middle income group country (based on World Bank 2004 criteria). The proportion of health budget to GDP is 5.5%. The per capita total expenditure on health is 356 international $, and the per capita government expenditure on health is 234 international $ (WHO, 2004).

The main language(s) used in the country is (are) Spanish. The largest ethnic group(s) is (are) Mestizo (half), and the other ethnic group(s) are (is) European (one-fourth) and native American. The largest religious group(s) is (are) Roman Catholic (95%).

The life expectancy at birth is 67.5 years for males and 76.3 years for females (WHO, 2004). The healthy life expectancy at birth is 58 years for males and 66 years for females (WHO, 2004).

EPIDEMIOLOGY

National surveys on mental health were conducted in 1993 and 2003. In the former study, SRQ (criteria DSM-III) and Zung Scale were applied to a random sample of 25135 adults. The lifetime prevalence for depression was 25.1%, anxiety disorders 9.6%, and alcohol abuse 7.8%. The latter study utilized the World Mental Health Survey methodology and applied CIDI 2000 (criteria DSM-IV) to 4596 adults and 1586 adolescents in a random sample of 5526 urban homes. The lifetime prevalence of mood disorders was 12.9%, anxiety disorders 24.0%, alcohol use disorders 9.2% and drug use disorders 1.7% (Ministry of Health, 2004). Torres de Galvis and Murrelle (1990) evaluated 2800 adults (12-64 years) from four cities and found the use of alcohol (56%), tobacco (29.7%), tranquilizers (6%), marijuana (1.1%), basuco (6%) and cocaine (3%) to be common. Approximately 8.1% of the subjects were dependent on alcohol and 7.3% were at risk of becoming dependent on alcohol. Drug use was associated with male gender (except tranquilizers), medium age groups and unmarried status. Differences in suicide rates between users and non-users were statistically significant in the population aged 15 to 54. Montoya and Chilcoat (1996) reported the integrated findings of a survey carried out in Bolivia, Colombia, Ecuador, Peru and Venezuela to estimate cocaine and coca use prevalence (n=24 108). The lifetime prevalence of cocaine or coca paste use was between 0.8 and 3.0% and it was associated with age (middle-age), class (middle), gender (male), education (high school), income (high) and residence (urban). In a cross-sectional study involving 512 schools, the prevalence of substance use was 59.4% in public schools and 40% in private schools. Alcohol, marijuana, cocaine were the commonly used drugs and family history of mental disorders and personal conflicts were associated with substance use (Bergonzoli et al, 1989). Brook et al (1999) interviewed more than 2800 adolescents and their mothers and found that factors like violence, drug availability, and machismo, family drug use, a distant parent-child relationship and unconventional behaviour are risk factors for adolescent illegal drug use. Jablensky et al (1992) reported the results of the WHO multi-country Determinants of Outcome of Severe Mental Disorders (DOS) that was carried out in a group of patients making their first treatment contact because of symptoms of a possibly schizophrenic illness. Better outcome was reported in patients living in developing countries. Significant differences were found between centres in the incidence of schizophrenia using a broad definition, although the rates ranged only from 1.5 to 4.2 per 100 000 population aged 15-54. In contrast, the incidence of schizophrenia using a narrow definition (category S+ of the CATEGO programme derived from the PSE-9 interview) was not significantly different between centres. Lima et al (1993) assessed 113 adult victims of a major Latin American disaster 1 and 5 years after the catastrophe with the Self-Reporting Questionnaire. The prevalence of emotional distress decreased from 65% in 1986 to 31% in 1990. A study conducted in three countries, Columbia, Ecuador and Venezuela (n=1946), showed that 53.4% of subjects had erectile dysfunction with 19.8% of all men reporting moderate to complete ED. Increasing age, hypertension, benign prostatic hyperplasia and diabetes mellitus were associated with the disorder (Morillo et al, 2002). In a general population sample of 1879 Spanish-speaking university students (mean age=24.0), the prevalence of self-reported stuttering was found to be 2% (Ardila et al, 1994). Giel et al (1981) assessed 925 children attending primary care centres in Columbia, India, Philippines and Sudan using a 2-stage design and found that the rate of psychiatric disorders varied between 12-29%. Pineda et al (1999) used multiple standardized rating scales, clinical interviews and neurological tests on large samples of preschool and school going children and reported the prevalence of ADHD to be more than 16.1%. But, the prevalence of subtypes differed in the two studies. Gender (male), age (school going) and economic status (lower) were significantly related to prevalence. Pinzon-Perez and Perez (2001) found that 21% of school students (n=1692) expressed suicidal ideation, 19% suicidal plans and 16% reported at least one attempt in the 30 days preceding the study.

MENTAL HEALTH RESOURCES

Mental Health Policy A mental health policy is present. The policy was initially formulated in 1979.

The components of the policy are advocacy, promotion, prevention, treatment and rehabilitation. The policy was reviewed in 1998, but it was not implemented. The policy is being reviewed again to make it consonant with the health system and the priorities emerging from the National Study of Mental Health, 2003.

Substance Abuse Policy A substance abuse policy is present. The policy was initially formulated in 1979. The policy was reformulated by the National Board of Economic and Social Policy in 2002 (CONPES 3078 of 2002). Currently, the 'Policy for the Reduction of the Demand for Consumption of Psychoactive Substances' is in final phase of consensus-building and implementation, under the leadership of the Ministry of the Social Protection.

National Mental Health Programme A national mental health programme is absent.
Under the guidelines defined by the Ministry of the Social Protection, each department is formulating plans of action in mental health that should be implemented within a period of 2 years.

National Therapeutic Drug Policy/Essential List of Drugs A national therapeutic drug policy/essential list of drugs is present. It was formulated in 1993.

Mental Health Legislation There is no comprehensive national mental health legislation, however, Law 715-2001 includes mental health functions in the regional-local levels, but it has not been enacted. The Ministerial Resolution No.2417 of 1992 allows for a charter of rights for mental health patients. Resolution 2358 of 1998 and Law 30 of 1986 relate to drug statutes.
Details about the year of enactment of the mental health legislation are not available.

Mental Health Financing There are budget allocations for mental health.
The country spends 0.08% of the total health budget on mental health.
The primary sources of mental health financing in descending order are tax based, social insurance, out of pocket expenditure by the patient or family and private insurances.
The country has disability benefits for persons with mental disorders. There is no mention to the proportion of the population entitled to get these benefits

Mental Health Facilities Mental health is not a part of primary health care system. Actual treatment of severe mental disorders is not available at the primary level. Despite some pilot projects, mental health services are not provided under the Primary Health Care scheme.
Regular training of primary care professionals is not carried out in the field of mental health.
There are community care facilities for patients with mental disorders. Mental health care is provided with different approaches according to users' affiliation with social security.

Psychiatric Beds and Professionals

Total psychiatric beds per 10 000 population	
Psychiatric beds in mental hospitals per 10 000 population	0.45
Psychiatric beds in general hospitals per 10 000 population	
Psychiatric beds in other settings per 10 000 population	
Number of psychiatrists per 100 000 population	2
Number of neurosurgeons per 100 000 population	
Number of psychiatric nurses per 100 000 population	
Number of neurologists per 100 000 population	
Number of psychologists per 100 000 population	
Number of social workers per 100 000 population	

20% of psychiatric beds are dedicated to long-stay patients. There are facilities in prison for offenders with mental disorders.

Non-Governmental Organizations NGOs are involved with mental health in the country. They are mainly involved in advocacy, promotion and prevention. These organizations participate in mental health activities related to displaced populations, women, children and domestic violence.

Information Gathering System There is mental health reporting system in the country. ICD-10 and DSM-IV criteria are used.
Information on ambulatory morbidity, admission and hospital discharge of mental disorders are recorded in the Individual Registries of Delivery of Services, however, this information is still not available with the opportunity, coverage and quality desired, which is in the process of standardization and implementation of the registry.
The country has data collection system or epidemiological study on mental health. The 'Asociación de Hospitales Mentales' (Psychiatric Hospitals Association) conducts specific surveys on mental health from time to time. There are 'Mental Health Groups' in charge of the data collection system for mental disorders both at regional and national levels. There are, in addition, records of data on injuries due to external cause such as accidents, homicides, domestic violence and other type of assaults, in routine registries of Forensic Medicine and through Observatories of Violence that operate in some departments.

Programmes for Special Population The country has specific programmes for mental health for minorities, refugees, disaster affected population, indigenous population, elderly and children.
Also, there are programmes for women and victims of domestic violence. Although specific programmes for indigenous populations are not present, they are provided comprehensive care through the Compulsory Plan of Health. Programmes for persons with mental disorders who are 'not criminally responsible' and psychological immaturity care have more than 250 places available.

Therapeutic Drugs The following therapeutic drugs are generally available at the primary health care level of the country: carbamazepine, phenobarbital, phenytoin sodium, sodium valproate, amitriptyline, chlorpromazine, diazepam, haloperidol, lithium, biperiden, carbidopa, levodopa.
The national therapeutic drug policy was revised in 2002 and the essential drug list was revised in 2002. Medicines are supplied as part of the benefits from compulsory health plan (POS) within the social security system.

Other Information Methods for assessing quality of care at primary, secondary and tertiary levels are available.

Additional Sources of Information

Ardila, A., Bateman, J. R., Nino, C. R., et al (1994) An epidemiologic study of stuttering. Journal of Communication Disorders, 27, 37-48.

Bergonzoli, P. G., Rico, O., Ramirez, A., et al (1989) Drug use among students in Cali, Colombia. Boletin de la Oficina Sanitaria Panamericana, 106, 22-31.

Brook, J. S., Brook, D. W., De La Rosa, M., et al (1999) The role of parents in protecting Colombian adolescents from delinquency and marijuana use. Archives of Pediatrics & Adolescent Medicine, 153, 457-464.

Giel, R., De Arango, M. V., Climent, C. E., et al (1981) Childhood mental disorders in primary health care: results of observations in four developing countries. A report from the WHO collaborative Study on Strategies for Extending Mental Health Care. Pediatrics, 68, 677-683.

Jablensky, A., Sartorius, N., Ernberg, G., et al (1992) Schizophrenia manifestations, incidence and course in different cultures. A World Health Organization ten-country study. Source Psychological Medicine, 22(Suppl. 20), 1-97.

Lima, B. R., Pai, S., Toledo, V., et al (1993) Emotional distress in disaster victims. A follow-up study. Journal of Nervous & Mental Disease, 181, 388-393.

Ministerio de Salud (1998) Politica Nacional de Salud Mental. Direccion General de Promocion y Prevencion Subdireccion de Promocion.

Ministerio de Salud (1998) Politica Nacional de Salud Mental, Resolucion Numero 2358.

Ministerio de Salud (1996) Resolucion Numero 4288.

Ministerio de Salud (1994) Decreto Numero 1292.

Ministerio de Salud (1986) Por la cual se adopta el Estatuto Nacional dfe Estupefacientes y se dictan otras disposiciones.

Montoya, I. D., Chilcoat, H. D., et al (1996) Epidemiology of coca derivatives use in the Andean region: a tale of five countries. Substance Use & Misuse, 31, 1227-1240.

Morillo, L. E., Diaz, J., Estevez, E., et al (2002) Prevalence of erectile dysfunction in Colombia, Ecuador, and Venezuela: a population-based study (DENSA). International Journal of Impotence Research, 14 (Suppl. 2), 10-18.

Pineda, D., Ardila, A., Rosselli, M., et al (1999) Prevalence of attention-deficit/hyperactivity disorder symptoms in 4- to 17-year-old children in the general population. Journal of Abnormal Child Psychology, 27, 455-462.

Pinzon-Perez, H., Perez, M. A., et al (2001) A study of suicide-related behaviors among Colombian youth: reflections on prevention and implications for health education. Journal of Health Education, 32, 288-292.

Torres de Galvis, Y., Murrelle, L., et al (1990) Consumption of dependence-producing substances in Colombia. SO – Bulletin of the Pan American Health Organization, 24, 12-21.

Comoros

GENERAL INFORMATION

Comoros is a country with an approximate area of 2 thousand sq. km. (UNO, 2001). The country is an archipelago with four main islands. Its population is 0.79 million, and the sex ratio (men per hundred women) is 101 (UNO, 2004). The proportion of population under the age of 15 years is 42% (UNO, 2004), and the proportion of population above the age of 60 years is 4% (WHO, 2004). The literacy rate is 63.5% for men and 49.1% for women (UNESCO/MoH, 2004).

The country is a low income group country (based on World Bank 2004 criteria). The proportion of health budget to GDP is 3.1%. The per capita total expenditure on health is 29 international $, and the per capita government expenditure on health is 17 international $ (WHO, 2004).

The main language(s) used in the country is (are) French, Arabic and Swahili. The largest ethnic group(s) is (are) Arab, and the other ethnic group(s) are (is) African, Malay-Indonesian and Creole. The largest religious group(s) is (are) Sunni Muslim (five-sixths), and the other religious group(s) are (is) Roman Catholic.

The life expectancy at birth is 61.6 years for males and 64.9 years for females (WHO, 2004). The healthy life expectancy at birth is 54 years for males and 55 years for females (WHO, 2004).

EPIDEMIOLOGY

There is a paucity of epidemiological data on mental illnesses in Comoros in internationally accessible literature.

MENTAL HEALTH RESOURCES

Mental Health Policy A mental health policy is absent.

Substance Abuse Policy A substance abuse policy is absent.

National Mental Health Programme A national mental health programme is absent.

National Therapeutic Drug Policy/Essential List of Drugs A national therapeutic drug policy/essential list of drugs is present. It was formulated in 1991.

Mental Health Legislation Details about the mental health legislation are not available.

Mental Health Financing There are no budget allocations for mental health.

Details about expenditure on mental health are not available.

The primary source of mental health financing is out of pocket expenditure by the patient or family.

The country does not have disability benefits for persons with mental disorders. Illness insurance has not been clearly defined by the Government, so benefits are not present.

Mental Health Facilities Mental health is not a part of primary health care system. Actual treatment of severe mental disorders is not available at the primary level. Patients are hospitalized in general hospitals.

Regular training of primary care professionals is not carried out in the field of mental health.

There are no community care facilities for patients with mental disorders. A centre was created but it is not operational even after 2 years. Patients are cared for by their families.

Psychiatric Beds and Professionals

Total psychiatric beds per 10 000 population	0
Psychiatric beds in mental hospitals per 10 000 population	0
Psychiatric beds in general hospitals per 10 000 population	0
Psychiatric beds in other settings per 10 000 population	0
Number of psychiatrists per 100 000 population	0
Number of neurosurgeons per 100 000 population	0
Number of psychiatric nurses per 100 000 population	0
Number of neurologists per 100 000 population	0.1
Number of psychologists per 100 000 population	0.4
Number of social workers per 100 000 population	0.15

One mental health student is in training.

Non-Governmental Organizations NGOs are not involved with mental health in the country.

Information Gathering System There is no mental health reporting system in the country. The reporting system has not worked for the last four years.

The country has no data collection system or epidemiological study on mental health. A survey had been done in 1998, but it has not been circulated.

Programmes for Special Population There are no special services for any population group.

Therapeutic Drugs The following therapeutic drugs are generally available at the primary health care level of the country: phenobarbital, chlorpromazine, diazepam.
If the drugs are not available in the PNAC they have to be bought from private pharmacies. Haloperidol may be ordered outside the PNAC by doctors. The essential list of drugs is presently being revised.

Other Information

Additional Sources of Information

Congo

C–D

GENERAL INFORMATION

Congo is a country with an approximate area of 342 thousand sq. km. (UNO, 2001). Its population is 3.818 million, and the sex ratio (men per hundred women) is 98 (UNO, 2004). The proportion of population under the age of 15 years is 47% (UNO, 2004), and the proportion of population above the age of 60 years is 5% (WHO, 2004). The literacy rate is 88.9% for men and 77.1% for women (UNESCO/MoH, 2004).
The country is a low income group country (based on World Bank 2004 criteria). The proportion of health budget to GDP is 2.1%. The per capita total expenditure on health is 22 international $, and the per capita government expenditure on health is 14 international $ (WHO, 2004).
The main language(s) used in the country is (are) French. The largest ethnic group(s) is (are) Kongo in the south and Sangha and M'Bochi in the north and in the center. The largest religious group(s) is (are) Christian, and the other religious group(s) are (is) indigenous groups.
The life expectancy at birth is 51.6 years for males and 54.5 years for females (WHO, 2004). The healthy life expectancy at birth is 45 years for males and 47 years for females (WHO, 2004).

EPIDEMIOLOGY

There is a paucity of epidemiological data on mental illnesses in Congo in internationally accessible literature. Salignon and Legros (2002) have reported on the physical and psychological impact of war on the population. Ibara et al (2002) found neuropsychiatric presentations in 49.7% of 175 hospitalized elderly HIV patients, and Hornabrook (1975) has reported on the occurrence of endemic cretinism in the region.

MENTAL HEALTH RESOURCES

Mental Health Policy A mental health policy is present. The policy was initially formulated in 1999.
The components of the policy are advocacy, promotion and rehabilitation.

Substance Abuse Policy A substance abuse policy is present. The policy was initially formulated in 1999.

National Mental Health Programme A national mental health programme is present. The programme was formulated in 2002.

National Therapeutic Drug Policy/Essential List of Drugs A national therapeutic drug policy/essential list of drugs is present. It was formulated in 1983.

Mental Health Legislation Till Independence, the French legislation was being used. Since Independence no legislation is in effect. Details about the year of enactment of the mental health legislation are not available.

Mental Health Financing There are no budget allocations for mental health.
Details about expenditure on mental health are not available.
The primary source of mental health financing is out of pocket expenditure by the patient or family.
The country does not have disability benefits for persons with mental disorders. Mental disorders are treated as any other disorder.

Mental Health Facilities Mental health is not a part of primary health care system. Actual treatment of severe mental disorders is not available at the primary level. There are no facilities for therapy.
Regular training of primary care professionals is not carried out in the field of mental health.
There are no community care facilities for patients with mental disorders.

Psychiatric Beds and Professionals

Total psychiatric beds per 10 000 population	0.06
Psychiatric beds in mental hospitals per 10 000 population	0
Psychiatric beds in general hospitals per 10 000 population	0.06
Psychiatric beds in other settings per 10 000 population	0
Number of psychiatrists per 100 000 population	0.03
Number of neurosurgeons per 100 000 population	0
Number of psychiatric nurses per 100 000 population	0.1
Number of neurologists per 100 000 population	0.03
Number of psychologists per 100 000 population	0.26
Number of social workers per 100 000 population	

There are 3000 social workers, but the specific number working in mental health is not available.

Non-Governmental Organizations NGOs are involved with mental health in the country.

Information Gathering System There is no mental health reporting system in the country.

The country has no data collection system or epidemiological study on mental health.

Programmes for Special Population There are no specific programmes for special population groups.

Therapeutic Drugs The following therapeutic drugs are generally available at the primary health care level of the country: carbamazepine, phenobarbital, phenytoin sodium, amitriptyline, chlorpromazine, diazepam, fluphenazine, haloperidol.

Other Information

Additional Sources of Information

Hornabrook, R. W. (1975) Endemic cretinism. Contemporary Neurology Series, 12, 91-108.

Ibara, J. R., Itoua, C., Gathse, A., et al (2002) Acquired immunodeficiency syndrome in elderly persons in a tropical zone. Apropos of 175 cases in the Congo. Bulletin de la Société de Pathologie Exotique, 95, 100-102.

Salignon, P., Legros, D. (2002) Impact of war on civilian population health. Republic of the Congo, December 1998-February 2000. Médecine Tropicale, 62, 433-437.

Cook Islands

GENERAL INFORMATION

Cook Islands is a country with an approximate area of 0.23 thousand sq. km. (UNO, 2001). The country consists of two main islands and many low-lying coral atolls. Its population is 0.018 million, and the sex ratio (men per hundred women) is 107 (UNO, 2004). The proportion of population under the age of 15 years is 36% (UNO, 2004), and the proportion of population above the age of 60 years is 7% (WHO, 2004).

The country is a high income group country (based on World Bank 2004 criteria). The proportion of health budget to GDP is 4.7%. The per capita total expenditure on health is 598 international $, and the per capita government expenditure on health is 404 international $ (WHO, 2004).

The main language(s) used in the country is (are) English and Maori. The largest ethnic group(s) is (are) Maori.

The life expectancy at birth is 69.2 years for males and 74.2 years for females (WHO, 2004). The healthy life expectancy at birth is 61 years for males and 63 years for females (WHO, 2004).

C–D

EPIDEMIOLOGY

There is a paucity of epidemiological data on mental illnesses in Cook Islands in internationally accessible literature.

MENTAL HEALTH RESOURCES

Mental Health Policy A mental health policy is absent.

Substance Abuse Policy A substance abuse policy is absent.

National Mental Health Programme A national mental health programme is absent.

National Therapeutic Drug Policy/Essential List of Drugs A national therapeutic drug policy/essential list of drugs is present. It was formulated in 1992.

Mental Health Legislation The mental health legislation is a part of the Crimes Act.
The latest legislation was enacted in 1969.

Mental Health Financing There are no budget allocations for mental health.
Details about expenditure on mental health are not available.
The primary source of mental health financing is tax based.
The country has disability benefits for persons with mental disorders. A monthly monetary benefit is made on recommendation of a physician to the social welfare department.

Mental Health Facilities Mental health is a part of primary health care system. Actual treatment of severe mental disorders is available at the primary level. Medications are provided by doctors and nurses.
Regular training of primary care professionals is not carried out in the field of mental health.
There are community care facilities for patients with mental disorders. Community care is the responsibility of public health nurses. A community-based programme has been started by an NGO with the agreement with the Ministry of Health.

Psychiatric Beds and Professionals

Total psychiatric beds per 10 000 population	0
Psychiatric beds in mental hospitals per 10 000 population	0
Psychiatric beds in general hospitals per 10 000 population	0
Psychiatric beds in other settings per 10 000 population	0
Number of psychiatrists per 100 000 population	0
Number of neurosurgeons per 100 000 population	0
Number of psychiatric nurses per 100 000 population	5.3
Number of neurologists per 100 000 population	0
Number of psychologists per 100 000 population	0
Number of social workers per 100 000 population	0

General physicians deal with psychiatry.

Non-Governmental Organizations NGOs are involved with mental health in the country. They are mainly involved in advocacy, treatment and rehabilitation.

Information Gathering System There is mental health reporting system in the country.
The country has no data collection system or epidemiological study on mental health. Information on known patients are collected.

Programmes for Special Population There are no special services available.

Therapeutic Drugs The following therapeutic drugs are generally available at the primary health care level of the country: carbamazepine, phenobarbital, phenytoin sodium, sodium valproate, amitriptyline, chlorpromazine, diazepam, fluphenazine, haloperidol, lithium, carbidopa, levodopa.

Other Information

Additional Sources of Information

Government document (2000) Cook Island Essential Drug List.

Costa Rica

GENERAL INFORMATION

Costa Rica is a country with an approximate area of 51 thousand sq. km. (UNO, 2001). Its population is 4.25 million, and the sex ratio (men per hundred women) is 103 (UNO, 2004). The proportion of population under the age of 15 years is 29% (UNO, 2004), and the proportion of population above the age of 60 years is 8% (WHO, 2004). The literacy rate is 95.7% for men and 95.9% for women (UNESCO/MoH, 2004).

The country is a higher middle income group country (based on World Bank 2004 criteria). The proportion of health budget to GDP is 7.2%. The per capita total expenditure on health is 562 international $, and the per capita government expenditure on health is 385 international $ (WHO, 2004).

The main language(s) used in the country is (are) Spanish. The largest ethnic group(s) is (are) European (descent). The largest religious group(s) is (are) Roman Catholic (three-fourths), and the other religious group(s) are (is) Evangelical Christian.

The life expectancy at birth is 74.8 years for males and 79.5 years for females (WHO, 2004). The healthy life expectancy at birth is 65 years for males and 69 years for females (WHO, 2004).

EPIDEMIOLOGY

Miguez (1984) found the prevalence of alcohol use disorder to be 14% in a sample of 469 subjects selected from a shanty town. Drug use was reported by 8% of the respondents. Escamilla et al (2001) recruited 110 subjects from two high-risk (for bipolar illness) Costa Rican pedigrees and 205 unrelated Costa Rican bipolar subjects and assessed them using structured interviews. Substance use disorders (primarily alcohol dependence) occurred in 17% of the bipolar patients from the population sample and 35% of the bipolar patients from the pedigree sample. Comorbid substance use disorder was strongly associated with gender but did not significantly alter the prevalence of psychosis or age of onset of mania in bipolar subjects. In comorbid subjects, alcohol dependence tended to predate the first manic episode. Sandi Esquivel and Avila (1990) did a case-control study in which they showed that patients with alcohol use disorder had greater likelihood of having noteworthy problems in family/social relations, work/finances and psychological status. A number of studies on substance use are available. Sandi et al (2002) used the Latin-American version of Drug Use Screening Inventory (DUSI) to interview randomly selected 304 students from rural schools. Results showed a high prevalence of past-year alcohol use for both males and females (56.6% and 47.4%, respectively), and a lower prevalence of past-year tobacco use (44.0% and 7.7%). In terms of illicit drugs, males preferred cocaine and marijuana whereas females preferred amphetamines. Costa Rica was one of the many countries involved in the Global Youth Tobacco Survey conducted by WHO and CDC, Atlanta, which showed that between 10-33% of adolescents used tobacco (Warren et al, 2000). The annual incidence of schizophrenia was reported to be 0.48/1000 population; however, the estimate was based on data on first time hospital admissions for schizophrenia (Handal & Dodds, 1997). De Lisi et al (2001) studied families of patients with schizophrenia in Costa Rica and the USA. Within multiplex families (both in the USA and Costa Rica), age of onset was found to have a familial component. There was significantly lower prevalence of affective symptoms (depression and mania) and drug abuse among the Costa Rican multiplex families by comparison with those from the USA. The families with only one ill member from Costa Rica had significantly more alcohol abuse than the multiply affected families. Maternal depression was assessed using the Center for Epidemiological Studies – Depression scale in three samples of women (total n=1256) in Chile and Costa Rica (Wolf et al, 2002). Lifetime prevalence of major depressive episodes was assessed in two Costa Rican samples by the Diagnostic Interview Schedule. Between 35% and 50% of all mothers had experienced at least one episode of major depression or were experiencing severe dysphoric mood at the time of the evaluation. In addition, one-third of the Costa Rican mothers had experienced dysphoric mood following delivery of a child. Lester (1995) reported that suicide rates are lower in Costa Rica than in the United States. Firearms are used less often and hanging more often as a method for suicide in Costa Rica. Suicide rates do not increase with age in Costa Rica, unlike the United States. A study on Tourette's disorder in a sample (n=85, aged 5-29 years) showed that the gender ratio (male: female) was 4.6:1 and that the mean age of onset was 6.1 years. However, many subjects denied any impairment or distress due to the disorder even when objectively impairment was evident (Mathews et al, 2001).

MENTAL HEALTH RESOURCES

Mental Health Policy A mental health policy is present. The policy was initially formulated in 1991.

The components of the policy are advocacy, promotion, prevention, treatment and rehabilitation. It was revised in 2001 and about 50% of its contents have been implemented. Currently, it is included within the National Policy of Health 2002-2006 and in the National Plan of Development. It emphasizes mental health care at the primary level, child and adolescent mental health and prevention of drug use disorders.

Substance Abuse Policy A substance abuse policy is present. The policy was initially formulated in 1986. It was revised in 2001. It has specific budget for its implementation and has been implemented to the extent of 25-50%.

National Mental Health Programme A national mental health programme is absent.

It exists within an intersectoral national plan of mental health, 2004-2010. There is no specific budget for its implementation. Its main components are strategy of services reform, promotion and prevention and specialized services.

National Therapeutic Drug Policy/Essential List of Drugs A national therapeutic drug policy/essential list of drugs is present. It was formulated in 1982.

Mental Health Legislation The mental health legislation focuses on promotion and prevention, human rights, regulation of mental health services, but it has no reference to regulation of involuntary treatment. Regular funds have not been allocated for its implementation and implementation is to the extent of 25 to 50%.
The latest legislation was enacted in 1995.

Mental Health Financing There are no budget allocations for mental health.
The country spends 8% of the total health budget on mental health.
The primary sources of mental health financing in descending order are social insurance and private insurances.
Approximately 10% of mental health funding is spent on general hospitals and 90% on psychiatric hospitals.
The country has disability benefits for persons with mental disorders. More than 90% of the eligible persons actually receive the benefits. Disability assessment is performed by a psychiatrist if it is for a short term period; if it is for a long term period, an expert committee is required. Any ICD-10 mental disorder that is associated with severe disability may avail public disability benefits. The department in charge is the 'Caja Costaricense del Seguro Social (CCSS)' (Social Security Department of Costa Rica).

Mental Health Facilities Mental health is a part of primary health care system. Actual treatment of severe mental disorders is available at the primary level. Although general health care through primary health care is available for most of the population, less than 25% of the population has mental health care provision in primary health care. The general staff structure is composed of primary health care doctors, auxiliary nurses and health care workers. General doctors are the main providers. Treatment for severe mental disorders is available at primary health care, mainly in the form of provision of anti-psychotic medications to patients discharged from psychiatric hospitals. A referral system is in place.
Regular training of primary care professionals is carried out in the field of mental health. In the last two years, about 500 personnel were provided training. A regular programme to train primary care professionals (general clinicians, auxiliary nurses and health care workers) in mental health started in 2001. The duration of the training is 2 days once a year.
There are community care facilities for patients with mental disorders. The community care based system for the mentally ill covers about 25% of the intended population and includes preventive/promotion interventions, home interventions, family interventions, residential facilities, vocational training and employment programmes.

Psychiatric Beds and Professionals

Total psychiatric beds per 10 000 population	2.6
Psychiatric beds in mental hospitals per 10 000 population	2.5
Psychiatric beds in general hospitals per 10 000 population	0.07
Psychiatric beds in other settings per 10 000 population	0
Number of psychiatrists per 100 000 population	2
Number of neurosurgeons per 100 000 population	0.8
Number of psychiatric nurses per 100 000 population	2
Number of neurologists per 100 000 population	1.1
Number of psychologists per 100 000 population	2
Number of social workers per 100 000 population	0.5

There are 2 psychiatric hospitals in the country, the larger one has 811 beds. These hospitals are managed by the Social Security Department (the Ministry of Health does not take care of the psychiatric hospitals). 60% of these beds are occupied by long stay patients.

Non-Governmental Organizations NGOs are involved with mental health in the country. They are mainly involved in advocacy, promotion, prevention, treatment and rehabilitation. These organizations participate in mental health activities related to women, children, consumers and domestic violence. Two-fifths of non-treatment related mental health activities (except psychiatric care), 5% of psychiatric care and 95% of care for drug abusers is provided by NGOs through 60 authorized programmes.

Information Gathering System There is mental health reporting system in the country. It is under the Social Security Department of Costa Rica. The mental health components reported are morbidity in emergencies and hospital admissions. It also conducts diagnostic evaluations on samples of outpatient consultations.
The country has data collection system or epidemiological study on mental health. The Department of Information and Health Services Statistics of the Social Security System is in charge of data collection.

Programmes for Special Population The country has specific programmes for mental health for elderly and children. AIDS patients receive psychiatric care from CCSS. The children's hospital provides services for children, whereas the geriatric hospital has a psychiatrist on its staff.
Also there are programmes for women, abused children and victims of domestic violence.

Therapeutic Drugs The following therapeutic drugs are generally available at the primary health care level of the country: carbamazepine, phenobarbital, phenytoin sodium, sodium valproate, amitriptyline, chlorpromazine, diazepam, fluphenazine, haloperidol, lithium, biperiden, carbidopa, levodopa.
The national therapeutic drugs policy was revised in 1989 and the essential drug list was revised in 2001. The information on medication is from the Social Security Department of Costa Rica.

Other Information

Additional Sources of Information

Caja Costarricense de Seguro Social, Direccion Tecnica Servicios de Salud, Seccion Trabajo Social (2000) Plan Annual Operativo Trabajo Social 2000.

DeLisi, L. E., Mesen, A., Rodriguez, C., et al (2001) Clinical characteristics of schizophrenia in multiply affected Spanish origin families from Costa Rica. Psychiatric Genetics, 11, 145-152.

Department of Pharmaceuticals (1999) List of Official Medicines.

Departamento de Salud Mental (1995) Bases Programaticas para la promocion de la salud mental y la atencion psiquiatrica.

Escamilla, M. A., Batki, S., Reus, V. I., et al (2001) Comorbidity of bipolar disorder and substance abuse in Costa Rica: pedigree- and population-based studies. Journal of Affective Disorders, 71, 71-83.

Government document (2000) Nuevo Modelo de Atencion en Salud Mental. Gerencia Medica, Gerencia de Modernizacion y Desarollo.

Government document (2000) El nuevo rol de la CCSS frente a las adiccions como problema de Salud Publica en Costa Rica.

Government document (1991) Iniciativa Intergerencial. Decreto Ejecutivo N 20665-S.

Handal, N., Dodds, J. H., et al (1997) Statistics for initial admission for schizophrenia in hospitals in Costa Rica. Pan American Journal of Public Health, 1, 426-434.

La Asamblea Legilativa de la Republica de Costa Rica (1996). Ley # 7600. Igualdad de oportunidades para las personas con discapacidad.

Lester, D. (1995) Suicide and homicide in Costa Rica. Source Medicine, Science & the Law, 35, 316-318.

Mathews, C. A., Herrera Amighetti, L. D., Lowe, T. L., et al (2001) Cultural influences on diagnosis and perception of Tourette syndrome in Costa Rica. Journal of the American Academy of Child & Adolescent Psychiatry, 40, 456-463.

Miguez, H. A.(1984) Drug dependence in poverty. Its prevalence in Costa Rica. Acta Psiquiatrica y Psicologica de America Latina, 30, 255-263.

Ministerio de Salud Caja Costarricense de Seguro Social (1991). Plan Nacional para la Atencion en Salud Mental y Psiquiatria.

Sandi Esquivel, L. E., Avila, C. K. (1990) Validity of the Addiction Severity Index (adapted version) in a Costa Rican population group. Bulletin of the Pan American Health Organization, 24, 70-76.

Sandi, L., Diaz, A., Uglade, F., et al (2002) Drug use and associated factors among rural adolescents in Costa Rica. Substance Use & Misuse, 37, 599-611.

Warren, C. W., Riley, L., Asma, S., et al (2000) Tobacco use by youth: a surveillance report from the Global Youth Tobacco Survey project. Bulletin of the World Health Organization, 78, 868-876.

Wolf, A. W., De Andraca, I., Lozoff, B., et al (2002) Maternal depression in three Latin American samples. Social Psychiatry & Psychiatric Epidemiology, 37, 169-176.

Côte d'Ivoire

GENERAL INFORMATION

Côte d'Ivoire is a country with an approximate area of 322 thousand sq. km. (UNO, 2001). Its population is 16.897 million, and the sex ratio (men per hundred women) is 104 (UNO, 2004). The proportion of population under the age of 15 years is 41% (UNO, 2004), and the proportion of population above the age of 60 years is 5% (WHO, 2004). The literacy rate is 59.5% for men and 37.2% for women (UNESCO/MoH, 2004).

The country is a low income group country (based on World Bank 2004 criteria). The proportion of health budget to GDP is 6.2%. The per capita total expenditure on health is 127 international $, and the per capita government expenditure on health is 20 international $ (WHO, 2004).

The main language(s) used in the country is (are) French, Akan and Mandés. The largest ethnic group(s) is (are) Akan, and the other ethnic group(s) are (is) Voltaiques, Northern Mandes, Krous and Southern Mandes. The largest religious group(s) is (are) indigenous groups and Muslim, and the other religious group(s) are (is) Christian.

The life expectancy at birth is 43.1 years for males and 48 years for females (WHO, 2004). The healthy life expectancy at birth is 38 years for males and 41 years for females (WHO, 2004).

EPIDEMIOLOGY

There is a paucity of epidemiological data on mental illnesses in Côte d'Ivore in internationally accessible literature.

MENTAL HEALTH RESOURCES

Mental Health Policy A mental health policy is present. The policy was initially formulated in 1962.
The components of the policy are treatment and rehabilitation.

Substance Abuse Policy A substance abuse policy is present. The policy was initially formulated in 1984.

National Mental Health Programme A national mental health programme is present. The programme was formulated in 1999.

National Therapeutic Drug Policy/Essential List of Drugs A national therapeutic drug policy/essential list of drugs is present. It was formulated in 1995.

Mental Health Legislation Details about the mental health legislation are not available.

Mental Health Financing There are budget allocations for mental health.
The country spends 0.1% of the total health budget on mental health.
The primary source of mental health financing is out of pocket expenditure by the patient or family.
The country has disability benefits for persons with mental disorders.

Mental Health Facilities Mental health is a part of primary health care system. Actual treatment of severe mental disorders is available at the primary level.
Regular training of primary care professionals is carried out in the field of mental health.
There are community care facilities for patients with mental disorders.

Psychiatric Beds and Professionals

Total psychiatric beds per 10 000 population	0.15
Psychiatric beds in mental hospitals per 10 000 population	0.13
Psychiatric beds in general hospitals per 10 000 population	0.02
Psychiatric beds in other settings per 10 000 population	0
Number of psychiatrists per 100 000 population	0.2
Number of neurosurgeons per 100 000 population	0.02
Number of psychiatric nurses per 100 000 population	0.2
Number of neurologists per 100 000 population	0.07
Number of psychologists per 100 000 population	0.07
Number of social workers per 100 000 population	0.03

There are 3 occupational therapists.

Non-Governmental Organizations NGOs are involved with mental health in the country. They are mainly involved in prevention and rehabilitation.

Information Gathering System There is mental health reporting system in the country. It exists as the Annual Report of Mental Health Activities.
The country has no data collection system or epidemiological study on mental health.

Programmes for Special Population There are no special services available.

Therapeutic Drugs The following therapeutic drugs are generally available at the primary health care level of the country: carbamazepine, phenobarbital, phenytoin sodium, sodium valproate, amitriptyline, chlorpromazine, diazepam, haloperidol, lithium.

Other Information

Additional Sources of Information

Croatia

GENERAL INFORMATION

Croatia is a country with an approximate area of 57 thousand sq. km. (UNO, 2001). Its population is 4.416 million, and the sex ratio (men per hundred women) is 93 (UNO, 2004). The proportion of population under the age of 15 years is 17% (UNO, 2004), and the proportion of population above the age of 60 years is 22% (WHO, 2004). The literacy rate is 99.3% for men and 97.1% for women (UNESCO/MoH, 2004).

The country is a higher middle income group country (based on World Bank 2004 criteria). The proportion of health budget to GDP is 9%. The per capita total expenditure on health is 726 international $, and the per capita government expenditure on health is 593 international $ (WHO, 2004).

The main language(s) used in the country is (are) Croatian. The largest ethnic group(s) is (are) Croatian (nine-tenths), and the other ethnic group(s) are (is) Serb. The largest religious group(s) is (are) Roman Catholic.

The life expectancy at birth is 71 years for males and 78.6 years for females (WHO, 2004). The healthy life expectancy at birth is 64 years for males and 69 years for females (WHO, 2004).

C–D

EPIDEMIOLOGY

Kozaric-Kovacic et al (2001) used the CAGE and Watson's Posttraumatic Stress Disorder (PTSD) Questionnaire to interview more than 350 displaced men and women. They found that PTSD (50.3% men, 36.5% women), alcohol dependence (60.5% men, 8.1% women) and comorbid alcohol dependence and PTSD (69.6% men, 11.7% women) were common. Comorbidity of alcohol dependence and PTSD in women was influenced by pre-war alcohol-related problems. Sakoman (2000) reviewed data from various registers and found that the number of patients with dependence on illicit drug (mostly heroin) increased from 1.0 per thousand population in 1991 to 2.7 in 1999. Kozumplik et al (2001) interviewed 582 school students and found that 23% had used drugs or alcohol (15.5% cigarettes, 3.3% alcohol and 2.6% drugs) and 17.9% used them periodically or continuously. Males and those with family or academic problems used drugs more often. Folnegovic et al (1990) found that the hospital based annual incidence rates (proxy variable for population rates) for schizophrenia ranged from 0.21 to 0.22 per 1000 population (0.26-0.29 per 1000 population aged over 15). Folnegovic et al (1992) found variable prevalence rates with a constant incidence rate of schizophrenia across various population groups in Croatia. Lemkau et al (1980) noted regional variation in the rate of psychoses in a representative community sample. Psychoses were more common in older age groups. Mollica et al (1999) interviewed 534 adults from a refugee camp using culturally validated measures for depression and posttraumatic stress disorder (PTSD) including the Hopkins Symptom Checklist 25, the Harvard Trauma Questionnaire and the Medical Outcomes Study Short-Form 20. Approximately 39.2% and 26.3% had a DSM-IV diagnosis of depression and PTSD, respectively. A total of 25.5% reported having a disability. Comorbidity (20.6%), older age, cumulative trauma and chronic medical illness were also associated with disability. In a follow-up study conducted after 3 years, Mollica et al (2001) found that almost 45% of the ill group continued to have these disorders and disability and another 16% developed depression or PTSD. Bosnar et al (2002) found that the suicide rate had increased from 16.2 to 19.1 per 100 000 population in the period between 1986-90 (pre-war period) and 1991-95 (war and post-war period). An increase in rate was noted particularly among those below 40 years and men. A fourfold increase in the use of firearms was also noted. Grubisic-Ilic et al (2002) examined 5349 suicides committed in the period 1993-1998. The suicide rate was significantly lower in the areas directly affected by war than in other areas. In war affected areas the number of suicides declined (more significantly in men). Suicide risk was higher in middle- and old-aged people in both areas. Firearms or explosive devices were used significantly more often in the areas directly affected by war, whereas hanging was significantly more frequent in other areas. Catipovic (2001) found that nearly 23.4% of suicides were committed by psychiatric patients (alcohol use disorders: 28.4%, depression: 25.4%, schizophrenia: 13.6%, personality disorders: 13.6% and neurosis: 11.9%). Males, single patients and those with physical comorbidity were significantly more likely and those with children less likely to commit suicide in the post-war period. Medical records of almost one third of the patients showed previous suicide attempts. Rudan et al (2002) found that the prevalence of learning disability (defined as the inability to attend the public school system which is mandatory in Croatia) ranged from 0.43% to 2.47% in isolate populations and that the prevalence was related to inbreeding. Hecimovic et al (2002) reported a rate of 3.5% for Fragile-X syndrome in a population of mentally retarded children attending a special school in Croatia (n=114) who were examined by molecular screening methods. In a study done on children injured during the war (n=322) using a structured interview in a clinical setting, Kocijan-Hercigonja (1996) found that PTSD correlated significantly with the degree of disability, social circumstances (displacement) and family situation (one or both parents killed).

MENTAL HEALTH RESOURCES

Mental Health Policy A mental health policy is absent.

A draft of the mental health policy and of the action plan was prepared in 2003. The Health Care Act of 2003 established the Croatian Mental Health Institute that has the responsibility of formalizing mental health policy and plans. The intention of health system is to rely on well-developed primary health care.

Substance Abuse Policy A substance abuse policy is present. The policy was initially formulated in 1996. The Commission for Narcotics is a permanent Government body, comprising representatives of health, education and social welfare authorities. A strategy on prevention of drug abuse has been accepted by the Croatian Parliament.

National Mental Health Programme A national mental health programme is absent.

A national mental health programme is in development. Several programmes that contain mental health elements are ongoing. An action plan for the implementation of a prevention programme on alcohol abuse was prepared by the Ministry of Health according to WHO guidelines in 2003.

National Therapeutic Drug Policy/Essential List of Drugs A national therapeutic drug policy/essential list of drugs is present. It was formulated in 2000.

Mental Health Legislation The Protection of the Rights of People with Mental Disorders Act has been approved by the Croatian Parliament in 1997 and revised in 1999. It defines the rights of people with mental disorders to protection and care, and to equality in health services. The law requires the use of the least restrictive alternative. Compulsory hospitalization is subject to court supervision. The law specifically prohibits discrimination of mental health patients concerning housing and employment. The Social Welfare Act includes provisions on vocational rehabilitation, employment consultation, and supported housing. Other relevant legislations are the Family Act (which protects the rights of family members without the means to support themselves) and the Family Violence Protection Act. National legislation restricts access to alcohol, nicotine and drugs.
The latest legislation was enacted in 1997.

Mental Health Financing There are budget allocations for mental health.
Details about expenditure on mental health are not available.
The primary sources of mental health financing in descending order are social insurance and tax based.
According to legal regulations in force since 2002, health insurance may be basic, supplementary and private. The basic health insurance is compulsory. The basic insurance is provided by CHII, while the additional may be provided by either CHII or other insurance companies. Within private insurance the CHII beneficiaries may insure themselves for other rights not included in the basic health insurance. All mental services for persons suffering from chronic mental disorders remain fully covered by obligatory insurance. The share of the private spending is estimated to be about 20%. All major classes of psychoactive drugs are covered by the obligatory health insurance. When co-payment exists, holders of supplementary health insurance are exempted from it. Chronic mentally ill patients are exempted from co-payment. Overall spending on psychoactive drugs was for a prolonged period among the top three therapeutic classes by spending. In 2002, it was the first therapeutic class by spending, because of inclusion of several novel drugs on the essential list.
The country has disability benefits for persons with mental disorders. Mental illness has the same status as other disabilities, i.e. compensations policy is regulated in a by-law regulating the issue of disabilities.

Mental Health Facilities Mental health is a part of primary health care system. Actual treatment of severe mental disorders is available at the primary level. The most numerous health care institutions owned by the state or counties, including the City of Zagreb, in Croatia are primary health care centres – amounting to 123. At present, mental health services are not uniformly provided at primary health care level. However, the new legislation defines creation of mental health units in primary health care centres.
Regular training of primary care professionals is carried out in the field of mental health. Training programmes to enable professionals to deal with trauma victims have also been held on a regular basis.
There are community care facilities for patients with mental disorders. A certain number of chronic patients is settled in institutions of social welfare system. Though these institutions are not formally dedicated for chronically ill mental patients, some institutions' capacities are almost entirely used for chronically mentally ill. In addition, some capacities of retirement homes are also used to treat mentally ill patients.

Psychiatric Beds and Professionals

Total psychiatric beds per 10 000 population	10.06
Psychiatric beds in mental hospitals per 10 000 population	8.02
Psychiatric beds in general hospitals per 10 000 population	0.98
Psychiatric beds in other settings per 10 000 population	1.06
Number of psychiatrists per 100 000 population	8.7
Number of neurosurgeons per 100 000 population	1.13
Number of psychiatric nurses per 100 000 population	
Number of neurologists per 100 000 population	3.76
Number of psychologists per 100 000 population	
Number of social workers per 100 000 population	

The number of psychiatrists has increased in the past decade by more than 50%. Social workers and clinical psychologists are present in all major psychiatric wards and hospitals. In Croatia, a considerable decrease (one quarter) in the total number of hospital beds took place between 1990 and 1996. However, large mental hospitals still represent the major share in overall inpatient capacities (four-fifths). Capacities for acute psychiatric care are present in 17 out of 23 general hospitals. About 50 beds are available for children and adolescents, but adolescents are also admitted to beds meant for adults. Specialization in child and adolescent psychiatry has been recognized by the Ministry since 1994. In paediatric clinics, mental health consultations are generally performed by psychologists.

Non-Governmental Organizations NGOs are involved with mental health in the country. They are mainly involved in advocacy, promotion and prevention. The Ministry of Health, is regularly co-operating with and sponsoring activities of various NGOs dealing with mental health programmes, including those of service providers and consumers. However, the number of NGOs is small, especially those of users.

Information Gathering System There is mental health reporting system in the country. Health morbidity and mortality data (including mental health) are regularly collected and analysed by the Croatian Institute of Public Health. The same institution maintains the Register of Psychoses that is operational since 1956. Mental health mortality accounts for 0.93% of total deaths in 2002. SDR from suicide and self-inflicted injuries in all ages was 17.38 per 100 000 and from selected alcohol related causes was reported 95.9 per 100 000. Among mental disorders, the most common disorders diagnosed in primary health care were neurotic/ stress and somatoform disorders, schizophrenia, alcohol related disorders, dementia, psychoactive substances abuse and mental retardation. There is a rise in incidence of alcohol and illegal drug use. Alcohol psychosis incidence per 100 000 is 23.41 in 2001.
The country has data collection system or epidemiological study on mental health.
The National Public Health Institute maintains a register on psychoses.

Programmes for Special Population The country has specific programmes for mental health for refugees, disaster affected population, elderly and children. Information about services for minorities and indigenous people are not known.
The country has specific programmes for substance dependencies and victims of war traumas. Child and adolescent mental health services are available in most cities, with two centres having day-treatment programmes. The social welfare system provides foster homes for abandoned and abused children and retirement homes for elderly.

Therapeutic Drugs The following therapeutic drugs are generally available at the primary health care level of the country: carbamazepine, ethosuximide, phenobarbital, phenytoin sodium, sodium valproate, amitriptyline, diazepam, fluphenazine, haloperidol, lithium, biperiden, carbidopa, levodopa.
The drug list is revised every year by the Croatian Health Insurance Institute.

Other Information Recent changes in health legislation will contribute to mental health awareness, to the development of community-based services in mental health and to enhancing cooperation between different sectors.

Additional Sources of Information

Bosanac, S.B. (2002) Involuntary hospitalisation and the rights of mental patients in recent Croatian legislation. Medicine and Law, 21, 87-106.

Bosnar, A., Stemberg, V., Zamolo, G., et al (2002) Increased suicide rate before and during the war in southwestern Croatia. Archives of Medical Research, 33, 301-304.

Catipovic, V. (2001) Suicide of psychiatrically treated patients in the bjelovar-bilogora county during the 1989-1999 period. Socijalna Psihijatrija, 29, 76-86.

Central Bureau of Statistics. Statistical information 2003. Zagreb: Central Bureau of Statistics. 2003.

Croatian Institute for Public Health. Croatian Health – Statistical Bulletin 2002. Croatian Institute for Public Health. 2003.

Folnegovic, Z., Folnegovic-Smalc, V. (1992) Schizophrenia in Croatia: interregional differences in prevalence and a comment on constant incidence. Journal of Epidemiology & Community Health, 46, 248-255.

Folnegovic, Z., Folnegovic-Smalc, V., Kulcar, Z. (1990) The incidence of schizophrenia in Croatia. British Journal of Psychiatry, 156, 363-365.

Grubisic-Ilic, M., Kozaric-Kovacic, D., Grubisic, F., et al (2002) Epidemiological study of suicide in the Republic of Croatia -- comparison of war and post-war periods and areas directly and indirectly affected by war. European Psychiatry: the Journal of the Association of European Psychiatrists, 17, 259-264.

Hecimovic, S., Petek Tarnik, I., Baric, I., et al (2002) Screening for Fragile X syndrome: Results from a school for mentally retarded children. Acta Paediatrica, 91, 535-539.

Kocijan-Hercigonja, D., Rijavec, M., Jones, W. P., et al (1996) Psychologic problems of children wounded during the war in Croatia. Nordic Journal of Psychiatry, 50, 451-456.

Kozaric-Kovacic D., Ljubin T., Grappe M. (2000) Comorbidity of posttraumatic stress disorder and alcohol dependence in displaced persons. Croatian Medical Journal, 41, 173-178.

Kozumplik, O., Cavlek, T., Jukic, V., et al (2001) Attitude towards addictive substances among the eighth-grade primary school students in Zagreb. Socijalna Psihijatrija, 29, 206-211.

Lemkau, P. V., Kulcar, Z., Kesic, B., et al (1980) Selected aspects of the epidemiology of psychoses in Croatia, Yugoslavia. IV. Representative sample of Croatia and results of the survey. American Journal of Epidemiology, 112, 661-674.

Mollica, R. F., McInnes, K., Sarajlic, N., et al (1999) Disability associated with psychiatric comorbidity and health status in Bosnian refugees living in Croatia. JAMA, 282, 433-439.

Mollica, R. F., Sarajlic, N., Chernoff, M., et al (2001) Longitudinal study of psychiatric symptoms, disability, mortality, and emigration among Bosnian refugees. JAMA, 286, 546-554.

Nikolic, S., Rudan, V., Vidovic, V. (1999) Child and adolescent psychiatry in Croatia. In: H. Remschmidt, H. van Engeland, H. (Eds). Child and Adolescent Psychiatry in Europe. Historical Development, Current Situation and Future Perspectives. Darmstadt, Steinkopff. pp41-54.

Rudan, I., Rudan, D., Campbell, H., et al (2002) Inbreeding and learning disability in Croatian island isolates. Collegium Antropologicum, 26, 421-428.

Sakoman, S. (2000) Substance abuse in the Republic of Croatia and National Program for Drug Control. Croatian Medical Journal, 41, 270-286.

The Health Care Act. Zagreb, Public Gazette, 2003.

The Health Protection Act. Zagreb, Public Gazette, 2003.

The Penal Act. Zagreb, Public Gazette, 110/97.

The Penal Procedure Act. Zagreb, Public Gazette, 110/97.

The Protection of the Rights of People with Mental Disorders Act. Zagreb, Public Gazzette, 111/97; 128/99.

The Social Welfare Act. Zagreb, Public Gazette, 1997.

Cuba

GENERAL INFORMATION

Cuba is a country with an approximate area of 111 thousand sq. km. (UNO, 2001). Its population is 11.328 million, and the sex ratio (men per hundred women) is 100 (UNO, 2004). The proportion of population under the age of 15 years is 19% (UNO, 2004), and the proportion of population above the age of 60 years is 14% (WHO, 2004). The literacy rate is 97% for men and 96.8% for women (UNESCO/MoH, 2004).
The country is a lower middle income group country (based on World Bank 2004 criteria). The proportion of health budget to GDP is 7.2%. The per capita total expenditure on health is 229 international $, and the per capita government expenditure on health is 198 international $ (WHO, 2004).
The main language(s) used in the country is (are) Spanish. The largest ethnic group(s) is (are) European (Spanish descent) and African (descent), and the other ethnic group(s) are (is) Asian and racially-mixed. The largest religious group(s) is (are) Roman Catholic (five-sixths), and the other religious group(s) are (is) Protestant, other Christian and traditional African (e.g. Yoruba).
The life expectancy at birth is 75 years for males and 79.3 years for females (WHO, 2004). The healthy life expectancy at birth is 67 years for males and 70 years for females (WHO, 2004).

EPIDEMIOLOGY

Libre et al (1999) interviewed a representative sample of almost 1140 people aged over 60 years from two regions using a two stage sampling technique. DSM-III-R and NINCDS-ADRDA criteria were used for the diagnosis of dementia. The authors found dementia in 8.2% of subjects, with rates of Alzheimer's disease and vascular type dementia being 5.1% and 1.9% respectively. Dementia was associated with older age, female sex and absence of spouse (due to widowhood or being single). De la Rosa et al (1998) used data from a natural survey of Cuban adult population to assess patterns of alcohol use. While 45.2% of the respondents reported themselves as drinkers, the overall prevalence of alcohol dependence in the population above 15 years was 8.8%. Higher prevalence rates were reported in the eastern areas and for men and older age groups. Smoking is significantly associated with heavy drinking. Data from the State Registry of Health suggest that in 1981 the rate of suicide for all ages was 21.7 per 100 000 population, which decreased in the year 2002 to 14.1 per 100 000. The rate of suicide was associated with age (elderly), gender (men), locality (rural). Regional variation was noted (MOH, 2004). Masso and Leon (1998) reported a retrospective case control study on suicide attempts in patients over 15 years of age. Suicide attempts were commoner in females, the age group between 15-25 years, housewife or unemployed category and in families that were incomplete/dysfunctional and less common in those who had stable partners. Reynaldo et al (2002) used psychometric tests and semi-structured interviews to assess the prevalence of psychiatric disorders in 150 patients with spinocerebellar disease type 2. They found that 88% manifested symptoms related to mental disorders which included – disorders involving adaptation, sleep, mood and sexual disorders. Mental retardation and dementia were also diagnosed.

MENTAL HEALTH RESOURCES

Mental Health Policy A mental health policy is present. The policy was initially formulated in 1986.
The components of the policy are advocacy, promotion, prevention, treatment and rehabilitation. It was revised in 2002 through a process that involved mental health professionals, civil servants and consumers. There are regular funds for its implementation. Between 85 to 90% of its original content has been put into practice.

Substance Abuse Policy A substance abuse policy is present. The policy was initially formulated in 2000. It has a specific budget for its implementation that follows the principles of decentralization of resources, and it has been implemented to the extent of 50 to 75%. A specific law on substance abuse is currently not in place, but the issues are discussed in various laws and statutes on general health.

National Mental Health Programme A national mental health programme is present. The programme was formulated in 1997. It was revised in 2001. There is to specific budget for its implementation, and it has been implemented to the extent of 85 to 90% by local, regional and national authorities. Its main components are strategy of services reform, promotion and prevention, integration of mental health services, health services in primary care and development of specialized services and community care.

National Therapeutic Drug Policy/Essential List of Drugs A national therapeutic drug policy/essential list of drugs is present. It was formulated in 1960.
Due to US sanctions and its pre-eminence in the pharmaceutical industry, nearly half of the new drugs on the market are not available in Cuba.

Mental Health Legislation The funds for the implementation are decentralized (provided by each province by its local Government). It has been implemented to the extent of over 90%. It focuses on human rights, regulation of mental health services, regulation of involuntary treatment, but it does not makes reference to advocacy, housing and regulation of mental health services. The latest legislation was enacted in 1997.

Mental Health Financing There are no budget allocations for mental health.
The country spends 5% of the total health budget on mental health.
The primary source of mental health financing is tax based.
Cuban constitution makes health care a right of every citizen and the responsibility of the Government. The national health care provides free preventive, curative and rehabilitation services. Medication and medical aids are charged for, but the prices are low and subsidized. Services are financed 80% by the Ministry of Health and 20% by Social Security from the Ministry of Labor. In the Cuban system, no other form of financing applies.
The country has disability benefits for persons with mental disorders. More than 90% of the eligible persons actually receive the benefits. It is not the type of mental disorder, but the associated impairment that is considered when a person is evaluated for disability benefits. The family doctor or the psychiatrist is in charge of evaluation for less than 6 months periods. Above that, a national expert within the Ministry of Labor and Social Security and Ministry of Health (health and mental health experts) makes the decision.

Mental Health Facilities Mental health is a part of primary health care system. Actual treatment of severe mental disorders is available at the primary level. Cuba has developed a system that prioritizes primary and preventive care. More than 75% of the population is covered by this kind of service. Mental health care is provided by primary health care physicians and psychiatrists. A system of referral is in place.
Regular training of primary care professionals is carried out in the field of mental health. In the last two years, about 120 personnel were provided training. The country has one doctor for just over 200 persons, the world's highest doctor-patient ratio. This makes the integration of mental health in primary care a little easier. Each year between 4 and 5% of primary care personnel from a wide range of disciplines receive training.
There are community care facilities for patients with mental disorders. The community care system for the mentally ill provides coverage for more than 75% of the treated population. Emphasis is made on preventive/promotion interventions, home interventions, family interventions and residential facilities. Vocational training and employment programmes are included. Each of the 14 regions have a 20-30 bedded psychiatric unit, attached to the general hospital. These centres are responsible for comprehensive mental health care including social rehabilitation. There are sheltered rehabilitation centres which are located near the place of employment of the patients. These are managed by a male nurse, an occupational therapist and a work instructor. There are different sheltered rehabilitation centres based on the occupational profile, sex and community location of the patient.

Psychiatric Beds and Professionals

Total psychiatric beds per 10 000 population	7.36
Psychiatric beds in mental hospitals per 10 000 population	5.72
Psychiatric beds in general hospitals per 10 000 population	1.54
Psychiatric beds in other settings per 10 000 population	1
Number of psychiatrists per 100 000 population	10
Number of neurosurgeons per 100 000 population	2.3
Number of psychiatric nurses per 100 000 population	2.7
Number of neurologists per 100 000 population	
Number of psychologists per 100 000 population	9
Number of social workers per 100 000 population	12

There are 1328 occupational therapists, logopedia and psychometrics. About 100 psychiatric beds are available in a private psychiatric hospital. Almost 15% of mental health beds are occupied by long stay patients. Specified beds for care of forensic psychiatry patients, patients with drug abuse exist. There are 200 child psychiatrists.

Non-Governmental Organizations NGOs are involved with mental health in the country. They are mainly involved in advocacy, promotion, prevention, treatment and rehabilitation.

Information Gathering System There is mental health reporting system in the country. ICD-10 system is used. The mental health components reported are morbidity, admission and discharge, suicide attempts and suicide, among others.
The country has data collection system or epidemiological study on mental health. The Department of Health System Statistics and the Health Tendencies Analysis Units is in charge of the data collection.

Programmes for Special Population The country has specific programmes for mental health for disaster affected population, elderly and children. There are no ethnic minorities, indigenous people or refugees for whom special mental health facilities should be present.
Also, there are programmes for women, victims of domestic violence, suicide, substance use problems, and social rehabilitation and reintegration of patients.

Therapeutic Drugs The following therapeutic drugs are generally available at the primary health care level of the country: carbamazepine, phenobarbital, sodium valproate, amitriptyline, chlorpromazine, diazepam, fluphenazine, haloperidol, lithium.
The national therapeutic drug policy was revised in 2001, and the essential drug list was released in 2001. Medicines are free for patients with chronic illnesses and for those entitled to public invalidity benefits. Others pay subsidized prices.

Other Information Mental health is integrated in one programme and several sub-programmes, all administered by the National Commission of Mental Health and the groups of psychiatry, child psychiatry and psychology and are present at the provincial level with a town hall person responsible. Psychiatry is being reoriented towards primary health care.
The country provides health tourism service through primary care in the form of physicians at hotels and international clinics, secondary care in clinics and hospitals offering specialized medical care, and a large number of medicines and medical aids. Among these clinics there are some that specialize in the management of drug and alcohol misuse and degenerative and neurological conditions. The health tourism industry also offers centres to improve the quality of life. These include thermal centres etc. where tourists can receive procedures that aid in stress control, sleep problems etc. The majority of health tourists are from Spanish-speaking countries, but the number from North America is increasing.

Additional Sources of Information

Collinson, S. R., Turner, T. H. (2002) Not just salsa and cigars: mental health care in Cuba. Psychiatric Bulletin, 26, 185-188.

De la Rosa, M. C., Canizares, P. M., Sandoval Ferrer, J. E., et al (1 A.D.) (1998) Characteristics of alcoholic consumption in the Cuban population. Revista del Hospital Psiquiatrico de la Habana, 39, 257-263.

Llibre, J.J., Guerra, M.A., Perez-Cruz, H., et al (1999) Dementia syndrome and risk factors in adults aged over 60 residing in La Habana. Revista de Neurologia, 29, 908-911.

Masso, A. S., Leon, C. P. (1 A.D.) (1998) Suicidal attempt psychosocials aspects in an area of health in Santiago de Cuba. Revista del Hospital Psiquiatrico de la Habana, 39, 160-163.

Ordaz, E. (1993) The Cuba Experience. Nursing RSA Verpleging, 8, 19-21, 44.

Reynaldo, A., Reynaldo-Hernandez, R., Paneque-Herrera, M., et al (2002) Mental disorders in patients with spinocerebellar ataxia type 2 in Cuba. Revista de Neurologia, 35, 818-821.

Cyprus

GENERAL INFORMATION

Cyprus is a country with an approximate area of 9 thousand sq. km. (UNO, 2001). Its population is 0.807 million, and the sex ratio (men per hundred women) is 100 (UNO, 2004). The proportion of population under the age of 15 years is 21% (UNO, 2004), and the proportion of population above the age of 60 years is 16% (WHO, 2004). The literacy rate is 98.6% for men and 95.1% for women (UNESCO/MoH, 2004).

The country is a high income group country (based on World Bank 2004 criteria). The proportion of health budget to GDP is 8.1%. The per capita total expenditure on health is 941 international $, and the per capita government expenditure on health is 449 international $ (WHO, 2004).

The main language(s) used in the country is (are) Greek, Turkish and English. The largest ethnic group(s) is (are) Greek, and the other ethnic group(s) are (is) Turkish. The largest religious group(s) is (are) Greek Orthodox Christian (four-fifths), and the other religious group(s) are (is) Sunni Muslim.

The life expectancy at birth is 75.5 years for males and 79.1 years for females (WHO, 2004). The healthy life expectancy at birth is 67 years for males and 68 years for females (WHO, 2004).

C–D

EPIDEMIOLOGY

There is substantial epidemiological data on mental illnesses in Cyprus in internationally accessible literature. No attempt was made to include this information here.

MENTAL HEALTH RESOURCES

Mental Health Policy A mental health policy is present. The policy was initially formulated in 1985.

The components of the policy are advocacy, promotion, prevention, treatment and rehabilitation. The mental health policy is concerned with updating legislation according to European standards, integrating mental health with community care and improving the living conditions of patients in the mental hospital in Nicosia.

Substance Abuse Policy A substance abuse policy is present. The policy was initially formulated in 1978.

National Mental Health Programme A national mental health programme is present. The programme was formulated in 1995.

National Therapeutic Drug Policy/Essential List of Drugs A national therapeutic drug policy/essential list of drugs is present. It was formulated in 1995.

Mental Health Legislation Cyprus has a Mental Health Act. The new law covers treatment, admission and care of the mentally ill. Human rights issues are also covered. Under this law, the mental hospital can admit voluntary patients, too. A new legislation envisaging a national anti-drug committee is under discussion in the parliament.

The latest legislation was enacted in 1997.

Mental Health Financing There are budget allocations for mental health.

The country spends 7% of the total health budget on mental health.

The primary sources of mental health financing in descending order are tax based, out of pocket expenditure by the patient or family, social insurance and grants.

The country has disability benefits for persons with mental disorders.

Mental Health Facilities Mental health is a part of primary health care system. Actual treatment of severe mental disorders is available at the primary level. There is an ongoing cooperation of the community psychiatrists with general practitioners, and there are regular workshops with the participation of WHO experts.

Regular training of primary care professionals is carried out in the field of mental health. In the last two years, about 60 personnel were provided training. Mental health services offer a three month training course for doctors trained as general practitioners.

There are community care facilities for patients with mental disorders. Community psychiatric nurses are present in all regions. In addition to regular services, they make home visits and provide crisis intervention. Nicosia has an Information and Counselling centre for drug abusers. Day care centres are available in 3 regions. These are run in cooperation with NGOs. A group home for 4 half-way patients and 3 hostels for ex-patients are available.

Psychiatric Beds and Professionals

Total psychiatric beds per 10 000 population	5.2
Psychiatric beds in mental hospitals per 10 000 population	4.5
Psychiatric beds in general hospitals per 10 000 population	0.6
Psychiatric beds in other settings per 10 000 population	0
Number of psychiatrists per 100 000 population	5
Number of neurosurgeons per 100 000 population	1.3
Number of psychiatric nurses per 100 000 population	45
Number of neurologists per 100 000 population	2.6
Number of psychologists per 100 000 population	19.3
Number of social workers per 100 000 population	25

Besides the mental hospital at Nicosia there are other psychiatric units and specialized units like the child psychiatry centres, detoxification centres, psychiatric units for geriatrics, mentally retarded, community centres, etc. Ongoing training has increased. Personnel are being trained locally and abroad in psychotherapy and other interventions. Workshops on research methodology are held.

Non-Governmental Organizations NGOs are involved with mental health in the country. They are mainly involved in promotion, prevention and rehabilitation.

Information Gathering System There is mental health reporting system in the country.
The country has no data collection system or epidemiological study on mental health. WHO support is being sought to develop a system.

Programmes for Special Population The country has specific programmes for mental health for minorities, refugees, disaster affected population, elderly and children.

Therapeutic Drugs The following therapeutic drugs are generally available at the primary health care level of the country: carbamazepine, phenobarbital, phenytoin sodium, sodium valproate, amitriptyline, chlorpromazine, diazepam, fluphenazine, haloperidol, lithium, biperiden, carbidopa, levodopa.

Other Information The National Five-Year Plan proposes to divide the country into five administrative sectors with each having their own mental health centre with most facilities for rehabilitation. Non-governmental organizations, church, other health services, local authorities and other interested bodies will help. Consultants from UNHCR have proposed that a bi-communal mental health services programme for the Greeks and Turks would help persons from both communities to share resources and professional expertise.

Additional Sources of Information

Annual Report (1999) Mental Health Services.

Sundel, M. (1996) Designing mental health services to improve ethnic relations. World Future, 47, 15-23.

Czech Republic

GENERAL INFORMATION

Czech Republic is a country with an approximate area of 79 thousand sq. km. (UNO, 2001). Its population is 10.226 million, and the sex ratio (men per hundred women) is 95 (UNO, 2004). The proportion of population under the age of 15 years is 15% (UNO, 2004), and the proportion of population above the age of 60 years is 19% (WHO, 2004). The literacy rate is 99% for men and 99% for women (UNESCO/MoH, 2004).

The country is a higher middle income group country (based on World Bank 2004 criteria). The proportion of health budget to GDP is 7.4%. The per capita total expenditure on health is 1129 international $, and the per capita government expenditure on health is 1031 international $ (WHO, 2004).

The main language(s) used in the country is (are) Czech. The largest ethnic group(s) is (are) Czech (four-fifths), and the other ethnic group(s) are (is) Slovak. The largest religious group(s) is (are) those without religious affiliation, and the other religious group(s) are (is) Roman Catholic.

The life expectancy at birth is 72.4 years for males and 79 years for females (WHO, 2004). The healthy life expectancy at birth is 66 years for males and 71 years for females (WHO, 2004).

EPIDEMIOLOGY

Dragomirecka et al (2002) assessed 1534 subjects aged 18 to 79 years using the Composite International Diagnostic Interview (CIDI). At least one mental disorder was detected in almost 27% of respondents (30% of women). The most frequently reported mental disorders were: neurotic disorders (18%), alcohol and tobacco use disorders (13%) and affective disorders (13%). Baudis et al (2002) reported findings on comorbidity from the same study. Lifetime comorbidity was found in 10.5% of respondents (8.6% men and 12.2% women) and 1-year comorbidity was found in 5.2% of the sample (5.0% men and 5.6% women). A significant association existed for the following sets of disorders: alcohol and tobacco use disorders, tobacco use disorders and affective disorders (mainly depression) and between affective disorders and neurotic disorders. Alcohol use disorders were correlated with all other groups of mental disorders in women. Psychiatric comorbidity was significantly associated with age and number of years of education. Koukolik (1996) reported a prevalence rate of 7.5% for Alzheimer's disease based on 2197 autopsies on patients aged 65 years and above. Beckova et al (1999) investigated drug use in over 550 university students. The most frequently used drug was marijuana (26.6%). Data from 142 treatment centres across the country showed that the commonest drugs being used were methamphetamine, heroin, marijuana and toluene. One-third of users were in the 15-19-year age group. Regional differences in prevalence and drug preferences and a trend towards an increase in intravenous drug was also noted (Polanecky et al, 1996). The current figure for drug misuse in the 15-39 years age range is 10.37/1000 (Polanecky et al, 2004). Sejda et al (1998) also reported that there was a gradual decrease in the average age of use and problematic use, especially in women. Consequently, the most affected age group was 15-19 years old and the male to female ratio stood at 2:1. Kubicka et al (1995) found an increase in alcohol use among 608 women interviewed twice in 1987 and 1992. Rate of heavy drinking increased from 7.2% to 14.0% and self-employed and independent women showed a greater increase in alcohol use. Topinkova and Neuwirth (1997) interviewed 1162 long-term residential elderly patients and found the prevalence of depression to be 47.7% (nearly 70% of the depressed individuals were more than 75 years old). Poor cognitive ability and physical disability was associated with depression. Jablensky et al (1992) discussed the results of the WHO Collaborative Study on the Determinants of Outcome of Severe Mental Disorders (DOS) in which Prague was one of the centers. The study showed that schizophrenia has similar incidence in different cultures but the outcomes were better in developing countries. In a six-country study in Europe, Wiersma et al (2000) assessed patients with schizophrenia at 1, 2 and 15 years intervals after the initial contact using the WHO Disability Assessment Schedule. Almost 83% of subjects had disability and 24% suffered from severe disability. A deteriorating course was more frequent than late improvement. Severity of disability at the first three assessments of the illness contributed significantly to the explanation of its variance at 15 years. In a study conducted on 981 adolescents, using standardized tools, bulimia nervosa (DSM-IV) was reported in 5.7% women with another 15% being at risk. None of the males met the criteria for eating disorders (Krch & Drabkova, 1996). Horazd'ovsky (1993) found a decline in the rate of suicides during 1975-1990 in a study based on statistical registers. Kvasnicova et al (1992) examined the records of 23 510 children from special schools and social care institutes and identified 510 with mental retardation (prevalence 2.2%). The prevalence of mental retardation was much higher in Gypsy children. Out of the 106 children in whom genetic analysis was done, 31.1% showed an evidence of chromosomal abnormality and a non-genetic etiology was found in 19.8%. The mean incidence of Down syndrome was 7.91 per 10 000 liveborn infants during 1961-1997 (Sipek et al, 1999). Gebhart et al (1990) screened 5080 children for minimal brain disorder in three districts by interviewing mothers. They found that 14.8% had minimal brain disorder and this was reflected in their poor academic performance.

MENTAL HEALTH RESOURCES

Mental Health Policy A mental health policy is present. The policy was initially formulated in 1953.

The components of the policy are advocacy, promotion, prevention, treatment and rehabilitation. The last amendment was in 2001. The policy in the field of mental health is formulated by the Psychiatric Society of the Czech Medical Association. This policy in the form of a programme document is presented to the Ministry of Health. The goals were published in 1997 and are known as Psychiatric Care in the Czech Republic – Programme Document and Mental Health Care Policy. This programme defines the status of psychiatry in the health care system and underlines requirements and conditions of modern trends in treatment, rehabilitation and social reintegration of mentally ill people.

Substance Abuse Policy A substance abuse policy is present. The policy was initially formulated in 1989. The policy is a part of a law amended in 1989 (Act No. 37/1989).

National Mental Health Programme A national mental health programme is present. The programme was formulated in 1953.

National Therapeutic Drug Policy/Essential List of Drugs A national therapeutic drug policy/essential list of drugs is present. It was formulated in 1997.
The national therapeutic drug policy/essential drug list was formed through the Act No. 48/1997 on Public Health Insurance, which defines 521 groups of pharmaceutical products.

Mental Health Legislation There is no specific law on mental health. The legislative regulation in the field of mental health is covered by the Law on Health Care for the Population (Act No.20/66 Coll.). This act, adopted in 1966, has been changed and amended by a series of health care reform legislation, most recently in 1999. More details can be obtained from the document: Health Care Systems in Transition – Czech Republic. European Observatory on Health Care Systems (WHO, 2000). There is another civil law bill on Involuntary Hospitalisation and Withdrawal of Legal Disposition, but it is yet to be passed.
The latest legislation was enacted in 1966.

Mental Health Financing There are budget allocations for mental health.
The country spends 3% of the total health budget on mental health.
The primary sources of mental health financing in descending order are social insurance, tax based, out of pocket expenditure by the patient or family and private insurances.
The country has disability benefits for persons with mental disorders.

Mental Health Facilities Mental health is a part of primary health care system. Actual treatment of severe mental disorders is available at the primary level. In principle, the primary health care is available for severe mental health disorders, but practically the preferred and common option is to use the services of ambulatory specialists.
Regular training of primary care professionals is carried out in the field of mental health. There are various options of training and education. Mental health care is a part of the training of general practitioners and nurses in primary care.
There are community care facilities for patients with mental disorders. There has been a substantial improvement in the quality of treatment provided in hospitals and also improvement in the living conditions of patients. Despite this positive changes, the current situation in rehabilitation and social reintegration of mentally ill patients is not satisfactory. The current status is partly due to limited financial resources. The costs of treatment are covered by health insurance fund, but for other interventions like social rehabilitation, coverage does not exist. The majority of work in this field is done by various non-governmental organizations and in few places by establishments supported by the churches, but they are unable to meet the demands. However, a number of very promising initiatives in day care (35 centres), sheltered housing, sheltered work and reintegration to the community have been started.

Psychiatric Beds and Professionals

Total psychiatric beds per 10 000 population	11.4
Psychiatric beds in mental hospitals per 10 000 population	9.8
Psychiatric beds in general hospitals per 10 000 population	1.5
Psychiatric beds in other settings per 10 000 population	0.2
Number of psychiatrists per 100 000 population	12.1
Number of neurosurgeons per 100 000 population	1.7
Number of psychiatric nurses per 100 000 population	33
Number of neurologists per 100 000 population	12.7
Number of psychologists per 100 000 population	4.9
Number of social workers per 100 000 population	

The total number of beds in residential facilities has decreased markedly within the last one and a half decade (by approximately one-fourth).

Non-Governmental Organizations NGOs are involved with mental health in the country. They are mainly involved in advocacy, promotion, prevention, treatment and rehabilitation. Sheltered housing is also provided by NGOs.

Information Gathering System There is mental health reporting system in the country. Mental health is reported as a part of the report of the health sector.

The country has data collection system or epidemiological study on mental health. The Institute for Health Information and Statistics is responsible for data collection in the health care sector. The information on psychiatric care are systematically collected and regularly published since 1963.

Programmes for Special Population The country has specific programmes for mental health for minorities, refugees, disaster affected population, elderly and children. There are also programmes for patients with eating disorders.
Development of the community mental health care led to the establishment of the Network of Crisis Services.

Therapeutic Drugs The following therapeutic drugs are generally available at the primary health care level of the country: carbamazepine, ethosuximide, phenobarbital, phenytoin sodium, sodium valproate, amitriptyline, chlorpromazine, diazepam, fluphenazine, haloperidol, lithium, biperiden, carbidopa, levodopa.

Other Information Socio-political changes in 1989 have started a process of rapid transformation of the whole society. The system of health care underwent a fundamental reform which affected the organizational structure of services as well as the system of funding and management. The major elements of the transformed health care system are 1) compulsory health insurance and establishment of health insurance funds; 2) decentralization, diversity and autonomy of service providers; and 3) the supervising and regulating role of the Government in negotiations between health insurance funds and health care providers on coverage and reimbursement issues. In the recent years, there were positive shifts in the attitudes of the public towards mentally ill persons and this continuing process will contribute to destigmatization and easier reintegration of patients to the community.

Additional Sources of Information

Bastecky, J., Boleloucky, Z. (1991) Psychosomatic medicine in Czechoslovakia: history, present state and perspectives. International Journal of Psychsomatics, 38, 63-67.

Baudis, P., Dragomirecka, E., Selepova, P., et al (2002) Comorbidity of psychic disorders. Part II: Results of investigation of the mental state of the population of the Czech Republic. Ceska a Slovenska Psychiatrie, 98, 261-267.

Beckova, I., Machackova, J., Stohr, J., et al (1999) Experience of university students from the eastern Czech region with substances inducing drug addiction, Hygiena, 44, 91-98.

Dragomirecka, E., Baudis, P., Smolova, E., et al (2002) Psychiatric morbidity of the population in the Czech Republic. Ceska a Sslovenska Psychiatrie, 98, 72-80.

European Observatory on Health Care Systems (2000) The Czech Republic. Health Care Systems in Transition. WHO, 2000.

Gebhart, J. A., Dytrych, Z., Tyl, J., et al (1990) Incidence of the minimal brain dysfunction syndrome in children. Ceskoslovenska Psychiatrie, 86, 1-6.

Horazd'ovsky, V. (1993) The suicide rate in Czechoslovakia 1975-1990. Ceskoslovenska Psychiatrie, 89, 233-238.

Jablensky, A., Sartorius, N., Ernberg, G., et al (1992) Schizophrenia manifestations, incidence and course in different cultures. A World Health Organization ten-country study. Psychological Medicine, 22 (SUPPL. 20), 1-97.

Kramarova, N. (1995) Legal regulations on admission of patients to in-patient care without their consent. Ceskoslovenska Psychiatrie, 91, 26-31.

Koukolik, F. (1996) Epidemiologic autopsy in Alzheimer's disease. Casopis Lekaru Ceskych, 135, 378-381.

Krch, F. D., Drabkova, H. (1996) Prevalence of anorexia nervosa and bulimia nervosa in the population of Czech adolescents. Ceskoslovenska Psychiatrie, 92, 237-247.

Kubicka, L., Csemy, L., Kozeny, J. (1995) Prague women's drinking before and after the 'velvet revolution' of 1989: a longitudinal study. Addiction, 90, 1471-1478.

Kvasnicova, M., Puskailerova, D., Csomoova, E., et al (1992) Genetic mental retardation in the district of Banska Bystrica. Ceskoslovenska Pediatrie, 47, 25-28.

Lorenc, J., Pec, O., Koblic, K., et al (2003) Crisis intervention and crisis services. Ceska.a Slovenska.Psychiatrie, 99, 27-30.

Pec, O., Koblic, K., Lorenc, J., et al (2003) Day clinics with psychotherapeutic care. Ceska.a Slovenska.Psychiatrie, 99, 10-16.

Polanecky, V., Sejda, J., Studnickova, B. (1996) Prevalence study of serious substance abusers in the Czech Republic. Central European Journal of Public Health, 4, 176-184.

Redaktor, V. (1997) Ceska A Slovenska Psychiatrie – Supplementum 2, Rocnik 93, Koncepce Psychiatrickè péce v CR (navrh) – Politika Péce o Dusveni Zdravi.

Sejda, J., Studnickova, B., Polanecky, V. (1998) Trends in the incidence of problematic drug addicts in the Czech Republic, 1995-1996. Central European Journal of Public Health, 6, 18-24.

Sipek, A., Gregor, V., Horacek, J., et al (1999) Down's syndrome in the Czech Republic 1961-1997. Ceska Gynekologie, 64, 173-179.

Student, V. (1995) Psychiatrists, lawyers and shamans in the care of the mentally ill. Ceskoslovenska Psychiatrie, 91, 35-44.

Topinkova, E., Neuwirth, J. (1997) Depressive syndrome in geriatric patients in long-term institutional care. Ceskoslovenska Psychiatrie, 93, 181-188.

Polanecký, V., Studniková, B., Klepetková, M., et al. (2004) Incidence, prevalence, health impact and trends of drug users in treatment. Annual Report CR 2002.

Wiersma, D., Wanderling, J., Dragomirecka, E. et al (2000) Social disability in schizophrenia: its development and prediction over 15 years in incidence cohorts in six European centres. Psychological Medicine, 30, 1155-1167.

Zdravotnicka rocenka Ceské republiky 1997 [Czech Health Statistics Yearbook 1997] (1998). IZIS CR, Praha.

Democratic People's Republic of Korea*

C–D

GENERAL INFORMATION

Democratic People's Republic of Korea is a country with an approximate area of 121 thousand sq. km. (UNO, 2001). Its population is 22.776 million, and the sex ratio (men per hundred women) is 100 (UNO, 2004). The proportion of population under the age of 15 years is 25% (UNO, 2004), and the proportion of population above the age of 60 years is 11% (WHO, 2004). The literacy rate is 99% for men and 99% for women (UNESCO/MoH, 2004).

The country is a low income group country (based on World Bank 2004 criteria). The proportion of health budget to GDP is 2.5%. The per capita total expenditure on health is 44 international $, and the per capita government expenditure on health is 32 international $ (WHO, 2004).

The main language(s) used in the country is (are) Korean. The largest ethnic group(s) is (are) Korean. The largest religious group(s) is (are) Buddhist, and the other religious group(s) are (is) Confucianist.

The life expectancy at birth is 64.4 years for males and 67.1 years for females (WHO, 2004). The healthy life expectancy at birth is 58 years for males and 60 years for females (WHO, 2004).

EPIDEMIOLOGY

There is a paucity of epidemiological data on mental illnesses in Democratic People's Republic of Korea in internationally accessible literature. In a multi-country study, involving Bahrain, Burma, DPR Korea, Egypt, Indonesia, Jordan, Sri Lanka, Thailand and Tunisia, Lamb (1996) assessed the quality of life of the non-institutionalized elderly population. Results showed that there were six profiles or types of disablement: functionally and emotionally healthy, functionally healthy with some depressive symptoms, some strength problems, severely depressed, mobility problems and functionally frail. The very depressed were more likely to be female, younger and single. Functional and emotional limitations were correlated with lower quality of life. Depressed profiles were associated with negative self-assessments of health, lower morale scores and low instrumental social support in terms of available kin. Country-specific patterns of elderly disablement indicate a possible disability transition such that as countries become more developed there may be an increase in the prevalence of disabled elderly. Mackinnon et al (1998) showed that the Center for Epidemiological Studies Depression (CES-D) scale could be used in the North Korean population.

MENTAL HEALTH RESOURCES

Mental Health Policy A mental health policy is present. Details about the year of formulation are not available.
The components of the policy are advocacy, promotion, prevention, treatment and rehabilitation.

Substance Abuse Policy A substance abuse policy is present. Details about the year of formulation are not available.

National Mental Health Programme A national mental health programme is present. Details about the year of formulation of the programme are not available.

National Therapeutic Drug Policy/Essential List of Drugs A national therapeutic drug policy/essential list of drugs is present. Details about the year of formulation are not available.

Mental Health Legislation There is a law on Regulation on Prevention of Mental Diseases.
Details about the year of enactment of the mental health legislation are not available.

Mental Health Financing There are budget allocations for mental health.
Details about expenditure on mental health are not available.
The primary source of mental health financing is tax based.
The country has disability benefits for persons with mental disorders.

Mental Health Facilities Mental health is a part of primary health care system. Actual treatment of severe mental disorders is available at the primary level.
Regular training of primary care professionals is carried out in the field of mental health.
There are community care facilities for patients with mental disorders.

Psychiatric Beds and Professionals

Total psychiatric beds per 10 000 population
Psychiatric beds in mental hospitals per 10 000 population
Psychiatric beds in general hospitals per 10 000 population
Psychiatric beds in other settings per 10 000 population
Number of psychiatrists per 100 000 population
Number of neurosurgeons per 100 000 population
Number of psychiatric nurses per 100 000 population
Number of neurologists per 100 000 population
Number of psychologists per 100 000 population
Number of social workers per 100 000 population

Non-Governmental Organizations NGOs are involved with mental health in the country. They are mainly involved in advocacy, promotion, prevention, treatment and rehabilitation.

Information Gathering System There is mental health reporting system in the country. There are annual mental health related tasks; periodic reports of these are prepared by the Ministry.
The country has data collection system or epidemiological study on mental health.

Programmes for Special Population The country has specific programmes for mental health for disaster affected population, elderly and children.

Therapeutic Drugs The following therapeutic drugs are generally available at the primary health care level of the country: chlorpromazine, diazepam, fluphenazine.

Other Information

* The verification of this country profile is still being awaited from the Ministry of Health of the Democratic People's Republic of Korea.

Additional Sources of Information

Lamb, V. L. (1996) A cross-national study of quality of life factors associated with patterns of elderly disablement. Social Science & Medicine, 42, 363-377.

Mackinnon, A., McCallum, J., Andrews, G., et al (1998) The Center for Epidemiological Studies Depression Scale in older community samples in Indonesia, North Korea, Myanmar, Sri Lanka, and Thailand. Journals of Gerontology Series B-Psychological Sciences & Social Sciences, 53, 343-352.

Democratic Republic of the Congo

GENERAL INFORMATION

Democratic Republic of the Congo is a country with an approximate area of 2345 thousand sq. km. (UNO, 2001). Its population is 54.417 million, and the sex ratio (men per hundred women) is 98 (UNO, 2004). The proportion of population under the age of 15 years is 47% (UNO, 2004), and the proportion of population above the age of 60 years is 4% (WHO, 2004). The literacy rate is 88.9% for men and 77.1% for women (UNESCO/MoH, 2004).

The country is a low income group country (based on World Bank 2004 criteria). The proportion of health budget to GDP is 3.5%. The per capita total expenditure on health is 12 international $, and the per capita government expenditure on health is 5 international $ (WHO, 2004).

The main language(s) used in the country is (are) French. The largest ethnic group(s) is (are) Bantu (the four largest tribes), and the other ethnic group(s) are (is) Mangbetu-Azande and about 350 tribes. The largest religious group(s) is (are) Roman Catholic, and the other religious group(s) are (is) Protestant, Kimbanguist, Muslim, Syncretic and indigenous groups.

The life expectancy at birth is 41 years for males and 46.1 years for females (WHO, 2004). The healthy life expectancy at birth is 35 years for males and 39 years for females (WHO, 2004).

EPIDEMIOLOGY

Chabwine and Mugabwa (2001) reported that mental disorders were common, especially in the urban population and during the active decades of life. Tashala et al (1999) used clinical tests, laboratory tests and epidemiological data to find the cause of a paralysis epidemic in a school population. Results showed that conversion of the somatic type were responsible for most of the cases with environmental factors playing an important role in the spread of the illness. Sebit (1995) estimated the prevalence and course of psychiatric and neuropsychological problems in patients with HIV-I. They found that symptomatic seropositive individuals were more depressed than matched seronegative controls. In another study done on a clinical sample of older (than 55 years) AIDS patients, Ibara et al (2002) found that neuropsychiatric disorders were present in a large proportion (49.7%). Lalive and Zivojinovic (1987) reported that nearly three-quarters of asylum seekers in Zaire had psychological dysfunction. Stanbury et al (1973) reported on issues related to endemic cretinism in the region.

MENTAL HEALTH RESOURCES

Mental Health Policy A mental health policy is present. The policy was initially formulated in 1999.

The components of the policy are advocacy, promotion, prevention, treatment and rehabilitation. Formation is also a component of the policy.

Substance Abuse Policy A substance abuse policy is present. The policy was initially formulated in 2002.

National Mental Health Programme A national mental health programme is present. The programme was formulated in 1999.

National Therapeutic Drug Policy/Essential List of Drugs A national therapeutic drug policy/essential list of drugs is present. It was formulated in 1998.

Mental Health Legislation A draft for a mental health legislation exists at the level of the parliament.

The latest legislation was enacted in 2000.

Mental Health Financing There are no budget allocations for mental health.

Details about expenditure on mental health are not available.

The primary source of mental health financing is out of pocket expenditure by the patient or family.

The cost of psychiatric treatment is considered to be high by the average earning capacity.

The country does not have disability benefits for persons with mental disorders.

Mental Health Facilities Mental health is a part of primary health care system. Actual treatment of severe mental disorders is available at the primary level. Mental health is being included in the primary health care and process charts are being defined for mental disorders.

Regular training of primary care professionals is carried out in the field of mental health. The Government also partially supports some charitable organizations like the Soins de Santé Mentale (SOSAME) that provide mental health services.

There are no community care facilities for patients with mental disorders. There is one mental health care centre.

Psychiatric Beds and Professionals

Total psychiatric beds per 10 000 population	0.17
Psychiatric beds in mental hospitals per 10 000 population	0.15
Psychiatric beds in general hospitals per 10 000 population	0.009
Psychiatric beds in other settings per 10 000 population	0.009
Number of psychiatrists per 100 000 population	0.04
Number of neurosurgeons per 100 000 population	0.004
Number of psychiatric nurses per 100 000 population	0.03
Number of neurologists per 100 000 population	0.04
Number of psychologists per 100 000 population	0.01
Number of social workers per 100 000 population	0.4

One occupational therapist is present.

Non-Governmental Organizations NGOs are involved with mental health in the country. They are mainly involved in advocacy, promotion, prevention and rehabilitation.

Information Gathering System There is no mental health reporting system in the country. Only epilepsy is reported.
The country has no data collection system or epidemiological study on mental health.

Programmes for Special Population The country has specific programmes for mental health for disaster affected population, elderly and children. There is a project for street children and also one for affected population.

Therapeutic Drugs The following therapeutic drugs are generally available at the primary health care level of the country: carbamazepine, phenobarbital, phenytoin sodium, amitriptyline, chlorpromazine, diazepam, haloperidol, levodopa.
The essential list of drugs was revised in 2001. The drugs mentioned are dispensed by the private sector and not by the Government.

Other Information

Additional Sources of Information

Chabwine, J. N., Mubagwa, K. (2001) Mental health problems in a population without a previous modern psychiatric care system. Tropical Doctor, 31, 206-208.

Ibara, J. R., Itoua, C., Gathse, A., et al (2002) Acquired immunodeficiency syndrome in elderly persons in a tropical zone. Apropos of 175 cases in the Congo. Bulletin de la Societe de Pathologie Exotique, 95, 100-102.

Lalive, J., Zivojinovic, S. (1987) Ethno-psychiatric crisis situation: the case of refugees seeking asylum in Black Africa. Annales Médico-Psychologiques, 145, 225-236.

Sebit, M. B. (1995) Neuropsychiatric HIV-1 infection study: in Kenya and Zaire cross-sectional phase I and II. Central African Journal of Medicine, 41, 315-322.

Stanbury, J. B., Delange, F., Ermans, A., et al (1973) The varied manifestations of endemic cretinism. Transactions of the American Clinical & Climatological Association, 85, 6-17.

Tshala, K., Nunga, M., Pukuta, S., et al (1999) Coexistence of mass hysteria, konzo and HTLV-1 virus in the Democratic Republic of the Congo. Médecine Tropicale, 59, 378-382.

Denmark

GENERAL INFORMATION

Denmark is a country with an approximate area of 43 thousand sq. km. (UNO, 2001). The country consists of more than 400 islands, of which about a quarter are inhabited. Its population is 5.375 million, and the sex ratio (men per hundred women) is 98 (UNO, 2004). The proportion of population under the age of 15 years is 19% (UNO, 2004), and the proportion of population above the age of 60 years is 20% (WHO, 2004). The literacy rate is 99% for men and 99% for women (UNESCO/MoH, 2004).
The country is a high income group country (based on World Bank 2004 criteria). The proportion of health budget to GDP is 8.4%. The per capita total expenditure on health is 2503 international $, and the per capita government expenditure on health is 2063 international $ (WHO, 2004).
The main language(s) used in the country is (are) Danish. The largest ethnic group(s) is (are) Scandinavian, and the other ethnic group(s) are (is) Inuit, Faeroese and German. The largest religious group(s) is (are) Lutheran Christian.
The life expectancy at birth is 74.8 years for males and 79.5 years for females (WHO, 2004). The healthy life expectancy at birth is 69 years for males and 71 years for females (WHO, 2004).

EPIDEMIOLOGY

There is substantial epidemiological data on mental illnesses in Denmark in internationally accessible literature. No attempt was made to include this information here.

MENTAL HEALTH RESOURCES

Mental Health Policy A mental health policy is present. The policy was initially formulated in 1991.
The components of the policy are prevention, treatment and rehabilitation. Since 1991, the policy has been implemented through three consecutive 3-year-period agreements between the Government and the counties dealing with priorities and agreements of financing. The Government makes an annual report concerning psychiatric facts and status.

Substance Abuse Policy A substance abuse policy is present. The policy was initially formulated in 1994.

National Mental Health Programme A national mental health programme is present. The programme was formulated in 1997.
Denmark has a comprehensive national suicide prevention programme.

National Therapeutic Drug Policy/Essential List of Drugs A national therapeutic drug policy/essential list of drugs is absent.

Mental Health Legislation The most recent legislation is a departmental order concerning imprisonment and other coercion in psychiatry. The other relevant departmental orders (laws) concern procedures for compulsory commitment and involuntary hospitalization; procedure for complaints regarding treatment in psychiatric departments; guidance about possible revision of the fundamental law of psychiatry; and the procedure for appointment and conduct of patients' advocates. The Danish Mental Health Act was introduced in 1989 and primarily regulates involuntary civil commitment, detainment and use of coercive measures in psychiatric hospitals and departments in Denmark, but also contains regulations relating to all hospitalized psychiatric patients. Certain sections of the Danish Penal Code pertain to issues related to forensic psychiatry. They established the type and extent of special provision orders for offenders with mental disorders.
The latest legislation was enacted in 2002.

Mental Health Financing There are budget allocations for mental health.
Details about expenditure on mental health are not available.
The primary source of mental health financing is tax based.
The country has disability benefits for persons with mental disorders. A mental health diagnosis makes it possible to have disability benefits.

Mental Health Facilities Mental health is a part of primary health care system. Actual treatment of severe mental disorders is available at the primary level. Patients are treated by specialists in general practice or by psychiatrists.
Regular training of primary care professionals is not carried out in the field of mental health.
There are community care facilities for patients with mental disorders. There is a decentralized system across the country.

Psychiatric Beds and Professionals

Total psychiatric beds per 10 000 population	7.1
Psychiatric beds in mental hospitals per 10 000 population	
Psychiatric beds in general hospitals per 10 000 population	
Psychiatric beds in other settings per 10 000 population	7.5
Number of psychiatrists per 100 000 population	16
Number of neurosurgeons per 100 000 population	2
Number of psychiatric nurses per 100 000 population	59
Number of neurologists per 100 000 population	3

Number of psychologists per 100 000 population 85
Number of social workers per 100 000 population 7

There are 450 occupational therapists and 3000 nursing aides.

Non-Governmental Organizations NGOs are involved with mental health in the country. They are mainly involved in advocacy, promotion, prevention and rehabilitation. NGOs also carry out research work.

Information Gathering System There is mental health reporting system in the country. There are Government yearly reports about psychiatric services.
The country has data collection system or epidemiological study on mental health. Details can be obtained from the Danish National Board of Health and the Psychiatric Demography Centre in Aarhus.

Programmes for Special Population The country has specific programmes for mental health for minorities, refugees, disaster affected population, elderly and children.
Treatment for forensic patients is provided in general inpatient or outpatient psychiatric facilities or in some cases in high security units. The Danish Medico-Legal Council provides consultative medical advice regarding legal cases to criminal cases as well as cases related to involuntary admission or detention.

Therapeutic Drugs The following therapeutic drugs are generally available at the primary health care level of the country: carbamazepine, ethosuximide, phenobarbital, phenytoin sodium, sodium valproate, amitriptyline, chlorpromazine, diazepam, fluphenazine, haloperidol, lithium, biperiden, carbidopa, levodopa.

Other Information During the last 10 years, there has been an increasing focus in Denmark on issues concerning mental illness and its care. This includes a growing political awareness of the problem, as well as an increasing political will and commitment in regard to the need for improving mental health services. It has led to the development of three consecutive 3-year period national agreements between the Government and the counties, who are responsible for the health care system, including mental health care. The first one was in 1997 and the third goes from 2003 – 2006. These agreements represent a nationwide strategy for development and improvement of care and treatment offered to patients suffering from mental disorders. These agreements also contain arrangements for the payment of accepted improvements. The planned improvements include education of doctors, nurses and other professional workers, new and modern hospital facilities (including single rooms for psychiatric patients), extension of community-based psychiatry, improvement in the treatment of children with mental illness, etc. Intersectoral co-operation is essential at all levels in the system. There is a significant degree of co-operation between the counties' social services and health service departments. Usually, the health department is the responsible authority for mental health care, however, in some counties, the social service department is responsible for the management and organization of the mental health care system. This arrangement demonstrates the focus of the last ten years on decentralization and the social psychiatric services. In respect of the individual patient, the major goal is interdisciplinary teamwork (between psychiatrist, psychologist, physiotherapist, occupational therapist, social worker, etc). The Ministry of Health and the Ministry of Social Affairs regularly sponsor activities concerning mental health. The Ministry of Health cooperates with the National Board of Health regarding mental health issues, as it does for other national health questions. Various consultative groups have been established concerning mental health, e.g. an advisory body with expert members within the framework of the National Board of Health. Statistical reviews and reports about mental illness are prepared continuously, e.g. dealing with objectives and treatment for different kinds of psychiatric problems and quality of care. National objectives in the next few years include: establishing databases of patients to permit quality assurance of psychiatric treatment; improving the conditions for those patients with chronic mental disorders; continuing education of mental health staff; improving the capacity of departments of child and adolescent psychiatry; and improving the quality of hospital accommodation for acute psychiatric patients. A recent study by the EPSILON Group on type of mental health services in Copenhagen for patients suffering from schizophrenia shows that there is comprehensive system of mental health services with the exception of outpatient and community emergency care.

Additional Sources of Information

Becker T., Hullsmann, S., Knudsen, H. C., et al & the EPSILON Group (2002). Provision of services for people with schizophrenia in five European regions. Journal of Social Psychiatry and Psychiatric Epidemiology, 37, 465-474.

Grasfisk, J. H. (1998) Bekendtgorelse af love om Frihedsberovelse of Anden Tvang I Psykiatrien.

Justitsministeriet, Socialministeriet and Sundhedsministeriet (1994) Rgeringens Narkotikapolitiske Redegorelse Til Folketinget.

Sestoft, D., Engberg, M. (2000) Law and mental health in Denmark. International Journal of Law and Psychiatry, 23, 533-540.

Socialmininsteriet (1999) Regeringens Statusrapport om Tilbuddene tile Sindslidende.

Djibouti

C–D

GENERAL INFORMATION

Djibouti is a country with an approximate area of 23 thousand sq. km. (UNO, 2001). Its population is 0.712 million, and the sex ratio (men per hundred women) is 99 (UNO, 2004). The proportion of population under the age of 15 years is 43% (UNO, 2004), and the proportion of population above the age of 60 years is 5% (WHO, 2004). The literacy rate is 75.6% for men and 54.4% for women (UNESCO/MoH, 2004).

The country is a lower middle income group country (based on World Bank 2004 criteria). The proportion of health budget to GDP is 7%. The per capita total expenditure on health is 90 international $, and the per capita government expenditure on health is 53 international $ (WHO, 2004).

The main language(s) used in the country is (are) Arabic and French. The largest ethnic group(s) is (are) Somali, and the other ethnic group(s) are (is) Afar. The largest religious group(s) is (are) Muslim.

The life expectancy at birth is 48.6 years for males and 50.7 years for females (WHO, 2004). The healthy life expectancy at birth is 42 years for males and 43 years for females (WHO, 2004).

EPIDEMIOLOGY

There is a paucity of epidemiological data on mental illnesses in Djibouti in internationally accessible literature. Mion and Oberti (1998) found that the prevalence of Khat use among 100 army recruits was 84% with a mean consumption of 400 grams per chew. Khat abuse is believed to be common and associated also with other mental disorders (Mohamed, 2004).

MENTAL HEALTH RESOURCES

Mental Health Policy A mental health policy is absent.

Substance Abuse Policy A substance abuse policy is absent.

National Mental Health Programme A national mental health programme is absent.
A national mental health programme is being formulated. This is expected to lead to the development of primary mental health care services, treatment facilities and human resources.

National Therapeutic Drug Policy/Essential List of Drugs A national therapeutic drug policy/essential list of drugs is present. It was formulated in 1997.

Mental Health Legislation An old French legislation forms the basis of legal action. New legislation needs to be formulated.
Details about the year of enactment of the mental health legislation are not available.

Mental Health Financing There are no budget allocations for mental health.
Details about expenditure on mental health are not available.
The primary source of mental health financing is grants.
The country does not have disability benefits for persons with mental disorders.

Mental Health Facilities Mental health is not a part of primary health care system. Actual treatment of severe mental disorders is not available at the primary level. Mental Health will be included with primary care in the new National Mental Health Programme.
Regular training of primary care professionals is not carried out in the field of mental health.
There are no community care facilities for patients with mental disorders. Ambulatory care is available following hospitalization and for those for whom hospitalization is not deemed necessary.

Psychiatric Beds and Professionals

Total psychiatric beds per 10 000 population	0.7
Psychiatric beds in mental hospitals per 10 000 population	0
Psychiatric beds in general hospitals per 10 000 population	0.7
Psychiatric beds in other settings per 10 000 population	0
Number of psychiatrists per 100 000 population	0
Number of neurosurgeons per 100 000 population	0
Number of psychiatric nurses per 100 000 population	0.16
Number of neurologists per 100 000 population	0
Number of psychologists per 100 000 population	0
Number of social workers per 100 000 population	0

There are 4 nursing attendants. A Chinese psychiatrist is providing services temporarily. Psychiatric assistance is concentrated to the psychiatry department of Peltier Hospital. Besides that, psychiatric services are non-existent.

Non-Governmental Organizations NGOs are not involved with mental health in the country.

Information Gathering System There is mental health reporting system in the country. Data of 1999 is available.
The country has no data collection system or epidemiological study on mental health.

Programmes for Special Population No specialized services exist. International organizations like the UNHCR provide help for refugees.

Therapeutic Drugs The following therapeutic drugs are generally available at the primary health care level of the country: carbamazepine, phenobarbital, phenytoin sodium, sodium valproate, amitriptyline, chlorpromazine, diazepam, haloperidol.
These drugs are available only at the general hospital and not at primary care level. None of the anti-parkinsonian drugs are available.

Other Information Magico-religious treatment is present to a great extent. General knowledge about mental disorders is very limited.

Additional Sources of Information

Mion, G., Oberti, M. (1998) Epidemiologic study of khat use in the National Army of Djibouti. Médecine Tropicale, 58, 161-164.

Mohamed, A. K. (2004) (Focal point for mental health, Djibouti, Personal Communication).

Dominica

C–D

GENERAL INFORMATION

Dominica is a country with an approximate area of 0.75 thousand sq. km. (UNO, 2001). Its population is 0.071 million, and the sex ratio (men per hundred women) is 103 (UNO, 2004). The proportion of population under the age of 15 years is 33% (UNO, 2004), and the proportion of population above the age of 60 years is 10% (WHO, 2004). The literacy rate is 76% for men and 82% for women (UNESCO/MoH, 2004).

The country is a higher middle income group country (based on World Bank 2004 criteria). The proportion of health budget to GDP is 6%. The per capita total expenditure on health is 312 international $, and the per capita government expenditure on health is 222 international $ (WHO, 2004).

The main language(s) used in the country is (are) English. The largest ethnic group(s) is (are) African, and the other ethnic group(s) are (is) Carib Amerindian. The largest religious group(s) is (are) Roman Catholic.

The life expectancy at birth is 71 years for males and 75.8 years for females (WHO, 2004). The healthy life expectancy at birth is 62 years for males and 66 years for females (WHO, 2004).

EPIDEMIOLOGY

There is a paucity of epidemiological data on mental illnesses in Dominica in internationally accessible literature.

MENTAL HEALTH RESOURCES

Mental Health Policy Details about the mental health policy are not available.

The protocol of the policy is not available. Lack of mental health personnel and stigma are constraints towards the development of the policy.

Substance Abuse Policy A substance abuse policy is present. Details about the year of formulation are not available. Lack of human resources and infrastructure hamper the development and implementation of the substance abuse policy.

National Mental Health Programme A national mental health programme is present. Details about the year of formulation of the programme are not available.

Staff development, mental health promotion and prevention along with evidence based practice are some of the components of the programme.

National Therapeutic Drug Policy/Essential List of Drugs Details about the national therapeutic drug policy/essential list of drugs are not available.

Mental Health Legislation There is a Mental Health Act.

The latest legislation was enacted in 1987.

Mental Health Financing There are budget allocations for mental health.

The country spends 2.9% of the total health budget on mental health.

The primary source of mental health financing is tax based.

The country has disability benefits for persons with mental disorders. Mental health is covered as other illnesses. The coverage is limited.

Mental Health Facilities Mental health is a part of primary health care system. Actual treatment of severe mental disorders available at the primary level. There is a need to develop primary and community care.

Regular training of primary care professionals is not carried out in the field of mental health. Psychiatrists and other mental health professionals function as an integral part of the primary health team.

Details about community care facilities in mental health are not available.

Psychiatric Beds and Professionals

Total psychiatric beds per 10 000 population
Psychiatric beds in mental hospitals per 10 000 population
Psychiatric beds in general hospitals per 10 000 population
Psychiatric beds in other settings per 10 000 population
Number of psychiatrists per 100 000 population
Number of neurosurgeons per 100 000 population
Number of psychiatric nurses per 100 000 population
Number of neurologists per 100 000 population
Number of psychologists per 100 000 population
Number of social workers per 100 000 population

The old mental hospital was destroyed in the hurricane of 1979 and was not rebuilt. A new inpatient psychiatric facility was created in the general hospital. There is a lack of multi-disciplinary approaches towards care.

Non-Governmental Organizations NGOs are not involved with mental health in the country. Efforts are under way to include NGOs in mental health.

Information Gathering System There is mental health reporting system in the country.
Details about data collection system or epidemiological study on mental health are not available.

Programmes for Special Population Details about any special mental health programmes are not available.

Therapeutic Drugs The following therapeutic drugs are generally available at the primary health care level of the country: unknown.
Availability of drugs is limited.

Other Information WHO could play a role in training and research development.

Additional Sources of Information

Camilleri, C. P., Kohn, R., Levav,, et al (2000) Attitudes towards mental illness in the Commonwealth of Dominica. Pan American Journal of Public Health, 7, 148-54.

La Grenade, L. (1998) Integrated primary Health care. West Indies Medical Journal, 47 (Suppl. 4), 31-33.

Dominican Republic

GENERAL INFORMATION

Dominican Republic is a country with an approximate area of 49 thousand sq. km. (UNO, 2001). Its population is 8.873 million, and the sex ratio (men per hundred women) is 103 (UNO, 2004). The proportion of population under the age of 15 years is 32% (UNO, 2004), and the proportion of population above the age of 60 years is 7% (WHO, 2004). The literacy rate is 84.3% for men and 84.4% for women (UNESCO/MoH, 2004).

The country is a lower middle income group country (based on World Bank 2004 criteria). The proportion of health budget to GDP is 6.1%. The per capita total expenditure on health is 353 international $, and the per capita government expenditure on health is 127 international $ (WHO, 2004).

The main language(s) used in the country is (are) Spanish (official). The largest religious group(s) is (are) Roman Catholic.

The life expectancy at birth is 64.9 years for males and 71.5 years for females (WHO, 2004). The healthy life expectancy at birth is 57 years for males and 62 years for females (WHO, 2004).

EPIDEMIOLOGY

Garcia et al (1996) asked mothers of 199 students to respond to the Wender Utah Rating Scale and found the prevalence of ADHD to be 6% with a male to female ratio of 3:1. The commonest age-group was 5-11 years. Sattler et al (2002) found that social support and personal resources were inversely associated with psychological distress after being affected by a hurricane in a sample of 697 college students from Dominican Republic, Puerto Rico, US Virgin Islands and USA. Da Costa e Silva and Koifman (1998) conducted a study measuring the prevalence of smoking across 14 Latin American countries. The prevalence in men varied from 24.1% (Paraguay) to 66.3% (Dominican Republic) and that in women, from 5.5% (Paraguay) to 26.6% (Uruguay). A wide variance in mortality patterns was also noted across the countries. Application of the point prevalence data to the stage model of the tobacco epidemic in developed countries suggested that the Latin American countries are in stage 2, i.e. with a clearly rising prevalence among men, a prevalence for women that is beginning to increase and mortality attributable to smoking among men still not reflecting peak prevalence.

MENTAL HEALTH RESOURCES

Mental Health Policy A mental health policy is absent.

The policy exists in the form of norms for action in mental health released by the Secretary of Health.

Substance Abuse Policy A substance abuse policy is present. The policy was initially formulated in 1998. It was revised in 2000. There is a regular budget for its implementation and it has been implemented to the extent of 50 to 75%. There is also a specific legislation for substance abuse from 1988.

National Mental Health Programme A national mental health programme is present. The programme was formulated in 1977. It was revised in 2001. There is a specific budget for its implementation and it has been implemented to the extent of 25 to 50% by local, regional and national authorities. Its main components are strategy of services reform, promotion and prevention, integration of mental health services at primary health care and development of specialized services.

National Therapeutic Drug Policy/Essential List of Drugs A national therapeutic drug policy/essential list of drugs is present. It was formulated in 1993.

Mental Health Legislation A proposal of law on Mental Health has been placed before the Senate and is pending its approval. Regular funds for its implementation have been proposed. It focuses on promotion and prevention, human rights, regulation of mental health services, but there is no reference to regulation of involuntary treatment.

The latest legislation was enacted in 2001.

Mental Health Financing There are no budget allocations for mental health.

The country spends 0.5% of the total health budget on mental health.

The primary sources of mental health financing in descending order are out of pocket expenditure by the patient or family, tax based, social insurance and private insurances.

The country does not have a separate budget line for mental health except for central expenses of the General Directorate of Mental Health. Approximately 40.0% of funds in mental health is spent on general hospitals, 40.0% in psychiatric hospitals, 10.0% in ambulatory clinics and 10.0% in community care.

The country has disability benefits for persons with mental disorders. Disabilities associated to mental health problems were included as conditions considered for getting state/public benefits in November 2002. Procedures are still to be worked out.

Mental Health Facilities Mental health is a part of primary health care system. Actual treatment of severe mental disorders is not available at the primary level. 25-50% of the population is covered by this kind of service. Mental health care in primary health care is provided by general doctors. Cases are identified and referred. Medication is supervised once they have been prescribed by specialists. Regular training of primary care professionals is carried out in the field of mental health. In the last two years, about 260 personnel were provided training. About 60 general physicians and 200 community workers have been trained.

There are community care facilities for patients with mental disorders. The community care system for the mentally ill includes preventive/promotion interventions family interventions, residential facilities, and vocational training. Current services cover about 25 to 50% of the treated population. Home interventions are available for 50 to 75%. Community center coordinators, psychologists, counsellors, physicians and health workers are provided training in mental health. A day hospital is functioning.

Psychiatric Beds and Professionals

Total psychiatric beds per 10 000 population	0.37
Psychiatric beds in mental hospitals per 10 000 population	0.3
Psychiatric beds in general hospitals per 10 000 population	0.07
Psychiatric beds in other settings per 10 000 population	0
Number of psychiatrists per 100 000 population	2
Number of neurosurgeons per 100 000 population	0.12
Number of psychiatric nurses per 100 000 population	0.4
Number of neurologists per 100 000 population	0.18
Number of psychologists per 100 000 population	2.2
Number of social workers per 100 000 population	

There are 25 assistants in psychiatry. The country has approximately 6000 psychologists, but all of them do not work in the mental health area. During the last 3 years, mental health units have started activities in 10 general hospitals. About 50% of beds are occupied by long stay patients. The SESPAS has 123 psychiatrists distributed in the eight sanitary regions, 60% of them in the National District (region 0), 15% in region II (Santiago) and the rest for the other six regions. At least two-thirds of mental health professionals from each discipline work in the public institutions.

Non-Governmental Organizations NGOs are involved with mental health in the country. They are mainly involved in advocacy, promotion, prevention, treatment and rehabilitation. These organizations participate in mental health activities related to women, children and domestic violence. The high participation of NGOs in most related activities in the country is noticeable.

Information Gathering System There is mental health reporting system in the country. Both ICD-10 and DSM-IV criteria are used in the reporting system. The mental health components reported are morbidity, treatment and discharge. Suicides are notified through the institute of forensic pathology. Violence and abuse against women are also notified.
The country has data collection system or epidemiological study on mental health. The 'Estadística de Salud General' (General Health Statistics) is in charge of the data collection system for mental disorders. Service data collection system is conducted for part of the mental health system (Psychiatric Hospital). Data from the only psychiatric hospital in the country indicate that affective disorders (particularly depression) are the main condition for seeking help in outpatient, inpatient and emergency mental health care. Other leading conditions are schizophrenia, drug abuse and dependence, mental retardation and epilepsy (Analisis de la Situación de la Salud Mental en la República Dominicana, Secretaria de Estado de Salud Publica y Asistencia Social, 2002).

Programmes for Special Population The country has specific programmes for mental health for disaster affected population, elderly and children. The country does not have any indigenous people or refugees. After the last hurricane, a mental health programme for victims of disaster was initiated, based on the experience of countries like Nicaragua and Honduras. There are some programmes with little coverage of the elderly population. There are institutions for children in the area of rights and duties of children, healthy child raising and prevention of child sexual abuse.
Also, there are programmes for women and victims of domestic violence.

Therapeutic Drugs The following therapeutic drugs are generally available at the primary health care level of the country: carbamazepine, phenobarbital, phenytoin sodium, amitriptyline, chlorpromazine, diazepam, haloperidol, lithium, biperiden, carbidopa, levodopa.
The essential drug list was revised in 1997. Diazepam is assigned to the first level, which means that it can be managed by that level without the due authorization of a specialist. All the medicines included in the listing are free.

Other Information Since 1997, a decentralization process has started, due to which the number of beds in mental hospitals have reduced by 50% and 15 general hospitals are receiving inpatients with acute disorders and also long term patients. Three psychology schools have started functioning with more than 100 students.

Additional Sources of Information

da Costae Silva,V. L., Koifman, S. (1998) Smoking in Latin America: a major public health problem. Cadernos de Saude Publica., 14 (Suppl. 3), 99-108.

Garcia, A. R., Quintero Lumbreras, F. J., Herrera Pino, J. A., et al (1996) Prevalence of attention-deficit, hyperactivity and disruptive behavior syndrome. Psiquis, 17, 19-32.

Sattler, D. N., Preston, A. J., Kaiser, C. F., et al (2002) Hurricane Georges: a cross-national study examining preparedness, resource loss, and psychological distress in the U.S. Virgin Islands, Puerto Rico, Dominican Republic, and the United States. Journal of Traumatic Stress, 15, 339-350.

Ecuador

GENERAL INFORMATION

Ecuador is a country with an approximate area of 284 thousand sq. km. (UNO, 2001). Its population is 13.193 million, and the sex ratio (men per hundred women) is 101 (UNO, 2004). The proportion of population under the age of 15 years is 32% (UNO, 2004), and the proportion of population above the age of 60 years is 7% (WHO, 2004). The literacy rate is 92.3% for men and 89.7% for women (UNESCO/MoH, 2004).

The country is a lower middle income group country (based on World Bank 2004 criteria). The proportion of health budget to GDP is 4.5%. The per capita total expenditure on health is 177 international $, and the per capita government expenditure on health is 89 international $ (WHO, 2004).

The main language(s) used in the country is (are) Spanish and Quichua. The largest ethnic group(s) is (are) Indian and Mestizo, and the other ethnic group(s) are (is) European. The largest religious group(s) is (are) Roman Catholic.

The life expectancy at birth is 67.9 years for males and 73.5 years for females (WHO, 2004). The healthy life expectancy at birth is 60 years for males and 64 years for females (WHO, 2004).

EPIDEMIOLOGY

Aguilar (1989, 1990) conducted a study on a probabilistic random sample of 6000 individuals, representative of the country's entire population, between the ages of 10 and 65, using questionnaires to assess the prevalence of alcohol, smoking and other illegal substance use and misuse. The rates of lifetime use reported were as follows: alcohol (75%), tobacco (54%), tranquilizers (16%), marijuana (4%), inhalants (2%), native plant drugs (1%), cocaine (1%) and cocaine base (1%). The highest prevalence of substance misuse corresponded to the consumption of alcohol and tobacco (13%), followed by tranquilizers (0.8%), opiates (0.4%), barbiturates and marijuana (0.2%) and cocaine base (0.11%). Ockene et al (1996) evaluated 800 subjects who were representative of the adult population of two cities and reported that one-third of the population smoked. Smoking was more common in males and in younger and educated subjects. Women smoked lesser number of cigarettes. Padgett et al (1998) assessed more than 2600 students from 40 communities spread across rural and urban settings. They found that 9% were current smokers and 61.1% had never smoked. Older boys and those with smokers in their families were more likely to smoke. Morillo et al (2002) conducted a population based study in Ecuador, Columbia and Venezuela to study the prevalence of erectile dysfunction (ED) in men aged 40 years and above. A 49-item questionnaire was completed by 1946 men and the age-adjusted combined prevalence of minimal, moderate and complete ED for all three countries was 53.4%, with 19.8% of all men reporting moderate to complete ED. People above 70 years and those with comorbid medical conditions suffered more compared to those below 50 years of age. Lima et al (1989, 1992) interviewed 150 patients attending a primary care centre 2 months after the 1987 earthquake. They found emotional disturbances in 40% of the population. The risk factors were – not being married, reporting poor physical or emotional health and having ill-defined physical complaints. In a gold-mining area, Counter et al (1998 a, b) found neurocognitive deficits in village children with chronic exposure to lead because of the ceramics industry. Gorenc et al (1999) found that suicides tended to be under-reported in Mexico (42 per 100 000) and Ecuador (3.6 per 100 000), especially in men using passive or soft methods.

MENTAL HEALTH RESOURCES

Mental Health Policy A mental health policy is present. The policy was initially formulated in 1980.
The components of the policy are promotion, prevention, treatment and rehabilitation. It was revised in 1999 by mental health professionals, civil servants and NGOs. There are no regular funds for its implementation and less than 10% of its original content was put into practice.

Substance Abuse Policy A substance abuse policy is present. Details about the year of formulation are not available. There is also specific legislation for substance abuse from 1997.

National Mental Health Programme A national mental health programme is present. The programme was formulated in 1980. It was revised in 1999. It was implemented less than 10.0% by regional and national authorities, probably because there was no specific budget for its implementation. Its main components are strategy of services reform, integration of mental health services at primary health care and development of specialized services.

National Therapeutic Drug Policy/Essential List of Drugs A national therapeutic drug policy/essential list of drugs is present. It was formulated in 1977.

Mental Health Legislation The Mental Health Act was revised in 2001. There are no regular funds for its implementation, and it has been implemented to the extent of 10 to 25 %. It focuses on promotion and prevention, human rights and regulation of mental health services, but there is no reference to regulation of involuntary treatment.
The latest legislation was enacted in 2000.

Mental Health Financing There are no budget allocations for mental health.
Details about expenditure on mental health are not available.
The primary source of mental health financing is out of pocket expenditure by the patient or family.
The country has disability benefits for persons with mental disorders. Mental disabilities are considered disabilities under Law 180. The evaluation is done by a psychiatrist and reviewed by the National Disability Council. Chronic psychosis, mental retardation, dementia and certain epilepsies are considered for disability benefits.

Mental Health Facilities Mental health is a part of primary health care system. Actual treatment of severe mental disorders is not available at the primary level. Less than 25% of the population is covered by this kind of service. Mental health care is provided by Primary Health Care doctors. A referral system is in place.
Regular training of primary care professionals is carried out in the field of mental health. In the last two years, about 250 personnel were provided training. General physicians, nurses, social workers and educators are provided a 30 hour training in mental health.
There are no community care facilities for patients with mental disorders. The community care system covers for one-fourth of the intended patient group. It includes preventive/promotion, home interventions and family interventions. Nurses are responsible for taking care of patients with mental disorders in the community.

Psychiatric Beds and Professionals

Total psychiatric beds per 10 000 population	1.69
Psychiatric beds in mental hospitals per 10 000 population	1.53
Psychiatric beds in general hospitals per 10 000 population	0.16
Psychiatric beds in other settings per 10 000 population	0
Number of psychiatrists per 100 000 population	2.1
Number of neurosurgeons per 100 000 population	
Number of psychiatric nurses per 100 000 population	0.5
Number of neurologists per 100 000 population	
Number of psychologists per 100 000 population	29.1
Number of social workers per 100 000 population	0.04

The personnel refer to those in the public sector only. Almost 50% of nurses, 80% of psychiatrists and 95% of psychologists work in the private sector.

Non-Governmental Organizations NGOs are involved with mental health in the country. They are mainly involved in prevention, treatment and rehabilitation. These organizations participate in mental health activities related to women, children and domestic violence.

Information Gathering System There is mental health reporting system in the country. Information is recorded utilizing ICD-10. The mental health components reported are morbidity, admission and discharge. Depression, suicide, psychosis, drug abuse and dependence, epilepsy, mental retardation, violence and child abuse are the conditions covered.
The country has data collection system or epidemiological study on mental health. The 'Departamento Nacional de Estatísticas' (National Department of Statistics) is in charge of the data collection system for mental disorders. It is stated that the main psychiatric problems are alcohol abuse and dependence (7.4 %), affective disorders, particularly depression (approximately 16 %), psychosocial problems like domestic violence and child abuse.

Programmes for Special Population The country has specific programmes for mental health for disaster affected population, indigenous population, elderly and children.
Also, there are programmes for victims of domestic violence.

Therapeutic Drugs The therapeutic drug policy was revised in 1996. An essential drug list was created in 1976 and revised in 1996. Prices of medication are subsidized.

Other Information

Additional Sources of Information

Aguilar, E. (1989) Prevalence of the improper use of alcohol, tobacco and drugs in the Ecuadorian population. Boletin de la Oficina Sanitaria Panamericana, 107, 510-513.

Aguilar, E. (1990) Prevalence of the improper use of alcohol, tobacco, and drugs in the Ecuadorian population. Bulletin of the Pan American Health Organization, 24, 35-38.

Bouwen, R., Craps, M., Santos, E. (1999) Multi-party collaboration: building generative knowledge and developing relationships among unequal partners in local community projects in Ecuador. Concepts & Transformation, 4, 133-51.

Counter, S. A., Buchanan, L. H., Laurell, G., et al (1998a) Blood mercury and auditory neuro-sensory responses in children and adults in the nambija gold mining area of Ecuador. Source Neurotoxicology, 19, 185-196.

Counter, S. A., Buchanan, L. H., Rosas, H. D., et al (1998b) Neurocognitive effects of chronic lead intoxication in Andean children. Journal of the Neurological Sciences, 160, 47-53.

Gorenc, K.-D., Flores, J. A., Peredo, S., et al (1999) Unregistered suicides in Mexico and Ecuador: a comparative study. Revista Mexicana de Sociologia, 61, 123-149.

Lima, B. R., Chavez, H., Samaniego, N., et al (1989) Disaster severity and emotional disturbance: implications for primary mental health care in developing countries. Acta Psychiatrica Scandinavica, 79, 74-82.

Lima, B. R., Chavez, H., Samaniego, N., et al (1992) Psychiatric disorders among emotionally distressed disaster victims attending primary mental health clinics in Ecuador. Bulletin of the Pan American Health Organization, 26, 60-66.

Morillo, L. E., Diaz, J., Estevez, E., et al (2002) Prevalence of erectile dysfunction in Colombia, Ecuador, and Venezuela: a population-based study (DENSA). International Journal of Impotence Research, 14 (Suppl. 2), 10-18.

Ockene, J. K., Chiriboga, D. E., Zevallos, J. C. (1996) Smoking in Ecuador: prevalence, knowledge, and attitudes. Tobacco Control, 5, 121-126.

Padgett, D. I., Selwyn, B. J., Kelder, S. H. (1998) Ecuadorian adolescents and cigarette smoking: a cross-sectional survey. Pan American Journal of Public Health, 4, 87-93.

Egypt

GENERAL INFORMATION

Egypt is a country with an approximate area of 1001 thousand sq. km. (UNO, 2001). Its population is 73.389 million, and the sex ratio (men per hundred women) is 100 (UNO, 2004). The proportion of population under the age of 15 years is 34% (UNO, 2004), and the proportion of population above the age of 60 years is 7% (WHO, 2004). The literacy rate is 67.2% for men and 43.6% for women (UNESCO/MoH, 2004).

The country is a lower middle income group country (based on World Bank 2004 criteria). The proportion of health budget to GDP is 3.9%. The per capita total expenditure on health is 153 international $, and the per capita government expenditure on health is 75 international $ (WHO, 2004).

The main language(s) used in the country is (are) Arabic. The largest ethnic group(s) is (are) Arab. The largest religious group(s) is (are) Sunni Muslim (nine-tenths), and the other religious group(s) are (is) Coptic Christian.

The life expectancy at birth is 65.3 years for males and 69 years for females (WHO, 2004). The healthy life expectancy at birth is 58 years for males and 60 years for females (WHO, 2004).

EPIDEMIOLOGY

Ghanem et al (2004) conducted a national household survey of prevalence of mental disorders in 5 governorates, using the Mini International Neuropsychiatric Interview-Plus (MINI-Plus). Almost 17% (11% to 25.4% in different governorates) of adults had mental disorders, with the common ones being mood disorders (6.4%), anxiety disorders (4.9%) and somatoform disorders (0.6%). Psychoses were seen in 0.3% of the population. Mental disorders were associated with gender (female), marital status (widow, divorced), occupation (housewife, unemployed), education (illiteracy), housing (overcrowding) and physical illnesses. Okasha et al (2001) assessed a sample of students, selected through multistage stratified random sampling with the General Health Questionnaire, the Arabic Obsessive Scale for obsessive traits and the Yale Brown Obsessive Compulsive Scale. They found that psychiatric morbidity was present in 51.7% and obsessive compulsive disorder (ICD 10) in 19.6%. Girls, younger adolescents and first-borns were likely to be affected to a greater extent. In a study on University students, Okasha et al (1985) found that almost 14% of students faced academic difficulties. Psychiatric disorders were diagnosed in 42% of male students with academic problems, compared to 9% of students with no such problems, with neuroses accounting for nearly half of the cases and schizophrenia for a quarter. Farrag et al (1988) examined 2000 elderly (above 60 years) subjects from a region in a 3-phase population-based study using a modified version of the MMSE and a standardized protocol for those who screened positive (MMSE score of 21 or below). The prevalence of dementia was 4.5% with Alzheimer in 2.2%, multi-infarct dementia in 0.9%, dementia of mixed type in 0.55% and secondary dementia in 0.45%. Age-specific prevalence tended to double every 5 years. Soueif et al (1982, 1990) reported on psychoactive drug use in a nationally representative sample (n=14 656) of male secondary school students, using standardized questionnaires. They found that between 8% (for alcohol) and 21.4% (for synthetic drugs) of experimenters continued their drug use and that the age of onset was between 12-16 years. A greater proportion of urban students used tobacco, alcohol and cannabis, and delinquency was associated with drug use. In another sample (n=5530), they noted that consistently more arts stream students in comparison to science stream students were immersed in the drug culture. In similar studies, Soueif et al (1986, 1987) examined the non-medical use of drugs among university students (n=2711), using standardized tools. They found that university students were more likely to use stimulants and continue with drug use (10%-31% for different drugs) compared to male secondary school students, but the age of starting drug use was later in this sample. In comparison to male university students using drugs, female university student (n=2366) who used drugs came from a higher socioeconomic background. They were less likely to use stimulants and narcotics or to smoke, and they started drug use later (usually after 16 years). Their preferred drugs were hypnotics, tranquilizers and alcohol. Nasser (1986, 1994) found lower rates of abnormal eating attitudes in college students in Cairo (12%) in comparison to those in London (22%). In the earlier study, no Arab student fulfilled criteria for an eating disorder, but in the later studies he found a prevalence rate of 1.2% for bulimia and 3.4% for partial syndrome of bulimia (Russel's criteria). Okasha and Lotaif (1979) estimated the rate of suicide attempts in Cairo to be 38.5/100 000 population based on their assessment of admissions for attempted suicide in one hospital. Among suicide attempters, those in the age group of 15-44 years and students were overrepresented. Depression, hysterical reactions and situational reactions were common psychiatric conditions associated with suicide. Overdosing was the commonest method (80%) used. Temtamy et al (1994) administered the Stanford-Binet test to 3000 randomly selected community subjects. The prevalence of mental retardation was 3.9% (higher rates were reported in rural areas). Parental consanguinity was established in 65%. Farrag et al (1998) assessed 2878 children from the 2nd and 3rd grades in elementary schools for their reading ability by means of standardized tests for linguistic ability and rate of letter identification. The 84 children (3%) with IQ 90 or more and no evidence of sensory or motor impairment identified as backward in their reading ability at this stage were reassessed after 3 years. Thirty seven (1%) children, who did not attain satisfactory reading skills even at this stage, were diagnosed to have specific reading disability. The male to female ratio was 2.7 to 1. Abou et al (1991) administered the Arabic version of the Children's Depression Inventory to 1561 preparatory school children selected through stratified random sampling and found the rate of depression to be 10.3%. Further testing in sub-samples revealed that depression scores were predicted by neuroticism, introversion, relationship with fathers, sibs and peers, scholastic performance and mothers' depression scores.

MENTAL HEALTH RESOURCES

Mental Health Policy A mental health policy is present. The policy was initially formulated in 1978.
The components of the policy are promotion, prevention and treatment. The objectives of the policy are to provide a basis for improving mental health and well-being of the population through provision of services to the population at risk, community care and family support.

Substance Abuse Policy A substance abuse policy is present. The policy was initially formulated in 1986. A President's Decree has established a National Fund for the Control of Drug Addiction and Abuse. The supreme Council for the Control of Drug Addiction and Abuse is chaired by the Prime Minister. Laboratories for detection of addictive substances in biological secretions have been established in most regions. The policy direction is towards harm reduction policy.

National Mental Health Programme A national mental health programme is present. The programme was formulated in 1986. A new mental health programme was adopted in 2002. The programme aims to integrate mental health into community care, develop health recording and information gathering system, provide essential drugs and develop human resources. The other areas earmarked for development are quality assurance, development of intermediate and alternative systems of proving mental health care, developing child and adolescent psychiatry services, analysing the role of NGOs, increasing awareness about mental health problems among the population and promoting mental health and preventing mental disorders.

National Therapeutic Drug Policy/Essential List of Drugs A national therapeutic drug policy/essential list of drugs is present. Details about the year of formulation are not available.

Mental Health Legislation There is a Mental Health Act from 1940's, that is being revised. There is also a more recent law on narcotics which was formulated in 1989. Currently, efforts are made to upgrade the law.
The latest legislation was enacted in 1944.

Mental Health Financing There are budget allocations for mental health.
The country spends 9% of the total health budget on mental health.
The primary sources of mental health financing in descending order are tax based, out of pocket expenditure by the patient or family, social insurance and private insurances.
The country has disability benefits for persons with mental disorders.

Mental Health Facilities Mental health is a part of primary health care system. Actual treatment of severe mental disorders is not available at the primary level. Psychiatry has been integrated in the primary health care services in line with the Health Reform adopted by the Ministry of Health. A system for referral between the different levels of care has been established.
Regular training of primary care professionals is carried out in the field of mental health. In the last two years, about 639 personnel were provided training. Manuals for mental health care for primary care physicians and basic health care units are available. Training facilities are present. Training courses have been organized for general practitioners, maternal child health physicians, social workers and nursing staff working at basic health units. Training courses have also been held for trainers. Evaluation of training programmes for general practitioners showed significant improvement in attitudes, knowledge and skills regarding mental disorders and drug misuse and their management.
There are community care facilities for patients with mental disorders. Intermediate services were started for both patients with chronic mental disorders and drug use disorders. Large mental hospitals are trying to place long-stay patients in and follow them up in the community.

Psychiatric Beds and Professionals

Total psychiatric beds per 10 000 population	1.3
Psychiatric beds in mental hospitals per 10 000 population	1.1
Psychiatric beds in general hospitals per 10 000 population	0.1
Psychiatric beds in other settings per 10 000 population	0.1
Number of psychiatrists per 100 000 population	0.9
Number of neurosurgeons per 100 000 population	0.2
Number of psychiatric nurses per 100 000 population	2
Number of neurologists per 100 000 population	0.5
Number of psychologists per 100 000 population	0.4
Number of social workers per 100 000 population	0.1

There are few occupational therapists. Almost four-fifths of psychiatric beds are in Cairo. Beds for treatment of drug abusers and forensic patients are available. Specific allocations of beds have not been made for child and adolescent mental health. In an effort to provide quality assurance in big mental hospitals, standards have been developed and quality assurance teams have been deployed. Most psychiatrists have their own private clinics. There is a permanent training centre for continuous in- service training of mental health professionals, particularly nurses, psychologist and social workers employed in mental health facilities.

Non-Governmental Organizations NGOs are involved with mental health in the country. They are mainly involved in advocacy, promotion, prevention and rehabilitation. The Child Mental Health Prevention Association, an NGO, was established in 1995, to spread the concept of mental health among families. There are also guidance and counselling centres at different governorates.

Information Gathering System There is mental health reporting system in the country.
The country has no data collection system or epidemiological study on mental health.
A new National Health Information System for Mental Health was developed by the Ministry of Health and Population. The General Secretariat of Mental Health is piloting a data collection system.

Programmes for Special Population The country has specific programmes for mental health for disaster affected population, elderly and children.
Outpatient clinics and day care centres for children and adolescents are present in some mental hospitals. Clinics for school and university students are available in 4 centres. Eight special schools for education and rehabilitation of mentally retarded children are available. Of these, one caters to girls. Under the aegis of the school mental health programme, training programmes for school teachers, school physicians and school supervisors are undertaken, orientation courses for adolescents are held and special clinics at district levels are conducted in the area of mental health and drug misuse.

Therapeutic Drugs The following therapeutic drugs are generally available at the primary health care level of the country: phenobarbital, amitriptyline, diazepam.
Imipramine is available in primary health care (commonest strength: 25 mg, approximate cost for 100 tablets: 9.45 USD).

Other Information Finland has provided support to the mental health programme in Egypt since 2002. The Programme addresses five main components: human resource development, functional development, structural development, community development and mental health prevention and promotion. UNODP supports some activities for improving treatment services and rehabilitation of drug abusers.

Additional Sources of Information

Abou Nazel, M. W., Fahmy, S. I., Younis, I. A., et al (1991) A study of depression among Alexandria preparatory school adolescents. Journal of the Egyptian Public Health Association, 66, 649-674.

Daoud, R., Atallah, S., Loza, N. (2002). Psychiatric services in Egypt – an update. International Psychiatry, 2, 12-14.

Farrag, A. F., el Behary, A. A., Kandil, M. R. (1988) Prevalence of specific reading disability in Egypt. Lancet, 2, 837-839.

Farrag, A., Farwiz, H. M., Khedr, E. H., et al (1998) Prevalence of Alzheimer's disease and other dementing disorders: Assiut-Upper Egypt study. Dementia & Geriatric Cognitive Disorders, 9, 323-328.

Ghanem, M., Gadallah, M., Mourad, S., et al (2004) National Survey of Prevalence of Mental Disorders in Egypt. WHO sponsored study (under publication).

Mental Health Programme in Egypt (2003) Country profile for mental health services. Mental Health programme in Egypt : heshmat1@egymen.com.

Mental Health Programme in Egypt (2003) Master plan for provision of mental health services in Egypt. Mental Health programme in Egypt : heshmat1@egymen.com.

Nasser, M. (1986) Comparative study of the prevalence of abnormal eating attitudes among Arab female students of both London and Cairo universities. Psychological Medicine, 16, 621-625.

Nasser, M. (1994) Screening for abnormal eating attitudes in a population of Egyptian secondary school girls. Social Psychiatry & Psychiatric Epidemiology, 29, 25-30.

Okasha, A. (1999) Mental Health in the Middle East: An Egyptian Perspective. Clinical Psychology Review, 19, 917-33.

Okasha, A., Fahmy, M., Haggag, W. et al. (2002) A psychiatric training programme for general practitioners in primary heatlh care in Egypt. Primary Care Psychiatry, 8, 9-16.

Okasha, A., Kamel, M., Khalil, A. H., et al (1985) Academic difficulty among male Egyptian university students. I. Association with psychiatric morbidity. British Journal of Psychiatry, 146, 140-144.

Okasha, A., Lotaif, F. (1979) Attempted suicide. An Egyptian investigation. Acta Psychiatrica Scandinavica, 60, 69-75.

Okasha, A., Ragheb, K., Attia, A. H., et al (2001) Prevalence of obsessive compulsive symptoms (OCS) in a sample of Egyptian adolescents. Encephale, 27, 8-14.

Soueif, M. I., Darweesh, Z. A., Hannourah, M. A., et al (1986) The extent of drug use among Egyptian male university students. Drug & Alcohol Dependence, 18, 389-403.

Soueif, M. I., el Sayed, A. M., Darweesh, Z. A., et al (1982) The extent of nonmedical use of psychoactive substances among secondary school students in Greater Cairo. Drug & Alcohol Dependence, 9, 15-41.

Soueif, M. I., Hannourah, M. A., Darweesh, Z. A., et al (1987) The use of psychoactive substances by female Egyptian university students, compared with their male colleagues on selected items. Drug & Alcohol Dependence, 19, 233-247.

Soueif, M. I., Youssuf, G. S., Taha, H. S., et al (1990) Use of psychoactive substances among male secondary school pupils in Egypt: a study on a nation-wide representative sample. Drug & Alcohol Dependence, 26, 63-79.

Temtamy, S. A., Kandil, M. R., Demerdash, A. M., et al (1994) An epidemiological/genetic study of mental subnormality in Assiut Governorate, Egypt. Clinical Genetics, 46, 347-351.

WHO, EMRO (1995) Intercountry Meeting on the Evaluation of the Progress of National Mental Health Programmes in the Eastern Mediterranean Region. World Health Organization, Regional Office for the Eastern Mediterranean.

WHO, EMRO (1997) Intercountry Consultation on Mental Health Legislation in Different Law Traditions. World Health Organization, Regional Office for the Eastern Mediterranean.

WHO, EMRO (1997) Intercountry Meeting on the Mental Health Needs Assessment at the Community, Health Services and Policy Levels in the Countries of the Eastern Mediterranean Region. World Health Organization, Regional Office for the Eastern Mediterranean.

El Salvador

E-I

GENERAL INFORMATION

El Salvador is a country with an approximate area of 21 thousand sq. km. (UNO, 2001). Its population is 6.614 million, and the sex ratio (men per hundred women) is 96 (UNO, 2004). The proportion of population under the age of 15 years is 34% (UNO, 2004), and the proportion of population above the age of 60 years is 8% (WHO, 2004). The literacy rate is 82.4% for men and 77.1% for women (UNESCO/MoH, 2004).

The country is a lower middle income group country (based on World Bank 2004 criteria). The proportion of health budget to GDP is 8%. The per capita total expenditure on health is 376 international $, and the per capita government expenditure on health is 175 international $ (WHO, 2004).

The main language(s) used in the country is (are) Spanish. The largest ethnic group(s) is (are) Mestizo. The largest religious group(s) is (are) Roman Catholic (five-sixths).

The life expectancy at birth is 66.5 years for males and 72.8 years for females (WHO, 2004). The healthy life expectancy at birth is 57 years for males and 62 years for females (WHO, 2004).

EPIDEMIOLOGY

Chocron et al (1995) conducted a two-phase study in a systematically selected primary care center sample (n=400) using the GHQ-28 (cut-off point 5/6) and Clinical Interview Schedule. The overall prevalence of psychopathology was 38.8%. Depression was found in 10.3% (major depression 6% and dysthymia 4.3%), anxiety in 13.8% (generalized 7.3%, panic 3% and obsessive/ compulsive 3%) and adjustment disorder in 9.5% of the sample. Barthauer and Leventhal (1999) have reported on the psychological effects of child sexual abuse on 83 rural women interviewed using Hopkins Symptom Checklist. Abused women showed more depressive pathology in comparison to non-abused women. After controlling for the number of relatives killed in the war, however, that difference failed to reach statistical significance. The lack of difference in psychological symptoms between abused and non-abused women may be related to the different characteristics of the abuse and perpetrators. It also may be secondary to adverse social conditions, e.g. poverty and war, which could obscure the long-term effects of childhood sexual abuse. Walton et al (1997) conducted an ecologically conceptualized study to assess the mental health impact of the Salvadoran Civil War on 12-year-olds (n=54) who were born during the war and had been exposed to different levels of war violence. Half of the students came from a repopulated country village and half from an industrial neighbourhood near the capital city. Interviews and some instruments were administered to children, mothers/caretakers and teachers. Children from the repopulated village reported higher war experience and lower mental health. The personal/social impact of the war was more important than family togetherness or war intensity in determining the mental health of the children. Children's intelligence was highly related to surviving with higher mental health. Higher socioeconomic status (SES) and education of parents was related to better mental health. Controlling for intelligence, children who experienced the highest personal-social impact of war showed the poorest mental health. Children with high war experience were most likely to have difficulty in imagining the future.

MENTAL HEALTH RESOURCES

Mental Health Policy A mental health policy is present. The policy was initially formulated in 2000.

The components of the policy are advocacy, promotion, prevention, treatment and rehabilitation. The policy was drafted through a process that involved professionals, NGOs and public servants. Between 10 to 25% of its original content have been put into practice. Mental health is included in the Government Programme 1999-2004 called 'the New Alliance', within the Solidarity Alliance, as one of its strategic areas of action and sets limits for the strategic borders. This structured programme includes six elements or 'alliances'- consolidation of economic stability, work alliance, solidarity alliance, security alliance, future alliance, participating and effective Government.

Substance Abuse Policy A substance abuse policy is present. The policy was initially formulated in 2001. The Ministry of Public Health and Welfare is responsible for it. Drug addiction is considered a priority area in mental health. There is the Salvadorean Anti-Drug Commission, which is made of four governmental and non-governmental institutions. Its purpose is to reduce drug demand. There is also a Commission against Drug-related Activities, which is made of four governmental institutions. Its aim is to reduce drugs offer. The National Plan Against Drugs, 2000-2005, is functional. The substance abuse policy has a specific budget for its implementation and has been implemented to the extent of 10 to 255 as yet. El Salvador also has a law on Substance Abuse established in 1998.

National Mental Health Programme A national mental health programme is present. The programme was formulated in 2000. It was revised in 2001 and has been implemented 10 to 25% by national authorities. There are no funds for its implementation. Its main components are strategy of services reform, promotion and prevention, integration of mental health care in primary care and development of specialized specialized services.

National Therapeutic Drug Policy/Essential List of Drugs A national therapeutic drug policy/essential list of drugs is present. It was formulated in 1997.

Currently, the seventh version of the essential drugs list is being used. The newly approved drugs list includes a lot of psychotropics for the first and second health care levels.

Mental Health Legislation There is no mental health legislation. During 1998, a proposal to modify the Health Code was made. It focuses on promotion, prevention and advocacy, but it makes no reference to human rights of patients or regulation of mental health services.
Details about the year of enactment of the mental health legislation are not available.

Mental Health Financing There are no budget allocations for mental health.
Details about expenditure on mental health are not available.
The primary sources of mental health financing in descending order are tax based, social insurance, out of pocket expenditure by the patient or family and private insurances.
The country has disability benefits for persons with mental disorders. Less than 10% of the population is entitled for receiving benefits as it applies only to those who are covered by social security.

Mental Health Facilities Mental health is a part of primary health care system. Actual treatment of severe mental disorders is available at the primary level. Primary care is carried out by the social security and is included in the proposal of the mental health programme. Less than 25% of the population is covered by this kind of service.
Regular training of primary care professionals is not carried out in the field of mental health.
There are no community care facilities for patients with mental disorders.

Psychiatric Beds and Professionals

Total psychiatric beds per 10 000 population	0.65
Psychiatric beds in mental hospitals per 10 000 population	0.65
Psychiatric beds in general hospitals per 10 000 population	0
Psychiatric beds in other settings per 10 000 population	0
Number of psychiatrists per 100 000 population	0.5
Number of neurosurgeons per 100 000 population	
Number of psychiatric nurses per 100 000 population	0
Number of neurologists per 100 000 population	
Number of psychologists per 100 000 population	31.2
Number of social workers per 100 000 population	

Three-fifths of the beds are occupied by long stay patients. Three mental health units in general hospitals are proposed in three different regions.

Non-Governmental Organizations NGOs are involved with mental health in the country. They are mainly involved in prevention and treatment. These organizations participate in mental health activities related to women, children, domestic violence and consumers.

Information Gathering System There is mental health reporting system in the country.
The country has data collection system or epidemiological study on mental health. Some figures related to mental health, such as drug addiction, physical violence, etc. are reported in the weekly epidemiological report.

Programmes for Special Population The country has specific programmes for mental health for disaster affected population, elderly and children. The Ministry of Health is working to include the mental health component in different programmes of comprehensive health care (children, adolescents, women, elderly).
Also there are programmes for women and children in vulnerable situations and for victims of domestic violence. Several of these activities are carried out with assistance of institutions like the Red Cross Federation, UNICEF and CICAD/OAS.

Therapeutic Drugs The following therapeutic drugs are generally available at the primary health care level of the country: carbamazepine, phenobarbital, phenytoin sodium, diazepam, haloperidol.
Some other drugs are also available but not at primary level.

Other Information The mental health team in the Health Ministry was created after the earthquake.

Additional Sources of Information

Barthauer, L. M., Leventhal, J. M. (1999) Prevalence and effects of child sexual abuse in a poor, rural community in El Salvador: a retrospective study of women after 12 years of civil war. Child Abuse & Neglect, 23, 1117-1126.

Chocron, B. L., Vilalta, F. J., Legazpi, R. I., et al (1995) Prevalence of psychopathology at a primary care center. Atencion Primaria, 16, 586-590.

Fernandes, J. D., Hurst, I. H., Oliveira, M. R., et al (1998) Psychiatric nursing research: concepts and expectations of nurses in psychiatric institutions. Revista Latinoamerica de Enfermagem, 6, 89-98.

Walton, J. R., Nuttall, R. L., Nuttall, E. V. (1997) The impact of war on the mental health of children: a Salvadoran study. Child Abuse & Neglect, 21, 737-749.

Equatorial Guinea

GENERAL INFORMATION

Equatorial Guinea is a country with an approximate area of 28 thousand sq. km. (UNO, 2001). The country consists of the mainland (Rio Muni) and several islands, the largest of which is Bioko. Its population is 0.507 million, and the sex ratio (men per hundred women) is 98 (UNO, 2004). The proportion of population under the age of 15 years is 44% (UNO, 2004), and the proportion of population above the age of 60 years is 6% (WHO, 2004). The literacy rate is 92.1% for men and 74.5% for women (UNESCO/MoH, 2004).

The country is a low income group country (based on World Bank 2004 criteria). The proportion of health budget to GDP is 2%. The per capita total expenditure on health is 106 international $, and the per capita government expenditure on health is 64 international $ (WHO, 2004).

The main language(s) used in the country is (are) Spanish, French, Ndowe, Bisio and Annobonés. The largest ethnic group(s) is (are) Fang, and the other ethnic group(s) are (is) Buby, Ndowe, Bisio and Annobonés. The largest religious group(s) is (are) Roman Catholic, and the other religious group(s) are (is) Protestant and indigenous groups.

The life expectancy at birth is 51.9 years for males and 54.8 years for females (WHO, 2004). The healthy life expectancy at birth is 45 years for males and 46 years for females (WHO, 2004).

EPIDEMIOLOGY

There is a paucity of epidemiological data on mental illnesses in Equatorial Guinea in internationally accessible literature.

MENTAL HEALTH RESOURCES

Mental Health Policy A mental health policy is absent.

Substance Abuse Policy A substance abuse policy is absent.

National Mental Health Programme A national mental health programme is present. The programme was formulated in 1997. The programme exists in a preliminary form.

National Therapeutic Drug Policy/Essential List of Drugs A national therapeutic drug policy/essential list of drugs is present. It was formulated in 1996.

Mental Health Legislation There is no mental health legislation.

Mental Health Financing There are budget allocations for mental health.
Details about expenditure on mental health are not available.
The primary sources of mental health financing in descending order are out of pocket expenditure by the patient or family, social insurance, private insurances and tax based.
Details about disability benefits for mental health are not available.

Mental Health Facilities Mental health is a part of primary health care system. Actual treatment of severe mental disorders is not available at the primary level. While mental health care is expected to cover for mental health, very limited care is actually available. Regular training of primary care professionals is not carried out in the field of mental health.
There are no community care facilities for patients with mental disorders. Only traditional healers offer treatment at community level.

Psychiatric Beds and Professionals

Total psychiatric beds per 10 000 population	0
Psychiatric beds in mental hospitals per 10 000 population	0
Psychiatric beds in general hospitals per 10 000 population	0
Psychiatric beds in other settings per 10 000 population	0
Number of psychiatrists per 100 000 population	0
Number of neurosurgeons per 100 000 population	0
Number of psychiatric nurses per 100 000 population	0
Number of neurologists per 100 000 population	0
Number of psychologists per 100 000 population	0
Number of social workers per 100 000 population	0.2

Non-Governmental Organizations NGOs are not involved with mental health in the country.

Information Gathering System There is no mental health reporting system in the country.
The country has no data collection system or epidemiological study on mental health.

Programmes for Special Population There are no specific programmes.

Therapeutic Drugs The following therapeutic drugs are generally available at the primary health care level of the country: carbamazepine, phenobarbital, phenytoin sodium, sodium valproate, chlorpromazine, diazepam, haloperidol, levodopa.
The essential drug list was revised in the year 2000.

Other Information The appointment of a Focal Point for mental health in the Ministry of Health is under consideration.

Additional Sources of Information

Eritrea

GENERAL INFORMATION

Eritrea is a country with an approximate area of 118 thousand sq. km. (UNO, 2001). Its population is 4.296 million, and the sex ratio (men per hundred women) is 99 (UNO, 2004). The proportion of population under the age of 15 years is 45% (UNO, 2004), and the proportion of population above the age of 60 years is 4% (WHO, 2004). The literacy rate is 67.3% for men and 44.5% for women (UNESCO/MoH, 2004).

The country is a low income group country (based on World Bank 2004 criteria). The proportion of health budget to GDP is 5.7%. The per capita total expenditure on health is 36 international $, and the per capita government expenditure on health is 23 international $ (WHO, 2004).

The main language(s) used in the country is (are) Tigrigna, Tigre, Saho, Afar, Bilen, Kunama, Nara, Hidarib and Arabic. The largest ethnic group(s) is (are) Tigrinya and Tigre. The largest religious group(s) is (are) Muslim, and the other religious group(s) are (is) Eritrean Orthodox Christian.

The life expectancy at birth is 55.8 years for males and 59.3 years for females (WHO, 2004). The healthy life expectancy at birth is 49 years for males and 51 years for females (WHO, 2004).

EPIDEMIOLOGY

There is a paucity of epidemiological data on mental illnesses in Eritrea in internationally accessible literature. Wolff and Fesseha (1998, 1999) followed a group of 4-7 year old war orphans and compared them to a group of refugee children living in a nearby camp with one or both parents. Behavioural problems were significantly more common among the orphans compared to the refugee children, but their cognitive performance was better. Though their behavioural manifestations had diminished at 5-years follow-up they continued to exhibit emotional distress. Their cognitive performance was at least as good as comparison groups from other residential settings (these children were not exposed to war). Orphans who lived in a setting where the entire staff participated in decisions affecting the children, and where the children were encouraged to become self-reliant through personal interactions with staff members, showed significantly fewer behavioural symptoms of emotional distress than orphans who lived in a setting where the director made decisions, daily routines were determined by explicit rules and schedules and interactions between staff members and the children were impersonal.

MENTAL HEALTH RESOURCES

Mental Health Policy A mental health policy is present. The policy was initially formulated in 1997.
The components of the policy are advocacy, promotion, prevention, treatment and rehabilitation.

Substance Abuse Policy A substance abuse policy is absent. The Government has issued a proclamation to provide for Tobacco Control in the Gazette of Eritrean Laws (Proclamation 143/2004, Vol. 13/2004 No. 7, August 23) in 2004.

National Mental Health Programme A national mental health programme is absent.

National Therapeutic Drug Policy/Essential List of Drugs A national therapeutic drug policy/essential list of drugs is present. It was formulated in 1997.

Mental Health Legislation The country has no mental health legislation except those mentioned in the penal code.
Details about the year of enactment of the mental health legislation are not available.

Mental Health Financing There are no budget allocations for mental health.
Details about expenditure on mental health are not available.
Details about sources of financing are not available.
The country does not have disability benefits for persons with mental disorders.

Mental Health Facilities Mental health is a part of primary health care system. Actual treatment of severe mental disorders is available at the primary level. Severe mental disorders are primarily treated at the tertiary level (at St. Mary's Psychiatric Hospital). However, limited care is available at secondary and primary levels.
Regular training of primary care professionals is carried out in the field of mental health. In the last two years, about 50 personnel were provided training. Training of primary care clinicians (physicians and nurses) started in 2004.
There are community care facilities for patients with mental disorders. The community-based rehabilitation programme run by the Ministry of Labour and Human Welfare gives the opportunity for priority rehabilitation and also referral for those severely ill patients who need active treatment.

Psychiatric Beds and Professionals

Total psychiatric beds per 10 000 population	0.64
Psychiatric beds in mental hospitals per 10 000 population	0.64
Psychiatric beds in general hospitals per 10 000 population	0
Psychiatric beds in other settings per 10 000 population	0
Number of psychiatrists per 100 000 population	0.03
Number of neurosurgeons per 100 000 population	0.03
Number of psychiatric nurses per 100 000 population	0.18
Number of neurologists per 100 000 population	0
Number of psychologists per 100 000 population	0
Number of social workers per 100 000 population	0

There are 2 psychiatrists (1 Dutch and 1 Eritrean). Both neurosurgeons are expatriates. Post basic training for psychiatric nursing (14 months full time) has started. Sixteen students are undergoing training.

Non-Governmental Organizations NGOs are not involved with mental health in the country.

Information Gathering System There is mental health reporting system in the country. The Health Management Information System collects data routinely from all health facilities.
The country has no data collection system or epidemiological study on mental health.

Programmes for Special Population There are no programmes for special populations.

Therapeutic Drugs The following therapeutic drugs are generally available at the primary health care level of the country: phenobarbital, chlorpromazine, diazepam.
The essential drug list is revised every 3 years. The next revision is due in January 2005.

Other Information

Additional Sources of Information

Wolff, P. H., Fesseha, G. (1998) The orphans of Eritrea: are orphanages part of the problem or part of the solution? American Journal of Psychiatry, 155, 1319-1324.

Wolff, P. H., Fesseha, G. (1999) The orphans of Eritrea: a five-year follow-up study. Journal of Child Psychology & Psychiatry & Allied Disciplines, 40, 1231-1237.

Estonia

GENERAL INFORMATION

Estonia is a country with an approximate area of 45 thousand sq. km. (UNO, 2001). Its population is 1.308 million, and the sex ratio (men per hundred women) is 85 (UNO, 2004). The proportion of population under the age of 15 years is 15% (UNO, 2004), and the proportion of population above the age of 60 years is 22% (WHO, 2004). The literacy rate is 99.8% for men and 99.8% for women (UNESCO/MoH, 2004).

The country is a higher middle income group country (based on World Bank 2004 criteria). The proportion of health budget to GDP is 5.5%. The per capita total expenditure on health is 562 international $, and the per capita government expenditure on health is 438 international $ (WHO, 2004).

The main language(s) used in the country is (are) Estonian. The largest ethnic group(s) is (are) Estonian (two-thirds), and the other ethnic group(s) are (is) Russian (one-fourth). The largest religious group(s) is (are) Lutheran Christian (four-fifths), and the other religious group(s) are (is) Orthodox Christian.

The life expectancy at birth is 65.1 years for males and 77.1 years for females (WHO, 2004). The healthy life expectancy at birth is 59 years for males and 69 years for females (WHO, 2004).

EPIDEMIOLOGY

A group of general practitioners used medical records and interviews using the Geriatric Depression Scale and MMSE to find the prevalence of physical and psychiatric disorders (especially depression and cognitive disorders) among a randomly selected elderly (65+ years) population in their practice. Psychiatric disorders were present in 5.7% with depression in 40.3% and cognitive disorders in 22.5% of the total respondents numbering 1000 (Saks et al, 2001). Parna et al (2002) did a nation wide cross-sectional survey to assess the prevalence of smoking. A stratified random sample of 2086 adults aged 30-59 was taken. The prevalence of current smoking was 57.9% among men and 25.7% among women. For both genders, smoking rates were lowest in the age group 50-59 years and highest in the age group 30-39 years. Smoking was significantly more common among divorced and widowed people. Education was associated with smoking among men but not among women. Pakriev et al (2001) evaluated a rural sample consisting of 232 respondents with unipolar depression. In this sample, 21.1% had single episodes, 62.5% had recurrent episodes and 16.4% had a chronic course. Being of local ethnicity and unmarried status were significantly associated with both recurrent and chronic course of depression. Comorbid dysthymia and poor family relationships were associated with chronic depression. Suicide attempts were associated with recurrent depression. Varnik et al (1994) presented their data on changing trends of suicide in the 3 Baltic states of Estonia, Latvia and Lithuania during the period 1968-90. Since 1986, the mean male suicide rate in Estonia fell by 26.6% from a high of 55.7 per 100 000 in the period 1968-84. Female suicide rates remained constant in both those periods (nearly 14.3 per 10 000). The male female ratio dropped to 3.1 from an earlier value of 3.9. In an earlier study by Varnik (1991) it was reported that suicide rates rose gradually since independence in 1922 till 1986 and then started to fall from 1986 onwards. Wasserman et al (1998) found that alcohol related suicides among women drinkers reduced by 19% in the period 1984-1990 in 8 republics (including Estonia) of the erstwhile USSR. This was attributed to the restrictions (in the form of increased prices) imposed on alcohol by the Government during that period.

MENTAL HEALTH RESOURCES

Mental Health Policy A mental health policy is present. The policy was initially formulated in 2002.
The mental health policy is contained in the Mental Health Basic Document. A mental health strategy document is under development.

Substance Abuse Policy A substance abuse policy is present. The policy was initially formulated in 1997. Details can be obtained about the drug policy from the website: www.narko.sm.ee

National Mental Health Programme A national mental health programme is absent.
Estonia does not have a comprehensive mental health plan but it has a national strategy on suicide prevention and a draft national programme.

National Therapeutic Drug Policy/Essential List of Drugs A national therapeutic drug policy/essential list of drugs is present. It was formulated in 1996.
Details can be obtained from the website: www.sam.ee

Mental Health Legislation There is a Mental Health Act. The main principles are: (1) Criteria are given for involuntary treatment (dangerousness to self or others due to mental disorder, other means of treatment not being effective); (2) Supervision over involuntary treatment is carried out both by the county medical officer and the administrative court; (3) The Mental Health Act also determines the basic requirements for psychiatric treatment, including responsibilities for the provision of services by the community and the state, the rights of patients and the basic regulations for forensic psychiatry.
The latest legislation was enacted in 1997.

Mental Health Financing There are no budget allocations for mental health.
Details about expenditure on mental health are not available.
The primary sources of mental health financing in descending order are social insurance, out of pocket expenditure by the patient or family and private insurances.
The country has disability benefits for persons with mental disorders.

Mental Health Facilities Mental health is a part of primary health care system. Actual treatment of severe mental disorders is available at the primary level.
Regular training of primary care professionals is carried out in the field of mental health.
There are community care facilities for patients with mental disorders. Community care training for nurses has begun. The Estonian Psychiatric Association has developed several proposals for the development of community services. It is expected that with the introduction of the Hospital Masterplan (www.sm.ee/develop.html) for the development of secondary health care services, the Government will develop more community-orientated services including services for the long-term mentally ill (see the development of special care: www.sm.ee/devspecialcare.html).

Psychiatric Beds and Professionals

Total psychiatric beds per 10 000 population	10.2
Psychiatric beds in mental hospitals per 10 000 population	8
Psychiatric beds in general hospitals per 10 000 population	2.1
Psychiatric beds in other settings per 10 000 population	0
Number of psychiatrists per 100 000 population	13
Number of neurosurgeons per 100 000 population	1
Number of psychiatric nurses per 100 000 population	0
Number of neurologists per 100 000 population	13
Number of psychologists per 100 000 population	
Number of social workers per 100 000 population	

Psychiatric hospitals and wards provide acute inpatient treatment, but the majority of long-term institutionalized patients are cared for in the psychiatric nursing homes of the social welfare system. The outpatient services are linked either to a psychiatric hospital or to the local general hospital. The Swedish East European Committee is supporting training of nurses.

Non-Governmental Organizations NGOs are involved with mental health in the country. They are mainly involved in advocacy, prevention and rehabilitation. There are several NGOs that are active in the field of mental health. Among them are organizations for consumers of the services or their families, professional societies and groups for the protection of consumer rights. At the level of local Government, the mental health services are mainly represented by day centres for psychiatric patients, crisis centres and telephone hotlines.

Information Gathering System There is mental health reporting system in the country.
The country has no data collection system or epidemiological study on mental health.

Programmes for Special Population There are no facilities for special population groups.

Therapeutic Drugs The following therapeutic drugs are generally available at the primary health care level of the country: carbamazepine, ethosuximide, phenobarbital, phenytoin sodium, sodium valproate, amitriptyline, chlorpromazine, diazepam, fluphenazine, haloperidol, lithium, biperiden, carbidopa, levodopa.
Details can be obtained about the drug policy from the website: www.narko.sm.ee

Other Information In Estonia, mental health services are provided by the medical facilities and practitioners, as well as by institutions from the social welfare sector. The state, the local level of services and private agencies are all represented in this field. Although cooperation between the different sectors is improving, there are still many steps to be taken to provide society with a well functioning network of services. Before the last decade, mental health services were characterized by: centralized provision, large institutions with poor material conditions, underdeveloped outpatient services, weak connections with primary health care, underdeveloped community care services for long-term severely ill patients, split between social and health care services, lack of relevant legislation, medical model dominating over psychosocial understanding of illness, lack of trained personnel (nurses, social workers) and the absence of psychotherapy training. The strategy of the Estonian Psychiatric Association are to: maintain and improve the links with the rest of the health care system, define responsibilities with the social welfare system, develop more community services for the long-term mentally ill, link the social services with health care, focus on legislation in order to meet European standards, improve training of mental health specialists and develop new structures for the provision of services like psychiatric wards in general hospitals and outpatient units with multidisciplinary teams.

Additional Sources of Information

Pakriev, S., Shlik, J., Vasar, V. (2001) Course of depression: findings from cross-sectional survey in rural Udmurtia. Nordic Journal of Psychiatry, 55, 185-189.

Parna, K., Rahu, K., Rahu, M. (2002) Patterns of smoking in Estonia. Addiction, 97, 871-876.

Saks, K., Kolk, H., Allev, R., et al (2001) Health status of the older population in Estonia. Croatian Medical Journal, 42, 663-668.

The provisional development plan of mental health services (in Estonian only): www.sm.ee/arengukavad/Psuhhiaatria.htm

Varnik, A. (1991) Suicide in Estonia. Acta Psychiatrica Scandinavica, 84, 229-232.

Varnik, A., Wasserman, D., Eklund, G. (1994) Suicides in the Baltic countries, 1968-1990. Scandinavian Journal of Social Medicine, 22, 166-169.

Wasserman, D., Varnik, A., Eklund, G. (1998) Female suicides and alcohol consumption during perestroika in the former USSR. Acta Psychiatrica Scandinavica, Supplementum 394, 26-33.

Ethiopia

GENERAL INFORMATION

Ethiopia is a country with an approximate area of 1104 thousand sq. km. (UNO, 2001). Its population is 72.42 million, and the sex ratio (men per hundred women) is 99 (UNO, 2004). The proportion of population under the age of 15 years is 45% (UNO, 2004), and the proportion of population above the age of 60 years is 5% (WHO, 2004). The literacy rate is 49.2% for men and 33.8% for women (UNESCO/MoH, 2004).

The country is a low income group country (based on World Bank 2004 criteria). The proportion of health budget to GDP is 3.6%. The per capita total expenditure on health is 14 international $, and the per capita government expenditure on health is 6 international $ (WHO, 2004).

The main language(s) used in the country is (are) Amharic, Oromo and Tigrinya. The largest ethnic group(s) is (are) Oromo and Amhara, and the other ethnic group(s) are (is) Tigre, Somale and Walayta. The largest religious group(s) is (are) Muslim, and the other religious group(s) are (is) Ethiopian Orthodox Christian.

The life expectancy at birth is 46.8 years for males and 49.4 years for females (WHO, 2004). The healthy life expectancy at birth is 41 years for males and 42 years for females (WHO, 2004).

EPIDEMIOLOGY

Alem et al (1999d) assessed 10 468 subjects from a rural and semi-urban community with the Self Reporting Questionnaire (SRQ). Psychiatric morbidity was found in 17% of the respondents (cut-off – 10/11). The rate was higher among women probably because they were more likely to be older, illiterate and widowed/divorced. Tafari et al (1991) used the SRQ (cut-off – 10/11, for psychotic symptoms – 2/3) and the Holmes-Rahe Social Readjustment Scale in another rural sample (n=2000) and found the prevalence of mental illness to be 17.2% (neurotic: 11.2% and psychotic: 6.0%). Prevalence of mental disorders was significantly associated with stress, family history of mental illness and with marital status (divorced, separated or widowed). Awas et al (1999) used the Ahmaric version of the CIDI (ICD-10 criteria) for assessing 501 respondents selected from a predominantly rural district by stratified random sampling. They found a lifetime prevalence rate of 31.8% (26.7% when substance dependence was not included). The most frequent specific diagnoses were: dissociative disorders (6.3%), mood disorders (6.2%), somatoform disorders (5.9%) and anxiety disorders (5.7%). Female gender was associated with increased risk of mood disorders and somatoform disorders. Cognitive and mood disorders were more common among the elderly. Kebede et al (1999) examined a sample from an urban community (n=10 203). They reported a probable diagnosis of psychosis in 5% of the sample (positive response to 2 out of 4 items of the SRQ) and of common mental disorders in 11.7% (using a cut-off of 6 out of 20 SRQ items). Age, female sex, lower educational level, unemployment, small family size and family history of mental illness were associated with high prevalence rates. Kebede and Alem (1999c, d, e) conducted a survey on a randomly selected urban community sample of 1420 individuals using the Ahmaric version of CIDI. Lifetime prevalence for severe cognitive deficits, schizophrenia, schizoaffective disorder, affective disorders, neurotic and somatoform disorders were 2.6%, 0.4%, 0.5%, 5.0% (overall: women 7.7% and men 3.2%, bipolar disorders: 0.3%, depressive episodes: 2.7%, recurrent depressive episodes: 0.2% and persistent mood disorders: 1.6%), 10.8% (phobic disorder: 4.8%, somatoform disorders: 2.7%, dissociative disorders: 0.8% and other anxiety disorders: 2.7%). The one month prevalence of schizophrenia, schizoaffective disorder, affective disorders, phobic anxiety disorders, other anxiety disorders, dissociative disorders, and somatoform disorders were 0.3%, 0.4%, 3.8% (women 5.9% and men 2.3%), 4.4%, 1.2%, 0.4% and 2.5%, respectively. Alem et al (1999b) and Kebede and Alem (1999b) reported that the overall prevalence of problem drinking (meeting 2 criteria on the CAGE questionnaire) was 3.7% in a rural (n=10 468) and 2.7% in an urban (n=10 203) sample. Age, gender (male), education (low), employment status (low), religion (Christian), ethnicity (non-Gurage) and smoking were associated with problem drinking in both sexes. Marital status, mental distress and income were associated with problem drinking only in men. Kebede et al (1999) reported that use of CIDI yielded a lifetime and one-month prevalence of alcohol dependence in 1.0% and 0.8% of the urban sample, respectively. Alcohol dependence was reported almost exclusively in males. Almost one third of the Ethiopean adult population uses or has used Khat. Alem et al (1999a) reported that 17.4% of subjects from a rural sample (n=19 468) used it daily. Habitual use was associated with gender (male), age (15-34 years), religion (Muslim), smoking, educational level (high), family functioning (better) and mental distress. De Jong et al (2001) assessed randomly selected post-conflict survivors in four countries – Algeria, Cambodia, Ethiopia (n=1200) and Gaza using the CIDI and Life Events and Social History Questionnaire. The prevalence rate of PTSD was 15.8% in Ethiopia. Conflict-related trauma after age 12 years, torture, psychiatric history and current illness were associated with PTSD in Ethiopia. Alem et al (1999c) and Kebede and Alem (1999a) reported the rate of suicide attempts to be 3.2% and 0.95% in rural (n=10 468) and urban (n=10 203) samples, respectively. In both studies hanging (among men) and poisoning (among women) were the preferred methods of attempting suicide. Suicide attempts were associated with young age (15-24 years), religion (Christianity), psychiatric morbidity and problem drinking. Kebede and Ketsela (1993) evaluated a representative sample of all high-school students in a city. Almost 14.3% of the adolescents reported having attempted suicide. Suicide attempts were strongly and linearly associated with hopelessness, grade and heavy alcohol intake. Mulatu (1995) interviewed mothers using the Child Behavior Problem Questionnaire to assess 611 randomly selected children from an urban community. They found that 21.5% of boys and 25.2% of girls had some behavioural problems. Tadesse et al (1999) used the Amharic version of the Reporting Questionnaire for Children in a community survey and found behavioural disorders in 17.7% of children. Childhood mental disorder was significantly associated with the subjects' own age (higher), gender, and parents' age (younger), marital status (not currently married) and psychopathology (neurosis in mothers). Ashenafi et al (2001) used an Amharic version of a Diagnostic Instrument for Children and Adolescents to interview parents in a rural community (n=1477) and found that 3.5% had at least one mental or behavioral disorder. The most frequent diagnoses were anxiety disorders (1.6%), attention deficit hyperactivity disorder (1.5%), disruptive behaviour disorders (1.5%), mood disorders (1%) and elimination disorders (0.8%).

MENTAL HEALTH RESOURCES

Mental Health Policy A mental health policy is absent.
A team of mental health professionals was assigned the task of drafting a mental health policy in 2004. The draft is expected to be submitted for approval in the same year.

Substance Abuse Policy A substance abuse policy is absent.

National Mental Health Programme A national mental health programme is absent.

National Therapeutic Drug Policy/Essential List of Drugs A national therapeutic drug policy/essential list of drugs is present. Details about the year of formulation are not available.
Shortage of essential drugs is a problem.

Mental Health Legislation There is no mental health legislation in the country. Currently, individual rights are seen in unison with the family. Involuntary treatment only requires informed consent from the escorts. Though a draft legislation was submitted for approval several years back, it has not yet been enacted. In 2004, the team working on mental health policy is also reviewing the draft legislation for re-submission.

Mental Health Financing There are budget allocations for mental health.
Details about expenditure on mental health are not available.
The primary sources of mental health financing in descending order are tax based, out of pocket expenditure by the patient or family, private insurances and grants.
The country has disability benefits for persons with mental disorders. Pension and transfer are allowed on the basis of psychiatric certification.

Mental Health Facilities Mental health is a part of primary health care system. Actual treatment of severe mental disorders is available at the primary level. Mental health has become part of primary health care in 42 units spread throughout the country. The number is gradually increasing as trained professionals are assigned to new sites every year. Thus, actual treatment of severe mental disorders at the primary level is steadily expanding.
Regular training of primary care professionals is carried out in the field of mental health. In the last two years, about 277 personnel were provided training. In the last two years, about 45 personnel were provided basic training, 160 primary mental health professionals participated in yearly refresher seminars and 72 on-the-job training programmes were conducted for those working at the different units in the country.
There are no community care facilities for patients with mental disorders.

Psychiatric Beds and Professionals

Total psychiatric beds per 10 000 population	0.07
Psychiatric beds in mental hospitals per 10 000 population	0.06
Psychiatric beds in general hospitals per 10 000 population	0.01
Psychiatric beds in other settings per 10 000 population	0
Number of psychiatrists per 100 000 population	0.02
Number of neurosurgeons per 100 000 population	0.003
Number of psychiatric nurses per 100 000 population	0.3
Number of neurologists per 100 000 population	0.006
Number of psychologists per 100 000 population	0.08
Number of social workers per 100 000 population	0.08

There are different medical assistants for other fields, around 10 000, but not for psychiatry. There are 36 regional and district mental health units besides the mental hospital in Addis Ababa. These hospitals are each staffed by at least 2 psychiatric nurses who are supervised by psychiatrists periodically. A system of referral and back-referral has been established. In some regional hospitals the psychiatric nurses admit and provide inpatient service to their cases in the medical wards when it is necessary. A postgraduate programme in psychiatry was started in Addis Ababa University with an initial intake of 7 residents in 2003.

Non-Governmental Organizations NGOs are not involved with mental health in the country. One indigenous NGO named 'Mental Health Society of Ethiopia' was established in 2004. The association is currently working on building up its membership but is already involved in supporting the only rehabilitation centre for mental health near Addis Ababa.

Information Gathering System There is mental health reporting system in the country. Hospitals send annual report to the Ministry of Health.

The country has data collection system or epidemiological study on mental health. The training and research division of the Amanvel Mental hospital has been established recently for this purpose.

Programmes for Special Population There are no programmes for special population.

Psychiatric services have been introduced to some police and army hospitals, one prison clinic, and some university and school clinics. Two substance abuse treatment units were opened in the capital city in 2004.

Therapeutic Drugs The following therapeutic drugs are generally available at the primary health care level of the country: carbamazepine, ethosuximide, phenobarbital, phenytoin sodium, sodium valproate, amitriptyline, chlorpromazine, diazepam, fluphenazine, haloperidol, lithium, carbidopa, levodopa.

The essential list of drugs was revised recently. Some other medicines like cloimipramine and fluoxetine are also a part of the list. All drugs in the essential list are available in major cities of the country but not in all areas at the primary health care level.

Other Information Traditional healers play a major role in the treatment of mental health; in one study (Alem et al 1999) it was found that 85% of emotionally disturbed people sought help from traditional healers.

Additional Sources of Information

Alem, A. (2000) Human rights and psychiatric care in Africa with particular reference to the Ethiopian situation. Acta Psychiatrica Scandinavica, Supplementum 399, 93-96.

Alem, A. (2001) Mental health services and epidemiology of mental health problems in Ethiopia. Ethiopean Medical Journal, 39, 153-165.

Alem, A. (2002) Community-based vs. hospital-based mental health care: the case of Africa. World Psychiatry, 1, 98-99.

Alem, A., Araya, M., Jacobsson, L., et al (1999) How are mental disorders seen and where is help sought in a rural Ethiopian community? A key informant study in Butajira, Ethiopia. Acta Psychiatrica Scandinavica, Supplementum 397, 40-47.

Alem, A., Kebede, D., Jacobsson, L., et al (1999c) Suicide attempts among adults in Butajira, Ethiopia. Acta Psychiatrica Scandinavica, Supplementum, 397, 70-76.

Alem, A., Kebede, D., Kullgren, G. (1999a) The prevalence and socio-demographic correlates of khat chewing in Butajira, Ethiopia. Acta Psychiatrica Scandinavica, Supplementum, 397, 84-91.

Alem, A., Kebede, D., Kullgren, G. (1999b) The epidemiology of problem drinking in Butajira, Ethiopia. Acta Psychiatrica Scandinavica, Supplementum, 397, 77-83.

Alem, A., Kebede, D., Woldesemiat, G., et al (1999d) The prevalence and socio-demographic correlates of mental distress in Butajira, Ethiopia. Acta Psychiatrica Scandinavica, Supplementum, 397, 48-55.

Ashenafi, Y., Kebede, D., Desta, M., et al (2001) Prevalence of mental and behavioural disorders in Ethiopian children. East African Medical Journal, 78, 308-311.

Awas, M., Kebede, D., Alem, A. (1999) Major mental disorders in Butajira, southern Ethiopia. Acta Psychiatrica Scandinavica, Supplementum, 397, 56-64.

de Jong, J. T., Komproe, I. H., Van Ommeren, M., et al (2001) Lifetime events and posttraumatic stress disorder in 4 postconflict settings. JAMA, 286, 555-562.

Giel, R. (1999). The prehistory of psychiatry in Ethiopia. Acta Psychiatrica Scandinavica. Supplementum 397, 2-4.

Kebede, D., Alem, A. (1999a) Suicide attempts and ideation among adults in Addis Ababa, Ethiopia. Acta Psychiatrica Scandinavica, Supplementum, 397, 35-39.

Kebede, D., Alem, A. (1999b) The epidemiology of alcohol dependence and problem drinking in Addis Ababa, Ethiopia. Acta Psychiatrica Scandinavica, Supplementum, 397, 30-34.

Kebede, D., Alem, A. (1999c) Major mental disorders in Addis Ababa, Ethiopia. III. Neurotic and somatoform disorders. Acta Psychiatrica Scandinavica, Supplementum, 397, 24-29.

Kebede, D., Alem, A. (1999d) Major mental disorders in Addis Ababa, Ethiopia. II. Affective disorders. Acta Psychiatrica Scandinavica, Supplementum, 397, 18-23.

Kebede, D., Alem, A. (1999e) Major mental disorders in Addis Ababa, Ethiopia. I. Schizophrenia, schizoaffective and cognitive disorders. Acta Psychiatrica Scandinavica, Supplementum, 397, 11-17.

Kebede, D., Alem, A., Rashid, E. (1999) The prevalence and socio-demographic correlates of mental distress in Addis Ababa, Ethiopia. Acta Psychiatrica Scandinavica, Supplementum, 99, 5-10.

Kebede, D., Ketsela, T. (1993) Suicide attempts in Ethiopian adolescents in Addis Abeba high schools. Ethiopian Medical Journal, 31, 83-90.

Mulatu, M. S. (1995) Prevalence and risk factors of psychopathology in Ethiopian children. Journal of the American Academy of Child & Adolescent Psychiatry, 34, 100-109.

Tadesse, B., Kebede, D., Tegegne, T., et al (1999) Childhood behavioural disorders in Ambo district, western Ethiopia. I. Prevalence estimates. Acta Psychiatrica Scandinavica, Supplementum, 397, 92-97.

Tafari, S., Aboud, F. E., Larson, C. P. (1991) Determinants of mental illness in a rural Ethiopian adult population. Social Science & Medicine, 32, 197-201.

Fiji

GENERAL INFORMATION

Fiji is a country with an approximate area of 18 thousand sq. km. (UNO, 2001). The country consists of more than 300 islands. Its population is 0.847 million, and the sex ratio (men per hundred women) is 104 (UNO, 2004). The proportion of population under the age of 15 years is 32% (UNO, 2004), and the proportion of population above the age of 60 years is 6% (WHO, 2004). The literacy rate is 94.5% for men and 91.4% for women (UNESCO/MoH, 2004).
The country is a lower middle income group country (based on World Bank 2004 criteria). The proportion of health budget to GDP is 4%. The per capita total expenditure on health is 224 international $, and the per capita government expenditure on health is 150 international $ (WHO, 2004).
The main language(s) used in the country is (are) Fijian, Hindi, English and Rotuman. The largest ethnic group(s) is (are) Fijian (more than half of the population), and the other ethnic group(s) are (is) Indian (two-fifths). The largest religious group(s) is (are) Christian, and the other religious group(s) are (is) Hindu and Muslim.
The life expectancy at birth is 64.6 years for males and 70.3 years for females (WHO, 2004). The healthy life expectancy at birth is 57 years for males and 61 years for females (WHO, 2004).

EPIDEMIOLOGY

Becker (1998) assessed the frequency of 'na tadoka ni vasucu', a somatic syndrome occurring among ethnic Fijian women. The authors assessed 85 consecutive newly delivered ethnic Fijian women within the first few postpartum days and then again after 2-5 months with translated structured interviews, the Kellner Symptom Questionnaire and visual analogy scales to assess social supports and occurrence of mood symptoms or an episode of 'na tadoka ni vasucu.' Semistructured ethnographic interviews were conducted with subjects who reported an episode of the latter. 'Na tadoka ni vasucu' occurred in 9% (n=7) of the sample. Both quantitative and narrative data demonstrated that this syndrome is associated with perceived inferior social supports. Aghanwa (2001a) compared characteristics of 51 unipolar mania patients with 31 bipolar patients in a hospital-based study. Diagnosis was confirmed using SCAN and ICD-10. Though the frequency of episodes, duration of affective illness, mean age at onset, gender distribution, marital status, employment status and race were not significantly different between the two groups, family history of major psychiatric morbidity was significantly more in the bipolar group (9.8% for the unipolar manic patients and 22.6% for the manic-depressive group). In other studies, Aghanwa (2000, 2001b) estimated the prevalence of attempted suicide to be 34.8 per 100 000 population based on a sample of 39 consecutive cases referred to psychiatric services at the main general hospital. Suicide formed 36.8% of all the cases referred to the psychiatric service. Social problems and/or psychiatric comorbidity were present in over 60% of cases. Suicide attempters were significantly more likely to be younger, single and unemployed. When 31 consecutive patients attending a hospital, with deliberate drug-overdose and 27 others with non-overdosed self-poisoning were compared, those with overdose were found to be older and to have a history of psychiatric disorder. Alcohol use was significantly more common in the other group, which also had a greater proportion of males. Pridmore et al (1995) assessed the prevalence of suicide and self-harm based on an unidentified data source. They reported that self-harm had become more common particularly among those of Indian ethnicity (in both males and females). Non-fatal injury by self was reported to be 8 times more common than suicide and it had a female preponderance. Disproportionately high rates of completed suicide was reported among Fijian Indians (women under 30 years and males above 30 years) based on police and medical records by Haynes (1984). Pridmore et al (1996) examined the hanging and poisoning autopsy reports from two distinct regions. The rate of autopsy (per 100 000 population per year) among Indians was significantly greater than among Fijians. Regional variation with respect to gender and method of attempting suicide were noted. Hanging remains the preferred option for all groups. Booth (1999) reported high suicide rates among 13 Pacific islands. Young women outnumbered men among Fiji Indians and Western Samoans. They noted that pesticides were a common method of attempting suicide. Fiji was one of the participating countries in the Global Youth Tobacco Survey (GYTS) project developed by the World Health Organization and the US Centers for Disease Control and Prevention to track tobacco use among youth in countries across the world (Warren et al, 2000).

MENTAL HEALTH RESOURCES

Mental Health Policy A mental health policy is present. The policy was initially formulated in 1994.
The components of the policy are advocacy, promotion, prevention, treatment and rehabilitation. The National Advisory Council in Mental Health is in the process of reviewing the National Mental Health Policy (National Mental Health Plan 2005-2008). NGOs are being consulted on this project. The draft policy focuses on development of community mental health services, development of mental health action volunteers to assist in rehabilitation, expansion of the mental health workforce, revision of the mental health legislation and mental health promotion.

Substance Abuse Policy A substance abuse policy is present. The policy was initially formulated in 1998.

National Mental Health Programme A national mental health programme is present. The programme was formulated in 1999.

National Therapeutic Drug Policy/Essential List of Drugs A national therapeutic drug policy/essential list of drugs is present. It was formulated in 1994.

Mental Health Legislation There are the Laws of Fiji – Chapter 113 – Mental Treatment Act. The Act was initially formulated in the 1940's and partly revised in 1978, but it is considered to be too narrow as it deals only with treatment issues. Based on a cabinet paper that was prepared with the assistance of WHO, the Cabinet has approved of review for MTA. Fiji Law Reform will draft the law and then consultations with various stakeholders will be held.
The latest legislation was enacted in 1978.

Mental Health Financing There are budget allocations for mental health.
The country spends 1.7% of the total health budget on mental health.
The primary sources of mental health financing in descending order are tax based, out of pocket expenditure by the patient or family and private insurances.
The entire mental health budget is spent on curative services.
The country has disability benefits for persons with mental disorders. They are able to apply for social welfare assistance.

Mental Health Facilities Mental health is a part of primary health care system. Actual treatment of severe mental disorders is not available at the primary level. There is a lack of sufficiently trained doctors or facilities to treat severely ill patients in the primary health centres.
Regular training of primary care professionals is carried out in the field of mental health. In the last two years, about 140 personnel were provided training. Training to primary health care workers is through workshops that are being held regularly since the last two years.
There are no community care facilities for patients with mental disorders. There are no community-based care facilities for the mentally ill. Discussions on establishing regional (in all 4 divisions) mental health units are under way. St. Giles Hospital has day care and occupational therapy facilities and the hospital staff provide limited community services in the greater Suva area. A community psychiatric nursing team has been established. The community service provided is largely a pre-discharge contact with the appropriate zone nurse and the sub-divisional medical officer to whom the details of the patient is provided. Medication required for the patients are sent every month to the nurse. A community team comprising of a doctor and nurses also make domiciliary visits and conduct counselling and education. This operates within a radius of about 10 km from the hospital.

Psychiatric Beds and Professionals

Total psychiatric beds per 10 000 population	2.34
Psychiatric beds in mental hospitals per 10 000 population	2.34
Psychiatric beds in general hospitals per 10 000 population	0
Psychiatric beds in other settings per 10 000 population	0
Number of psychiatrists per 100 000 population	0.25
Number of neurosurgeons per 100 000 population	0.1
Number of psychiatric nurses per 100 000 population	0
Number of neurologists per 100 000 population	0
Number of psychologists per 100 000 population	0.25
Number of social workers per 100 000 population	0

There is one occupational therapist. There are 23 nurses working in mental health care settings. The clinical psychologists are in private practice and other psychologists work in the university (academic psychology) setting. There are about 10 000 social workers, but they are not trained in mental health.

Non-Governmental Organizations NGOs are involved with mental health in the country. They are mainly involved in advocacy, promotion, prevention and rehabilitation.

Information Gathering System There is mental health reporting system in the country. The main source of information collection is through annual reports of the St. Giles Hospital at Suva (these are submitted to the MOH). A patient Information System (PATIS) is being established in the general health sector. The mental health services are yet to be linked to the PATIS.
The country has data collection system or epidemiological study on mental health. The Statistics Department collects information from hospitals.

Programmes for Special Population The Fiji Council for Social Services attends to the needs of the elderly in the community.

Therapeutic Drugs The following therapeutic drugs are generally available at the primary health care level of the country: carbamazepine, ethosuximide, phenobarbital, phenytoin sodium, sodium valproate, amitriptyline, chlorpromazine, diazepam, fluphenazine, haloperidol, lithium, carbidopa, levodopa.
Olanzapine has been added to the essential list. The supply is limited to 1000 (10 mg) tablets per month. The approximate cost of 100 tablets of a generic brand (10 mg – commonest strength) is 14.25 USD. It is, however, not available at the primary care level.

Other Information

Additional Sources of Information

Aghanwa, H. S. (2000) The characteristics of suicide attempters admitted to the main general hospital in Fiji Islands. Journal of Psychosomatic Research, 49, 439-445.

Aghanwa, H. S. (2001a) Recurrent unipolar mania in a psychiatric hospital setting in the Fiji Islands. Psychopathology, 34, 312-317.

Aghanwa, H. S. (2001b) Attempted suicide by drug overdose and by poison-ingestion methods seen at the main general hospital in the Fiji islands: a comparative study. General Hospital Psychiatry, 23, 266-271.

Becker, A. E. (1998) Postpartum illness in Fiji: a sociosomatic perspective. Psychosomatic Medicine, 60, 431-438.

Booth, H. (1999) Pacific Island suicide in comparative perspective. Journal of Biosocial Science, 31, 433-448.

Cruz, M. (2004) A review of existing functions and responsibilities of the Fiji Ministry of Health in relation to the care, treatment and rehabilitation of mentally ill people in Fiji (Draft).

Government document (1978) Laws of Fiji. Mental Treatment, Chapter 113.

Government document (1998) Substance Abuse Advisory Council Act.

Haynes, R. H. (1984) Suicide in Fiji: a preliminary study. British Journal of Psychiatry, 145, 433-438.

Khan, S. (1998) Community Psychiatric Nursing Annual Report.

Medical Superintendent (1998) Report on the St. Giles Staff Activities in the Western Division.

Narayan, S. (2003) Country report on mental health issues for the Regional Report on Mental Health from the Western Pacific Region.

Narayan, S., Plange, N-K. (2003) Project: Mental Health Policy project. Country Fiji (Draft).

Pridmore, S., Ryan, K., Blizzard, L. (1995) Victims of violence in Fiji. Australian & New Zealand. Journal of Psychiatry, 29, 666-670.

Pridmore, S., Lawler, A., Couper, D. (1996) Hanging and poisoning autopsies in Fiji. Australian & New Zealand Journal of Psychiatry, 30, 685-687.

St. Giles Hospital Annual Report (1999) Mental Health, Non-Communicable Diseases.

St. Giles Hospital Annual Report (1997) Community Mental Health Team.

Warren, C. W., Riley, L., Asma, S., et al (2000) Tobacco use by youth: a surveillance report from the Global Youth Tobacco Survey project. Bulletin of the World Health Organization, 78, 868-876.

Finland

GENERAL INFORMATION

Finland is a country with an approximate area of 338 thousand sq. km. (UNO, 2001). Its population is 5.216 million, and the sex ratio (men per hundred women) is 96 (UNO, 2004). The proportion of population under the age of 15 years is 17% (UNO, 2004), and the proportion of population above the age of 60 years is 20% (WHO, 2004). The literacy rate is 99% for men and 99% for women (UNESCO/MoH, 2004).
The country is a high income group country (based on World Bank 2004 criteria). The proportion of health budget to GDP is 7%. The per capita total expenditure on health is 1845 international $, and the per capita government expenditure on health is 1395 international $ (WHO, 2004).
The main language(s) used in the country is (are) Finnish and Swedish. The largest ethnic group(s) is (are) Finn. The largest religious group(s) is (are) Lutheran Christian (five-sixths), and the other religious group(s) are (is) Orthodox Christian.
The life expectancy at birth is 74.8 years for males and 81.5 years for females (WHO, 2004). The healthy life expectancy at birth is 69 years for males and 74 years for females (WHO, 2004).

EPIDEMIOLOGY

There is substantial epidemiological data on mental illnesses in Finland in internationally accessible literature. No attempt was made to include this information here.

E–I

MENTAL HEALTH RESOURCES

Mental Health Policy A mental health policy is present. The policy was initially formulated in 1993.
The components of the policy are advocacy, promotion, prevention, treatment and rehabilitation. Finland has a health policy document (Health 2015) where mental health is included as an integrated component (a specific mental health policy paper is not there). In health policy, the main priorities are basic services and outpatient services. The Ministry of Social Affairs and Health produced quality guidelines for mental health services in 2001 and is working on quality guidelines for supportive housing regarding people with mental health problems.

Substance Abuse Policy A substance abuse policy is present. The policy was initially formulated in 1997. The substance abuse policy is known as Drug Strategy. The Government has adopted a Drug Policy Action Programme for the period 2004-2007. An Alcohol Programme was formulated in 2004.

National Mental Health Programme A national mental health programme is present. The programme was formulated in 1999. Finland was the first country in the world to adopt a comprehensive national suicide prevention programme (in 1992).

National Therapeutic Drug Policy/Essential List of Drugs A national therapeutic drug policy/essential list of drugs is absent.

Mental Health Legislation There is a Mental Health Act. An amendment was made in 1997 regarding involuntary treatment of persons with criminal records and in 2000 regarding coercive actions. The other laws are Specialized Health Care Act, Public Health Act, Social Welfare Act and The Law of Patient's Rights. In Finland, there are two national laws that deal with the forensic psychiatric services: the Penal Code (1889, amended 2003) and the Mental Health Act (1990) with the Mental Health Decree (1990). While the Mental Health Act defines when and how patients can be committed into mental hospitals involuntarily, according to the Finnish Law, the courts decide if a forensic psychiatric evaluation should be conducted. In many cases of violent acts, the court asks the National Authority of Medicolegal Affairs to arrange for an evaluation.
The latest legislation was enacted in 1990.

Mental Health Financing There are budget allocations for mental health.
Details about expenditure on mental health are not available.
The primary sources of mental health financing in descending order are tax based, social insurance, out of pocket expenditure by the patient or family and private insurances.
One special feature of the Finnish health care system, since the state subsidy reform in 1993, is that its financing is much decentralized. The financial units are the municipalities which total 450, with an average size of 6000 people. The biggest municipality is Helsinki, with half a million people, but the smallest have only a few hundred inhabitants. Despite this, every municipality has the responsibility to provide all health care, including the most specialized, to their inhabitants, either by organizing this themselves or by buying it from health care districts, other municipalities or private providers. The municipalities have the right to collect their own taxes. The other part of the needed money comes to municipalities as a state subsidy, but without any specific earmarking for health. This has led to increasing regional and local differences in the provision of mental health care, e.g. the differences between health care districts in the annual prevalence of hospital treated patients was twofold in 2002. The differences between municipalities were even greater. The same is true for the numbers of outpatient personnel: the difference between the districts was three-fold in this respect in 1999.
The country has disability benefits for persons with mental disorders.

Mental Health Facilities Mental health is a part of primary health care system. Actual treatment of severe mental disorders is available at the primary level. Mainly, emergency treatment of severe mental disorders is available at the primary level.
Regular training of primary care professionals is not carried out in the field of mental health. Mental health is a part of basic training for physicians and nurses, however, systematic further education is not provided to primary care workers in mental health.
There are community care facilities for patients with mental disorders. Mental health services are primarily organized as community-based outpatient services. According to available data, the deinstitutionalization process was in the balance during the 1980s. The decrease in the number of psychiatric beds was compensated for by increasing outpatient resources and by developing community-based care, e.g. the personnel in outpatient care doubled from 1982 to 1992. The main problem in implementing community care is the scarcity of supporting services for long-term patients living in general communities. There is a need for more supported housing, day centres, support persons and guided leisure activities; patients' families also need more help and support. In recent years, there has in fact been a slight increase in these services. Extramural rehabilitative facilities used to be provided mainly by the public health sector and a few semi-private foundations. In the 1990s, a large number of private complimentary services were founded, and now they provide nearly 90% of all extramural residential services. Currently, nearly as many patients stay in such facilities as in psychiatric hospitals. However, the standard of care in such facilities is variable as the control of authorities over such institutions is weak.

Psychiatric Beds and Professionals

Total psychiatric beds per 10 000 population	10
Psychiatric beds in mental hospitals per 10 000 population	0
Psychiatric beds in general hospitals per 10 000 population	9
Psychiatric beds in other settings per 10 000 population	1
Number of psychiatrists per 100 000 population	22
Number of neurosurgeons per 100 000 population	1
Number of psychiatric nurses per 100 000 population	180
Number of neurologists per 100 000 population	4
Number of psychologists per 100 000 population	79
Number of social workers per 100 000 population	150

Mental health services are organized around the concept of catchment areas, which are currently governed by health care districts (HCD). Roughly two-fifths of psychiatric services, mostly outpatient care, has been moved administratively to primary care in many districts. Most psychiatric wards belong to the administration of general hospitals. Other settings include state hospital beds for forensic psychiatry, prisoners, military psychiatric wards, psychiatric wards in primary care and in private hospitals. Traditionally, the mental health care system has been hospital-centred, and the deinstitutionalization process started later than in many other developed countries. At the beginning of the 1980s, Finland still had about 20 000 psychiatric beds, almost all situated in separate psychiatric hospitals. A specific feature of the Finnish situation, however, was that there never were really big hospitals; beds are spread between 60 hospitals located all over the country, and no hospital has more than 300 beds. During the last two decades, a substantial (75%) reduction in the number of beds in psychiatric institutions has occurred. The 1990 Mental Health Act forbade the treatment of minors in the same wards as adults, so the Health Care districts had to build separate units for adolescents run by adolescent psychiatrists. Hospital services for adolescents and children are separated, though they may be provided together with outpatient services. The Finnish mental health care system is characterized by teamwork (usual outpatient team comprises of psychiatrist, psychologist, psychiatric nurses and social worker). One prerequisite for this cooperation is the high standard of training among all personnel, so that all staff groups can participate in this cooperation on an equal basis. For instance, many nurses have received formal training in psychotherapy, especially family therapy. At the municipality level, local mental health work is often organized on a multidisciplinary basis. Currently there is a shortfall of psychiatrists by about one-third of the requirement, despite the intensified programme for training of psychiatrists since 1980s. Four psychiatric specialities are recognized: general psychiatry, child psychiatry, adolescent psychiatry and forensic psychiatry. About one-fifth of psychiatrists work as private practitioners only and one-third of psychiatrists working in the public sector have part-time private practice.

Non-Governmental Organizations NGOs are involved with mental health in the country. They are mainly involved in advocacy, promotion, prevention, treatment and rehabilitation. The Finnish Mental Health Association is the world's oldest NGO in the mental health field.

Information Gathering System There is mental health reporting system in the country. The Ministry of Social Affairs and Health biannually sends a social and health report to the parliament and mental health is incorporated in it.
The country has data collection system or epidemiological study on mental health. A large national epidemiological health examination study (Health 2000) was conducted in 2000. A central finding was that the prevalence of mental disorders is at present the same as twenty years before. Finland has a care register for institutional social and health care, including mental health, for service data collection.

Programmes for Special Population The country has specific programmes for mental health for refugees, disaster affected population, elderly and children.

The Finnish National Schizophrenia Project, which was carried out in the 1980s, recommended that 'acute psychosis' teams should be established in every catchment area. Their task would be to take care of new psychotic patients in the area by active initial intervention which, whenever possible, includes family participation. The 10-year follow-up of the Project, focusing on the year 1992, verified that most of the catchment areas had established these multi-disciplinary teams. In the last few years, the Government has allocated special resources for the development of services for children and adolescents. Financing of psychotherapy for children and adolescents has also increased. Specialized outpatient departments and a few wards in mental hospitals have been created for substance abuse patients. In the last few years, the Government has allocated funds for expanding such services and extending it also to primary care. There is still, however, a shortage of rehabilitative services for chronic drug users. For forensic patients, who are judged to be not criminally responsible and in need of treatment, hospitalization usually starts at either of the two state mental hospitals. After discharge the patient is under supervision for the initial 6 months and is assessed regularly at a municipal psychiatric centre, since there are no specific forensic psychiatric outpatient treatment facilities in Finland. After this period he has no other obligations to the judicial system and can continue treatment, if required, as any other psychiatric patient.

Therapeutic Drugs The following therapeutic drugs are generally available at the primary health care level of the country: carbamazepine, ethosuximide, phenytoin sodium, sodium valproate, amitriptyline, chlorpromazine, diazepam, fluphenazine, haloperidol, lithium, biperiden, carbidopa, levodopa.

Fluphenazine is available only as a decanoate injection. Medicines for outpatients are dispensed from private pharmacies and not by the Government or institutions.

Other Information Social welfare and health care are integrated at the national and provincial levels. At the national level, the Ministry of Social Affairs and Health has the highest administrative responsibility, and STAKES (National Research and Development Centre for Welfare and Health) is the active agent in the field of research and development activities. In every provincial administration, there is a Department for Social Affairs and Health. At municipal level, the models and degree of cooperation vary. In some, the social welfare and primary health care services are joined both at the administrative as well as at the practical level. In others, they still work separately from each other, although there has been, especially during the 1990s, an increasing tendency to achieve stronger integration. One practical example of increasing multi-sectoral cooperation in the area of mental health work has been the development programme called 'Meaningful Life'. This nation-wide programme from 1998-2002, the aim of which was to improve the quality of life for people suffering from mental disorders or their consequences, operated at national, regional and local levels. It has a genuinely multi-sectoral approach, as almost all ministries are participating in its steering group. The main target areas in the field of mental health promotion have been: enhancement of the value and visibility of mental health; development of mental health indicators; promotion of mental health in children and adolescents; in old age; in relation to working life and employment policy and the use of telematics in mental health promotion and substance abuse prevention. Mental health and its promotion have been stressed both in the new health strategy 'Health for 2015', as well in the governmental Goal and Action Plan for Social Welfare and Health Care 2004-2007. A national project to secure the future of health care services started in 2002 and a national development project for social services started in 2003. Both projects are financed and coordinated by the Ministry of Social Affairs and Health. The main priority is regional development of mental health work.

Additional Sources of Information

Eronen, M. Repo, E., Vartiainen, H., et al (2000) Forensic psychiatric organization in Finland. International Journal of Law and Psychiatry, 23, 541-546.

Korkeila, J. (1998) Perspectives on the Public Psychiatric Services in Finland – Evaluating the Deinstitutionalization Process. National Research and Development Centre for Welfare and Health – Finland.

Lahtinen, E., Lehtinen, V., Riikonen, E., et al (1999) Framework for Promoting Mental Health in Europe. National Research and Development Centre for Welfare and Health – Finland.

Lavikainen J, Lahtinen E, Lehtinen V. (2000) Public Health Approach to Mental Health in Europe – A Report Prepared Within the EU-Funded Project on Putting Mental Health on the European Agenda. Ministry of Social Affairs and Health.

Ministry of Social Affairs and Health (1987) Health for All by the Year 2000 – The Finnish National Strategy.

Ministry of Social Affairs and Health (1993) Health for All by the Year 2000 – Revised Strategy for Cooperation.

Ministry of Social Affairs and Health (1997) Finnish Drug Policy Committee.

Ministry of Social Affairs and Health (1998) Third Evaluation of Progress Towards Health for All – Finland.

Ministry of Social Affairs and Health (2001) Government Resolution on the Health 2015 Public Health Programme

Ministry of Social Affairs and Health (2004) Government Resolution on a drug Policy Action Program in Finland 2004-2007.

National Board of Medicolegal Affairs (1997) Amending the Mental Health Act.

Quality Recommendations for Mental Health Services (2001) Ministry of Social Affairs and Health.

Salokangas, R. K. R. (2004) Psychiatric specialist care in Finland-achievements and challenges. Journal of Mental Health, 13, 47-54.

France

GENERAL INFORMATION

France is a country with an approximate area of 552 thousand sq. km. (UNO, 2001). Its population is 60.434 million, and the sex ratio (men per hundred women) is 95 (UNO, 2004). The proportion of population under the age of 15 years is 18% (UNO, 2004), and the proportion of population above the age of 60 years is 20% (WHO, 2004). The literacy rate is 99% for men and 99% for women (UNESCO/MoH, 2004).

The country is a high income group country (based on World Bank 2004 criteria). The proportion of health budget to GDP is 9.6%. The per capita total expenditure on health is 2567 international $, and the per capita government expenditure on health is 1951 international $ (WHO, 2004).

The main language(s) used in the country is (are) French. The largest ethnic group(s) is (are) Celtic, Latin and Teutonic., and the other ethnic group(s) are (is) Slavic, North African and Southeast Asian. The largest religious group(s) is (are) Roman Catholic.

The life expectancy at birth is 76 years for males and 83.6 years for females (WHO, 2004). The healthy life expectancy at birth is 69 years for males and 75 years for females (WHO, 2004).

EPIDEMIOLOGY

There is substantial epidemiological data on mental illnesses in France in internationally accessible literature. No attempt was made to include this information here.

MENTAL HEALTH RESOURCES

Mental Health Policy A mental health policy is present. The policy was initially formulated in 1960.

The components of the policy are advocacy, promotion, prevention, treatment and rehabilitation. Details can be obtained from the circulars of 1960, 1990 and 1992.

Substance Abuse Policy A substance abuse policy is present. The policy was initially formulated in 1970.

National Mental Health Programme A national mental health programme is present. The programme was formulated in 1985. France has a comprehensive national suicide prevention programme and more recently a programme titled 'Actions against Depression.'

National Therapeutic Drug Policy/Essential List of Drugs A national therapeutic drug policy/essential list of drugs is present. Details about the year of formulation are not available.

Mental Health Legislation The latest legislation deals with admission under constraints in psychiatric hospitals. The law is due for modification in 2005 following a thorough evaluation.

The latest legislation was enacted in 1990.

Mental Health Financing There are budget allocations for mental health.

The country spends 8% of the total health budget on mental health.

The primary sources of mental health financing in descending order are social insurance and tax based.

Much of mental health care including psychotherapy of long duration is financed by social security system. Patients have free access to private or public mental health professionals of their choice. The cost of private treatment is partly financed by the social security system (fully for severe mentally ill and severely deprived patients) and partly through private insurance. However, psychotherapy by psychologists and many psychoanalysts working in the private sector are not financed by social security.

The country has disability benefits for persons with mental disorders. There are allowances for handicapped people under the law from 1975. There are also some housing benefits for them.

Mental Health Facilities Mental health is a part of primary health care system. Actual treatment of severe mental disorders is available at the primary level.

Regular training of primary care professionals is carried out in the field of mental health.

There are community care facilities for patients with mental disorders.

Psychiatric Beds and Professionals

Total psychiatric beds per 10 000 population	12
Psychiatric beds in mental hospitals per 10 000 population	7
Psychiatric beds in general hospitals per 10 000 population	3
Psychiatric beds in other settings per 10 000 population	2
Number of psychiatrists per 100 000 population	22
Number of neurosurgeons per 100 000 population	
Number of psychiatric nurses per 100 000 population	98
Number of neurologists per 100 000 population	
Number of psychologists per 100 000 population	5
Number of social workers per 100 000 population	

The public sector is responsible for sectorization and includes more than 80% of the inpatient facilities. However, there is a 5-10 fold variation in the manpower and structural resources between sectors. The private sector is also involved in sectorization but to a much smaller degree. Bed reduction is proceeding. In the 1990s, 20% of beds were reduced. General physicians manage most of the minor psychiatric illnesses, with psychiatrists providing expert opinions whenever consulted. Though psychiatrists work in close cooperation with other doctors a true liaison service involving multidisciplinary treatment approach is not yet fully developed. More than half of the psychiatrists have a private practice or are working in private institutions. A large proportion of private psychiatrists are exclusively practicing psychotherapy. Psychiatrists are concentrated in big cities, with posts lying vacant in rural areas and in northern regions. There is likely to be reduction in the number of psychiatrists due to a decrease in the number of medical students allowed to train in psychiatry. Most psychologists work in the private sector.

Non-Governmental Organizations NGOs are involved with mental health in the country. They are mainly involved in advocacy, promotion, prevention, treatment and rehabilitation. Families began to take an active role in psychiatric management and programme development since 1970 and are involved in advocacy, prevention and promotion and participation in different boards as representatives of consumers.

Information Gathering System There is mental health reporting system in the country.
The country has data collection system or epidemiological study on mental health.
A new information system collecting data on hospital activity is currently being implemented (PMSI, Programme de Médicalisation des Systèmes d'Information). Psychiatric diagnoses of adult patients are made according to ICD-10 criteria, but patients younger than 20 years are still categorized according to French classification of child psychiatry.

Programmes for Special Population The country has specific programmes for mental health for disaster affected population, elderly and children.
A national programme 'Mental health: the user at the core of an organization in need of renovation' was launched in 2001 to promote campaigns against stigma, reinforce patients' rights, improve professional practices, prevention and rehabilitation programmes and community psychiatry.

Therapeutic Drugs The following therapeutic drugs are generally available at the primary health care level of the country: carbamazepine, ethosuximide, phenobarbital, sodium valproate, amitriptyline, chlorpromazine, diazepam, fluphenazine, haloperidol, lithium, biperiden, carbidopa, levodopa.

Other Information Psychiatric services in France have been defined according to the legislation of 1838, when it was decided to have one hospital per Département. The first open unit was set up in 1920 and the first outpatient unit in 1930. The concept of sectorization, where one team would be responsible for both inpatient and outpatient care of persons within its parameters, was conceptualized during the second world war, but was fully implemented only after necessary laws were passed in 1986. Each sector (there are about 1000 sectors in France) consists of inpatient, outpatient, community care and sheltered workshops. There are different sectors for adult psychiatry, child and adolescent psychiatry and forensic psychiatry.

Additional Sources of Information

Jaeger, M. (1995) Inflections in France's Mental Health Policy. Santé Mentale au Quebec, 20, 77-87.

Provost, D., Bauer, A. (2001) Trends and developments in public psychiatry in France since 1975. Acta Psychiatrica Scandinavica, 104 (suppl. 410), 63-68.

Verdoux, H. (2003) Psychiatry in France. International Journal of Social Psychiatry, 49, 83-86.

Gabon

GENERAL INFORMATION

Gabon is a country with an approximate area of 268 thousand sq. km. (UNO, 2001). Its population is 1.352 million, and the sex ratio (men per hundred women) is 99 (UNO, 2004). The proportion of population under the age of 15 years is 40% (UNO, 2004), and the proportion of population above the age of 60 years is 6% (WHO, 2004). The literacy rate is 74% for men and 53% for women (UNESCO/MoH, 2004).

The country is a higher middle income group country (based on World Bank 2004 criteria). The proportion of health budget to GDP is 3.6%. The per capita total expenditure on health is 197 international $, and the per capita government expenditure on health is 94 international $ (WHO, 2004).

The main language(s) used in the country is (are) French (official), Fang, Punu and Nzèbi. The largest ethnic group(s) is (are) Fang, and the other ethnic group(s) are (is) Shira-Punu, Nzèbi-Duma, Mbede-Teke, Kota-Kele and Myène. The largest religious group(s) is (are) Roman Catholic (more than half), and the other religious group(s) are (is) Protestant and Muslim.

The life expectancy at birth is 57.3 years for males and 61.4 years for females (WHO, 2004). The healthy life expectancy at birth is 50 years for males and 53 years for females (WHO, 2004).

EPIDEMIOLOGY

There is a paucity of epidemiological data on mental illnesses in Gabon in internationally accessible literature. In a hospital based study, Mboussou and Milebou-Aubusson (1989) reported 39 cases of suicides and 208 attempted suicides. No gender difference was observed in those completing suicide, but the male to female ratio among those who attempted suicide was 3:1. Ingestion of chloroquin was the commonest method of committing suicide.

MENTAL HEALTH RESOURCES

Mental Health Policy A mental health policy is absent.

Substance Abuse Policy A substance abuse policy is absent.

National Mental Health Programme A national mental health programme is absent.

National Therapeutic Drug Policy/Essential List of Drugs A national therapeutic drug policy/essential list of drugs is present. It was formulated in 1983.

Mental Health Legislation There is no existing mental health legislation, but one is being formulated.
Details about the year of enactment of the mental health legislation are not available.

Mental Health Financing There are budget allocations for mental health.
The country spends 0.3% of the total health budget on mental health.
The primary sources of mental health financing in descending order are tax based, out of pocket expenditure by the patient or family, private insurances, social insurance and grants.
The country does not have disability benefits for persons with mental disorders. No benefits are present except where mental disorders result from industrial accidents.

Mental Health Facilities Mental health is a part of primary health care system. Actual treatment of severe mental disorders is available at the primary level. Treatment for the unemployed villagers is present.
Regular training of primary care professionals is not carried out in the field of mental health.
There are community care facilities for patients with mental disorders.

Psychiatric Beds and Professionals

Total psychiatric beds per 10 000 population	0.7
Psychiatric beds in mental hospitals per 10 000 population	0.6
Psychiatric beds in general hospitals per 10 000 population	0
Psychiatric beds in other settings per 10 000 population	0.06
Number of psychiatrists per 100 000 population	0.3
Number of neurosurgeons per 100 000 population	0.2
Number of psychiatric nurses per 100 000 population	1
Number of neurologists per 100 000 population	0.4
Number of psychologists per 100 000 population	0.5
Number of social workers per 100 000 population	2

There is a need to have training centres for health workers in the field of mental health.

Non-Governmental Organizations NGOs are involved with mental health in the country. They are mainly involved in advocacy, promotion, prevention and rehabilitation.

Information Gathering System There is no mental health reporting system in the country. The national health reporting system is being finalized.
The country has no data collection system or epidemiological study on mental health. There is a lack of logistics to allow such data collection.

Programmes for Special Population The country has specific programmes for mental health for indigenous population. Due to a lack of technical people and resources it is not possible to have services for all special groups of population.

Therapeutic Drugs The following therapeutic drugs are generally available at the primary health care level of the country: carbamazepine, phenobarbital, phenytoin sodium, amitriptyline, chlorpromazine, diazepam, fluphenazine, haloperidol.

Other Information

Additional Sources of Information

Mboussou, M., Milebou-Aubusson, L. (1989) Suicides and attempted suicides at the Jeanne Ebori Foundation, Libreville (Gabon). Médecine Tropicale, 49, 259-264.

Gambia

GENERAL INFORMATION

Gambia is a country with an approximate area of 11 thousand sq. km. (UNO, 2001). Its population is 1.462 million, and the sex ratio (men per hundred women) is 98 (UNO, 2004). The proportion of population under the age of 15 years is 40% (UNO, 2004), and the proportion of population above the age of 60 years is 6% (WHO, 2004). The literacy rate is 43.7% for men and 29.7% for women (UNESCO/MoH, 2004).

The country is a low income group country (based on World Bank 2004 criteria). The proportion of health budget to GDP is 6.4%. The per capita total expenditure on health is 78 international $, and the per capita government expenditure on health is 39 international $ (WHO, 2004).

The main language(s) used in the country is (are) English. The largest religious group(s) is (are) Muslim, and the other religious group(s) are (is) Christian.

The life expectancy at birth is 55.4 years for males and 58.9 years for females (WHO, 2004). The healthy life expectancy at birth is 48 years for males and 50 years for females (WHO, 2004).

EPIDEMIOLOGY

There is a paucity of epidemiological data on mental illnesses in Gambia in internationally accessible literature. There are two studies on Sierra Leonean (Fox & Tang, 2000) and Senegalese (Tang & Fox, 2001) refugees living in Gambian refugee camps. The Harvard Trauma Questionnaire and the Hopkins Symptom Checklist-25 were used as survey instruments. High prevalence of anxiety, depression and PTSD was found among the exposed population.

MENTAL HEALTH RESOURCES

Mental Health Policy A mental health policy is absent.

The Department of State for Health and Social Welfare in collaboration with the WHO is in the process of developing a national mental health policy. The draft of the policy document is now ready for a final review by an expert committee, prior to its final submission for approval of the cabinet.

Substance Abuse Policy A substance abuse policy is absent.

National Mental Health Programme A national mental health programme is present. The programme was formulated in 1992. The national mental health programme was developed with the technical assistance of the Voluntary Services Overseas (Country Office) through the support of the British Government.

National Therapeutic Drug Policy/Essential List of Drugs A national therapeutic drug policy/essential list of drugs is present. It was formulated in 1996.

Mental Health Legislation There is a Mental Health Act. It was last amended in 1964. There is a need for an updated legislation. The latest legislation was enacted in 1924.

Mental Health Financing There are no budget allocations for mental health.

Details about expenditure on mental health are not available.

The primary source of mental health financing is grants.

The country has disability benefits for persons with mental disorders.

Mental Health Facilities Mental health is a part of primary health care system. Actual treatment of severe mental disorders is available at the primary level. Treatment is available and mental health is being integrated into the primary health system.

Regular training of primary care professionals is carried out in the field of mental health. A good number of doctors and nurses were trained on the diagnosis, treatment and management of mental health disorders through WHO support last year. Some traditional healers have also been trained.

There are community care facilities for patients with mental disorders. There is a community mental health service that conducts country wide mental health promotional activities.

Psychiatric Beds and Professionals

Total psychiatric beds per 10 000 population	0.78
Psychiatric beds in mental hospitals per 10 000 population	0.78
Psychiatric beds in general hospitals per 10 000 population	0
Psychiatric beds in other settings per 10 000 population	0
Number of psychiatrists per 100 000 population	0.08
Number of neurosurgeons per 100 000 population	0.06
Number of psychiatric nurses per 100 000 population	0
Number of neurologists per 100 000 population	0
Number of psychologists per 100 000 population	0
Number of social workers per 100 000 population	0.08

There are 2 assistant occupational therapists.

Non-Governmental Organizations NGOs are involved with mental health in the country. They are mainly involved in promotion and prevention.

Information Gathering System There is no mental health reporting system in the country.
The country has no data collection system or epidemiological study on mental health.

Programmes for Special Population The country has specific programmes for mental health for children.

Therapeutic Drugs The following therapeutic drugs are generally available at the primary health care level of the country: carbamazepine, phenobarbital, phenytoin sodium, amitriptyline, chlorpromazine, diazepam, fluphenazine, haloperidol, biperiden.
The essential drug list was formulated in 2001, and it will be reviewed again in 2004-2005. Some of the drugs are not always available at primary level, but these are always available at the secondary and tertiary levels.

Other Information

Additional Sources of Information

Fox, S. H., Tang, S. S. (2000) The Sierra Leonean refugee experience: traumatic events and psychiatric sequelae. Journal of Nervous & Mental Disease, 188, 490-495.

Tang, S. S., Fox, S. H. (2001) Traumatic experiences and the mental health of Senegalese refugees. Journal of Nervous & Mental Disease 189, 507-512.

Georgia

GENERAL INFORMATION

Georgia is a country with an approximate area of 70 thousand sq. km. (UNO, 2001). Its population is 5.074 million, and the sex ratio (men per hundred women) is 91 (UNO, 2004). The proportion of population under the age of 15 years is 14% (UNO, 2004), and the proportion of population above the age of 60 years is 19% (WHO, 2004). The literacy rate is 100% for men and 98% for women (UNESCO/MoH, 2004).

The country is a lower middle income group country (based on World Bank 2004 criteria). The proportion of health budget to GDP is 3.6%. The per capita total expenditure on health is 108 international $, and the per capita government expenditure on health is 41 international $ (WHO, 2004).

The main language(s) used in the country is (are) Georgian. The largest ethnic group(s) is (are) Georgian (seven-tenths), and the other ethnic group(s) are (is) Armenian and Russian. The largest religious group(s) is (are) Georgian Orthodox Christian (two-thirds), and the other religious group(s) are (is) Russian Orthodox Christian and Muslim.

The life expectancy at birth is 68.4 years for males and 75 years for females (WHO, 2004). The healthy life expectancy at birth is 62 years for males and 67 years for females (WHO, 2004).

EPIDEMIOLOGY

There is a paucity of epidemiological data on mental illnesses in Georgia in internationally accessible literature. Tchanturia et al (2002) held focus groups of various health professionals to establish how eating disorders present in Georgia and to identify groups perceived to be at high risk of having an eating disorder. They assessed 245 women from these identified high risk groups with translated versions of a number of standardized questionnaires (measuring eating and general psychopathology) and a sub-sample with a structured clinical interview. They estimated from the responses to the questionnaires that as many as 5% of the sample may have clinically significant bulimia nervosa, 7% fell in the weight range for anorexia nervosa with a further 7% in the weight range for obesity. Interviews with the high scoring group confirmed the presence of clinically significant eating pathology in the majority of those identified as possible cases. Georgia was one of the countries included in the study to assess changing patterns of suicide in different countries of erstwhile USSR during the period 1984-90 (Wasserman et al, 1998). There was wide variation in suicide rates across the countries with a decrease in rate after 1986. The suicide rates in the Caucasus (Georgia, Azerbaijan and Armenia) region was 3.5 cases per 100 000 inhabitants during 1984-1990 with the rates for men and women being 4.9 and 2.1 per 100 000 inhabitants, respectively. Chubarovskii and Loginova (1986) did a comparative clinico-epidemiological study to assess borderline mental disorders in adolescents living in Moscow and Batumi. Borderline disorders were correlated with maladaptive schooling. Cultural factors were found to affect the severity and direction of adolescent reactions.

MENTAL HEALTH RESOURCES

Mental Health Policy A mental health policy is present. The policy was initially formulated in 1999.
The components of the policy are prevention, treatment and rehabilitation. Mental health is one of the priorities of Georgia's National Health Policy document of 1999. Various issues pertinent to mental health policy are discussed in other documents like the 1999 presidential decree 'Improving Psychiatric Services in Georgia'.

Substance Abuse Policy A substance abuse policy is present. The policy was initially formulated in 1996.

National Mental Health Programme A national mental health programme is present. The programme was formulated in 1995. The Strategic Health Plan for 2000-2009 outlined specific measures for mental health care development. Georgia also has a national suicide prevention initiative. The implementation of the Strategic Plan was limited by the lack of resources.

National Therapeutic Drug Policy/Essential List of Drugs A national therapeutic drug policy/essential list of drugs is present. It was formulated in 1995.

Mental Health Legislation The mental health legislation is known as Law on Mental Health Assistance. Enforcement of the law is impeded at times due to funding shortfalls. Georgia has elected to enforce participation in continuing medical education programmes on the part of physicians through law to help speed up the implementation process.
The latest legislation was enacted in 1995.

Mental Health Financing There are budget allocations for mental health.
Details about expenditure on mental health are not available.
The primary source of mental health financing is tax based.
Psychiatric services are jointly financed by the health insurance programme and central budget transfers. State funding is supposed to provide for the inpatient treatment of mentally ill offenders, acute psychotics, patients with posttraumatic stress disorders and those without a family, for the outpatient treatment of psychotic patients and those with chronic disorders prone to frequent exacerbations. In reality, state funding is limited and provides for a few cheap medicines from the essential drug list. Limited funding has impeded the provision of even the inpatient services, where shortage of food is also known to occur. Between 1991 and 1995 about

800 psychiatric patients died in mental hospitals due to lack of food, medication and/or care as a result of the civil war and the economic crisis. Even now the premature death rate of inpatients is as high as in other low income countries.
The country has disability benefits for persons with mental disorders.

Mental Health Facilities Mental health is not a part of primary health care system. Actual treatment of severe mental disorders is not available at the primary level. Actual treatment is carried out in hospitals and outpatient clinics.
Regular training of primary care professionals is not carried out in the field of mental health. Primary care is mainly provided by specialists. An integrated model of family medicine is not operational.
There are no community care facilities for patients with mental disorders.

Psychiatric Beds and Professionals

Total psychiatric beds per 10 000 population	2.1
Psychiatric beds in mental hospitals per 10 000 population	2
Psychiatric beds in general hospitals per 10 000 population	0
Psychiatric beds in other settings per 10 000 population	0.1
Number of psychiatrists per 100 000 population	6
Number of neurosurgeons per 100 000 population	0.6
Number of psychiatric nurses per 100 000 population	24
Number of neurologists per 100 000 population	13
Number of psychologists per 100 000 population	
Number of social workers per 100 000 population	0

There are no institutions for training of social workers. Between 1990 and 1995, the bed strength was brought down from 5000 to about 1000 due to shortage of resources. However, even now most of the beds are housed in old asylums, often distant from families and homes. Some beds have been earmarked for drug addiction and forensic services. Staff remunerations are extremely poor (a psychiatrist's monthly salary is the equivalent of $30-50 and a nurse's about $17-20). About 15 child psychiatrists are available. Psychotherapists, occupational therapists and social workers are not officially recognized by the Government and are not registered. Every physician has to pass a CME course lasting 3-4 months every five years.

Non-Governmental Organizations NGOs are involved with mental health in the country. They are mainly involved in advocacy, promotion, prevention and rehabilitation. A few community-based services have been established by NGOs and donors from abroad. NGOs receive only occasional and very limited support from the Government. International humanitarian aid organizations provide some support through the supply of medicines (International Red Cross), food (World Food Programme) and other means (e.g. operational repairs by the Investment Fund of Georgia).

Information Gathering System There is mental health reporting system in the country.
The country has no data collection system or epidemiological study on mental health. No epidemiological research has been carried out over the last 6 years due to lack of funds.

Programmes for Special Population The country has specific programmes for mental health for refugees and children.

Therapeutic Drugs The following therapeutic drugs are generally available at the primary health care level of the country: carbamazepine, amitriptyline, chlorpromazine, diazepam, fluphenazine, haloperidol, lithium, biperiden.
The medicines are distributed free of charge under the State Programme on Mental Health Assistance.

Other Information

Additional Sources of Information

Chubarovskii, V. V., Loginova, M. S. (1986) Clinico-epidemiologic characteristics of borderline mental disorders comparison of the Moscow and Batumi populations of students of specialized educational institutions. Zhurnal Nevropatologii i Psikhiatrii Imeni S-S-Korsakova, 86, 1203-1208.

Sharashidze, M., Naneishvili, G., Silagadze, T., et al (2004) Georgia mental health profile. International Review of Psychiatry, 16, 107-116.

Tchanturia, K., Katzman, M., Troop, N. A., et al (2002) An exploration of eating disorders in a Georgian sample. International Journal of Social Psychiatry, 48, 220-230.

Wasserman, D., Varnik, A., Dankowicz, M. (1998) Regional differences in the distribution of suicide in the former Soviet Union during perestroika, 1984-1990. Acta Psychiatrica Scandinavica, Supplementum 394, 5-12.

Germany

GENERAL INFORMATION

Germany is a country with an approximate area of 357 thousand sq. km. (UNO, 2001). Its population is 82.526 million, and the sex ratio (men per hundred women) is 96 (UNO, 2004). The proportion of population under the age of 15 years is 15% (UNO, 2004), and the proportion of population above the age of 60 years is 24% (WHO, 2004). The literacy rate is 99% for men and 99% for women (UNESCO/MoH, 2004).

The country is a high income group country (based on World Bank 2004 criteria). The proportion of health budget to GDP is 10.8%. The per capita total expenditure on health is 2820 international $, and the per capita government expenditure on health is 2113 international $ (WHO, 2004).

The main language(s) used in the country is (are) German and English. The largest ethnic group(s) is (are) German, and the other ethnic group(s) are (is) Turkish and Russian. The largest religious group(s) is (are) Protestant, and the other religious group(s) are (is) Roman Catholic, Muslim and Jew.

The life expectancy at birth is 75.6 years for males and 81.6 years for females (WHO, 2004). The healthy life expectancy at birth is 70 years for males and 74 years for females (WHO, 2004).

EPIDEMIOLOGY

There is substantial epidemiological data on mental illnesses in Germany in internationally accessible literature. No attempt was made to include this information here.

MENTAL HEALTH RESOURCES

Mental Health Policy A mental health policy is present. The policy was initially formulated in 1975.

The components of the policy are advocacy, promotion, prevention, treatment and rehabilitation. Mental health policy in Germany is essentially based on two important documents. In 1975, a relevant Study Commission submitted to the German Parliament, the Bundestag, a report (Psychiatrie Enquête) about the situation of psychiatry in the Federal Republic of Germany, which pointed out the main targets of a psychiatry reform. In 1988, an Expert Commission reported on the first results of the reform and formulated further needs to go on with the reform process of mental health services. Coordinating psychiatric services, an orientation towards community-based care, the availability of mental health services for all those in need and policies to give mental disorders the same status as somatic illnesses were the main requirements. As a consequence, the Federal Government initiated a huge pilot programme in the field of psychiatry. Based on the results of this pilot programme, in which a host of individual projects were financed by the Federal Government until the end of 2002, mental health policy nowadays intends to provide a networked treatment which caters to the individual needs of the patient. In 2002, the Federal Ministry of Health and Social Security re-established a working group for the further development of psychiatric care in Germany. It consists of representatives of all the main players in the field of psychiatry, including physicians, professional associations, 'users' and family representatives as well as competent institutions and representatives of health insurances.

Substance Abuse Policy A substance abuse policy is present. The policy was initially formulated in 1990. In June 2003, the Federal Cabinet approved the 'Action Plan on Drugs and Addiction', presented by the Federal Drug Commissioner. Devised to serve as a framework for addiction policy for the next 5-10 years, it replaced the 'Plan to combat drugs' of 1990. It is meant to contribute 'to changing health awareness and to avoiding harmful consumption or at least reduce it'. It is based on the four pillars of the national drug and addiction policy (prevention of drug consumption, offering advice and treatment to consumers, survival assistance and harm reduction, repression and supply reduction). Compared to the plan of 1990, legal drugs have been taken more into consideration and that new elements of care (internet offers, consumption rooms) have been included. Alongside a number of targets that involve influencing the consumption of illegal drugs indirectly by preventing tobacco use, the plan relates also specifically to drugs. For instance, it includes the demand to avoid, or at least reduce, the consumption of illegal drugs by referring to the special risks of infection – especially Hepatitis C – and possible damages to the brain through synthetic drugs. Moreover, individual target groups (children of addicted parents, high-risk groups, car drivers, polydrug users) are to be treated specifically.

National Mental Health Programme A national mental health programme is absent.

Due to the decentralized German health system, a national mental health programme in the narrower sense does not exist. However, boards for coordinating and planning mental health services and policy are in place on the federal, state and local levels. The key players in mental health policy are the States (Länder). Most of them have formulated a central psychiatric planning document (Psychiatrie-Plan). A 'National Programme for the Prevention of Suicide exacerbations' was launched in 2002 by the German Society for Suicide Prevention. In addition, a national programme for the destigmatization of mental illness is currently being planned jointly by the German Ministry of Health and Social Security, the German Association for Psychiatry, Psychotherapy and Neurology and the initiative 'Open the Doors' of the WPA.

National Therapeutic Drug Policy/Essential List of Drugs Details about the national therapeutic drug policy/essential list of drugs are not available.

Mental Health Legislation The Federal Government has an important frame-setting role, especially by providing the social and welfare legislation laid down in several Social Code Books. Some provisions deal with the special needs of mentally ill persons, others, while crucial for the interests of psychiatric patients interests, are of a general nature and not specific to this group (e.g. referring to rehabilitation, nursing care or welfare legislation). Special legislation as well as planning and coordinating mental health policy is mainly the responsibility of the States, and they have mental health legislations of their own. These also contain provisions on compulsory referral and involuntary treatment.
The latest legislation was enacted in 1999.

Mental Health Financing There are budget allocations for mental health.
Details about expenditure on mental health are not available.
The primary sources of mental health financing in descending order are social insurance, private insurances, tax based and out of pocket expenditure by the patient or family.
Specific budget allocations do not exist for the field of health in general. The health system is financed in a concerted system, in which all services that are medically necessary and are performed in a cost-effective manner are covered by the statutory or private health insurance. In this regard, the social law as the legal basis of this principle does not distinguish between the treatment of somatic diseases and mental illnesses. Rehabilitation is financed by the health insurance or the statutory pension insurance or – if necessary – by the social welfare system. Self-employed psychiatrists are paid on a fee-for-service basis in a strictly regulated market with semi-statutory professional associations exerting stringent control and negotiating fees with health insurance organizations.
The country has disability benefits for persons with mental disorders. There are Disability IDs, disability compensation schemes, compensations for accidents, schemes for tax reductions, free transportation and other rehabilitation facilities.

Mental Health Facilities Mental health is a part of primary health care system. Actual treatment of severe mental disorders is available at the primary level.
Regular training of primary care professionals is not carried out in the field of mental health.
There are community care facilities for patients with mental disorders. Community-based care is provided as a part of the psychiatric reforms. The crucial step towards its implementation was taken with the creation of the Expert Commission on mental health care in 1970 to 1975. This effort was encouraged further by the recommendations of the Central Institute of Mental Health of Baden-Württemberg and the expert commission for the Federal Republic of Germany. Funding came from by the Federal Government as well as States and local bodies. At present, there are almost 9000 places in nearly 360 day-clinics and more than 15 000 beds for rehabilitative services. Currently, the population of people with mental illness in sheltered homes is approximately equal to the number of beds in psychiatric inpatient services. Implementation of the programme, however, varies across different regions. The involvement of family members and ex-users, newly organized in groups to design several forms of activity, has proven extremely useful. However, there is no one agency that has overall responsibility for community mental health care in a given catchment area. Since 2000, pilot projects involving mental health services in 35 catchment areas, covering 10% of the population, have pursued the comprehensive care planning for individual patients involving local authority social services which fund approximately half of mental health care.

Psychiatric Beds and Professionals

Total psychiatric beds per 10 000 population	7.5
Psychiatric beds in mental hospitals per 10 000 population	4.5
Psychiatric beds in general hospitals per 10 000 population	2.9
Psychiatric beds in other settings per 10 000 population	
Number of psychiatrists per 100 000 population	11.8
Number of neurosurgeons per 100 000 population	1.5
Number of psychiatric nurses per 100 000 population	52
Number of neurologists per 100 000 population	3.4
Number of psychologists per 100 000 population	51.5
Number of social workers per 100 000 population	477

The figure for psychiatrists includes specialists in psychosomatics and psychotherapy. The figure for psychologists is an estimate of only employees. The figure for social workers refers to all related professions, not only social workers in a narrow sense (only employees). Since the late 1960s, psychiatric hospitals have reduced their beds by about 50 % and one psychiatric hospital was closed. A 15% reduction was recorded even after 1999. More than 220 general psychiatry units have opened. There is, however, significant regional variation in the number of beds. Staffing and funding of inpatient facilities is now based on the type of patients in a given service. This system was audited in more than half of such centres and the results showed an increase in staff by 24% (doctors +43%, nurses +18%, psychologists +33%, occupational therapists +41% and social workers +84%) in such institutions. Along with increased staffing, there came the obligation to implement quality assurance. There are about 7000 beds in 65 forensic psychiatry clinics.

Non-Governmental Organizations NGOs are involved with mental health in the country. They are mainly involved in advocacy, promotion, prevention, treatment and rehabilitation. On the federal level there is an association of family members (Familienselbsthilfe Psychiatrie) and one of the 'users' (Bundesverband Psychiatrie-Erfahrener). Their importance and influence has grown in the last decades, meanwhile they are involved in relevant bodies and decision-making processes.

Information Gathering System There is mental health reporting system in the country. Reporting is done under the Health Reporting and Data of Health Services.
The country has data collection system or epidemiological study on mental health. There is a data analysis system with respect to services provided for chronic mental diseases.

Programmes for Special Population The country has specific programmes for mental health for minorities, refugees, disaster affected population, indigenous population, elderly and children.
Due to the federal system in Germany and given responsibilities there are no specific programmes on the federal level for special populations as far as only the aspect of 'mental health' is affected. Within more general programmes, as for the elderly or for children the issue of mental health within those groups is taken into account. On-state level programmes for special groups as minorities, refugees, disaster-affected populations etc. do exist.

Therapeutic Drugs The following therapeutic drugs are generally available at the primary health care level of the country: carbamazepine, ethosuximide, phenobarbital, phenytoin sodium, odium valproate, amitriptyline, chlorpromazin, diazepam, fluphenazine, haloperidol, lithium, biperiden, carbidopa, levodopa.

Other Information Hospital treatment has been improved thanks to the Psychiatrie-Personalverordnung (1991) – a federal staffing directive which has brought an additional 6500 multidisciplinary staff members to inpatient treatment since 1991. In Germany, the trend has been to reduce the size of psychiatric hospitals without closing them down while simultaneously developing general hospital services and community care.

Additional Sources of Information

Aktion Psychisch Kranke. Mental Health Care in the Federal Republic of Germany – Summary of the Report Submitted by an Expert Commission to Parliament (Bundestag).

Bauer, M., Kunze, H., von Cranach, M., et al (2001) Psychiatric reform in Germany. Acta Psychiatrica Scandinavica 104 (suppl. 410), 27-34.

Bock, T. (1994) Long-term mental illness in Germany. International Journal of Social Psychiatry, 40, 276-282.

Bramesfeld A., Wismar M. (2003) The third pillar of psychiatric health care reform – structures for coordinating a planning of psychiatric health care in Germany. Psychiatrische Praxis, 30, 318-325.

Brand,U. (2001) Mental health care in Germany: carer's perspective. Acta Psychiatrica Scandinavica, 104 (suppl. 410), 35-40.

Hafner, H. (1997) A quarter of a century of rehabilitation of psychiatric patients in Germany. Gesundheitswesen, 59, 69-78.

Kallert, T. W., Leisse, M. (1999) Occupational status of Saxony social psychiatry service clients as a result of the reunification of Germany. Psychiatrische Praxis, 26, 133-138.

Kunze, H., Becker, T., Priebe, S. (2004) Reform of psychiatric services in Germany: hospital staffing directive and commissioning of community care. Psychiatric Bulletin, 28, 218-221.

Muller-Isberner, R., Freese, R., Jockel, D., et al (2000) Forensic psychiatric assessment and treatment in Germany. International Journal of Law and Psychiatry, 23, 467-480.

Rossler, W., Salize, H.J., Reicher-Rossler, A. (1996) Changing Patterns of Mental Health Care in Germany. International Journal of Law and Psychiatry, 19, 391-411.

Wolfersdorf, M., Kukla, R. (2004) Clinics for psychiatry and psychotherapy in Germany in July 2003. An overview on numbers of beds and day-clinic places. Krankenhauspsychiatrie, 15, 12-15.

Ghana

GENERAL INFORMATION

Ghana is a country with an approximate area of 239 thousand sq. km. (UNO, 2001). Its population is 21.377 million, and the sex ratio (men per hundred women) is 99 (UNO, 2004). The proportion of population under the age of 15 years is 39% (UNO, 2004), and the proportion of population above the age of 60 years is 5% (WHO, 2004). The literacy rate is 81.9% for men and 65.9% for women (UNESCO/MoH, 2004).

The country is a low income group country (based on World Bank 2004 criteria). The proportion of health budget to GDP is 4.7%. The per capita total expenditure on health is 60 international $, and the per capita government expenditure on health is 36 international $ (WHO, 2004).

The main language(s) used in the country is (are) English. The largest ethnic group(s) is (are) African. The largest religious group(s) is (are) Christian, and the other religious group(s) are (is) indigenous groups and Muslim.

The life expectancy at birth is 56.3 years for males and 58.8 years for females (WHO, 2004). The healthy life expectancy at birth is 49 years for males and 50 years for females (WHO, 2004).

EPIDEMIOLOGY

Affinnih (1999) found that heroin and cocaine were the common drugs of abuse in a sample of 117 current and former drug users. The typical drug user was a 30-year old, who belonged to the working or lower socioeconomic class. Petty theft was common among male drug users. Community-based studies on chronic psychosis (Field, 1968) and schizophrenia (Sikanartey & Eaton, 1984) are also available. Turkson and colleagues have published a series of studies on psychiatric outpatients. In a sample of 131 depressed female outpatients, Turkson and Dua (1996) reported that the majority of patients were in the 20-40 years age group, were married with 5-8 children but with poor financial support from husbands and had limited education or employment opportunities. They often presented with somatic symptoms like headache and insomnia. Social stress was one of the causes for onset of depression. Turkson (1996) reviewed 7-year (1987-94) outpatient data on adolescents (n=454). Results indicated that only 59.3% had a psychiatric illness. In the subgroup with psychiatric disorders (n= 269), 32.7% had functional psychoses (more than half of these were depression), neurotic disorders (23.4%), personality disorders (20.4%) and organic psychosis (10%) were the other common disorders. Turkson and Asamoah (1997) did a retrospective assessment of 35 elderly (more than 60 years) outpatients seen between 1989-93. The commonest presentations were depression, dementia and paranoid disorders. Dementia was associated with the history of alcohol use and paranoid disorders with female sex, past history of a similar disorder and hearing and visual impairment. Turkson (1998) studied the prevalence of psychiatric disorders in patients referred to the psychiatry outpatient clinics of a teaching hospital. Out of the 96 patients referred in 1988, 62.8% were referred by physicians and 14.9% by surgeons. Nearly half of these patients suffered from affective, neurotic and stress related disorders, 13.2% from schizophrenia, schizotypal and delusional disorders. Behavioural disorders and drug use were common among the adolescent group. About 2/3 of the patients were treated as outpatients in the centre, whereas the remaining required admission in specialized centres or general hospitals. Turkson and Asante (1997) reviewed records of 130 criminal offenders seen as outpatients and found that the commonest diagnoses were psychotic states related to drug use, schizophrenia and drug use disorders (without psychosis).

MENTAL HEALTH RESOURCES

Mental Health Policy A mental health policy is present. The policy was initially formulated in 1994.
The components of the policy are advocacy, promotion, prevention, treatment and rehabilitation. The mental health policy has been revised in 2000.

Substance Abuse Policy A substance abuse policy is present. The policy was initially formulated in 1990. On substance abuse there are three laws. The Narcotic Drugs (Control, Enforcement and Sanctions) Law 1990, PNDC Law 236 and Pharmacy and Drugs Act 1961.

National Mental Health Programme A national mental health programme is present. The programme was formulated in 1994. The national mental health programme was revised in 2000.

National Therapeutic Drug Policy/Essential List of Drugs A national therapeutic drug policy/essential list of drugs is present. It was formulated in 1986.
Risperidone, olanzapine and fluoxetine are available in the open market but they are expensive.

Mental Health Legislation The NRC Decree (1972) is the current mental health law. Plans to revise this law to conform with changes in mental health delivery, particularly community mental care and human rights concerns are in an advanced stage.
The latest legislation was enacted in 1972.

Mental Health Financing There are budget allocations for mental health.
The country spends 0.5% of the total health budget on mental health.
The primary source of mental health financing is tax based.
The World Health Organization contributes to Ghana's mental health budget. Admission to hospital is free to all patients, medication and tests are subsidized, but these are provided free to very poor patients.
The country has disability benefits for persons with mental disorders. The benefits are primarily available to those employed in the public sector. Treatment, boarding and lodging in Government institutions are free.

Mental Health Facilities Mental health is a part of primary health care system. Actual treatment of severe mental disorders is available at the primary level. Trained community psychiatric nurses have been posted to regions and most districts.
Regular training of primary care professionals is carried out in the field of mental health. In the last two years, about 250 personnel were provided training. Community psychiatric nurses (CPN) have been trained since 1952. The Danish International Development Assistance provided additional support for the training of CPNs and medical assistants in the northern region. This programme significantly improved primary care psychiatry in the north. With WHO assistance, 228 volunteers and 160 providers have been trained for community care.
There are community care facilities for patients with mental disorders. Community psychiatric nurses are available. Trained volunteers are being considered. There are also 'healing churches' which help in community care; few halfway houses and charitable institutions also help in community care. Informal community care plays an important role in psychiatric management.

E–I

Psychiatric Beds and Professionals

Total psychiatric beds per 10 000 population	1.03
Psychiatric beds in mental hospitals per 10 000 population	1
Psychiatric beds in general hospitals per 10 000 population	0.01
Psychiatric beds in other settings per 10 000 population	0.2
Number of psychiatrists per 100 000 population	0.08
Number of neurosurgeons per 100 000 population	0.01
Number of psychiatric nurses per 100 000 population	2
Number of neurologists per 100 000 population	0.01
Number of psychologists per 100 000 population	0.04
Number of social workers per 100 000 population	0.03

One qualified occupational therapist and six assistants are present. The first asylum for mental health was opened in Accra in 1906. By 1960, it housed 1700 patients. There are 10 to 20 beds for psychiatric patients in three regional hospitals, but all other regional hospitals can admit and manage less severe mentally ill patients. Some patients are also managed in district hospitals. The military and police hospitals have no beds allocated to psychiatric persons. Patients are treated in medical wards or transferred to the Accra Psychiatric Hospital. The special wards meant for the mentally ill offenders are crowded and often lack proper infrastructure to support such a large number of patients. Many professionals who were sent for training abroad have not returned. There is also an efflux of locally trained staff to more lucrative work abroad.

Non-Governmental Organizations NGOs are involved with mental health in the country. They are mainly involved in advocacy. BasicNeeds, a British NGO, provides services in the northern region of Ghana. It supports quarterly outreach consultant clinical services and rehabilitation of patients. A club house for the mentally ill has also been provided in Tamale by this NGO.

Information Gathering System There is mental health reporting system in the country. However, the data collected are not very reliable and are not utilized for system development.
The country has data collection system or epidemiological study on mental health. Data is collected but not processed.

Programmes for Special Population The country has specific programmes for mental health for refugees. Mental health professionals are invited occasionally to manage such groups of population.
A couple of private establishments provide rehabilitation and training for learning disability.

Therapeutic Drugs The following therapeutic drugs are generally available at the primary health care level of the country: carbamazepine, phenobarbital, phenytoin sodium, amitriptyline, chlorpromazine, diazepam, fluphenazine, haloperidol.
Benztropine and benzhexol are available.

Other Information Traditional practices and spirituality play an important role in psychiatric care and are a source of community involvement. In February 2000, the Traditional Medical Practice Act was passed to regulate and codify the practice of traditional medicine. Ghana has also introduced a postgraduate Bachelor of Science Degree in Herbal Medicine.

Additional Sources of Information

Affinnih, Y. H. (1999) Drug use in greater Accra, Ghana: pilot study. Substance Use & Misuse, 34, 157-169.

Ewusi-Mensah. (2001) Post colonial psychiatric care in Ghana. Psychiatric Bulletin, 25, 228-229.

Field, M. J. (1968) Chronic psychosis in rural Ghana. British Journal of Psychiatry, 114, 31-33.

Kyei-Faried, S., Hermans, M. (1995) Primary health care in Ghana: no pay no cure? Nederlands Tijdschrift voor Geneeskunde, 139, 2321-2325.

Laugharne, R., Burns, T. (1999) Mental health services in Kumasi, Ghana. Psychiatric Bulletin, 23, 361-363.

Osei, Y. (1994) Psychiatric services in a developing country – the case of Ghana. Curare, 17, 39-43.

Roberts, H. (2001). A way forward for mental health care in Ghana? Lancet, 357, 1859.

Roberts, H. (2001) Mental health in Ghana. Research Report. The Ghana Mental Health Association. Accra-North.

Sikanartey, T., Eaton, W. W. (1984) Prevalence of schizophrenia in the Labadi District of Ghana. Acta Psychiatrica Scandinavica, 69, 156-161.

Tsey, K. (1997) Traditional medicine in contemprory Ghana: a public policy analysis. Social Science and Medicine, 45, 1065-1074.

Turkson, S. N. (1996) Psychiatric disorder among adolescents attending a psychiatric out-patient clinic in Accra, Ghana: a seven year review study (1987-1994). West African Journal of Medicine, 15, 31-35.

Turkson, S. N. (1998) Psychiatric diagnosis among referred patients in Ghana. East African Medical Journal, 75, 336-338.

Turkson, S. N., Asamoah, V. (1997) Common psychiatric disorders among the elderly attending a general psychiatric out patient clinic in Accra, Ghana: a five year retrospective study (1989-1993). West African Journal of Medicine, 16, 146-149.

Turkson, S. N., Asante, K. (1997) Psychiatric disorders among offender patients in the Accra Psychiatric Hospital. West African Journal of Medicine, 16, 88-92.

Turkson, S. N., Dua, A. N. (1996) A study of the social and clinical characteristics of depressive illness among Ghanaian women--(1988-1992). West African Journal of Medicine, 15, 85-90.

Greece

GENERAL INFORMATION

Greece is a country with an approximate area of 132 thousand sq. km. (UNO, 2001). Its population is 10.977 million, and the sex ratio (men per hundred women) is 97 (UNO, 2004). The proportion of population under the age of 15 years is 14% (UNO, 2004), and the proportion of population above the age of 60 years is 24% (WHO, 2004). The literacy rate is 98.5% for men and 95.9% for women (UNESCO/MoH, 2004).

The country is a high income group country (based on World Bank 2004 criteria). The proportion of health budget to GDP is 9.4%. The per capita total expenditure on health is 1522 international $, and the per capita government expenditure on health is 852 international $ (WHO, 2004).

The main language(s) used in the country is (are) Greek (official). The largest ethnic group(s) is (are) Greek. The largest religious group(s) is (are) Greek Orthodox (official religion, 98% of the population), and the other religious group(s) are (is) Muslim (1.5%).

The life expectancy at birth is 75.8 years for males and 81.1 years for females (WHO, 2004). The healthy life expectancy at birth is 69 years for males and 73 years for females (WHO, 2004).

EPIDEMIOLOGY

There is substantial epidemiological data on mental illnesses in Greece in internationally accessible literature. No attempt was made to include this information here.

MENTAL HEALTH RESOURCES

Mental Health Policy A mental health policy is present. The policy was initially formulated in 1983.

The components of the policy are advocacy, promotion, prevention, treatment and rehabilitation. A ten-year National Plan for Mental Health that was submitted for financial assistance to the EU in 1997 (Psychoargos). The main points of this plan were: the continuation of deinstitutionalization and di-stigmatization; sectorization of the psychiatric services throughout the country; continuation of the development of primary health care units and psychiatric units in general hospitals; continuation and intensification of the development of rehabilitation facilities; establishment and development of patient co-operatives in order to promote the social, economic and occupational reintegration into society of patients with severe psychiatric problems; establishment of detailed guarantees and procedures for the protection of patients' rights. The ten-year National Mental Health Plan was revised in 2001 and henceforth the revisions will be done every five years. The latest plan anticipates the closure of five out of the nine psychiatric hospitals by 2006 and the rest by 2015 (the first psychiatric hospital was closed under this plan in January 2004). During the period 2000 – 2006, there will also be a special emphasis on the areas of child psychiatry and psychogeriatrics.

Substance Abuse Policy A substance abuse policy is present. The policy was initially formulated in 1970.

National Mental Health Programme A national mental health programme is present. The programme was formulated in 1984.

National Therapeutic Drug Policy/Essential List of Drugs A national therapeutic drug policy/essential list of drugs is present. It was formulated in 1998.

Mental Health Legislation The Act 2716 deals with mental health. The new Mental Health Act (Law 2716/99) is based on and informed by the Mental Health Plan. All the essential points are included in the Act; in particular, the sectorization of mental health services is elaborated in considerable detail. The passing of the Mental Health Act constitutes a comprehensive policy document for the further development of psychiatric services in Greece, including its emphasis on the sectorization of mental health services and the priority it gives to primary health care and community-based psychiatry.

The latest legislation was enacted in 1999.

Mental Health Financing There are no budget allocations for mental health.

Details about expenditure on mental health are not available.

The primary sources of mental health financing in descending order are tax based, social insurance, out of pocket expenditure by the patient or family and private insurances.

Under current laws, it is forbidden to have separate budget for mental health. The social security system covers 95% of the population. Clients on social security can use the services of private practitioners for which part-payment is often made through private insurance. Psychological services are not included in private insurance plans.

The country has disability benefits for persons with mental disorders. Special pensions, tax deductions and therapeutic benefits are provided.

Mental Health Facilities Mental health is a part of primary health care system. Actual treatment of severe mental disorders is available at the primary level. Primary care is available in some areas only.

Regular training of primary care professionals is not carried out in the field of mental health. General practitioners spend three months in psychiatry during their specialist training. Training of other primary care professionals is not carried out systematically in the field of mental health. However, for the last three years an annual 3-day seminar on communication and diagnostic skills has been run by psychiatrists for general physicians. There were 30 participants each year. Psychiatrists are currently visiting and providing consultation in about one-third of primary care centres.

There are community care facilities for patients with mental disorders. Community care is available through visiting psychiatrists at the health centres, through hostels, sheltered accommodation and sheltered workshops. Community care facilities changed considerably during the period 1981-1996. The developments have changed substantially the pattern of provision of psychiatric services in Greece with more emphasis on care provided through general hospitals and mental health centres. The EU, through the 'Psychoargos' programme, has already approved the development of many hostels and rehabilitation centres. By 1996, 388 new psychiatric settings in the community were in operation and the regional distribution was reasonably even, although there are particular problems in developing services in remote mountainous and small island areas. For these areas, Act 2716/99 provides for mental health mobile units, and currently four such units are in operation in the Cyclades and the Dodecanese. The momentum of establishing community care facilities during the period 1991-1996, has been accelerated in recent years. As a result, 31 mental health centres, 60 psychiatric units in general hospitals, 12 day centres, 27 child guidance clinics, 302 rehabilitation units (hostels, boarding houses, sheltered flats) and 69 vocational rehabilitation centres were in operation by 2004.

Psychiatric Beds and Professionals

Total psychiatric beds per 10 000 population	8.7
Psychiatric beds in mental hospitals per 10 000 population	4.3
Psychiatric beds in general hospitals per 10 000 population	0.3
Psychiatric beds in other settings per 10 000 population	4.1
Number of psychiatrists per 100 000 population	15
Number of neurosurgeons per 100 000 population	2
Number of psychiatric nurses per 100 000 population	3
Number of neurologists per 100 000 population	4
Number of psychologists per 100 000 population	14
Number of social workers per 100 000 population	56

Since 1984, there has been a reduction in psychiatric beds in almost all regions. Almost all psychiatrists are working in urban areas and most are in western and central regions. Licensing/certification is required to work as a psychologist but there is no further additional legal provision to practice as a clinical psychologist. There is also no requirement for continuing education in the field of psychology. Most psychologists work in the private sector. Psychologists do not have prescription privileges.

Non-Governmental Organizations NGOs are involved with mental health in the country. They are mainly involved in advocacy, promotion, prevention, treatment and rehabilitation.

Information Gathering System There is no mental health reporting system in the country.
The country has no data collection system or epidemiological study on mental health.

Programmes for Special Population The country has specific programmes for mental health for minorities, refugees, disaster affected population, elderly and children.
There are extensive health programmes targeted at the use of narcotic drugs. A programme for depression, with particular emphasis on the elderly is in the initial stages. Services for children and adolescents and elderly are being expanded.

Therapeutic Drugs The following therapeutic drugs are generally available at the primary health care level of the country: carbamazepine, ethosuximide, phenobarbital, phenytoin sodium, sodium valproate, amitriptyline, chlorpromazine, diazepam, haloperidol, lithium, biperiden, carbidopa, levodopa.

Other Information In 1983, Greece enacted the legislation aimed at the formation of a national health service and psychiatric legislation became a part of the NHS. There is very close cooperation between the Ministry of Health and the Ministry of Labour and Social Security concerning management and support for the National Mental Health Plan. The Ministry of Health also works closely with the Ministry of Internal Affairs and Public Administration to achieve approval of new posts within the Health Sector in general and mental health in particular. There is variable cooperation at the local level between mental health units and County authorities. Telepsychiatry in the form of internet and helpline, based on the success of similar exercises in cardiology and radiology is being developed. This e-facility is linked with the psychiatry department of the University of Athens.

Additional Sources of Information

Constantopoulos, A., Yannulatos, P. (2004) Greek psychiatric reform: difficulties, achievements and perspectives. In: J. Kyriopoulos (Ed.). Health Systems in the World: From Evidence to Policy. Athens: Papazisis Publishers.

Lambousis, E., Politis, A., Markidis, M., et al (2002) Development and use of online mental health services in Greece. Journal of Telemedicine and Telecare, 8 (suppl. 2), 51-52.

Madianos, M. G., Zacharakis, C., Tsitsa, C., et al. (1999) The mental health care delivery system in Greece: regional variation and socioeconomic correlates. Journal of Mental health Policy and Economics, 2, 169-176.

Macri, I. (2001) Medical psychology in Greece. Journal of Clinical Psychology in Medical Settings, 8, 27-30.

Strutti, C., Rauber, S. (1994) Leros and the Greek mental health system. International Journal of Social Psychiatry, 40, 306-312.

Yfantopoulos, J. (1994) Economic and legal aspects of mental health policies in Greece. International Journal of Social Psychiatry, 40, 296-305.

Grenada*

GENERAL INFORMATION

Grenada is a country with an approximate area of 0.34 thousand sq. km. (UNO, 2001). Its population is 0.103 million, and the sex ratio (men per hundred women) is 98 (UNO, 2004). The proportion of population above the age of 60 years is 10% (WHO, 2004). The literacy rate is 98% for men and 98% for women (UNESCO/MoH, 2004).

The country is a higher middle income group country (based on World Bank 2004 criteria). The proportion of health budget to GDP is 5.3%. The per capita total expenditure on health is 445 international $, and the per capita government expenditure on health is 320 international $ (WHO, 2004).

The main language(s) used in the country is (are) English. The largest ethnic group(s) is (are) African. The largest religious group(s) is (are) Roman Catholic, and the other religious group(s) are (is) Anglican and Protestant.

The life expectancy at birth is 65.9 years for males and 68.8 years for females (WHO, 2004). The healthy life expectancy at birth is 58 years for males and 60 years for females (WHO, 2004).

EPIDEMIOLOGY

There is a paucity of epidemiological data on mental illnesses in Grenada in internationally accessible literature.

MENTAL HEALTH RESOURCES

Mental Health Policy A mental health policy is absent.

Substance Abuse Policy A substance abuse policy is absent.

National Mental Health Programme A national mental health programme is present. The programme was formulated in 1985.

National Therapeutic Drug Policy/Essential List of Drugs A national therapeutic drug policy/essential list of drugs is present. Details about the year of formulation are not available.

Mental Health Legislation There is a mental health legislation which is being upgraded.
Details about the year of enactment of the mental health legislation are not available.

Mental Health Financing There are budget allocations for mental health.
The country spends 10% of the total health budget on mental health.
The primary source of mental health financing is tax based.
The country does not have disability benefits for persons with mental disorders.

Mental Health Facilities Mental health is a part of primary health care system. Actual treatment of severe mental disorders is available at the primary level. Mental health care services are offered within primary care set-ups.
Regular training of primary care professionals is not carried out in the field of mental health.
There are community care facilities for patients with mental disorders. There are weekly community mental health clinics.
Community health workers and social workers also render community care services. The community health worker pays regular visits to patients' houses to ensure compliance to treatment. They were also trained to pick up early signs of deterioration and to intervene where necessary in order to prevent re-hospitalization. The public health nurse supports the community mental health worker.

Psychiatric Beds and Professionals

Total psychiatric beds per 10 000 population	10.8
Psychiatric beds in mental hospitals per 10 000 population	8.6
Psychiatric beds in general hospitals per 10 000 population	2.2
Psychiatric beds in other settings per 10 000 population	0
Number of psychiatrists per 100 000 population	1
Number of neurosurgeons per 100 000 population	
Number of psychiatric nurses per 100 000 population	5.4
Number of neurologists per 100 000 population	
Number of psychologists per 100 000 population	1
Number of social workers per 100 000 population	3

There is one occupational therapist. There is an urgent demand for trained psychiatric nurses and social workers to meet the demands of the increasing mental health population.

Non-Governmental Organizations NGOs are not involved with mental health in the country. There is a need for involvement of NGOs in mental health.

Information Gathering System There is mental health reporting system in the country. There is not much emphasis on collection of mental health data, and the information gathering system requires improvement.

The country has no data collection system or epidemiological study on mental health. Only patients' charts are available for collecting data related to health services.

Programmes for Special Population The country has specific programmes for mental health for elderly and children. Weekly outpatient clinics are carried out for children.
Psychiatrists and the psychiatric nurses pay regular visits to the prisons to assess any psychiatric problems among the prisoners.

Therapeutic Drugs The following therapeutic drugs are generally available at the primary health care level of the country: carbamazepine, phenobarbital, phenytoin sodium, amitriptyline, chlorpromazine, diazepam, haloperidol, lithium.

Other Information Since 1855, psychiatric care has largely been provided by the island's only mental hospital. Mental health had low priority and the main patients, till the late 1950s, were the 'wandering lunatics'. In 1970, an acute psychiatric unit was opened adjacent to the general hospital. After the US intervention, US aids facilitated the reconstruction of the destroyed psychiatric hospital and the development of psychiatry. Project HOPE was launched in 1985 to help in establishing diagnostic facilities, treatment and rehabilitation programmes and community care facilities. There is a need to establish policy and legislation for mental health and substance abuse. Additional mental health services need to be incorporated into the programme, such as day hospitals and psychogeriatric facilities.
* The verification of this country profile is still being awaited from the Ministry of Health of Grenada.

Additional Sources of Information

DeVooght, J, Walker, K. (1989) Community mental health Care in Grenada. International Nursing Review, 36, 22-24.

Fisher, F. D., Griffith, E., May, G. (1998) Recent developments in the Grenada Mental Health Program. Hospital and Community Psychiatry, 39, 980-85.

Guatemala

GENERAL INFORMATION

Guatemala is a country with an approximate area of 109 thousand sq. km. (UNO, 2001). Its population is 12.661 million, and the sex ratio (men per hundred women) is 101 (UNO, 2004). The proportion of population under the age of 15 years is 42% (UNO, 2004), and the proportion of population above the age of 60 years is 5% (WHO, 2004). The literacy rate is 77.3% for men and 62.5% for women (UNESCO/MoH, 2004).

The country is a lower middle income group country (based on World Bank 2004 criteria). The proportion of health budget to GDP is 4.8%. The per capita total expenditure on health is 199 international $, and the per capita government expenditure on health is 96 international $ (WHO, 2004).

The main language(s) used in the country is (are) Spanish and Indian (Maya). The largest ethnic group(s) is (are) indigenous (Maya, more than two-fifths of the population), and the other ethnic group(s) are (is) Mestizo. The largest religious group(s) is (are) Roman Catholic, and the other religious group(s) are (is) Protestant and Mayan.

The life expectancy at birth is 63.1 years for males and 69 years for females (WHO, 2004). The healthy life expectancy at birth is 55 years for males and 60 years for females (WHO, 2004).

EPIDEMIOLOGY

There is a paucity of epidemiological data on mental illnesses in Guatemala in internationally accessible literature. In a report from the Ministry of Health from Guatemala, in Chiquimula, a province with 300 thousand habitants, the percentage of outpatient consultations by diagnosis was: Depression (25.5%), Chronic Psychosis (21.9%), Epilepsy(10.4%), Bipolar Disorder (5.2%), Somatoform Disorders (11.4%), Mental Retardation (4.4%) and Anxiety Disorders (8.3%) (La Salud Mental en Guatemala: Ideas y Reflexiones, 1999). Berganza and Aguilar (1992) used a modified version of the Center for Epidemiological Studies Depression Scale for Children (CES-DC-M) in 339 adolescent school children belonging to three different social strata to identify the prevalence of depression. The prevalence was 35.1%. Gender rather than social class was related to depression. Weller et al (1991) described clinical characteristics of a folk illness called 'empacho' which manifested as diarrhea, headache, vomiting and lack of appetite. It differed from other gastrointestinal illnesses in that headaches were more likely and stomach-aches were less likely to be reported. Though empacho was frequently diagnosed by residents both in adults and children, folk healers were rarely consulted for it. Nevertheless, a strong association exists between a household diagnosis of empacho and the use of folk healers by those households.

MENTAL HEALTH RESOURCES

Mental Health Policy A mental health policy is present. The policy was initially formulated in 1997.

The components of the policy are promotion, prevention, treatment and rehabilitation. It was revised in 2000 by mental health professionals and public servants. There are regular funds for its implementation Between 50 to 75% of its original content has been implemented.

Substance Abuse Policy A substance abuse policy is present. The policy was initially formulated in 1998. The substance abuse policy does not have a specific budget for its implementation and has been implemented to the extent of 25 to 50%. Guatemala also has a law on Substance Abuse from 2000, 'Decreto Ley 50-2000 (Reformas al Código de Salud)', aiming to control and to reduce alcohol and tobacco use. The national mental health programme has a sub-programme for the prevention of alcoholism and other addictions, which in turn is considered within the National Steering Plan prepared by the Secretariat against addictions and illicit drug trafficking.

National Mental Health Programme A national mental health programme is present. The programme was formulated in 1997. It was revised in 2000. There are regular funds for its implementation and it has been implemented 50 to 75% by local, regional and national authorities. Its main components are strategy of services reform, promotion and prevention, mental health services at primary health care and specialized services.

National Therapeutic Drug Policy/Essential List of Drugs A national therapeutic drug policy/essential list of drugs is present. It was formulated in 1984.

Mental Health Legislation The decree 50/2000 (Reforms to the Health Code) is an anti-tobacco legislation and was enacted in 2000.

Details about the year of enactment of the mental health legislation are not available.

Mental Health Financing There are budget allocations for mental health.

The country spends 0.9% of the total health budget on mental health.

The primary sources of mental health financing in descending order are tax based, social insurance, out of pocket expenditure by the patient or family and private insurances.

Psychiatric hospitals receive 85% of the budget, community care 10%. General hospitals receive 5% of the funding.

The country has disability benefits for persons with mental disorders. Only 18% of the population have social security coverage, which is the portion that could be entitled to social benefit.

Mental Health Facilities Mental health is a part of primary health care system. Actual treatment of severe mental disorders is available at the primary level. This is possible in some primary health units (10/22) where the national mental health programme has been implemented.25-50% of the population is covered by this kind of service. Mental health care is provided by Primary Health Care doctors.

Regular training of primary care professionals is not carried out in the field of mental health. In the last two years, about 9980 personnel were provided training.

There are community care facilities for patients with mental disorders. Community care system for the mentally ill includes preventive/promotion interventions and covers 25 to 50% of the population. Home interventions, family interventions, vocational training and employment programmes are also available, but cover less than 25% of the treated population. The major part of community care facilities exist in the capital. The church plays a major role in providing community care services.

Psychiatric Beds and Professionals

Total psychiatric beds per 10 000 population	0.35
Psychiatric beds in mental hospitals per 10 000 population	0.32
Psychiatric beds in general hospitals per 10 000 population	0.03
Psychiatric beds in other settings per 10 000 population	0
Number of psychiatrists per 100 000 population	0.54
Number of neurosurgeons per 100 000 population	
Number of psychiatric nurses per 100 000 population	0.04
Number of neurologists per 100 000 population	0.009
Number of psychologists per 100 000 population	0.7
Number of social workers per 100 000 population	0.07

These professionals include those in public services and Guatemalan Mental Health Services. No information from the private sector is available. There are 4 other workers in mental health. Two-thirds of the beds are occupied by long stay patients. All mental health professionals are employed in public institutions.

Non-Governmental Organizations NGOs are involved with mental health in the country. They are mainly involved in advocacy, promotion, prevention, treatment and rehabilitation. These organizations participate in mental health activities related to women, children, domestic violence and consumers. These activities include treatment (psychiatric care), promotion (community work with children, women and human rights), prevention (at risk populations), rehabilitation (for victims of armed conflicts and disasters) and advocacy (education and information). The Ministry is working with NGOs on psychosocial recovery of war victims.

Information Gathering System There is mental health reporting system in the country. ICD-10 is used to record information. Besides psychiatric diagnoses, the other mental health component reported is family violence.

The country has data collection system or epidemiological study on mental health. An epidemiological assessment of the mental disorders is included. The department in charge of service data collection system is the National Program of Mental Health and the 'Departamento del Sistema Único de Información' both from the Ministry of Health. Data is collected only in the areas where the Mental Health Program is implemented. Only data coming from the public health system is available. The system is not very reliable.

Programmes for Special Population The country has specific programmes for mental health for refugees, disaster affected population, indigenous population and children. There is a school care system. Several NGOs are working in areas affected by war and Hurricane Mitch.

In addition, there are programmes for women, children in vulnerable situation and for domestic violence. There is an Inter-institutional Working Group in Mental Health composed by the Ministry of Health, Guatemalan Institute of Social Security, Psychiatric Association of Guatemala, Psychologist Association of Guatemala, Neurological Association of Guatemala, Alzheimer of Guatemala with support from PAHO and UNICEF. It is not functional as yet; efforts are being made by Ministry to get the collaboration of multiple sectors.

Therapeutic Drugs The following therapeutic drugs are generally available at the primary health care level of the country: carbamazepine, phenobarbital, phenytoin sodium, amitriptyline, chlorpromazine, diazepam, fluphenazine, haloperidol, lithium, biperiden. Some drugs are subsidized in state owned pharmacies and others are available only at normal prices. Free medication is provided to outpatients, but not in community centres where there are limitations. As the prices are high the Ministry of Health is establishing a network of national (popular) pharmacies which have reduced prices. Free service through primary health centres is being attempted.

Other Information Its reported that about 40% of the country has no mental health services and in the remaining part there are inadequate numbers of mental health professionals. The hospitals are in a poor state due to the lack of resources, and a large number of residents are institutionalized for a number of years.

Additional Sources of Information

Berganza, C. E., Aguilar, G. (1992) Depression in Guatemalan adolescents. Adolescence, 27, 771-782.

Republica de Guatemala Ministerio de salud publica y asistencia social (1999). Programa Nacional de salud mental memoria de labores.

Roberts, H. (2002). Mental health, truth and justice in Guatemala. Lancet, 359, 953.

Weller, S. C., Ruebush, T. K., Klein, R. E. (1991) An epidemiological description of a folk illness: a study of empacho in Guatemala. Medical Anthropology, 13, 19-31.

Guinea

GENERAL INFORMATION

Guinea is a country with an approximate area of 246 thousand sq. km. (UNO, 2001). Its population is 8.62 million, and the sex ratio (men per hundred women) is 101 (UNO, 2004). The proportion of population under the age of 15 years is 44% (UNO, 2004), and the proportion of population above the age of 60 years is 4% (WHO, 2004). The literacy rate is 50% for men and 22% for women (UNESCO/MoH, 2004).

The country is a low income group country (based on World Bank 2004 criteria). The proportion of health budget to GDP is 3.5%. The per capita total expenditure on health is 61 international $, and the per capita government expenditure on health is 33 international $ (WHO, 2004).

The main language(s) used in the country is (are) French. The largest ethnic group(s) is (are) Peuhl, and the other ethnic group(s) are (is) Malinke and Susu. The largest religious group(s) is (are) Muslim.

The life expectancy at birth is 50.9 years for males and 53.7 years for females (WHO, 2004). The healthy life expectancy at birth is 44 years for males and 46 years for females (WHO, 2004).

EPIDEMIOLOGY

There is a paucity of epidemiological data on mental illnesses in Guinea in internationally accessible literature.

MENTAL HEALTH RESOURCES

Mental Health Policy A mental health policy is present. The policy was initially formulated in 1995.

The components of the policy are advocacy, promotion, prevention, treatment and rehabilitation. Integration and decentralization are also components of the policy.

Substance Abuse Policy A substance abuse policy is present. The policy was initially formulated in 1999.

National Mental Health Programme A national mental health programme is present. The programme was formulated in 2000.

National Therapeutic Drug Policy/Essential List of Drugs A national therapeutic drug policy/essential list of drugs is present. Details about the year of formulation are not available.

Mental Health Legislation Measures related to prevention, protection and treatment have been taken (chapter 11, article 209-221 of the public health code) as part of the mental health legislation.

The latest legislation was enacted in 1997.

Mental Health Financing There are no budget allocations for mental health.

Details about expenditure on mental health are not available.

The primary source of mental health financing is out of pocket expenditure by the patient or family.

The country does not have disability benefits for persons with mental disorders.

Mental Health Facilities Mental health is a part of primary health care system. Actual treatment of severe mental disorders is not available at the primary level. Mental health in primary care is to be introduced.

Regular training of primary care professionals is not carried out in the field of mental health.

There are no community care facilities for patients with mental disorders. Traditional medicine is available at the community level.

Psychiatric Beds and Professionals

Total psychiatric beds per 10 000 population	0.05
Psychiatric beds in mental hospitals per 10 000 population	0.05
Psychiatric beds in general hospitals per 10 000 population	0
Psychiatric beds in other settings per 10 000 population	0
Number of psychiatrists per 100 000 population	0.04
Number of neurosurgeons per 100 000 population	0.03
Number of psychiatric nurses per 100 000 population	0
Number of neurologists per 100 000 population	0.04
Number of psychologists per 100 000 population	0
Number of social workers per 100 000 population	0

Psychologists and social workers are present in the Ministry of Social Affairs.

Non-Governmental Organizations NGOs are involved with mental health in the country. They are mainly involved in advocacy, prevention, treatment and rehabilitation.

Information Gathering System There is no mental health reporting system in the country. It is proposed to start a form of reporting system for mental health.
The country has no data collection system or epidemiological study on mental health. Data is collected only at the hospital level. No epidemiological survey exists.

Programmes for Special Population There are no programmes for special population.

Therapeutic Drugs The following therapeutic drugs are generally available at the primary health care level of the country: carbamazepine, phenobarbital, phenytoin sodium, amitriptyline, chlorpromazine, diazepam, fluphenazine, haloperidol, lithium.
Only phenobarbital, chlorpromazine and diazepam are available at the primary care level. Other drugs are on the list but are not available at the primary care level.

Other Information

Additional Sources of Information

Guinea-Bissau

GENERAL INFORMATION

Guinea-Bissau is a country with an approximate area of 36 thousand sq. km. (UNO, 2001). Its population is 1.537 million, and the sex ratio (men per hundred women) is 98 (UNO, 2004). The proportion of population under the age of 15 years is 47% (UNO, 2004), and the proportion of population above the age of 60 years is 5% (WHO, 2004). The literacy rate is 54.1% for men and 23.5% for women (UNESCO/MoH, 2004).

The country is a low income group country (based on World Bank 2004 criteria). The proportion of health budget to GDP is 5.9%. The per capita total expenditure on health is 37 international $, and the per capita government expenditure on health is 20 international $ (WHO, 2004).

The main language(s) used in the country is (are) Portuguese (official). The largest religious group(s) is (are) indigenous groups, and the other religious group(s) are (is) Muslim.

The life expectancy at birth is 45.7 years for males and 48.7 years for females (WHO, 2004). The healthy life expectancy at birth is 40 years for males and 42 years for females (WHO, 2004).

EPIDEMIOLOGY

There is a paucity of epidemiological data on mental illnesses in Guinea-Bissau in internationally accessible literature. A study by de Jong (1996) described the community mental health programme set-up in Guinea-Bissau. An epidemiological study was a part of the programme. A two-stage design was used to screen 351 consecutive adults and 100 children attending general health care set-ups in both rural and urban areas. Psychiatric disorders were present in 12% of the adults and 13% of the children attending a primary care centre. The commonest presentations were neuroses (74%). Psychoses were also common. Residence in rural/urban or war/no war zones was not significantly associated with occurrence of disorder. Overall, the programme showed a profitable cost/benefit ratio and a high sustainability over a 10-year period.

MENTAL HEALTH RESOURCES

Mental Health Policy A mental health policy is absent.

Substance Abuse Policy A substance abuse policy is absent.

National Mental Health Programme A national mental health programme is absent.
All documents related to the national mental health programme were destroyed during the military conflict. A national mental health programme is being formulated with WHO support. It is likely to be ready for adoption in 2004-2005.

National Therapeutic Drug Policy/Essential List of Drugs A national therapeutic drug policy/essential list of drugs is present. It was formulated in 1984.
After the introduction of the World Bank and International Monetary Fund Programme, the Essential Drug List Policy has suffered in more recent years.

Mental Health Legislation Details about the mental health legislation are not available.

Mental Health Financing There are budget allocations for mental health.
The country spends 2.3% of the total health budget on mental health.
The primary source of mental health financing is out of pocket expenditure by the patient or family.
The country does not have disability benefits for persons with mental disorders. Government employees with a medical attestation issued by the National Medical Committee receive their salaries.

Mental Health Facilities Mental health is not a part of primary health care system. Actual treatment of severe mental disorders is not available at the primary level. Patients with problems are sent to the mental health centre for treatment and follow-up.
Regular training of primary care professionals is carried out in the field of mental health. A nation-wide intervention programme with training of health workers and repetitive supervisory visits was initiated. In 1984 itself, 150 health workers were trained in 5-day seminars. It was followed by the evaluation of the programme. By 1985, Guinea-Bissau was the first third world country to succeed in integrating a social-psychiatric programme into its basic health care services on a national level. In the next three years, 600 health workers were trained in order to compensate for transfers, deaths and emigration. Over 10 years, it sustained these efforts. In 1997, a programme was started to train primary care doctor and nurses in mental health, but it was interrupted due to the war.
There are no community care facilities for patients with mental disorders. No community care exists due to lack of training and integration among workers. However, before the war, a community mental health programme was set up in 1983-84. The first part concentrated on epidemiological aspects. Subsequently, 850 primary health care workers were trained and supervised nationwide on their ability to manage mental disorders in patients.

E–I

Psychiatric Beds and Professionals

Total psychiatric beds per 10 000 population	0
Psychiatric beds in mental hospitals per 10 000 population	0
Psychiatric beds in general hospitals per 10 000 population	0
Psychiatric beds in other settings per 10 000 population	0
Number of psychiatrists per 100 000 population	0
Number of neurosurgeons per 100 000 population	0
Number of psychiatric nurses per 100 000 population	0
Number of neurologists per 100 000 population	0
Number of psychologists per 100 000 population	0
Number of social workers per 100 000 population	0

There are psychologists and social workers but they do not work in the area of mental health. In fact, two psychologists work in the Ministry of Health but not in the area of mental health. With support of WHO, one doctor initiated his specialization in Psychiatry in Cuba. The training will finish in October 2006. There was one mental health centre with 60 beds, but it was destroyed during the military conflict. After the Military Conflict, WHO helped in refurbishing two pavilions, which are being used for outpatient consultation and for inpatient care (2 rooms with 5 beds each and 2 other rooms for acute/emergency cases). Unfortunately the hospitalization unit is not functioning fully because of the inadequate support from the Government (electricity, water and security).

Non-Governmental Organizations NGOs are not involved with mental health in the country.

Information Gathering System There is no mental health reporting system in the country.
The country has no data collection system or epidemiological study on mental health. The Work Plan for 2004/05 has suggested the inclusion of mental disorders in studies on the prevalence of non-communicable diseases.

Programmes for Special Population The country has specific programmes for mental health for refugees, disaster affected population, elderly and children. The Government, international organizations and NGOs help whenever there is a crisis and the situation demands activities for a special group of population.

Therapeutic Drugs The following therapeutic drugs are generally available at the primary health care level of the country: carbamazepine, phenobarbital, phenytoin sodium, amitriptyline, chlorpromazine, diazepam, fluphenazine, haloperidol, biperiden, carbidopa, levodopa.
Hospital drugstores provide the drugs free. Other drugs are available from private pharmacies. Mental health centres obtain drugs from the central warehouse. The central drug deposit provides phenobarbital, haloperidol, amitriptylline, chlorpromazine and diazepam. Following the implementation of the Work Plan of 2002/03 and 2004/05 (supported by WHO) it is expected that the situation with regard to availability of psychotropics will improve.

Other Information

Additional Sources of Information

de Jong, J. T. (1996). A comprehensive public mental health program in Guinea-Bissau: a useful model for African, Asian and Latin-American countries. Psychological Medicine, 26, 97-108.

Guyana

GENERAL INFORMATION

Guyana is a country with an approximate area of 215 thousand sq. km. (UNO, 2001). Its population is 0.767 million, and the sex ratio (men per hundred women) is 94 (UNO, 2004). The proportion of population under the age of 15 years is 29% (UNO, 2004), and the proportion of population above the age of 60 years is 7% (WHO, 2004). The literacy rate is 98.9% for men and 98.1% for women (UNESCO/MoH, 2004).

The country is a lower middle income group country (based on World Bank 2004 criteria). The proportion of health budget to GDP is 5.3%. The per capita total expenditure on health is 215 international $, and the per capita government expenditure on health is 171 international $ (WHO, 2004).

The main language(s) used in the country is (are) English. The largest ethnic group(s) is (are) East Indian, and the other ethnic group(s) are (is) African. The largest religious group(s) is (are) Christian (half), and the other religious group(s) are (is) Hindu and Muslim.

The life expectancy at birth is 61.5 years for males and 66.9 years for females (WHO, 2004). The healthy life expectancy at birth is 53 years for males and 57 years for females (WHO, 2004).

EPIDEMIOLOGY

There is a paucity of epidemiological data on mental illnesses in Guyana in internationally accessible literature. Affonso et al (2000) conducted a study to identify the characteristics of postpartum depression (PPDS) in almost 900 women across 9 countries. The Edinburgh Postnatal Depression Scale (EPDS) and the Beck Depression Inventory (BDI) were used to assess PPDS among a convenience sample of primiparae with no obstetrical complications and having a healthy baby. On both the scales, European and Australian women had the lowest levels of PPDS, women from the USA were at the midpoint and women from Asia and South America had the highest levels of PPDS.

E–I

MENTAL HEALTH RESOURCES

Mental Health Policy A mental health policy is absent.

Substance Abuse Policy A substance abuse policy is absent.

National Mental Health Programme A national mental health programme is absent.
The national mental health programme is currently in development.

National Therapeutic Drug Policy/Essential List of Drugs A national therapeutic drug policy/essential list of drugs is present. It was formulated in 1997.

Mental Health Legislation Details about the mental health legislation are not available.

Mental Health Financing There are budget allocations for mental health.
Details about expenditure on mental health are not available.
The primary source of mental health financing is tax based.
The budget allocations are mainly made for psychiatric institutions and departments.
The country has disability benefits for persons with mental disorders.

Mental Health Facilities Mental health is a part of primary health care system. Actual treatment of severe mental disorders is not available at the primary level. Treatment is available in hospitals and psychiatric clinics.
Regular training of primary care professionals is not carried out in the field of mental health.
There are no community care facilities for patients with mental disorders.

Psychiatric Beds and Professionals

Total psychiatric beds per 10 000 population	3
Psychiatric beds in mental hospitals per 10 000 population	2.6
Psychiatric beds in general hospitals per 10 000 population	0.4
Psychiatric beds in other settings per 10 000 population	0
Number of psychiatrists per 100 000 population	0.2
Number of neurosurgeons per 100 000 population	14
Number of psychiatric nurses per 100 000 population	0.6
Number of neurologists per 100 000 population	14
Number of psychologists per 100 000 population	0
Number of social workers per 100 000 population	0.4

The numbers represent those working in the public health sector.

Non-Governmental Organizations NGOs are involved with mental health in the country. NGOs are also involved with substance abuse programmes.

Information Gathering System There is no mental health reporting system in the country.
The country has no data collection system or epidemiological study on mental health.

Programmes for Special Population There are no special programmes.

Therapeutic Drugs The following therapeutic drugs are generally available at the primary health care level of the country: carbamazepine, phenobarbital, phenytoin sodium, sodium valproate, amitriptyline, chlorpromazine, diazepam, fluphenazine, haloperidol, carbidopa, levodopa.
The essential drug list was updated in 2004.

Other Information

Additional Sources of Information

Affonso, D. D., De, A. K., Horowitz, J. A., et al (2000) An international study exploring levels of postpartum depressive symptomatology. Journal of Psychosomatic Research, 49, 207-216.

Government document (1998) Essential Drug List of Guyana. Government Pharmacy Programme, 1

Haiti

GENERAL INFORMATION

Haiti is a country with an approximate area of 28 thousand sq. km. (UNO, 2001). Its population is 8.437 million, and the sex ratio (men per hundred women) is 98 (UNO, 2004). The proportion of population under the age of 15 years is 38% (UNO, 2004), and the proportion of population above the age of 60 years is 6% (WHO, 2004). The literacy rate is 53.8% for men and 50% for women (UNESCO/MoH, 2004).

The country is a low income group country (based on World Bank 2004 criteria). The proportion of health budget to GDP is 5%. The per capita total expenditure on health is 56 international $, and the per capita government expenditure on health is 30 international $ (WHO, 2004).

The main language(s) used in the country is (are) French and Creole. The largest ethnic group(s) is (are) African (descent). The largest religious group(s) is (are) indigenous groups, and the other religious group(s) are (is) Roman Catholic.

The life expectancy at birth is 49.1 years for males and 51.1 years for females (WHO, 2004). The healthy life expectancy at birth is 44 years for males and 44 years for females (WHO, 2004).

EPIDEMIOLOGY

There is a paucity of epidemiological data on mental illnesses in Haiti in internationally accessible literature.

MENTAL HEALTH RESOURCES

Mental Health Policy A mental health policy is absent.
Discussions between various stakeholder groups are being held on the development of a national mental health policy.

Substance Abuse Policy A substance abuse policy is absent. Discussions between various stakeholder groups are being held on the development of a substance abuse policy.

National Mental Health Programme A national mental health programme is absent.

National Therapeutic Drug Policy/Essential List of Drugs A national therapeutic drug policy/essential list of drugs is present.
Details about the year of formulation are not available.

Mental Health Legislation Details about the mental health legislation are not available.

Mental Health Financing Details about disability benefits for mental health are not available.
Details about expenditure on mental health are not available.
Details about sources of financing are not available.
Details about disability benefits for mental health are not available.

Mental Health Facilities Details about mental health facilities at the primary care level are not available.
Details about training facilities are not available.
Details about community care facilities in mental health are not available.

Psychiatric Beds and Professionals

Total psychiatric beds per 10 000 population
Psychiatric beds in mental hospitals per 10 000 population
Psychiatric beds in general hospitals per 10 000 population
Psychiatric beds in other settings per 10 000 population
Number of psychiatrists per 100 000 population
Number of neurosurgeons per 100 000 population
Number of psychiatric nurses per 100 000 population
Number of neurologists per 100 000 population
Number of psychologists per 100 000 population
Number of social workers per 100 000 population

Non-Governmental Organizations Details about NGO facilities in mental health are not available.

Information Gathering System Details about mental health reporting systems are not available.
Details about data collection system or epidemiological study on mental health are not available.

Programmes for Special Population Details about special programmes are not available.

Therapeutic Drugs The following therapeutic drugs are generally available at the primary health care level of the country: carbamazepine, phenobarbital, phenytoin sodium, chlorpromazine, diazepam, haloperidol, biperiden.
The PAHO/WHO list has been adapted to serve as the national essential drug list.

Other Information

Additional Sources of Information

Hohner, J. A., Hughes, D. A., Jones, J. (1998) Mental health nursing support during Operation Sea Signal: Cuban/Haitian humanitarian mission. Military Medicine, 163, 353-57.

Honduras

GENERAL INFORMATION

Honduras is a country with an approximate area of 112 thousand sq. km. (UNO, 2001). Its population is 7.1 million, and the sex ratio (men per hundred women) is 102 (UNO, 2004). The proportion of population under the age of 15 years is 40% (UNO, 2004), and the proportion of population above the age of 60 years is 5% (WHO, 2004). The literacy rate is 79.8% for men and 80.2% for women (UNESCO/MoH, 2004).

The country is a lower middle income group country (based on World Bank 2004 criteria). The proportion of health budget to GDP is 6.1%. The per capita total expenditure on health is 153 international $, and the per capita government expenditure on health is 81 international $ (WHO, 2004).

The main language(s) used in the country is (are) Spanish. The largest ethnic group(s) is (are) Mestizo (nine-tenths). The largest religious group(s) is (are) Roman Catholic.

The life expectancy at birth is 64.2 years for males and 70.4 years for females (WHO, 2004). The healthy life expectancy at birth is 56 years for males and 60 years for females (WHO, 2004).

EPIDEMIOLOGY

There is a paucity of epidemiological data on mental illnesses in Honduras in internationally accessible literature. Kohn et al examined 800 victims of Hurricane Mitch. They were stratified from high, medium and low class areas and high and low exposure subgroups. Current DSM-IV major depressive episode was diagnosed in 18.3% of the population and PTSD in 11.2%. Co-morbidity between PTSD and major depressive episode was high. Prevalence of both disorders were associated with exposure. Other risk factors for PTSD included lower SES, increasing age and 'general nervousness' before the disaster. Quirk and Casco (1994) described the effect of forced disappearance on the physical and psychological health of family members. The families of the disappeared were compared with two control groups: (1) families who lost a member due to accident or illness, and (2) families where no one had died within the past 10 years. Constellations of stress-related symptoms commonly seen in post-traumatic stress disorder and other anxiety disorders were approximately 2 times more prevalent in families of the disappeared as compared to the other two groups, indicating that families of the disappeared suffer over and above that due to normal grieving. Meza (1988) found that the presence of mental disorders in parents was associated with serious malnutrition in children. The commonest mental disorders in his sample were neurosis and alcohol use disorders. Wittig et al (1997) reported on the use of drugs by street children (n=1244) and found that family relations, length of time on the street and delinquency were associated with drug use, especially with sniffing glue.

MENTAL HEALTH RESOURCES

Mental Health Policy A mental health policy is present. The policy was initially formulated in 2004.

Substance Abuse Policy A substance abuse policy is present. The policy was initially formulated in 1989. In 1988, the National Government created the Institute for the Prevention of Alcoholism, Drug Addiction and Pharmaceutical Dependence, with the fundamental objective to prevent the consumption of alcohol, tobacco products and other drugs especially in children and young adults. The substance abuse policy has a specific budget for its implementation. It focuses on drinking and driving, prohibition of selling alcohol to underage subjects and regulation of advertisement. More than 90% of the policy has been already implemented. There is legislation on substance abuse in place since 2001.

National Mental Health Programme A national mental health programme is present. Details about the year of formulation of the programme are not available.

There is a national programme under the Secretary of Mental Health. The objective is to have community participation.

National Therapeutic Drug Policy/Essential List of Drugs A national therapeutic drug policy/essential list of drugs is present. It was formulated in 1985.

Mental Health Legislation There is no mental health legislation. Although, there is a law against domestic violence which was passed in 1998.

Details about the year of enactment of the mental health legislation are not available.

Mental Health Financing There are budget allocations for mental health.

The country spends 2.3% of the total health budget on mental health.

Details about sources of financing are not available.

More than 90% of funds for mental health services goes to the psychiatric hospitals.

The country has disability benefits for persons with mental disorders. However, only a minority of the eligible population get the benefits (less than 10%).

Mental Health Facilities Mental health is a part of primary health care system. Actual treatment of severe mental disorders is available at the primary level. Less than 25 % of the population is covered by this kind of service. Psychiatrists are responsible for treatment of mental disorders at primary care level. Medication is the only therapy available.
Regular training of primary care professionals is not carried out in the field of mental health.
There are no community care facilities for patients with mental disorders.

Psychiatric Beds and Professionals

Total psychiatric beds per 10 000 population	0.6
Psychiatric beds in mental hospitals per 10 000 population	0.53
Psychiatric beds in general hospitals per 10 000 population	0.07
Psychiatric beds in other settings per 10 000 population	0
Number of psychiatrists per 100 000 population	0.76
Number of neurosurgeons per 100 000 population	0.36
Number of psychiatric nurses per 100 000 population	0
Number of neurologists per 100 000 population	0.17
Number of psychologists per 100 000 population	0.5
Number of social workers per 100 000 population	0.26

90% of the beds are occupied by long stay patients. There are no psychiatric beds in general hospitals and prisons. There is one day care centre for mental health patients.

Non-Governmental Organizations NGOs are involved with mental health in the country. They are mainly involved in advocacy, promotion, prevention, treatment and rehabilitation. They participate in activities related to women, children, domestic violence and consumers.

Information Gathering System There is mental health reporting system in the country. ICD-10 is used for recording information. The country has data collection system or epidemiological study on mental health. The data is collected at regional level and sent to the Department of Statistics, but mental health data are not processed.

Programmes for Special Population The country has specific programmes for mental health for elderly. There are facilities for counselling on family violence and on HIV.
Also there are programmes for domestic violence. These programmes are managed by multidisciplinary personnel and have been developed under the National Program of Mental Health. There are 15 distributed councils of family in all the country. Also, a programme of Council in VIH/SIDA exists.

Therapeutic Drugs The essential drug list was revised in 2001. There is almost no availability of the medications listed below at primary health care level. Medicines in the primary health care are free and in some cases subsidized for those in need based on economic and social graph anchors and according to the availability of financing and to prices in the market for the following medications: carbamazepine, phenobarbital, phenytoin sodium, diazepan, flufenazin, cloropromazin, biperiden and levodopa. Ethosuximide, chlorpromazine, biperiden and lithium carbonate are available only at the Ministry of Health.

Other Information

Additional Sources of Information

Meza, J. M. (1988) Prevalence of mental health problems in parents of children with malnutrition in one area of Tegucigalpa, Honduras. Acta Psiquiatrica y Psicologica de America Latina, 34, 145-148.

Quirk, G. J., Casco, L. (1994) Stress disorders of families of the disappeared: a controlled study in Honduras. Social Science & Medicine, 39, 1675-1679.

Wittig, M. C., Wright, J. D., Kaminsky, D. C. (1997) Substance use among street children in Honduras. Substance Use & Misuse, 32, 805-827.

Hungary

GENERAL INFORMATION

Hungary is a country with an approximate area of 93 thousand sq. km. (UNO, 2001). Its population is 9.831 million, and the sex ratio (men per hundred women) is 91 (UNO, 2004). The proportion of population under the age of 15 years is 16% (UNO, 2004), and the proportion of population above the age of 60 years is 20% (WHO, 2004). The literacy rate is 99.5% for men and 99.2% for women (UNESCO/MoH, 2004).

The country is a higher middle income group country (based on World Bank 2004 criteria). The proportion of health budget to GDP is 6.8%. The per capita total expenditure on health is 914 international $, and the per capita government expenditure on health is 686 international $ (WHO, 2004).

The main language(s) used in the country is (are) Modern Hungarian. The largest ethnic group(s) is (are) Hungarian (nine-tenths), and the other ethnic group(s) are (is) Roma, German and Slovak. The largest religious group(s) is (are) Roman Catholic (three-fourths).

The life expectancy at birth is 68.4 years for males and 76.8 years for females (WHO, 2004). The healthy life expectancy at birth is 62 years for males and 68 years for females (WHO, 2004).

EPIDEMIOLOGY

Kopp and Csoboth (2001) studied a national representative sample of 12640 people and found that just less than half of men and more than a quarter of women smoked. In a community sample of 2953 randomly selected adults, Szadoczky et al (1998, 2000) found that the lifetime prevalence of major depressive disorder (MDD), bipolar disorder (BD) and dysthymia were 15.1% (male to female ratio of 2.7), 5.1%, and 4.5%, respectively. The 1-year and 1-month prevalence rates were 7.1% and 2.6% for MDD, 0.9% and 0.5% for manic episodes and 0.8%, and 0.5% for dysthymia. The highest risk for the development of MDD, dysthymia and BD was in 15-19 years, but in MDD and dysthymia another peak was found in the forties. MDD was associates with higher rates of dysthymia and all anxiety disorders, BD was associated with the occurrence of generalized anxiety disorder and panic disorder and dysthymia was associated with MDD and anxiety disorders. Zonda et al (2000) used the Diagnostic Interview Schedule and Beck's Depression Inventory to interview a representative sample from a region (n=750) and found the point and lifetime prevalence of affective disorders to be: major depression 3.7% and 10.9%, dysthymia 2.9% and 5.3% and bipolar disorders zero and 1.07%. The risk of suicide was high in those with major depression and dysthymia. Kopp et al (2000) conducted a survey on depression in nationally representative samples of 21 000 adults in 1988 and 12 370 adults in 1995 using a modified version of Beck's Depression Inventory. In surveys done in 1988 and 1995, 2.9% and 7.1% suffered from severe depression requiring treatment. Between 1988 and 1995 depression increased among the socially deprived, i.e. those with low education, unemployed and elderly. Rihmer et al (2001) assessed 2953 adults regarding comorbidity between anxiety and affective disorders using the Diagnostic Interview Schedule. The prevalence of generalized anxiety disorder, agoraphobia and simple phobia was highest among bipolar II patients (20.8%, 37.5% and 16.7%, respectively); social phobia was most prevalent in major depression (17.6%) and panic disorder was equally prevalent in the major depressive and bipolar II subgroups (12.4% and 12.5%, respectively). Women had a higher risk for comorbidity between anxiety disorders and MDD. Szabo and Tury (1991) conducted a two-stage survey to determine the prevalence of bulimia in two non-clinical samples. In an adolescent sample no bulimic subjects were found. In the college sample 1.3% of females and 0.8% of males met DSM-III-R diagnostic criteria for bulimia nervosa. La Vecchia et al (1994) analysed suicide data from the World Health Organization mortality database. Hungary had the highest rate of suicide for men (52.1 per 100 000) and the second highest rate for women (17.6 per 100 000). The high rate of suicide in Hungary is probably related to similarly high rates in Eastern Europe (Sartorius, 1995). Toero et al (2001) reported that Hungary has the highest suicide rate among children and adolescents. Zonda (1999) found that suicide rate was associated with locality (rural), gender (male/female ratio was 4:1), age (elderly), marital status (divorced/widowed) and psychiatric (60.1%) and multiple somatic illnesses (8.8%). In a community sample, Szadoczky et al (2000) found that suicide attempts occurred more frequently among women and divorced/widowed persons. The presence of any lifetime anxiety and/or affective disorder, comorbidity, recurrence and chronicity were significant predictors of suicide attempts. Osvath et al (2001) reported that chronic physical and mental problems were frequent among suicide attempters and many of them were on medication. Czeizel et al (1990) assessed 1276 school age children with mental retardation and estimated that 3% of school age children had an IQ of less than 50 and that low IQ was associated with 58 years of life lost.

MENTAL HEALTH RESOURCES

Mental Health Policy A mental health policy is absent.

A mental health policy constitutes an important chapter of the National Public Health Strategy voted for by the government and to be submitted for the Parliament in 2001.

Substance Abuse Policy A substance abuse policy is present. The policy was initially formulated in 2000.

National Mental Health Programme A national mental health programme is present. The programme was formulated in 2001. Some national mental health programmes including one against drug misuse have been elaborated/reframed during the last five years. A new version of the national mental health programme is in preparation, taking into account the shift in the concept of health (e.g. the Ottawa and Jakarta Declarations) and the priorities of the World Health Organization. The National Mental Health

Programme constitutes one of the 20 sub-programmes of the recently initiated National Public Health Programme which is to be implemented over the next 10 years.

National Therapeutic Drug Policy/Essential List of Drugs A national therapeutic drug policy/essential list of drugs is present. It was formulated in 2000.

Mental Health Legislation The Health Act (No CL IV) of 1997 relates to mental health. A new Health Act, voted by the Parliament in 1998, came into effect in 1999. There is no special law on mental health, but this Act contains a chapter on mental disorders and their treatment, including hospitalization and compulsory measures. The legislation on mental health issues, with the protection of human rights of mental patients, conforms to EU requirements. The legislation was modified with more precision on coercive measures in 2001 and in 2004.
The latest legislation was enacted in 1997.

Mental Health Financing There are budget allocations for mental health.
The country spends 8% of the total health budget on mental health.
The primary sources of mental health financing in descending order are social insurance and tax based.
The health service is based on insurance system. Due to this, emphasis is more on short term medical treatment and psychotherapy has lost out. As outpatient care is financed to a lesser degree than inpatient care, institutions have tended to develop their inpatient facilities to a greater extent. The American mechanism of 'diagnostic related groups' was adopted to finance hospital services. In outpatient care, the 'German score system' was introduced. Care of handicapped children is financed by the social welfare budget. The country has disability benefits for persons with mental disorders.

Mental Health Facilities Mental health is a part of primary health care system. Actual treatment of severe mental disorders is not available at the primary level. There are mental health centres all over the country to cater to primary care.
Regular training of primary care professionals is carried out in the field of mental health. In the last two years, about 500 personnel were provided training. Training facilities for primary care doctors are present. Family doctors treat a significant proportion of psychiatry patients.
There are community care facilities for patients with mental disorders. Community care is mainly provided by some mental health centres and universities. The development of community care and primary care facilities is dependent on grants and is occurring at a gradual pace. A few halfway institutions are in operation.

Psychiatric Beds and Professionals

Total psychiatric beds per 10 000 population	9.6
Psychiatric beds in mental hospitals per 10 000 population	2.3
Psychiatric beds in general hospitals per 10 000 population	7.2
Psychiatric beds in other settings per 10 000 population	0.1
Number of psychiatrists per 100 000 population	9
Number of neurosurgeons per 100 000 population	1
Number of psychiatric nurses per 100 000 population	19
Number of neurologists per 100 000 population	7
Number of psychologists per 100 000 population	2
Number of social workers per 100 000 population	1

There are 3080 other kind of mental health professionals. Over the last decade, substantial reduction (one-third) in psychiatry hospital beds has occurred. A reform of psychiatric institutions offering care to chronic psychotic patients is also under way and many of them now offer rehabilitative services. The private sector is small and is limited to outpatient care. About 160 beds are available with child and adolescent psychiatry departments. There is a system of psychiatric outpatient services staffed by psychiatrists, clinical psychologists, social workers, psychiatric nurses, etc. Though the significance of multidisciplinary teamwork seems to be generally acknowledged, the health system is medically dominated, and non-medical professionals play a secondary role. There are very few psychologists and almost no social workers or occupational therapists. Within psychiatry, however, specialized qualifications like addictology, forensic psychiatry, psychotherapy and child psychiatry are available. A full fledged child psychiatry training programme was started as a part of TEMPUS project funded by the European Union.

Non-Governmental Organizations NGOs are involved with mental health in the country. They are mainly involved in advocacy, promotion, prevention and rehabilitation. There are different self-help groups.

Information Gathering System There is mental health reporting system in the country. Mental health forms part of the statistical reports of the National Institute of Statistics.
The country has data collection system or epidemiological study on mental health. Annual reports of services are collected at the state mental hospitals.

Programmes for Special Population The country has specific programmes for mental health for refugees, elderly and children. Child psychiatry is underdeveloped and dependent on outpatient facilities. There are some child and youth guidance centres, which are usually run by psychologists. Larger schools employ psychologists. A separate school network deals with developmental disorders and learning difficulties. Substance abuse, forensic psychiatry services are also developing. There are regional drug outpatient departments all over the country and all psychiatry wards are obliged to admit patients in withdrawal. Churches also help in management of patients of drug dependence. A Government programme of mental hygiene was established to support and coordinate local initiatives. The forensic psychiatric institution is under the charge of Ministry of Justice.

Therapeutic Drugs The following therapeutic drugs are generally available at the primary health care level of the country: carbamazepine, ethosuximide, phenobarbital, phenytoin sodium, sodium valproate, amitriptyline, chlorpromazine, diazepam, fluphenazine, haloperidol, lithium, biperiden, carbidopa, levodopa.
The costs of most important drugs are reimbursed by the social insurance. All modern anti-psychotics and anti-depressants are available and are covered by social insurance. The full cost of anti-psychotics and 90% of the cost of anti-depressants is covered.

Other Information Before the 19th century there were no psychiatric care facilities, and monasteries took care of mentally ill patients. The first psychiatric institution was founded in 1840. From the beginning of the 20th century mental departments were being established in general hospitals and some psychiatric hospitals were being transformed into general hospitals. Psychiatry and neurology remained united till 1960. Psychiatry begun in universities in the middle of the 19th century. Hungary has contributed a lot to the development of psychiatry through the works of many psychiatrists. It developed under the influence of the German school of psychopathology. Psychiatric research is funded by a National Research Fund (Tringer, 1999).

E-I

Additional Sources of Information

Czeizel, A., Sankaranarayanan, K., Szondy, M. (1990) The load of genetic and partially genetic diseases in man. III. Mental retardation. Mutation Research, 232, 291-303.

Kopp, M., Csoboth, C. (2001) Smoking and alcohol abuse in the Hungarian population. Fogorvosi Szemle, 94, 177-182.

Kopp, M. S., Skrabski, A., Szedmak, S. (2000) Psychosocial risk factors, inequality and self-rated morbidity in a changing society. Social Science & Medicine, 51, 1351-1361.

La Vecchia C., Lucchini, F., Levi, F. (1994) Worldwide trends in suicide mortality, 1955-1989. Acta Psychiatrica Scandinavica, 90, 53-64.

Maylath, E. (2000) Diagnosis-related group financing and its influence on hospital financing – a comparison with Hungary: Could this be a useful model for German conditions? Gesundheitswesen, 62, 633-645.

Osvath, P., Fekete, S., Abraham, I. (2001) Physical illness and suicidal behavior. Review of results at the Pecs Center of the WHO/EURO Multicenter Study of Parasuicide. Orvosi Hetilap, 142, 127-131.

Rihmer, Z., Szadoczky, E., Furedi, J., et al (2001) Anxiety disorders comorbidity in bipolar I, bipolar II and unipolar major depression: results from a population-based study in Hungary. Journal of Affective Disorders, 67, 175-179.

Sartorius, N. (1995) Recent changes in suicide rates in selected Eastern European and other European countries. International Psychogeriatrics, 7, 301-308.

Szabo, P., Tury, F. (1991) The prevalence of bulimia nervosa in a Hungarian college and secondary school population. Psychotherapy & Psychosomatics, 56, 43-47.

Szadoczky, E., Papp, Z., Vitrai, J., et al (1998) The prevalence of major depressive and bipolar disorders in Hungary. Results from a national epidemiologic survey. Journal of Affective Disorders, 50, 153-162.

Szadoczky, E., Rihmer, Z., Papp, Z., et al (2000) Epidemiology of dysthymic disorder. Psychiatria Hungarica, 15, 66-75.

Szadoczky, E., Vitrai, J., Rihmer, Z., et al (2000) Suicide attempts in the Hungarian adult population. Their relation with DIS/DSM-III-R affective and anxiety disorders. European Psychiatry: the Journal of the Association of European Psychiatrists, 15, 343-347.

Toero, K., Nagy, A., Sawaguchi, T., et al (2001) Characteristics of suicide among children and adolescents in Budapest. Pediatrics International, 43, 368-371.

Tringer, L. (1999) Focus on psychiatry in Hungary. British Journal of Psychiatry, 174, 81-85.

van Benium, M.E., McGuiness, D., Csik. V. et al (1998) Contrasting child and adolescent psychiatry services in Szeged, Hungary and Glasgow, Scotland.

Vetro, A. (1999) Child and adolescent psychiatry in hungary. In: H. Remschmidt, H. van Engeland (Eds). Child and Adolescent Psychiatry in Europe. Historical Development, Current Situation and Future Perspectives. Darmstadt, Steinkopff. pp151-164.

Zonda, T. (1999) Suicide in Nograd County, Hungary, 1970-1994. Crisis: Journal of Crisis Intervention & Suicide, 20, 64-70.

Zonda, T., Bartos, E., Nagy, G. (2000) Affective disorders in a district of Budapest. Hungarian. Orvosi Hetilap, 141, 1443-1447.

Iceland

GENERAL INFORMATION

Iceland is a country with an approximate area of 103 thousand sq. km. (UNO, 2001). Its population is 0.291 million, and the sex ratio (men per hundred women) is 101 (UNO, 2004). The proportion of population under the age of 15 years is 22% (UNO, 2004), and the proportion of population above the age of 60 years is 15% (WHO, 2004). The literacy rate is 99% for men and 99% for women (UNESCO/MoH, 2004).
The country is a high income group country (based on World Bank 2004 criteria). The proportion of health budget to GDP is 9.2%. The per capita total expenditure on health is 2643 international $, and the per capita government expenditure on health is 2192 international $ (WHO, 2004).
The main language(s) used in the country is (are) Icelandic. The largest ethnic group(s) is (are) Icelandic (Norwegian and Celtic descent). The largest religious group(s) is (are) Christian.
The life expectancy at birth is 78.4 years for males and 81.8 years for females (WHO, 2004). The healthy life expectancy at birth is 72 years for males and 74 years for females (WHO, 2004).

EPIDEMIOLOGY

There is substantial epidemiological data on mental illnesses in Iceland in internationally accessible literature. No attempt was made to include this information here.

MENTAL HEALTH RESOURCES

Mental Health Policy A mental health policy is absent.
No specific mental health policy is being implemented but mental health is regarded as one of 7 identified key areas in long-term health planning in Iceland. Important developments in mental health care in the first years of the 21st century include stronger advocacy groups, mental health promotion schemes, more focus on prevention, evidence-based treatment and more active rehabilitation.

Substance Abuse Policy A substance abuse policy is present. The policy was initially formulated in 1974. Amendments to the policy are due to be discussed in Parliament, partly reflecting EU-law and practices in other countries within the European Economic Area.

National Mental Health Programme A national mental health programme is present. The programme was formulated in 2001. The Icelandic Ministry of Health and the Health Committee of the Icelandic Parliament put forward a plan for national health targets in 2001 extending to the year 2010. This plan emphasizes long-term objectives in health. Among the main objectives is a 25% reduction in suicide rates. However, no specific budget is set aside in order to try and implement this plan.

National Therapeutic Drug Policy/Essential List of Drugs A national therapeutic drug policy/essential list of drugs is absent.

Mental Health Legislation Iceland has mental health legislation. The law concerning care, treatment and rehabilitation of mental patients is mainly included in the legislation for health services; the legislation for social security and the legislation for national health insurance is included in the law no 97/1990 relating to health services; law no 59/1992 is related to the disabled; law no 117/1993 is related to social and health insurance; law no 39/1964 is related to treatment of alcoholics and people under the influence of alcohol. There is no separate Mental Health Act in Iceland. The necessary legislation, e.g. for involuntary hospital admission, is included under the law on legal capacity. This ensures, among other things, the rights of patients to an appeal and an independent medical review.
The latest legislation was enacted in 1997.

Mental Health Financing There are no budget allocations for mental health.
Details about expenditure on mental health are not available.
The primary sources of mental health financing in descending order are tax based and out of pocket expenditure by the patient or family.
There are no separate budget allocations for mental health, the costs being covered as part of overall expenditure on health services. Inpatient treatment is free, but patients pay a modest fee for outpatient treatment; psychiatrist consultations in outpatient settings are subsidized by the Ministry of Health.
The country has disability benefits for persons with mental disorders. Iceland provides rehabilitation benefits for up to 18 months and disability benefits both short- and long-term for persons suffering from psychiatric disorders.

Mental Health Facilities Mental health is a part of primary health care system. Actual treatment of severe mental disorders is available at the primary level. Mental health services work in close liaison with primary health care system. The primary health service is mainly run from health centres which have no beds and admissions are only made at specialist wards in the major hospitals. Regular training of primary care professionals is carried out in the field of mental health. Training opportunities for primary care professionals are on offer through the Departments of Psychiatry at the two hospitals in Iceland. The Ministry of Education is responsible for the training of health care workers.

There are community care facilities for patients with mental disorders. Non-governmental organizations and local authorities are gradually developing psychiatric care and other support services in the community, although this development has still not been fully achieved.

Psychiatric Beds and Professionals

Total psychiatric beds per 10 000 population	5
Psychiatric beds in mental hospitals per 10 000 population	0
Psychiatric beds in general hospitals per 10 000 population	5
Psychiatric beds in other settings per 10 000 population	0
Number of psychiatrists per 100 000 population	25
Number of neurosurgeons per 100 000 population	2
Number of psychiatric nurses per 100 000 population	33
Number of neurologists per 100 000 population	6
Number of psychologists per 100 000 population	60
Number of social workers per 100 000 population	110

The psychiatric services have been deinstitutionalized in recent decades and all psychiatric beds are now within general hospitals although in separate buildings on site or on special sites. The number of acute beds has decreased by about 25% since 1997 but day-patient and outpatient facilities have expanded at the same time. Psychiatric care is primarily provided by multidisciplinary teams. In recent years, the numbers of psychiatrists, psychologists and social workers have followed the growth of the population, but there continues to be a relative shortage of psychiatric nurses.

Non-Governmental Organizations NGOs are involved with mental health in the country. They are mainly involved in promotion, prevention and treatment. The role of NGOs is of growing importance, e.g. in terms of residential care, treatment facilities for substance abusers and as promoters of patients' rights. In addition to residential support, NGOs have important roles in non-hospital care.

Information Gathering System Details about mental health reporting systems are not available.
Details about data collection system or epidemiological study on mental health are not available.
There is no ongoing systemic mental health reporting taking place at present in the country. In recent years, requirement for collecting and storing personal data on subjects have become much tighter than they used to be, even to the degree where this may hamper epidemiological studies into sensitive subjects like mental health.

Programmes for Special Population The country has specific programmes for mental health for refugees, disaster affected population, elderly and children.
Specialized psychiatric services for children and adolescents have improved over the last decade and are currently expanding further. This is regarded a priority to facilitate multidisciplinary early assessment, intervention and treatment.

Therapeutic Drugs The following therapeutic drugs are generally available at the primary health care level of the country: carbamazepine, ethosuximide, phenobarbital, phenytoin sodium, sodium valproate, amitriptyline, chlorpromazine, diazepam, fluphenazine, haloperidol, lithium, biperiden, levodopa.

Other Information There is considerable intersectoral cooperation at Government level, e.g. among the Ministries of Health, Social Affairs and Education as well as local authorities. NGOs, the Surgeon General of Health and others with the help of the media have promoted awareness in the public of mental health through publications and other activities.

Additional Sources of Information

India

GENERAL INFORMATION

India is a country with an approximate area of 3287 thousand sq. km. (UNO, 2001). Its population is 1.081 billion, and the sex ratio (men per hundred women) is 106 (UNO, 2004). The proportion of population under the age of 15 years is 32% (UNO, 2004), and the proportion of population above the age of 60 years is 8% (WHO, 2004). The literacy rate is 68.4% for men and 45.4% for women (UNESCO/MoH, 2004).

The country is a low income group country (based on World Bank 2004 criteria). The proportion of health budget to GDP is 5.1%. The per capita total expenditure on health is 80 international $, and the per capita government expenditure on health is 14 international $ (WHO, 2004).

The main language(s) used in the country is (are) Hindi, English and 14 other official languages. The largest ethnic group(s) is (are) Indo-Aryan, and the other ethnic group(s) are (is) Dravidian. The largest religious group(s) is (are) Hindu, and the other religious group(s) are (is) Muslim, Sikh and Christian.

The life expectancy at birth is 60.1 years for males and 62 years for females (WHO, 2004). The healthy life expectancy at birth is 53 years for males and 54 years for females (WHO, 2004).

EPIDEMIOLOGY

A meta-analysis of 13 psychiatric epidemiological studies (n=33 572) yielded an estimated prevalence rate of 5.8% (Reddy & Chandrashekar, 1998). Organic psychosis (0.04%), alcohol/drug dependence (0.69%), schizophrenia (0.27%), affective disorders (1.23%), neurotic disorders (2.07%), mental retardation (0.69%) and epilepsy (0.44%) were commonly diagnosed. Psychiatric morbidity was associated with residence (urban), gender (females), age group (35-44 years), marital status (married/widowed/divorced), socioeconomic status (lower) and family type (nuclear). Epilepsy and hysteria were significantly more common in rural communities. Nandi et al (2000) reported that psychiatric morbidity decreased from 11.7% to 10.5% over 20 years in a rural setting. Rao (1993) reported that mental morbidity was present in 8.9% of the elderly (above 60 years), with depression being the most common disorder (6%). Psychiatric morbidity was associated with physical diseases. Many studies (e.g. Vas et al, 2001) have evaluated large samples (n=2077 to 24 488) of subjects above the age of 55 years with standardized instruments (e.g. Mini Mental State Examination, Clinical Dementia Rating Scale) and diagnostic criteria (e.g. DSM-IV, NINCDS-ADRDA) using a two/three stage procedure. The rate of dementia was reported to be in the range of 0.8% to 3.4% and that of Alzheimer's disease in the range of 0.6% to 1.5%. Gender (female) and age were associated with higher prevalence rates. The incidence rates per 1000 person-years for Alzheimer's disease was 3.2 for those over 65 years and 1.7 for those over 55 years (Chandra et al, 2001). Mohan et al (2002) assessed 10 312 urban subjects with an instrument based on DSM-III-R criteria at two points of time one year apart. The prevalence of tobacco, alcohol, cannabis and opioids use among males was 27.6%, 12.6%, 0.3% and 0.4%, respectively. The annual incidence rates among males for any drug use and use of alcohol, tobacco, cannabis and opioids were 5.9%, 4.2%, 4.9%, 0.02% and 0.04%, respectively. Among females, incidence of any drug use was 1.2%. Gupta (1996) assessed 99 598 individuals above 35 years of age. Almost 69.3% of men and 57.5% of women reported current use of tobacco (23.6% of men smoked, most women consumed smokeless tobacco). Educational level was inversely associated with tobacco use of all kinds except cigarette smoking. Based on quantity/frequency index analysis, Mohan et al (1984) reported that almost 4.2% of their sample of rural subjects was dependent on alcohol. Kartikeyan et al (1992) assessed 9863 subjects from an urban slum. The prevalence of drug dependence was 1.1% (83.7% heroin, 10.7% cannabis and 5.8% opium). Chandran et al (2002) assessed 359 women in the last trimester of pregnancy and 6-12 weeks after delivery. The incidence of post-partum depression was 11%. Rate of post-partum depression was associated with low income, birth of a daughter, relationship difficulties, adverse life events during pregnancy and lack of practical help. Lester et al (1999) reported that in 1991, the national suicide rate was 9.2 per 100 000 per year (males: 10.6 and females: 7.9). The most common methods for suicide were poisoning and hanging. The only predictor of the regional variation in suicide rates was population density, while the time-series suicide rate was predicted by female participation in labour force and fertility. Mayer and Ziaian (2002) reported that there was an increase in the rate of suicide over six years. The incidence of suicides was highest in the 30-44 year-old category. Suicide rates were nearly equal for young women and men. Vijayakumar and Rajkumar (1999) conducted psychological autopsies on 100 suicide victims and 100 controls and found that the presence of a personal or family history of mental disorder and recent life events were significant risk factors for suicide. Bhatia et al (2000) reviewed records of patients who had suicidal ideations (n=260), had made suicide attempts (n=58) or had completed suicide (n=55). Suicidal phenomena were associated with depression and adjustment disorder, previous suicide attempts (6.9%-18.2% in various subgroups) and a family history of depression. Organophosphorus poisoning and hanging were the commonest methods of attempting suicide. Siwach and Gupta (1995) reported that in a sample of 559 cases of acute poisoning, suicidal attempt was suspected to be the cause in 91.4% of cases. A number of studies (e.g. Shenoy et al, 1998) have evaluated large samples of children and adolescents (n=348 to 1535) with standardized instruments (e.g. Children's Behaviour Questionnaire, Child Behaviour Checklist) using a two stage procedure. The prevalence of psychiatric morbidity was in the range of 14.4% to 31.7%. Higher rates were obtained on parent reports in comparison to teacher reports. Boys manifested more externalizing problems and girls more internalizing problems. Hackett et al (1999) assessed 1403 children and found the prevalence of psychiatric disorders to be 9.4% as per ICD-10. Psychiatric morbidity was associated with gender (male), socioeconomic status (low), parental education (poor), attainment in school (impaired) and life events. Malhotra et al (2002) examined 933 urban school children using the Rutter-B Scale (teachers' assessment) and the Childhood

Psychopathology Measurement Schedule. Psychiatric disorders according to ICD-10 were diagnosed in 6.3% of subjects. Hackett et al (2001) reported that the 1-year prevalence of enuresis and encopresis was 18.6% and 4.3%, respectively. Chopra et al (1999) administered the Disability Screening Schedule (DSS) to 3560 children (0-6 years) from urban slums. Almost 6.9% of children were assessed as having disabilities. Mathur et al (1995) assessed 1545 children through a two stage procedure and found that the rate of mental disability was 2.7%.

MENTAL HEALTH RESOURCES

Mental Health Policy A mental health policy is absent.
The National Health Policy – 2002 incorporates most of the suggestions made in the draft of the National Mental Health Policy, hence the latter was not pursued as a separate document. The National Mental Health Programme (NMHP), launched in 1982, was restrategized during 2002 for implementation during the 10th Five Year Plan (2002-2007) with a quantum increase in fiscal allocation (Rs 190 crore, up from Rs 28 crore during the 9th Plan). It forms the basis for public health initiatives in the field of mental health. The restrategized national mental health programme under implementation aims to provide a balanced mix of closely networked services, with dedicated budgetary support for modernization of the Government mental hospitals, strengthening of medical college departments of psychiatry, implementation of the district mental health programme in 100 districts across the country in the first phase, focussed information, education, communication (IEC) strategies, training and research.

Substance Abuse Policy A substance abuse policy is absent. A national master plan for substance abuse (1994) focused on the establishment of treatments and rehabilitation centres, human resource development, intersectoral collaboration and public education. These programmes are guided by the Ministry of Health and Family Welfare and the Ministry of Social Justice and Empowerment. Many Indian states have now banned smoking in public places and on public transport (e.g. Delhi Prohibition of Smoking and Non-Smokers Health Protection Act – 1996).

National Mental Health Programme A national mental health programme is present. The programme was formulated in 1982. Pilot projects have been undertaken to look at the feasibility of extending mental health services to the community and primary care levels. A review of the national mental health programme by the Central Council in 1995 led to the launch of the District Mental Health Programme (it covers 24 districts currently, with plans for expansion to 100 districts in the near future and to all districts by 2020).

National Therapeutic Drug Policy/Essential List of Drugs A national therapeutic drug policy/essential list of drugs is present. Details about the year of formulation are not available.
A large, mostly indigenous, pharmaceutical industry ensures that most psychotropic drugs are available in India, often at a fraction of their cost in high-income countries.

Mental Health Legislation The Mental Health Act of 1987 simplified admission and discharge procedures, provided for separate facilities for children and drug abusers and promoted human rights of the mentally ill. In 2002, it was implemented in 25 out of 30 states and Union Territories from which information was available. Other acts relevant to the mental health field are: the Juvenile Justice Act, the Persons with Disabilities Act and the Narcotic Drugs and Psychotropic Substances Act (amended in 2001).
The latest legislation was enacted in 1987.

Mental Health Financing There are budget allocations for mental health.
The country spends 2.05% of the total health budget on mental health.
The primary sources of mental health financing in descending order are tax based, out of pocket expenditure by the patient or family, private insurances and social insurance.
Government funding for health services are provided both by the states and the centre. Services provided at Government health centres are free. Certain industrial/governmental organizations provide health care schemes for their employees. In the 10th Five Year Plan estimates, mental health constitutes 2.05% of the total plan outlay for health.
The country has disability benefits for persons with mental disorders. Disability benefits have become available recently and in a limited way.

Mental Health Facilities Mental health is a part of primary health care system. Actual treatment of severe mental disorders is available at the primary level. Mental health care in primary care is available in 22 districts out of about 600 districts. It will be extended to over 100 districts in the next few years.
Regular training of primary care professionals is carried out in the field of mental health. In the last two years, about 600 personnel were provided training. Many workshops for the sensitization/training of programme officers, voluntary agencies, health directorate personnel and mental health professionals, have been undertaken. A range of training materials were developed and field tested. However, training facilities are available in some districts of the country only.

There are community care facilities for patients with mental disorders. Mental health facilities in community care is available in some designated districts. In addition, various non-governmental organizations provide different types of services ranging from telephone hotlines to residential rehabilitative services.

Psychiatric Beds and Professionals

Total psychiatric beds per 10 000 population	0.25
Psychiatric beds in mental hospitals per 10 000 population	0.2
Psychiatric beds in general hospitals per 10 000 population	0.05
Psychiatric beds in other settings per 10 000 population	0.01
Number of psychiatrists per 100 000 population	0.2
Number of neurosurgeons per 100 000 population	0.06
Number of psychiatric nurses per 100 000 population	0.05
Number of neurologists per 100 000 population	0.05
Number of psychologists per 100 000 population	0.03
Number of social workers per 100 000 population	0.03

There are 200 mental health workers of other types. One third of mental health beds are in one state (Maharashtra) and several states have no mental hospitals. Some mental hospitals have more than 1000 beds and several still have a large proportion of long-stay patients. During the past two decades, many mental hospitals have been reformed through the intervention of the voluntary organizations (e.g. Action Aid India), media, National Human Rights Commission and judiciary (courts), and yet a survey in 2002 showed that about a quarter had shortages in terms of drugs/treatment modalities and three quarters in terms of staff. The current emphasis is on general health psychiatry units that support voluntary admissions and encourage family members to stay with the patient. Some beds are allocated to treatment of drug abuse and for child psychiatry. Very few mental health professionals are based in rural areas. Most states allow public sector psychiatrists to have private clinics. Many mental health professionals have emigrated. In 2003 itself, more than 82 psychiatrists sought short-term and long-term employment in the United Kingdom in response to the latter's international recruitment drive. Psychologists do not have prescription privileges, and there is no formal system of licensing clinical psychologists.

Non-Governmental Organizations NGOs are involved with mental health in the country. They are mainly involved in advocacy, promotion, prevention, treatment and rehabilitation. NGOs are involved in counselling, suicide prevention, training of lay counsellors and provision of rehabilitation programmes through day care, sheltered workshops, halfway homes, hostels for recovering patients and long-term care facilities. Parents and other family members of mentally ill persons have recently come together to form self-help groups.

Information Gathering System There is mental health reporting system in the country. Mental health is reported, but in a limited manner only by mental hospitals.
The country has no data collection system or epidemiological study on mental health. A major multi-site study on the epidemiology of mental disorders, using WMH-2000 (Revised/updated), is nearing completion at 11 geographically widely distributed sites, and the data emerging from this project are likely to substantially augment the evidence-base in this regard.

Programmes for Special Population The country has specific programmes for mental health for disaster affected population and elderly. Services for special population are provided in few places.
In the 1980s, the Government with the help of the UNDCP set up 68 drug dependence treatment centres and trained about one thousand psychiatrists and medical officers in the treatment of substance use disorders. Simultaneously, the Ministry of Welfare supported the establishment of 341 counselling and rehabilitation centres in the voluntary sector under its Community Drug Rehabilitation and Workplace Drug Prevention Programmes. No formal school mental health programme exists, but some academic centres and NGOs participate in school health initiatives. Residential facilities are available for mentally challenged and mentally ill children.

Therapeutic Drugs The following therapeutic drugs are generally available at the primary health care level of the country: carbamazepine, phenobarbital, phenytoin sodium, sodium valproate, amitriptyline, chlorpromazine, diazepam, fluphenazine, haloperidol, lithium, carbidopa, levodopa.
None of these drugs are routinely distributed by the Government at the primary health care level except for some designated districts where a special programme is operational.

Other Information The National Human Rights Commission has published its report on Quality Assurance in Mental Health relating to mental hospitals in the country.

The traditional Indian medical systems of Ayurved and Unani recognized mental illness and provided necessary treatment. Recently, a document 'Mental Health: An Indian Perspective (1946-2003)' that summarizes mental health initiatives with relevance to public mental health in India was released by the Ministry for Health and Family Welfare.

Additional Sources of Information

Agarwal, S. P. (2004) Mental Health: An Indian Perspective (1946-2003). New Delhi: Directorate General of Health Services, Ministry of Health and Family Welfare.

Bhatia, M. S., Aggarwal, N. K., Aggarwal, B. B. (2000) Psychosocial profile of suicide ideators, attempters and completers in India. International Journal of Social Psychiatry, 46, 155-163.

Central Council of Health and Family Welfare (1999) Notes from Proceedings & Resolutions of the South Conference on Central Council of Health and Family Welfare.

Chandra, V., Pandav, R., Dodge, H. H., et al (2001) Incidence of Alzheimer's disease in a rural community in India: the Indo-US study. Neurology, 57, 985-989.

Chandran, M., Tharyan, P., Muliyil, J., et al (2002) Post-partum depression in a cohort of women from a rural area of Tamil Nadu, India. Incidence and risk factors. British Journal of Psychiatry, 181, 499-504.

Chisholm, D., Sekar, K., Kumar, K., et al. (2000). Integration of mental health care into primary care: demonstration cost-outcome study in India and Pakistan. British Journal of Psychiatry, 176, 581-588.

Chopra, G., Verma, I. C., Seetharaman, P. (1999) Development and assessment of a screening test for detecting childhood disabilities. Indian Journal of Pediatrics, 66, 331-335.

Drug Dependence Treatment Centre and Ministry of Health and Family Welfare (1997) Summary and Recommendations of the National Workshop on Alcohol Policy.

Ganju, V. (2000) The mental health system in India: history, current system, and prospects. International Journal of Law & Psychiatry, 23, 393-402.

Gupta, P. C. (1996) Survey of sociodemographic characteristics of tobacco use among 99,598 individuals in Bombay, India using handheld computers. Tobacco Control, 5, 114-120.

Hackett, R., Hackett, L., Bhakta, P., et al (1999) The prevalence and associations of psychiatric disorder in children in Kerala, South India. Journal of Child Psychology & Psychiatry & Allied Disciplines, 40, 801-807.

Hackett, R., Hackett, L., Bhakta, P., et al (2001) Enuresis and encopresis in a south Indian population of children. Child: Care, Health & Development, 27, 35-46.

Isaac, M. (2000) Bridging the Gap. Health Action, 6-9.

Issac, M., Thara, R., Nagpal, J., et al. (2004) Mental health and substance abuse control programmes in India: Role of World Health Organization. New Delhi: WHO (SEARO).

Kartikeyan, S. K., Chaturvedi, R. M., Bhalerao, V. R. (1992) Role of the family in drug abuse. Journal of Postgraduate Medicine, 38, 5-7.

Khandelwal, S. K., Jhingan, H. P., Ramesh, S. (2004) India mental health country profile. International Review of Psychiatry, 16, 126-141.

Lester, D., Agarwal, K., Natarajan, M. (1999) Suicide in India. Archives of Suicide Research, 5, 91-96.

Malhotra, S., Kohli, A., Arun, P. (2002) Prevalence of psychiatric disorders in school children in Chandigarh, India. Indian Journal of Medical Research, 116, 21-28.

Mathur, G. P., Mathur, S., Singh, Y. D., et al (1995) Detection and prevention of childhood disability with the help of Anganwadi workers. Indian Pediatrics, 32, 773-777.

Mayer, P., Ziaian, T. (2002) Suicide, gender, and age variations in India. Are women in Indian society protected from suicide? Crisis: Journal of Crisis Intervention & Suicide, 23, 98-103.

Mellor D. (2003) Commentary: Recruitment is ethical. British Medical Journal, 327, 928.

Mohan, D., Chopra, A., Sethi, H. (2002) Incidence estimates of substance use disorders in a cohort from Delhi, India. Indian Journal of Medical Research, 115, 128-135.

Mohan, D., Sundaram, K. R., Advani, G. B., et al (1984) Alcohol abuse in a rural community in India. Part II: characteristics of alcohol users. Drug & Alcohol Dependence, 14, 121-128.

Nandi, D. N., Banerjee, G., Mukherjee, S. P., et al (2000) Psychiatric morbidity of a rural Indian community. Changes over a 20-year interval. British Journal of Psychiatry, 176, 351-356.

National Human Rights Commission (1999) Quality Assurance in Mental Health – Report of the National Human Rights Commission Project, New Dehli, NHRC.

Patel V, Saxena S. (2002) Psychiatry in India. International Psychiatry, 1, 16-18.

Prasadarao, P. S. D. V., Sudhir, P. M. (2001) Clinical psychology in India. Journal of Clinical Psychology in Medical Settings, 8, 31-38.

Ramana R., Saxena, S. (1991) India: quality and access are the priorities. In: L. Appleby, R. Araya (Eds). Mental Health Services in the Global Village, 3-13, London, Gaskell: The Royal College of Psychiatrists.

Rao, A. V. (1993) Psychiatry of old age in India. International Review of Psychiatry, 5, 165-170.

Reddy, M. V., Chandrashekar, C. R. (1998) Prevalence of mental and behavioral disorders in India: a meta-analysis. Indian Journal of Psychiatry, 40, 149-157.

Shenoy, J., Kapur, M., Kaliaperumal, V. G. (1998) Psychological disturbance among 5- to 8-year-old school children: a study from India. Social Psychiatry & Psychiatric Epidemiology, 33, 66-73.

Siwach, S. B., Gupta, A. (1995) The profile of acute poisonings in Harayana-Rohtak Study. Journal of the Association of Physicians of India, 43, 756-759.

The Narcotic Drugs and Psychotropic Substances Act (1985) Universal Law Publishing Co. Pvt. Ltd.

Vas, C. J., Pinto, C., Panikker, D., et al (2001) Prevalence of dementia in an urban Indian population. International Psychogeriatrics, 13, 439-450.

Vijayakumar, L., Rajkumar, S. (1999) Are risk factors for suicide universal? A case-control study in India. Acta Psychiatrica Scandinavica, 99, 407-411.

Weiss, M. G., Issac, M., Parkar, S. R., et al (2001) Global, national and local approaches to mental health: examples from India. Tropical Medicine & International Health, 6, 4-23.

Indonesia

GENERAL INFORMATION

Indonesia is a country with an approximate area of 1905 thousand sq. km. (UNO, 2001). Indonesia is an archipelago with five big islands and 13 669 small islands. Its population is 222.611 million, and the sex ratio (men per hundred women) is 100 (UNO, 2004). The proportion of population under the age of 15 years is 29% (UNO, 2004), and the proportion of population above the age of 60 years is 8% (WHO, 2004). The literacy rate is 92.5% for men and 83.4% for women (UNESCO/MoH, 2004).
The country is a lower middle income group country (based on World Bank 2004 criteria). The proportion of health budget to GDP is 2.4%. The per capita total expenditure on health is 77 international $, and the per capita government expenditure on health is 19 international $ (WHO, 2004).
The main language(s) used in the country is (are) Bahasa Indonesia. The largest ethnic group(s) is (are) Javanese, and the other ethnic group(s) are (is) Sundanese, Batak, Minang, Maduranese and coastal Malays. The largest religious group(s) is (are) Muslim (nine-tenths), and the other religious group(s) are (is) Christian, Hindu and Buddhist.
The life expectancy at birth is 64.9 years for males and 67.9 years for females (WHO, 2004). The healthy life expectancy at birth is 57 years for males and 59 years for females (WHO, 2004).

EPIDEMIOLOGY

E-I

Bahar et al (1992) administered the Bahasa version of the 30-item General Health Questionnaire to a probability sample of 1670 adults. The Present State Examination was conducted on a weighted sub-sample of 100. Overall morbidity rates were similar to those in industrialized countries. A strong association was found between psychological symptoms and poverty. A mental health household survey conducted in 11cities by the Indonesian Psychiatric Epidemiologic Network suggested that the prevalence of mental disorders in adults was 18.5% (Personal Communication, 2004). Another study conducted in 16 cities (n=1600) using proportional sampling and CIDI (Composite International Diagnostic Interview) found that among those with mental disorders, the following diagnoses were common: drug abuse (44.0%), mental retardation (34.9%), mental dysfunction (16.2%) and mental disintegration (5.8%) (Personal Communication, 2004). Suryani et al (1990) noted a relatively high prevalence (about 40%) of excessive alcohol consumption in a less developed village compared to a more developed one. Narendra et al (1990) noted an increase in risk taking behaviours like drug use among adolescents in Indonesia. Smet et al (1999) conducted a study on a random sample of schools (n=149) in Semarang (population 1.5 million) using a stratified sampling procedure (strata based on type of school and district). Within the schools, 186 classes were selected, targeting the 11, 13, 15 and 17 year olds. An anonymous, self-administered questionnaire was filled in by all students present at the day of the survey (n=6276). Among male students, smoking increased dramatically between the ages of 11 and 17, from 8.2% to 38.7%. Best friends' smoking behaviour and attitudes towards smoking and older brothers' smoking behaviour were important determinants of smoking. The variance explained by the regression model increased from 19.8% for 11 year olds to 53% for 17 year olds. Kurihara et al (2000) compared patients with schizophrenia in Bali and Tokyo during a 5-year follow-up study using standardized tools. They found that the clinical outcome was similar in the two sites. Waluyo et al (1996) found a high prevalence of musculoskeletal symptoms in assembly workers from Sweden and Indonesia. Greater stress and psychosomatic symptoms were reported by the Swedish group. Tanner and Chamberland (2001) found that the symptoms of Latah, a syndrome manifesting increased startle response, echolalia and echopraxia were similar to those described 100 years ago. Wignyosumarto et al (1992) examined 5120 children for non-verbal intelligence, social maturity behaviour or adaptive skills and autistic features (with the Bryson's screening scale). Sixty-six children who scored above 16 were assessed with CARS. The prevalence rate of autism within the birth cohort was 0.12%. Bleichrodt et al (1980) administered an extensive test battery to all children and adolescents in two village populations: one village in an area with severe iodine deficiency and a control village in a non-iodine-deficient area. No evidence of significant mental retardation was detected in the non-cretin group in the severely iodine-deficient area.

MENTAL HEALTH RESOURCES

Mental Health Policy A mental health policy is present. The policy was initially formulated in 1999.
The components of the policy are advocacy, promotion, prevention, treatment and rehabilitation. Mental health policy forms a part of the general health policy. A national training workshop focusing on planning and budgeting for service delivery and organization of services (Mental Health Policy Project) was held in 2003. Twelve trainers (senior mental health personnel) and 24 planners were trained.

Substance Abuse Policy A substance abuse policy is present. The policy was initially formulated in 1997. Two laws form the core of the substance abuse policy: Narcotic Law and Psychotropic Law (both were enacted in 1997). The National Narcotic Board that answers to the President coordinates the functioning of governmental and non-governmental activities in this area.

National Mental Health Programme A national mental health programme is present. The programme was formulated in 1995. The new national mental health programme has been developed in the year 2001.

National Therapeutic Drug Policy/Essential List of Drugs A national therapeutic drug policy/essential list of drugs is present. It was formulated in 1998.
Shortages in the supply of the psychotropic drugs to some primary health centres and general hospitals have been noted and are probably due to underreporting of need by district /municipal health officials.

Mental Health Legislation The current mental health legislation is integrated into General Health Law. A specific mental health legislation has now been developed and awaits the approval of the Government.
The latest legislation was enacted in 1992.

Mental Health Financing There are budget allocations for mental health.
The country spends 1% of the total health budget on mental health.
The primary sources of mental health financing in descending order are out of pocket expenditure by the patient or family, tax based, social insurance, private insurances and grants.
The country has disability benefits for persons with mental disorders. Destitute psychotics and mentally retarded are considered as socially disabled, and the Government provides social institutional care in a limited way.

Mental Health Facilities Mental health is a part of primary health care system. Actual treatment of severe mental disorders is available at the primary level. Training programmes for primary care physicians in treating mental disorders are present, and anti-psychotics (chlorpromazine and haloperidol) are available. Severe and disturbed psychotics are referred to mental hospitals, and families tend to bring the patients to traditional healers.
Regular training of primary care professionals is carried out in the field of mental health. In the last two years, about 300 personnel were provided training.
There are no community care facilities for patients with mental disorders. No systematic approach is present as limited facilities are available. However, traditional healers and nurses from Government mental hospitals make occasional visits.

Psychiatric Beds and Professionals

Total psychiatric beds per 10 000 population	0.4
Psychiatric beds in mental hospitals per 10 000 population	0.38
Psychiatric beds in general hospitals per 10 000 population	0.02
Psychiatric beds in other settings per 10 000 population	0.02
Number of psychiatrists per 100 000 population	0.21
Number of neurosurgeons per 100 000 population	0.01
Number of psychiatric nurses per 100 000 population	0.9
Number of neurologists per 100 000 population	0.06
Number of psychologists per 100 000 population	0.3
Number of social workers per 100 000 population	1.5

State mental hospitals are available in 24 out of 32 provinces. Private mental hospitals account for about 8% of all beds. Fifty beds are allocated for a drug abuse treatment centre.

Non-Governmental Organizations NGOs are involved with mental health in the country. They are mainly involved in advocacy, promotion, prevention, treatment and rehabilitation.

Information Gathering System There is mental health reporting system in the country. Mental health reporting is a part of hospital reporting system and primary health centre reporting system.
The country has no data collection system or epidemiological study on mental health. In the past epidemiological data had been collected with the support of the USA, but since 1996 it has not been done due to budget constraints.
The data for mental health planning comes from the National Health Household Survey – Section on Mental Health, which is done every five years. The last survey was in 1995.

Programmes for Special Population The country has specific programmes for mental health for refugees, disaster affected population, elderly and children.
Specific services are also available for drug abusers, HIV/AIDS patients, prisoners and workers.

Therapeutic Drugs The following therapeutic drugs are generally available at the primary health care level of the country: carbamazepine, phenobarbital, phenytoin sodium, amitriptyline, chlorpromazine, diazepam, haloperidol.
The most common anti-parkinsonian drug is trihexiphenidyl. The essential drug list is updated every year.

Other Information

Additional Sources of Information

Bahar, E., Henderson, A. S., Mackinnon, A. J. (1992) An epidemiological study of mental health and socioeconomic conditions in Sumatera, Indonesia. Acta Psychiatrica Scandinavica, 85, 257-263.

Bleichrodt, N., Drenth, P. J., Querido, A. (1980) Effects of iodine deficiency on mental and psychomotor abilities. American Journal of Physical Anthropology, 53, 55-67.

Kurihara, T., Kato, M., Reverger, R., et al (2000) Outcome of schizophrenia in a non-industrialized society: comparative study between Bali and Tokyo. Acta Psychiatrica Scandinavica, 101, 148-152.

Narendra, M., Basuki, P. S., Soeharjono, L. B., et al (1990) Risk taking behavior of adolescents in Indonesia (country report). Paediatrica Indonesiana, 30, 319-324.

Smet, B., Maes, L., De Clercq, L., et al (1999) Determinants of smoking behaviour among adolescents in Semarang, Indonesia. Tobacco Control, 8, 186-191.

Suryani, L. K., Adnyana, T. A., Jensen, G. D. (1990) Palm wine drinking in a Balinese village: environmental influences. International Journal of the Addictions, 25, 911-920.

Tanner, C. M., Chamberland, J. (2001) Latah in Jakarta, Indonesia. Movement Disorders, 16, 526-529.

Waluyo, L., Ekberg, K., Eklund, J. (1996) Assembly work in Indonesia and in Sweden--ergonomics, health and satisfaction. Ergonomics, 39, 199-212.

Wignyosumarto, S., Mukhlas, M., Shirataki, S. (1992) Epidemiological and clinical study of autistic children in Yogyakarta, Indonesia. Kobe Journal of Medical Sciences, 38, 1-19.

Iran, Islamic Republic of

GENERAL INFORMATION

Iran, Islamic Republic of is a country with an approximate area of 1648 thousand sq. km. (UNO, 2001). Its population is 69.789 million, and the sex ratio (men per hundred women) is 103 (UNO, 2004). The proportion of population under the age of 15 years is 31% (UNO, 2004), and the proportion of population above the age of 60 years is 6% (WHO, 2004). The literacy rate is 83.5% for men and 70.4% for women (UNESCO/MoH, 2004).

The country is a lower middle income group country (based on World Bank 2004 criteria). The proportion of health budget to GDP is 6.3%. The per capita total expenditure on health is 422 international $, and the per capita government expenditure on health is 183 international $ (WHO, 2004).

The main language(s) used in the country is (are) Persian, Azari, Gilaki, Kurdish, Mazandarani, Baluchi, Arabic, Turkmani, Armenian and Ashuri. The largest ethnic group(s) is (are) Persian (half), and the other ethnic group(s) are (is) Azerbaijani, Gilaki, Kurd and Mazandarani. The largest religious group(s) is (are) Muslim (Shia), and the other religious group(s) are (is) Muslim (Sunni).

The life expectancy at birth is 66.5 years for males and 71.7 years for females (WHO, 2004). The healthy life expectancy at birth is 56 years for males and 59 years for females (WHO, 2004).

EPIDEMIOLOGY

According to the most recent epidemiologic survey (Noorbala et al, 2004) that used the General Health Questionnaire (GHQ-28) (n=35 014), 21% of the population (25.9% of the women and 14.9% of the men) were detected as likely to be suffering from mental illness. Interview of families by general practitioners revealed that the rates of mental retardation, epilepsy and psychosis were 1.4%, 1.2% and 0.6%respectively. Bash and colleagues (Bash & Bash-Liecht, 1978; Bash 1984) reported on psychiatric-epidemiological surveys (based partly on census studies, partly on random samples) that sampled rural, urban, tribal subjects above 6 years. The surveys employed questionnaires and tests in the screening phase and individual psychiatric examinations of all possible cases in the confirmation phase. Prevalence in various settings for any psychiatric disorder was: rural (14.9%), urban (16.6%), tribal (2.1%); for all psychoreactive cases (included in the foregoing): rural (8.7%), urban (9.8%), tribal (1.2%); for all psychosomatic cases (included in the psychoreactive): rural (1.7%), urban (2.3%), tribal (0.9%). Significant sex differences were found only in the poor strata. Alemi (1978) found the prevalence of opium use disorders in a survey of randomly chosen households from a rural community to be 6.9% in comparison to the rate of 1.1% estimated for the population based on registry of patients. Merchant et al (1976) found that 24% of the university students (n=607) reported life time use of drugs with 11% reporting use more than three times in their lives. The majority of drug users had used marijuana (54%). Use of drugs was significantly associated with sex, age, number of years of university attended, and father's education. In another study on university students (n=501), Ahmadi and Yazdanfur (2002) reported that the prevalence of regular current use of various substances was: cigarettes (36.1%), alcohol (21.4%), opium (7.6%) and cannabis (3.0%). Substance use was significantly higher among males. Ahmadi and Javadpour (2001) found that among randomly selected health care students (n=346), 34.7% used substances at some point in time. Almost 6.9% of the students were current regular users of substances (cigarettes: 5.5%, alcohol: 1.7%, opium: 1.4%, cannabis: 1.2%, heroin: 0.3% and LSD: 0.3%). Use of substances was significantly related to gender (11.3% of males and 1.4% of females were current regular users). Agahi and Spencer (1982) found that among 712 students aged 14-18 years, 11% had used some drugs of which opium was the commonest, followed by marijuana and heroin. Thornicroft and Sartorius (1993) reported the ten-year follow-up data of the WHO Collaborative Study on Depression (n=439). Almost 18% had very poor clinical outcome, 24% had severe social impairment for more than half of the follow-up period and 21% had no full remissions. The best clinical course (one or two reasonably short episodes of depression with complete remission between episodes) was more common in endogenous depression (65%) in comparison to psychogenic depression (29%). A fifth (22%) had at least one episode lasting for more than 1 year, and 10% had an episode lasting over 2 years during follow-up. Death by suicide occurred in 11% of patients, with a further 14% making unsuccessful suicide attempts. Shokrollahi et al (1999) administered a sexual function questionnaire to 300 healthy married women (16-53 years old) attending a family planning centre. Approximately 38% of the women had at least one sexual dysfunction; the common ones were inhibited desire (15%), inhibited orgasm (26%), lack of lubrication (15%), vaginismus (8%) and dyspareunia (10%). There were significant correlations between sexual dysfunction in women and their knowledge (low) and attitude (conservative) towards sexuality and their husbands' sexual dysfunction. Nobakht and Dezhkam (2000) conducted a two-stage study to assess eating disorders in 3100 schoolgirls in the age group of 15-18 years using the Persian translation of the Eating Attitudes Test (EAT-26), the Eating Disorder Diagnostic Inventory and a supplementary clinical interview. The lifetime prevalence of anorexia nervosa, bulimia nervosa and partial syndrome was 0.9%, 3.2% and 6.6%, respectively. Zarghami and Khalilian (2002) conducted interviews and/or psychological autopsies on 318 cases of self-burning. Self-immolation was associated with young age (average: 27 years), female gender (83%), housewife status, high school education, psychiatric (95%, mostly adjustment disorder) and chronic physical illnesses (30%) and high mortality (79%).

MENTAL HEALTH RESOURCES

Mental Health Policy A mental health policy is present. The policy was initially formulated in 1986.

The components of the policy are advocacy, promotion, prevention, treatment and rehabilitation. Community education is a component of the policy.

Substance Abuse Policy A substance abuse policy is present. The policy was initially formulated in 1987. Alcohol is prohibited by both religion and legislation.

National Mental Health Programme A national mental health programme is present. The programme was formulated in 1986.
The national mental health programme was evaluated in 1995 and 1997 and changes were made based on suggestions. In 1995, it was evaluated jointly by the WHO and the Teheran Psychiatric Institute. Recently, different sub-programmes on service delivery in urban areas, prevention and promotion have been added to the main body in accordance with the population shift and change of priorities. Other related programmes are Integration of Substance Abuse Prevention within the Primary Health Care and a Harm Reduction Programme.

National Therapeutic Drug Policy/Essential List of Drugs A national therapeutic drug policy/essential list of drugs is present. It was formulated in 1988.
The essential drugs list was last updated in 2001.

Mental Health Legislation Though there are different laws regarding the mentally ill, there is no modern mental health legislation. Since last year, a team has been working on a draft for a new legislation. A mandate by the Minister of Health has been issued in 1997 to allocate 10% of all general hospitals to psychiatry beds. The Mental Health Department has recently started a nation-wide advocacy campaign to implement this mandate.
Details about the year of enactment of the mental health legislation are not available.

Mental Health Financing There are budget allocations for mental health.
The country spends 3% of the total health budget on mental health.
The primary sources of mental health financing in descending order are tax based, out of pocket expenditure by the patient or family, social insurance and private insurances.
The national health service in Iran is funded by the Government and health insurance. If covered by health insurance, patients pay 25% of the fee for outpatient and 10% of the fee for inpatient treatment (consultation, laboratory investigations or medicines). Fees do not vary across age ranges. All emergencies are treated immediately without prior payment. The private sector can accept patients without insurance but it provides a limited range of services and the fees are high. Psychologists cannot send bills to insurance companies directly.
The country has disability benefits for persons with mental disorders. Since 2001, the disabled mentally ill patients are entitled to a stipend of about $30 per month if they do not receive other free services. Already, about 10 000 disabled patients are receiving disability benefits and the number is increasing. Institutional care is free of charge for the disabled mentally ill.

Mental Health Facilities Mental health is a part of primary health care system. Actual treatment of severe mental disorders is available at the primary level. Mental health delivery for severe illnesses is one of the objectives in rural and deprived areas.
Regular training of primary care professionals is carried out in the field of mental health. In the last two years, about 20185 personnel were provided training. Mental health services at the primary care level are available to more than one-fifth of urban and more than four-fifths of the rural population. Behvarz (multipurpose health workers), who are selected from the target community have a pivotal role in the country's primary health care network. Their training lasts two years and equips them for active case finding, appropriate referral to the GP and active follow-up of the patients. Psychologists are playing a vital role at the level of primary health care and supervision of health houses. Postgraduate training facilities for medical and nursing graduates are available. Training facilities for general physicians and mental health workers (or Behvarz) is also present. Manuals for the training of medical doctors and Behvarz are available. A difficulty noted in the provision of primary mental health care was the rapid turnover of doctors at this level (average stay of 3-6 months), which often led to many of the posted doctors not having specific mental health training. To keep up with the urban shift in population, neighbourhood health volunteers are being trained for preventive and promotive activities and appropriate referral.
There are community care facilities for patients with mental disorders. Mental health is integrated into the primary care system whose basis is community care. Community participation is sought through involvement of NGOs and religious establishments in mental health care and public education (e.g. during mental health week).

Psychiatric Beds and Professionals

Total psychiatric beds per 10 000 population	1.6
Psychiatric beds in mental hospitals per 10 000 population	1.4
Psychiatric beds in general hospitals per 10 000 population	0.2
Psychiatric beds in other settings per 10 000 population	0.04
Number of psychiatrists per 100 000 population	1.9
Number of neurosurgeons per 100 000 population	0.4
Number of psychiatric nurses per 100 000 population	0.5
Number of neurologists per 100 000 population	0.6
Number of psychologists per 100 000 population	2
Number of social workers per 100 000 population	0.6

Among the other 325 professionals are occupational therapists and medical assistants. Facilities for treatment of drug abusers (300 beds) and re-orientation centres for drug abusers with criminal and social problems are available. At least 100 beds are available for children with behavioural disorders. Board certification in child psychiatry with a two-year additional training period is available. There is no requirement for licensure or certification of clinical psychologists and they do not have prescription privileges. There are numerous psychologists working outside the mental health sector. Guidelines have been developed and refresher/training workshops have been held for physicians, nurses and social workers on demand-reduction issues.

Non-Governmental Organizations NGOs are involved with mental health in the country. They are mainly involved in advocacy and promotion. In 2004, many joint activities between the Department of Mental Health and NGOs were started on prevention, promotion and homecare for mentally ill patients.

Information Gathering System There is mental health reporting system in the country. There is a simple information system for mental disorders like psychosis, depression, epilepsy, mental retardation, etc.
The country has no data collection system or epidemiological study on mental health. The Department of Mental Health in the MOH has recently started collecting national data on mental health with collaboration of the National Health Research Center. A national epidemiological study on mental health was done in 1999 (Noorbala, 2004) as an adjunct to the periodic National Health Survey.

Programmes for Special Population The country has specific programmes for mental health for disaster affected population and children. Though the mental health programme caters to all populations, since 2003, children and adolescents have been receiving more attention.
There are special facilities for child and adolescent psychiatry in the form of special departments, training facilities, school mental health programmes. Special projects on school mental health and on prevention of child abuse and violence against women (in collaboration with UNICEF and WHO) are under way. Life skills training has gained impetus and cascade training of main focal points in all provinces was accomplished in 2003. Four foundations provide special services ranging from consultation to rehabilitation to populations affected by war. Under the national programme on mental health interventions in natural disasters, more than 70 000 survivors received planned interventions during the 8 months after Bam earthquake and over 400 psychiatrists/psychologists and 1500 teachers were trained. Pilot projects on suicide prevention, under way in 4 cities have shown promising results. Integration of substance abuse prevention within primary health care and harm reduction activities including methadone maintenance and outreach activities for street drug users has been launched with collaboration of MOH and NGOs.

Therapeutic Drugs The following therapeutic drugs are generally available at the primary health care level of the country: carbamazepine, phenobarbital, phenytoin sodium, sodium valproate, chlorpromazine, diazepam, fluphenazine, haloperidol, lithium, biperiden.
In 2003, the list was amended to include 32 medications, e.g. nortryptiline, fluoxetine, trihexiphenedyl, risperidone, etc.

Other Information

Additional Sources of Information

Agahi, C., Spencer, C. (1982) Patterns of drug use among secondary school children in post-revolutionary Iran. Drug & Alcohol Dependence, 9, 235-242.

Ahmadi, J., Benrazavi, L. (2002) Substance use among Iranian nephrologic patients. American Journal of Nephrology, 22, 11-13.

Ahmadi, J., Javadpour, A. (2001) Assessing substance use among Iranian healthcare students. Journal of Substance Use, 6, 196-198.

Ahmadi, J., Yazdanfar, F. (2002) Current substance abuse among Iranian university students. Addictive Disorders & Their Treatment, 1, 61-64.

Alemi, A. A. (1978) The iceberg of opium addiction. An epidemiological survey of opium addiction in a rural community. Drug & Alcohol Dependence, 3, 107-112.

Bash, K. W. (1984) Epidemiology of psychosomatic disorders in Iran. Psychotherapy & Psychosomatics, 42, 182-186.

Bash, K. W., Bash-Liechti, J. (1978) Psychiatric resurvey of a central Iranian village thirteen years later. Nervenarzt, 49, 713-719.

Ghobari, B., Bolhari, J. (2001) The current state of medical psychology in Iran. Journal of Clinical Psychology in Medical Settings, 8, 39-43.

Hashemi, N., London, M. (2003) Psyciatric practice in Iran and the UK. Psychiatric Bulletin, 27, 190-191.

Merchant, N. M., Pournadeali, E., Zimmer, S. P., et al (1976) Factors related to drug abuse among Iranian university students. Pahlavi Medical Journal, 7, 516-528.

Nobakht, M., Dezhkam, M. (2000) An epidemiological study of eating disorders in Iran. International Journal of Eating Disorders, 28, 265-271.

Noorbala, A. A., Bagheri Yazdi, S. A., Yasamy, M. T.,et al (2004) Mental health survey of the adult population in Iran. British Journal of Psychiatry, 184, 70-73.

Shadpour K. (2000) Primary health care networks in the Islamic Republic of Iran. Eastern Mediterranean Health Journal, 6, 822-825.

Shokrollahi, P., Mirmohamadi, M., Mehrabi, F., et al (1999) Prevalence of sexual dysfunction in women seeking services at family planning centers in Tehran. Journal of Sex & Marital Therapy, 25, 211-215.

Thornicroft, G., Sartorius, N. (1993) The course and outcome of depression in different cultures: 10-year follow-up of the WHO Collaborative Study on the Assessment of Depressive Disorders. Psychological Medicine, 23, 1023-1032.

Yasamy, M. T., Shahmohammadi, D., Bagheri Yazdi, S. A., et al. (2001). Mental health in the Islamic Republic of Iran: achievements and the areas of need. Eastern Mediterranian Health Journal, 7, 381-391.

Zarghami, M., Khalilian, A. (2002) Deliberate self-burning in Mazandaran, Iran. Burns, 28, 115-119.

Iraq

GENERAL INFORMATION

Iraq is a country with an approximate area of 438 thousand sq. km. (UNO, 2001). Its population is 25.856 million, and the sex ratio (men per hundred women) is 103 (UNO, 2004). The proportion of population under the age of 15 years is 41% (UNO, 2004), and the proportion of population above the age of 60 years is 5% (WHO, 2004). The literacy rate is 54.9% for men and 23.3% for women (UNESCO/MoH, 2004).

The country is a lower middle income group country (based on World Bank 2004 criteria). The proportion of health budget to GDP is 3.2%. The per capita total expenditure on health is 97 international $, and the per capita government expenditure on health is 31 international $ (WHO, 2004).

The main language(s) used in the country is (are) Arabic and Kurdish. The largest ethnic group(s) is (are) Arab (four-fifths), and the other ethnic group(s) are (is) Kurdish. The largest religious group(s) is (are) Muslim.

The life expectancy at birth is 59.1 years for males and 63.1 years for females (WHO, 2004). The healthy life expectancy at birth is 49 years for males and 52 years for females (WHO, 2004).

EPIDEMIOLOGY

Ahmad et al (1998, 2000a) developed the Posttraumatic Stress Symptoms in Children (PTSS-C) and applied it to a group of children affected by a mass-escape tragedy in Kurdistan; they found the prevalence rate of PTSD to be 20% according to DSM-III-R criteria. PTSD symptoms reduced at 4 month follow-up but were again high at 14 and 26 month follow-up. Dyregrov et al (2002) interviewed a group of 94 children, who had been exposed to a bombing that killed more than 750 people, at 6 months, 1 year and 2 years intervals with the help of selected items from different inventories, including the Impact of Event Scale (IES). The children continued to experience sadness and remained afraid of losing their family. Although there was no significant decline in intrusive and avoidance reactions as measured by the IES from 6 months to 1 year following the war, reactions were reduced 2 years after the war. However, the scores were still high, indicating that symptoms persist, with somewhat diminished intensity over time. Ahmed et al (2000b) interviewed randomly selected 45 pairs of children and their caregivers (mostly mothers) in two displacement camps in Kurdistan with the help of PTSS-C and the Harvard Trauma Questionnaire (HTQ). PTSD was reported in 87% of children and 60% of their caregivers. Childhood PTSD was significantly predicted by child trauma score and the duration of captivity, but was unaffected by maternal PTSD. It did not disappear after the reunion with the PTSD-free father. In a 1-year follow up study, Ahmad and Mohamad (1996) found that children in orphanages showed greater behavioural symptoms and PTSD compared to children in foster care. Yasseen and Al-Musawi (2001) and Hamamy et al (1990) performed karyotypic analyses on children suffering from severe mental retardation and Down's syndrome. The former study showed that while two-thirds of patients had chromosomal abnormalities, only 10% had recognizable syndromes. In the latter study, 81.9% of children with Down's syndrome were shown to have trisomy 21 and 18.1% to have 46/47 + G type of mosaic. Examination for parental consanguinity revealed that 77.9%, 16.2% and 5.9% of the trisomy 21 cases and 53.3%, 26.7% and 20.0% of the mosaic cases were from non-consanguineous, first-cousin and second-cousin marriages, respectively. Amin-Zaki et al (1978, 1979) studied 32 infants exposed to methylmercury exposure over a 5 year period. In nine cases of cerebral palsy, methylmercury exposure occurred only during the last trimester or post-natally via suckling. Whereas the mother's symptoms usually improved, the damage to the fetal nervous system appears to be permanent. Milder cases (minimal brain damage syndrome) previously not identified in other studies were also reported. The syndrome consists of varying degrees of developmental retardation in addition to exaggerated tendon reflexes and the pathologic extensor plantar reflex.

MENTAL HEALTH RESOURCES

Mental Health Policy A mental health policy is present. The policy was initially formulated in 1981.
The components of the policy are advocacy, promotion, prevention, treatment and rehabilitation.

Substance Abuse Policy A substance abuse policy is present. The policy was initially formulated in 1965.

National Mental Health Programme A national mental health programme is present. The programme was formulated in 1987. The national mental health programme was started in 1989 and is concerned primarily with the integration of mental health with primary care leading to improvement of the mental health status of the country. Promotion of proper research facilities and information gathering systems are also a part of the programme. Coordination of mental health is done by the Iraqi Committee for Mental Health Promotion, an advisory body to the Minister of Health. In 2004, an advisory body called the National Council for Mental Health has been established in the MOH, which is working to formulate/implement a mental health policy, a mental health legislation, a substance abuse policy and a national mental health programme.

National Therapeutic Drug Policy/Essential List of Drugs A national therapeutic drug policy/essential list of drugs is present. It was formulated in 1986.

Mental Health Legislation There is a Public Health Act (No. 89/1981). This includes mental health issues. A draft of the mental health legislation has recently been submitted to the Government for approval.
The latest legislation was enacted in 1981.

Mental Health Financing There are budget allocations for mental health.
Details about expenditure on mental health are not available.
The primary sources of mental health financing in descending order are tax based and out of pocket expenditure by the patient or family.
The country has disability benefits for persons with mental disorders. The services provided by the Government are free, though payment has to be made for private services.

Mental Health Facilities Mental health is a part of primary health care system. Actual treatment of severe mental disorders is available at the primary level. Drugs are supplied to needy patients at the primary care level after confirmation of the diagnosis by specialists.
Regular training of primary care professionals is carried out in the field of mental health. Postgraduation in psychology and training for paramedical staff is also present. Training is also provided to teachers, social workers employed in special schools, primary care physicians and nurses. General practitioners in the primary health centres are being trained in psychiatry in order to deliver better psychiatric services at the primary level. Short training courses for orientation are provided.
There are community care facilities for patients with mental disorders. Care is provided through the facilities of the Ministry of Social Welfare.

Psychiatric Beds and Professionals

Total psychiatric beds per 10 000 population	0.63
Psychiatric beds in mental hospitals per 10 000 population	0.55
Psychiatric beds in general hospitals per 10 000 population	0.06
Psychiatric beds in other settings per 10 000 population	0.02
Number of psychiatrists per 100 000 population	0.7
Number of neurosurgeons per 100 000 population	0.09
Number of psychiatric nurses per 100 000 population	0.1
Number of neurologists per 100 000 population	0.04
Number of psychologists per 100 000 population	0.05
Number of social workers per 100 000 population	0.2

There are approximately 300 beds for forensic psychiatry and 15 beds for treatment of drug dependence. Approximately half of mental health professionals are based in Baghdad. Most psychiatrists have private clinics.

Non-Governmental Organizations NGOs are involved with mental health in the country. They are mainly involved in advocacy, prevention, treatment and rehabilitation. Training facilities are also provided by NGOs. The Iraqi Society of Psychiatrists, which is an NGO, is actively involved in the promotion of mental health. The Iraqi Mental Health foundation UK focuses on training and academic liaison in the post-war situation. The Red Cross helped in the rehabilitation of Al-Rashad Mental Hospital in Baghdad, which had been seriously damaged by mobs during the War.

Information Gathering System There is mental health reporting system in the country.
The country has data collection system or epidemiological study on mental health.
There is a lack of proper information gathering system and monitoring of existing mental health services is not possible due to lack of operational data and other information.

Programmes for Special Population The country has specific programmes for mental health for refugees, disaster affected population, elderly and children. Special services are limited in scope.
There are 12 schools for the mentally challenged. In addition, some homes for the elderly and institutes for homeless children and orphans are available.

Therapeutic Drugs The following therapeutic drugs are generally available at the primary health care level of the country: carbamazepine, phenobarbital, phenytoin sodium, sodium valproate, amitriptyline, chlorpromazine, diazepam, fluphenazine, haloperidol, levodopa.
The drug supply is erratic and new generation drugs are lacking.

Other Information One of the earliest psychiatric centres was set up in Baghdad, but since 1990, mental health facilities have suffered due to the war and embargo.

Additional Sources of Information

Ahmad, A., Mohamad, K. (1996) The socioemotional development of orphans in orphanages and traditional foster care in Iraqi Kurdistan. Child Abuse & Neglect, 20, 1161-1173.

Ahmad, A., Mohamed, H. T., Ameen, N. M. (1998) A 26-month follow-up of posttraumatic stress symptoms in children after the mass-escape tragedy in Iraqi Kurdistan. Nordic Journal of Psychiatry, 52, 357-366.

Ahmad, A., Sundelin-Wahlsten, V., Sofi, M. A., et al (2000a) Reliability and validity of a child-specific cross-cultural instrument for assessing posttraumatic stress disorder. European Child & Adolescent Psychiatry, 9, 285-294.

Ahmad, A., Sofi, M. A., Sundelin-Wahlsten, V., et al (2000b) Posttraumatic stress disorder in children after the military operation 'Anfal' in Iraqi Kurdistan. European Child & Adolescent Psychiatry, 9, 235-243.

Amin-Zaki, L., Majeed, M. A., Clarkson, T. W., et al (1978) Methylmercury poisoning in Iraqi children: clinical observations over two years. British Medical Journal, 1, 613-616.

Amin-Zaki, L., Majeed, M. A., Elhassani, S. B., et al (1979) Prenatal methylmercury poisoning. Clinical observations over five years. American Journal of Diseases of Children, 133, 172-177.

Dyer, O. (2003) British Iraqi doctors set up charity to support Iraq's mental health services. British Medical Journal, 327, 832-833.

Dyregrov, A., Gjestad, R., Raundalen, M. (2002) Children exposed to warfare: a longitudinal study. Journal of Traumatic Stress, 15, 59-68.

Hamamy, H. A., al Hakkak, Z. S., al Taha, S. (1990) Consanguinity and the genetic control of Down syndrome. Clinical Genetics, 37, 24-29.

Yasseen, A. A., Al-Musawi, T. A. (2001) Cytogenetics study in severely mentally retarded patients. Saudi Medical Journal, 22, 444-449.

Ireland

GENERAL INFORMATION

Ireland is a country with an approximate area of 70 thousand sq. km. (UNO, 2001). Its population is 3.999 million, and the sex ratio (men per hundred women) is 99 (UNO, 2004). The proportion of population under the age of 15 years is 21% (UNO, 2004), and the proportion of population above the age of 60 years is 15% (WHO, 2004). The literacy rate is 99% for men and 99% for women (UNESCO/MoH, 2004).

The country is a high income group country (based on World Bank 2004 criteria). The proportion of health budget to GDP is 6.5%. The per capita total expenditure on health is 1935 international $, and the per capita government expenditure on health is 1470 international $ (WHO, 2004).

The main language(s) used in the country is (are) English and Irish. The largest religious group(s) is (are) Roman Catholic.

The life expectancy at birth is 74.4 years for males and 79.8 years for females (WHO, 2004). The healthy life expectancy at birth is 68 years for males and 72 years for females (WHO, 2004).

EPIDEMIOLOGY

There is substantial epidemiological data on mental illnesses in Ireland in internationally accessible literature. No attempt was made to include this information here.

MENTAL HEALTH RESOURCES

Mental Health Policy A mental health policy is present. The policy was initially formulated in 1984.

The components of the policy are advocacy, promotion, prevention, treatment and rehabilitation. An Expert Group on Mental Health Policy to prepare a national policy framework for the further modernization of the mental health services, updating the 1984 policy document, Planning for the Future, was established on 4th August 2003. The Group has completed an extensive consultation process which included consultation initiatives with various stakeholders, including users of the mental health services. The Group is expected to complete its work in 2005.

Substance Abuse Policy A substance abuse policy is present. The policy was initially formulated in 1983. A National Drugs Strategy was published in 2001 and runs to 2008. This Strategy covers the four pillars of prevention and education, supply reduction, treatment and rehabilitation and research.

National Mental Health Programme A national mental health programme is absent.

Further to the publication of the Report of the National Task Force on Suicide in 1998, work has commenced on a new Strategic Action Plan for Suicide Reduction which is expected to be completed by June 2005. All measures aimed at reducing the number of deaths by suicide will be considered in the context of the preparation of this action plan.

National Therapeutic Drug Policy/Essential List of Drugs A national therapeutic drug policy/essential list of drugs is present. Details about the year of formulation are not available.

Mental Health Legislation The Mental Health Act, which was enacted in July 2001, will significantly improve safeguards for mentally disordered persons who are involuntarily admitted for psychiatric care and treatment. The Act will bring Irish law in this area into conformity with the European Convention for the Protection of Human Rights and Fundamental Freedoms. The Act provided for the establishment of an independent agency known as the Mental Health Commission whose primary function is to promote and foster high standards and good practices in the delivery of mental health services and to ensure that the interests of detained persons are protected.

The latest legislation was enacted in 2001.

Mental Health Financing There are budget allocations for mental health.

The country spends 6.8% of the total health budget on mental health.

The primary sources of mental health financing in descending order are tax based, private insurances, social insurance and out of pocket expenditure by the patient or family.

About one-third of the population invests in voluntary health insurance, although all are entitled to public services.

The country has disability benefits for persons with mental disorders.

Mental Health Facilities Mental health is a part of primary health care system. Actual treatment of severe mental disorders is available at the primary level. Primary care is provided by general physicians, community care and primary care nurses and family doctors.

Regular training of primary care professionals is carried out in the field of mental health.

There are community care facilities for patients with mental disorders. There are community care facilities for the patients with mental disorders. There are community psychiatry nursing services, community residences, day hospitals and day care centres, voluntary associations and other rehabilitation facilities.

Psychiatric Beds and Professionals

Total psychiatric beds per 10 000 population	9.43
Psychiatric beds in mental hospitals per 10 000 population	7.45
Psychiatric beds in general hospitals per 10 000 population	1.86
Psychiatric beds in other settings per 10 000 population	1.28
Number of psychiatrists per 100 000 population	6.82
Number of neurosurgeons per 100 000 population	0.23
Number of psychiatric nurses per 100 000 population	136
Number of neurologists per 100 000 population	0.46
Number of psychologists per 100 000 population	12.71
Number of social workers per 100 000 population	47.7

Within each health authority/board, mental health services are organized in catchment areas, of which there are 33 in total. Thus, each health authority/board has from 2 to 11 catchment areas, whose populations range from 50 000 to over 270 000. Catchment areas are in turn divided into sectors. Sectors have a population of 13 000 to 80 000. Each sector has a mental health team, led by a consultant psychiatrist. Psychiatric beds are available for every catchment area in either psychiatric hospitals or in acute admission units attached to general hospitals. Catchments are generally self-contained with respect to community-based services such as day hospitals, day centres, rehabilitation workshops and community residences. Outpatient care is delivered from mental health centres.

Non-Governmental Organizations NGOs are involved with mental health in the country. They are mainly involved in advocacy, promotion, prevention and rehabilitation. The increase in community-based care requires cooperation and good communication between the many different agencies involved in providing medical care, training and rehabilitation, day care and accommodation. Much of the success and effectiveness of the policy of successive Governments to deliver mental health services in a more acceptable manner to communities has been and will continue to be dependent on the active involvement of voluntary organizations such as Schizophrenia Ireland, which offers support to both people with schizophrenia and their carers and relatives. Funding has been made available to support groups and organizations such as Schizophrenia Ireland, Mental Health Ireland, GROW, AWARE and the Irish Advocacy Network to heighten awareness and develop services which include carers' support groups. This partnership approach has also extended to the provision of extensive rehabilitation programmes including Back to Work programmes for people suffering from mental illness. It is intended to continue to develop this co-operation and to provide a comprehensive range of services to both patients and their families.

Information Gathering System There is mental health reporting system in the country. Details can be obtained from 'Irish Psychiatric Services Activities' which is published annually by the Health Research Board.
The country has data collection system or epidemiological study on mental health.

Programmes for Special Population The country has specific programmes for mental health for elderly and children. Special services are also available for homeless and forensic populations.
Child and adolescent psychiatry operates from Child and Family Centres as a separate service from adult psychiatry; it seldom uses beds and is, in the main, not hospital-based. In recent years, significant resources have been made available for this purpose. Each health board now has a minimum of two child and adolescent consultant-led multi-disciplinary teams in place. A number of in-patient facilities for children and adolescents are planned. Attention has been given in recent years to the development of specialist hospital and community services for the care of the elderly mentally ill and infirm. All health board regions now have such a service in their area. In recent years, there has been considerable reinforcement of various sub-specialities, with the appointment since 1998 of a total of 72 additional consultant psychiatrists in Later-Life Psychiatry, Child and Adolescent Psychiatry, Forensic Psychiatry, Rehabilitation Psychiatry and Liaison psychiatry in general hospitals.

Therapeutic Drugs The following therapeutic drugs are generally available at the primary health care level of the country: carbamazepine, ethosuximide, phenobarbital, phenytoin sodium, sodium valproate, amitriptyline, chlorpromazine, diazepam, fluphenazine, haloperidol, lithium, biperiden, carbidopa, levodopa.

Other Information The Mental Health Act 2001 is designed to be implemented on a phased basis. The Commission has indicated that one of its priorities is to put in place the structures required for the operation of the Mental Health Tribunals. The Mental Health Tribunals, operating under the aegis of the Mental Health Commission, will conduct a review of each decision on involuntary detention within 21 days of the detention/extension order being signed. The Commission will also operate a scheme to provide legal aid to patients whose detention is being reviewed by a tribunal. Under the provisions of the Mental Health Act, 2001 the Commission has appointed an Inspector of Mental Health Services. The Minister will be empowered to make regulations specifying the standards to be maintained in all approved centres, and these will be enforced by the inspector.

Additional Sources of Information

Daly A., Walsh D. (2001) Irish Psychiatric Hospitals and Units Census. The Health Research Board.

Daly A., Walsh, D. (2002) Activities of Irish Psychiatric Services. The Health Research Board.

Ministry of Health. (2001) Mental Health Act.

Department of Health and Children (1998) Report of the National Task Force on Suicide

Department of Health and Children (2001) A National Drugs Strategy.

Department of Health and Children (2001) First Report of the Working Group on Child and Adolescent Psychiatric Services; Second Report (2003).

Department of Health and Children (2001) Health Strategy Quality and Fairness – A Health System for You.

Department of Health and Children (2004). Report of the Inspector of Mental Hospitals for the year ending 31st December, 2003.

McClelland, R., Webb, M., Mock, G. (2000) Mental health services in Ireland. International Journal of Law and Psychiatry, 23, 309-328.

Mental Health Commission, Annual Report (2003).

National Suicide Review Group, Annual Report (2003).

The Psychiatric Services – Planning for the Future: Report of a Study Group on the Development of Psychiatric Services. The Stationery Office (1984).

Israel

GENERAL INFORMATION

Israel is a country with an approximate area of 21 thousand sq. km. (UNO, 2001). Its population is 6.56 million, and the sex ratio (men per hundred women) is 98 (UNO, 2004). The proportion of population under the age of 15 years is 28% (UNO, 2004), and the proportion of population above the age of 60 years is 13% (WHO, 2004). The literacy rate is 97.3% for men and 93.4% for women (UNESCO/MoH, 2004).

The country is a high income group country (based on World Bank 2004 criteria). The proportion of health budget to GDP is 8.7%. The per capita total expenditure on health is 1839 international $, and the per capita government expenditure on health is 1272 international $ (WHO, 2004).

The main language(s) used in the country is (are) Hebrew and Arabic. The largest ethnic group(s) is (are) Jew, and the other ethnic group(s) are (is) Arab. The largest religious group(s) is (are) Jew (four-fifths), and the other religious group(s) are (is) Muslim.

The life expectancy at birth is 77.3 years for males and 81.4 years for females (WHO, 2004). The healthy life expectancy at birth is 70 years for males and 72 years for females (WHO, 2004).

EPIDEMIOLOGY

There is substantial epidemiological data on mental illnesses in Israel in internationally accessible literature. No attempt was made to include this information here.

MENTAL HEALTH RESOURCES

Mental Health Policy A mental health policy is present. The policy was initially formulated in 1991.

The components of the policy are advocacy, promotion, prevention, treatment and rehabilitation. The national mental health policy is not found in a single document. Besides the features mentioned above, the policy focuses on human resource training and safe-guarding patients' rights. It is guided by community principles and great efforts are made to expand the network of community-based clinics and rehabilitation facilities. Integration of general health and mental health and constant pursuit of high quality and effective care provision are also a part of the basic principles of the policy.

Substance Abuse Policy A substance abuse policy is present. The policy was initially formulated in 1999.

National Mental Health Programme A national mental health programme is absent.

Guidelines on a national mental health programme are present. A draft programme was formulated in 1995. Once adopted, the plan will be based on the following policy objectives, which are endorsed by almost all stakeholders: to promote the mental health of the population, to integrate mental health care within the general health system, to ensure equity of access to services in all parts of the country, to provide high-quality evidence-based and cost-effective care to persons with mental disorders, to promote the psychosocial rehabilitation of persons with mental disability, to strengthen and expand community-based care and reduce both hospital admission rates and length of stay, and to ensure the availability of emergency and crisis services, specially in security-related situations.

National Therapeutic Drug Policy/Essential List of Drugs A national therapeutic drug policy/essential list of drugs is present. It was formulated in 1994.

Mental Health Legislation Mental health legislation has been advanced in recent years, e.g. The Community-Based Rehabilitation of the Mentally Disabled Act (2000); Patients' Rights Act (1996); The Treatment of the Mentally Ill Act (1991); The Forensic Unit of the Mental Health Services Department of the Ministry of Health examines all subjects regarding compulsory admission, and along with the Ministry of Justice supervises some aspects of the work of the district psychiatric committees. The concept of diminished responsibility is reflected in the legislation – Law of Punishment (1977) and its amendment in 1995. There is also a provision for compulsory outpatient care. The 1996 Israel Law for Patients' Rights introduces to the field of health legislation two new entities: internal examination committees and quality-control committees. The former investigates unusual, irregular or exceptional events related to diagnosis and/or treatment and shares its findings to the patient (or representatives). The Community-Based Rehabilitation of the Mentally Disabled Act (2000) grants all consumers whose degree of mental disability reaches 40%, as established by the National Insurance Institute, full entitlement to receive a set of rehabilitation services in the community.

The latest legislation was enacted in 2000.

Mental Health Financing There are budget allocations for mental health.

The country spends 6.2% of the total health budget on mental health.

The primary sources of mental health financing in descending order are tax based, social insurance, out of pocket expenditure by the patient or family and private insurances.

By law, all residents are insured for health care and contribute to a national fund according to income. Most of the population is served by one of the four health maintenance organizations, the largest of which was established in the pre-State years (before 1948) by the labour unions. Importantly, the law that established this health system did not include either psychiatric care or geriatric and nursing services. In 2002, the Government decided to transfer all responsibility for mental health care to the health maintenance organizations; implementation of this decision is expected in 2005. Care provided by a general practitioner is free while a visit to a specialist (other than a psychiatrist) carries a nominal fee (less than US$5). Visits to a psychiatric clinic, care in a psychiatric hospital or hostel and drugs in the 'basket of drugs' are free of charge. The insurance schemes cover for a limited number of hours of psychotherapy, thus most patients needing psychotherapy pay for it privately. Preventive maternal and child health services are provided free by the municipalities and by the Ministry of Health. The budget for psychiatric community services is 29.4% of the budget allocated to mental health. The responsibility for psychosocial rehabilitation services is shared with the welfare services and, especially, with the National Insurance Institute. Disabled and dependent people are entitled to up to 95% of their rent (up to a certain level). Rental payments are provided to eligible individuals by the Ministry of Housing.

The country has disability benefits for persons with mental disorders.

Mental Health Facilities Mental health is a part of primary health care system. Actual treatment of severe mental disorders is available at the primary level.

Regular training of primary care professionals is carried out in the field of mental health.

There are community care facilities for patients with mental disorders. The rehabilitation facilities (about 224 in number) include sheltered housing, hostels, vocational rehabilitation units, employment services, social clubs and home care. The hostels are intended for those patients requiring intensive 24 hour care and assistance. Comprehensive hostels are for those with low level of functioning, but not requiring inpatient care. Sheltered housing are for those individuals who can live in the community, but still require some support in specific areas of their life. Other areas of community psychiatry (e.g. the rehabilitation of deviant youth, care for rape victims) are covered by ministries other than health or by NGOs, which may or may not have governmental financial support.

Psychiatric Beds and Professionals

Total psychiatric beds per 10 000 population	8.1
Psychiatric beds in mental hospitals per 10 000 population	7.6
Psychiatric beds in general hospitals per 10 000 population	0.4
Psychiatric beds in other settings per 10 000 population	0.1
Number of psychiatrists per 100 000 population	13.7
Number of neurosurgeons per 100 000 population	0.8
Number of psychiatric nurses per 100 000 population	10.7
Number of neurologists per 100 000 population	3.6
Number of psychologists per 100 000 population	35.6
Number of social workers per 100 000 population	5.18

There are 2476 occupational therapists and 1742 creativity and self-expression therapists. About 6.6%, 16.3% and 2.6% of beds are for child and adolescents, geriatric and forensic services, respectively. Geographical inequality exists, thus central regions have many more beds than do northern and southern regions. A decline in the number of beds has occurred over the last two decades, but this has been more pronounced in the private sector. Private psychiatric hospitals mainly provide long-term care and are often similar to nursing homes. Their fee structure and management is regulated by the Government. In addition to psychiatric clinics in different settings, there are other clinics that provide outpatient care and rehabilitation facilities. Presently, most of the psychiatric care in the public sector is gratis and patients' rights are embodied in special legislation. The six district offices are responsible for service planning, development, coordination and supervision of standards of work including those at general hospitals. About 156 psychiatrists specialize in child and adolescent practice. A postgraduate training programme for forensic psychiatry was initiated in 1997. About 67 psychiatrists have completed their diploma and 23 will complete it this year. A cadre of clinical criminologists, with training in academic criminology and sociology, psychology and health sciences also exists. Most psychologists working in the public sector supplement their income through private practice. Psychologists are not allowed to prescribe medication.

Non-Governmental Organizations NGOs are involved with mental health in the country. They are mainly involved in advocacy, promotion, prevention, treatment and rehabilitation. There are a number of self-help groups which are involved in activities related to mental health promotion and prevention of mental disorders. They also lobby with the Government on policy and service issues and provide support for families. In addition, several non-government organizations are active in mental health care, such as ERAN, which offers telephone first-aid assistance nationally, and another one that provides initial guidance to foreign workers. Eshet collaborates with the Ministry of Health for occupational rehabilitation of mentally ill people. Volunteers' activities in psychiatric institutions is expanding.

Information Gathering System There is mental health reporting system in the country.
The country has data collection system or epidemiological study on mental health.
A psychiatric case register that has been in operational since 1950. It records data related to psychiatric inpatient and day care facilities. More recently, the database has included information from most outpatient services. The confidentiality of the database is specifically protected by law.

Programmes for Special Population The country has specific programmes for mental health for minorities, disaster affected population, elderly and children. Services that cater to the needs of new immigrants are available.
There are community centres and day-care centres for the treatment of autistic children and children with selected developmental disorders. There are psychological services in the school system as well. The Ministry of Education has a programme for promoting healthy life skills. The national strategies on drug abuse, including health promotion and prevention activities, is coordinated by an autonomous council. The services, such as methadone supply, however, are the responsibility of the Ministry of
Health, in association with the welfare system. Special inpatient facilities are available for the treatment of adolescents with drug abuse and for patients with dual diagnosis. The Ministry of Social Affairs' Division for Mental Retardation is in contact with approximately 23 000 persons of all ages. Residential care is provided to about 6000 persons in 54 institutions countrywide. In addition, 2000 persons receive residential care in hostels or protected apartments within the community. More than 50 other settings provide vocational and educational services to 15 000 persons (day-care kindergartens, day-treatment centres, sheltered workshops or integrated care within the community). Secure facilities for treatment of mentally ill offenders are available. During the current wave of terrorist attacks, the Ministry of Health and several NGOs have established mental health activities that are provided as early as possible in the emergency rooms and wards of general hospitals that treat casualties. The Ministry has trained several teams of mental health specialists that are attached to general hospitals. Half of them are trained to care for children and adolescents. Trained personnel in outpatient clinics are entrusted with the care of persons affected by acute stress disorders or post-traumatic stress disorder. At the time of a national emergency, these outpatient clinics are open 24 hours a day.

Therapeutic Drugs The following therapeutic drugs are generally available at the primary health care level of the country: carbamazepine, ethosuximide, phenobarbital, phenytoin sodium, sodium valproate, amitriptyline, chlorpromazine, diazepam, fluphenazine, haloperidol, lithium, biperiden, carbidopa, levodopa.

Other Information The Division of Mental Health Services of the Ministry of Health is advised by two intersectoral advisory boards – one on mental health care and one responsible for psychosocial rehabilitation. Both boards include representatives from users of services and their families. The Division includes a special unit responsible for substance abuse that coordinates activities with the National Council against Drug Use. Since 1950, the Division cumulatively records all psychiatric admissions to inpatient facilities. Intersectoral cooperation has been facilitated by the social welfare orientation of the country. Primarily, the Ministry of Health coordinates with the Ministry of Labour and Welfare, the National Insurance Institute, the Judicial system and others. This cooperation operates at both the central and peripheral level. There has been a revamping of mental health services in Israel since the report by the Netanyahu Commission (1990) and the report of the State Comptroller's office (1991). Details can be obtained from the document Mental Health in Israel (2000).

Additional Sources of Information

Barak, P., Gordon, H. (2002) Forensic psychiatry in Israel. Psychiatric Bulletin, 26, 143-145.

Laufer, N., Jecsmien, P., Hermesh, H., et al (1998) Application of models of working at the interface between primary care and mental health services in Israel. Israel Journal of Psychiatry & Related Sciences, 35, 120-127.

Mark, M., Rabinowitz, J., Feldman, D. (1997) Revampign mental health care in Israel: from the Netanyahu Commission to National Health Insurance Law. Social Work in Health Care, 25, 119-129.

Ministry of Health (2000) Mental Health in Israel. Annual Statistics 2000. Ministry of Health, Mental Health Services, Department of Information and Evaluation, Jerusalem.

Ministry of Health (1990) Report of the State Commission of Inquiry into the Operation and Efficiency of the Health Care System in Israel, Jerusalem.

Levav, I., Grinshpoon, A. (2004) Mental health services in Israel. International Psychiatry, 4, 10-14.

Merrick, J., Kandel, I. (2003) Medical services for persons with intellectual disability in Israel. Public Health Reviews, 31, 45-68.

Mester, R., Mozes, T., Spivak, B., et al (2000) The patient's right to know, in the 1996 Israel law for the rights of the patient: the pains of progress. Israel Journal of Psychiatry & Related Sciences, 37, 95-102.

Italy

GENERAL INFORMATION

Italy is a country with an approximate area of 301 thousand sq. km. (UNO, 2001). Its population is 57.346 million, and the sex ratio (men per hundred women) is 94 (UNO, 2004). The proportion of population under the age of 15 years is 14% (UNO, 2004), and the proportion of population above the age of 60 years is 24% (WHO, 2004). The literacy rate is 98.9% for men and 98% for women (UNESCO/MoH, 2004).

The country is a high income group country (based on World Bank 2004 criteria). The proportion of health budget to GDP is 8.4%. The per capita total expenditure on health is 2204 international $, and the per capita government expenditure on health is 1660 international $ (WHO, 2004).

The main language(s) used in the country is (are) Italian. The largest ethnic group(s) is (are) Italian. The largest religious group(s) is (are) Roman Catholic.

The life expectancy at birth is 76.8 years for males and 82.5 years for females (WHO, 2004). The healthy life expectancy at birth is 71 years for males and 75 years for females (WHO, 2004).

EPIDEMIOLOGY

There is substantial epidemiological data on mental illnesses in Italy in internationally accessible literature. No attempt was made to include this information here.

MENTAL HEALTH RESOURCES

Mental Health Policy A mental health policy is present. The policy was initially formulated in 1994.

The components of the policy are advocacy, promotion, prevention, treatment and rehabilitation. The mental health policy is broadly defined in the National Plan for Mental Health. The first such plan was launched in 1994-96 and was essentially directed at the process of deinstitutionalization and the creation of community care facilities. The plan of 1998-2000, provided objectives and intervention strategies in order to monitor the progress and maintain uniform levels of care. The latest official policy is a part of the National Plan for Health (2003-2005) that includes a specific section about mental health.

Substance Abuse Policy A substance abuse policy is present. The policy was initially formulated in 1990.

National Mental Health Programme A national mental health programme is present. The programme was formulated in 1999.

National Therapeutic Drug Policy/Essential List of Drugs Details about the national therapeutic drug policy/essential list of drugs are not available.

Mental Health Legislation In Italy, the national laws are generally a wide framework of norms, the application of which is defined at local level by regional laws. Each region has a certain degree of autonomy. The most recent law is the 'Target Project 1998-2000'; the first important approach was included in the Laws No. 180/1978 and No. 833/1978 (articles 33, 34, 35 and 64), the latter included the former. The reform law was then incorporated into a more comprehensive legislation setting up the National Health Service, which aimed to provide sectorized community based integrated services. Other than these, there are a number of articles under the Penal Code that guide forensic psychiatrists in criminal cases. Offenders suffering from mental disorders that make them liable to dangerous offenses are required to undergo treatment at a forensic psychiatry hospital and the others are treated in the community set-ups or general hospitals.

The latest legislation was enacted in 1998.

Mental Health Financing There are budget allocations for mental health.

Details about expenditure on mental health are not available.

The primary sources of mental health financing in descending order are tax based, out of pocket expenditure by the patient or family and private insurances.

The amount for mental health budget is defined by each regional programme and then more precisely at the level of local health units. Taxes are the primary source of financing for public services and out of pocket payments and private insurances for private services. Each citizen is registered with a primary care doctor under the National Health Service. Citizens have unlimited coverage, but need to contribute some proportions of the drug prescriptions, laboratory charges and diagnostic tests. There are local health districts catering to the needs of the catchment population, but it is not compulsory for residents to go to their local doctors only. Each local district has its own budget and is free to access services provided by non-governmental centres on payment of predetermined cost.

The country has disability benefits for persons with mental disorders.

Mental Health Facilities Mental health is a part of primary health care system. Actual treatment of severe mental disorders is available at the primary level. Mental health services are considered to be primary care services. Referral from primary care doctors is not required.
Details about training facilities are not available. Training of medical doctors provide special emphasis on community care and they are trained to work in close contact with primary care doctors.
There are community care facilities for patients with mental disorders. Mental Health Departments provide actual treatment for persons with mental disorders. These departments include and coordinate four different services: community facilities, day care facilities, residential facilities, and general hospital psychiatry wards. Though the implementation of community care in mental health has made mental health accessible to all, the quality of care is not uniform across the country. At present, there were 707 CMHC operating in the country. There are more than more than 1552 residential facilities (17 101 beds) and 612 day care facilities. There are also more than 13 000 vocational organizations operating in the social sector that involve over 260 000 participants. Regional distribution of these facilities, however, is uneven, with only 20% located in the south. Territorial Pacts for Mental health is a new strategy promoting the functional integration of health, social, economic and vocational resources (both public and private) available in a given catchment area. The community itself is also expected to play a crucial role through vocational and self-help organizations.

Psychiatric Beds and Professionals

Total psychiatric beds per 10 000 population	4.63
Psychiatric beds in mental hospitals per 10 000 population	0
Psychiatric beds in general hospitals per 10 000 population	0.92
Psychiatric beds in other settings per 10 000 population	3.7
Number of psychiatrists per 100 000 population	9.8
Number of neurosurgeons per 100 000 population	
Number of psychiatric nurses per 100 000 population	32.9
Number of neurologists per 100 000 population	
Number of psychologists per 100 000 population	3.2
Number of social workers per 100 000 population	6.4

There are 120 sociologists and 171 psychiatric rehabilitation therapists associated directly with mental health facilities. Also, there are more than 3700 workers (non mental health professionals) working in the social sector and the field of rehabilitation. All mental hospitals were gradually phased out with the last one being closed in 1999. General hospital psychiatry wards have a maximum of 15 beds. Non-residential medium and long-term facilities now account for more beds than the hospital sector. The service providing units are the mental health centre, psychiatric services for diagnosis and care, day hospital, day centre, residential facilities. The district services vary from region to region and also from centre to centre. Private care facilities have more than 50% of the acute short term beds in the country. Patients requiring long-term residential care are catered by non-hospital residential facilities (NHRFs).

Non-Governmental Organizations NGOs are involved with mental health in the country. They are mainly involved in advocacy, promotion, prevention, treatment and rehabilitation. Families are fundamental stakeholders in health administration and their associations have become very influential on national and regional mental health policies. They are involved in 60% of the organizations working in the mental health sector. There are twice as many voluntary organizations in the north as in the south.

Information Gathering System There is no mental health reporting system in the country. A national mental health reporting system is being developed. This system will become operational in 2006. However, six regional reporting systems that record data on mental health departments already exist.
The country has data collection system or epidemiological study on mental health. These operate at regional level.

Programmes for Special Population The country has specific programmes for mental health for minorities, elderly and children. Substance misuse disorders, mental disorders in children and adolescents and forensic psychiatric sector are managed by specialist services which are not under the department of mental health. In the past, these facilities rarely contacted mental health, but now there is better integration of services.

Therapeutic Drugs The following therapeutic drugs are generally available at the primary health care level of the country: carbamazepine, ethosuximide, phenobarbital, phenytoin sodium, sodium valproate, amitriptyline, chlorpromazine, diazepam, fluphenazine, haloperidol, lithium, biperiden, carbidopa, levodopa.
Atypical anti-psychotics like risperidone, clozapine, olanzapine and quetiapine are also available.

Other Information The deinstitutionalization movement was started by the psychiatrist Franco Basaglia in the state hospital of Gorizia and later this was modelled upon to formulate Law 180 in 1978. The 1990s witnessed the development of a comprehensive community care network. A recent study by the EPSILON Group showed that in Verona there were limited provisions for long stay residential services for patients suffering from schizophrenia and community care was the mainstay.

Additional Sources of Information

Barbato, A. (1998) Psychiatry in Transition: Outcomes of Mental Health Policy Shift in Italy. Australian and New Zealand Journal of Psychiatry, 32, 673-679.

Becker T., Hullsmann, S., Knudsen, H. C. et al & the EPSILON Group (2002) Provision of services for people with schizophrenia in five European regions. Journal of Social Psychiatry and Psychiatric Epidemiology, 37, 465-474.

Burti, L. (2001) Italian psychiatric reform 20 years plus years after. Acta Psychiatrica Scandinavica, 104 (suppl. 410), 41-46.

Crepet, P. (1990) A transition period in psychiatric care in Italy ten years after the reform. British Journal of Psychiatry, 156, 27-36.

De Salvia, D., Barbato, A. (1993) Recent trends in mental health services in Italy. Canadian Journal of Psychiatry, 38, 185-186.

de Girolamo, G., Cozza, M. (2000) The Italian psychiatric reform. International Journal of Law and Psychiatry, 23, 197-214.

de Girolamo, G., Picardi, A., Micciolo, R., et al for the PROGRES Group (2002) Residential care in Italy. British Journal of Psychiatry, 181, 220-225.

Fioritti, A., Bassi, M., de Girolamo, G. (2003) Italian psychiatry – 25 years of change. International Psychiatry, 2, 14-17.

Gazzetta Ufficiale Della Republica Italiana (1998) Approvazione del Piano Sanitario Nazionale per il Triennio 1998 – 2000.

Government document (1999) Mental Health Act Review – Mental Health Care in Italy.

Liffredo, C., Callegaro, D., Gallino, G. et al (1993) The role of the professional nurse in mental health service. Minerva Psichiatrica, 34, 117-120.

Piccinelli, M., Politi, P., Barale, F. (2002) Focus on psychiatry in Italy. British Journal of Psychiatry, 181, 538-544.

Traverso, G. B., Ciappi, S., Ferracuti, S. (2000) The treatment of the criminally insane in Italy. International Journal of Law and Psychiatry, 23, 493-508.

Jamaica

GENERAL INFORMATION

Jamaica is a country with an approximate area of 11 thousand sq. km. (UNO, 2001). Its population is 2.676 million, and the sex ratio (men per hundred women) is 97 (UNO, 2004). The proportion of population under the age of 15 years is 30% (UNO, 2004), and the proportion of population above the age of 60 years is 10% (WHO, 2004). The literacy rate is 83.8% for men and 91.4% for women (UNESCO/MoH, 2004).

The country is a lower middle income group country (based on World Bank 2004 criteria). The proportion of health budget to GDP is 6.8%. The per capita total expenditure on health is 253 international $, and the per capita government expenditure on health is 106 international $ (WHO, 2004).

The main language(s) used in the country is (are) English and Jamaican Creole. The largest ethnic group(s) is (are) African, and the other ethnic group(s) are (is) Afro-European. The largest religious group(s) is (are) Protestant.

The life expectancy at birth is 71.1 years for males and 74.6 years for females (WHO, 2004). The healthy life expectancy at birth is 64 years for males and 66 years for females (WHO, 2004).

EPIDEMIOLOGY

In a sample of 89 physically healthy subjects who were administered the Psychiatric Assessment Schedule, Hilton et al (1997) found that the prevalence of psychiatric disorder was 14% in men and 36% in women. Psychiatric disorders were associated with female gender, unemployment, difficulties with social adjustment and number of episodes of physical illness in the 6 months prior to the interview. Eldemire (1996) conducted a community based study in subjects over 60 years using the Mini Mental State Examination (MMSE) and identified 2.3% as severely impaired and 11.8% as having borderline impairment. Soyibo and Lee (1999) conducted a survey of more than 2400 high school children in 26 schools and found that drug use was common. The following drugs were used by the students: alcohol (50.2%), tobacco (16.6%), marijuana (10.2%), cocaine (2.2%), heroin (1.5%) and opium (1.2%). Illicit drug use was associated with gender (male), locality (urban) and parental occupation (professionals). Hickling and Rodgers-Johnson (1995) used the Present State Examination (PSE) to find the incidence of schizophrenia in the population by locating first contact patients (n=355). The incidence was found to be 1.2/10 000 population. The age adjusted (15-54 years) rate was 2.1/10 000 population. Hickling et al (2001) followed first contact patients with schizophrenia identified by the Present Status Examination (n=317) for one year. In this period, almost 38% were admitted to hospital for treatment, 83% were still being seen and only 43% were employed. The relapse rate was 13% and it was associated with hospital admission, being brought into care by the police or mental health officers, gainful employment and poor intramuscular medication compliance. Crijnen et al (1999) administered the parent version of the Child Behaviour Checklist for 13 697 children and adolescents aged 6 -17 years in 12 countries (including Jamaica). The researchers concluded that age and gender variations were cross-culturally consistent, although clinical cut-off points varied across all cultures. Medium effect sizes for cross-cultural variations were noted in total problem, externalizing and internalizing scores, but great cross-cultural consistency was seen in the decline of total and externalizing scores with age and increase in internalizing scores with age. Boys obtained higher total and externalizing scores but lower internalizing scores than girls. Lambert et al (1989) compared parent-reported behaviour problems of 360 Jamaican and 946 U.S. children aged 6 to 11 and found few differences in individual, total, internalizing (e.g. depression) and externalizing (e.g. fighting) problem scores as a function of nationality, gender or age. Thorburn et al (1992) used a modification of the International Classification of Impairments, Disabilities and Handicaps assessment to identify six types of disabilities (visual, hearing, speech, motor, cognitive and fits) in children (2-9 years) in a population-based survey. The estimated prevalence of all types of disabilities was 9.4% and for serious disability 2.5%. Cognitive disabilities were seen in 8.1%. Of the disabled children, 23% had two and 6% had three or four disabilities (Paul et al, 1992). Readett et al (1991) assessed 477 primary school children for nocturnal enuresis. If nocturnal enuresis was defined as 2 wet nights per week, it occurred in 62%, 48%, 42% and 40% of children at 2, 3, 4 and 5 years of age, respectively. If enuresis was defined as 1 wet night per month, it occurred in 68%, 58%, 53% and 52%, respectively. Though there was no significant differences between sexes, girls with family history of nocturnal enuresis were at significantly higher risk. Studies in two children's homes in Jamaica showed that 33% and 66% of children had pica (Wong et al, 1988).

MENTAL HEALTH RESOURCES

Mental Health Policy A mental health policy is present. The policy was initially formulated in 1994.
The components of the policy are advocacy, promotion, prevention, treatment and rehabilitation. Integration of mental health into primary health care is a component of the policy.

Substance Abuse Policy A substance abuse policy is present. The policy was initially formulated in 1997.

National Mental Health Programme A national mental health programme is present. The programme was formulated in 1999.

National Therapeutic Drug Policy/Essential List of Drugs A national therapeutic drug policy/essential list of drugs is present. It was formulated in 1998.

Mental Health Legislation Jamaica has a Mental Health Act. Under the new Mental Health Bill, provisions have been made for the admissions of patients, whether voluntary or involuntary, and the designation of psychiatric facilities for the mentally ill. The provisions relate to the establishment of the Mental Health Appeal Tribunal, the consent of patients to treatment and the discharge of patients among others. Community care and role of urbanisation on mental health are also discussed.
The latest legislation was enacted in 1997.

Mental Health Financing There are budget allocations for mental health.
The country spends 5% of the total health budget on mental health.
The primary sources of mental health financing in descending order are tax based, out of pocket expenditure by the patient or family and private insurances.
Social security arrangements are limited. Destitute mentally ill people are issued food stamps under the Poor Law, but the registration process is cumbersome.
The country has disability benefits for persons with mental disorders. Relief for the poor and food stamps are provided to the indigent mentally ill and the National Fund subsidizes medication.

Mental Health Facilities Mental health is a part of primary health care system. Actual treatment of severe mental disorders is available at the primary level. Primary care is traditionally performed by mental health officers and psychiatrists. These functions are now being handed over to medical practitioners (about 1200) and nurses in primary health care. They refer the more serious patients to psychiatrists, but within the community they are responsible to a substantial degree to modify drug dosages and carry out other therapies for which they are trained initially. They also liaise with the police and forensic experts and other community services linked to mental health. They also hold meetings and give lectures within their parishes to educate people about the role of mental health.
Regular training of primary care professionals is carried out in the field of mental health. Training in psychiatry is provided to all medical practitioners and nurses. The most experienced nurses were called mental health officers and given further training in psychopharmacology and psychotherapy. Besides these, there are psychiatric aides, paraprofessionals trained in basic mental health and supposed to help the mental health officers in the community and enrolled assistant nurses, nurses with shorter training periods with the function of helping the registered nurses in hospitals and clinics.
There are community care facilities for patients with mental disorders. Despite several changes in the Government over the past 30 years, continuity of public policy and fiscal support has allowed ongoing development of the island's community mental health service. The National Community Mental Health Service relies on specially trained psychiatric nurse practitioners who provide crisis management, medication, supportive psychotherapy and make home visits and carry out treatment plans formulated by the psychiatrist. More patients are treated within the community based services than in hospitals. This has led to a decrease in psychiatric hospital admissions by almost 50%. Many patients of schizophrenia receive depot neuroleptics at 'Modecate Clinics' run by general nurses with psychiatric training. However, there are few rehabilitation units and they are not well resourced. Also, there is little support for destitute mentally ill people in the community.

Psychiatric Beds and Professionals

Total psychiatric beds per 10 000 population	5
Psychiatric beds in mental hospitals per 10 000 population	4
Psychiatric beds in general hospitals per 10 000 population	
Psychiatric beds in other settings per 10 000 population	
Number of psychiatrists per 100 000 population	1.6
Number of neurosurgeons per 100 000 population	0.2
Number of psychiatric nurses per 100 000 population	8
Number of neurologists per 100 000 population	
Number of psychologists per 100 000 population	0.7
Number of social workers per 100 000 population	0.4

There are 10 occupational therapists. The Bellevue Hospital (bed strength 900) offers the broad range of psychiatric services including (limited) rehabilitation services. Two general hospital psychiatric units provide just over 50 acute care beds. Psychotic patients are admitted to all general hospitals' medical wards also. The University Hospital also has a small unit for alcohol and drug abuse patients. In the 1970s, as a step to educate the public, the Bellevue Hospital had started a novel programme where on one particular day the public were encouraged to come to the hospital and participate in cultural and sports activities with the patients. Weekly call-in programmes on the radio and sociodrama process was also started in 1978. These resulted in the publication of a large number of studies on mental health by the lay press and stigma was reduced. Many general nurses working in the mental health field have received 9 month training in psychiatric nursing. They deal with routine care of patients with psychotic illness and are the mainstay of mental health care. Some work almost independently of psychiatrists, and in rural areas may initiate treatment, including medication.

Non-Governmental Organizations NGOs are involved with mental health in the country. They are mainly involved in advocacy, treatment and rehabilitation. There are self-help groups providing help to schizophrenics and persons with attention-deficit disorder and also shelter for the homeless. The university hospital collaborates with the Alcoholic Anonymous.

Information Gathering System There is mental health reporting system in the country. The Annual Report has a mental health section.
The country has data collection system or epidemiological study on mental health.

Programmes for Special Population The country has specific programmes for mental health for disaster affected population and children.

Therapeutic Drugs The following therapeutic drugs are generally available at the primary health care level of the country: carbamazepine, phenobarbital, phenytoin sodium, sodium valproate, amitriptyline, chlorpromazine, diazepam, fluphenazine, haloperidol, lithium.

Other Information

Additional Sources of Information

Bellevue Hospital Task Force Implementation Plan.

Crijnen, A. A. M., Achenbach, T. M., Verhulst, F. C. (1999) Problems reported by parents of children in multiple cultures: the Child Behavior Checklist syndrome constructs. American Journal of Psychiatry, 156, 569-574.

Eldemire, D. (1996) Level of mental impairment in the Jamaican elderly and the issues of screening levels, caregiving, support systems, carepersons, and female burden. Molecular & Chemical Neuropathology, 28, 115-120.

Government document (1999) Mental Health Plan Year.

Government document (1999) National Health Plan for Children and Adolescents.

Government document (1997) The Mental Health Act.

Hickling, F. W. (1993) Psychiatry in Jamaica: growth and development. International Review of Psychiatry, 5, 193-203.

Hickling, F. W. (1994) Community psychiatry and deinstitutionalization in Jamaica. Hospital and Community Psychiatry, 45, 1122-26.

Hickling, F. W. (1999) Transforming mental health legislation. Psychiatric Bulletin, 23, 115.

Hickling, F. W., McCallum, M., Nooks, L., et al (2001) Outcome of first contact schizophrenia in Jamaica. West Indian Medical Journal, 50, 194-197.

Hickling, F. W., Rodgers-Johnson, P. (1995) The incidence of first contact schizophrenia in Jamaica. British Journal of Psychiatry, 167, 193-196.

Hilton, C., Osborn, M., Serjeant, G. (1997) Psychiatric disorder in young adults in Jamaica. International Journal of Social Psychiatry, 43, 257-268.

Hilton, C. (1996) Psychiatry in Jamaica. Psychiatric Bulletin, 20, 437-39.

Integration of Mental Health Services into Primary Health Care. Health Centres in all Regions (Government document).

La Grenade, J. (1998) Integrated primary mental health care. West Indian Medical Journal, 47 (Suppl. 4), 31-33.

Lambert, M. C., Weisz, J. R., Knight, F. (1989) Over- and undercontrolled clinic referral problems of Jamaican and American children and adolescents: the culture general and the culture specific. Journal of Consulting & Clinical Psychology, 57, 467-472.

Ministry of Health (1998) List of Vital Essential and Necessary Drugs and Medical Sundries.

National Council on Drug Abuse, Ministry of Health (1997). National/Master Drug Abuse Prevention and Control Plan.

National Mental Health Policy (Government document).

Paul, T. J., Desai, P., Thorburn, M. J. (1992) The prevalence of childhood disability and related medical diagnoses in Clarendon, Jamaica. West Indian Medical Journal, 41, 8-11.

Readett, D. R., Bamigbade, T., Serjeant, G. R. (1991) Nocturnal enuresis in normal Jamaican children. Implications for therapy. West Indian Medical Journal, 40, 181-184.

Soyibo, K., Lee, M. G. (1999) Use of illicit drugs among high-school students in Jamaica. Bulletin of the World Health Organization, 77, 258-262.

The Mental Health Amendment Bill (Government document).

The New Mental Health Bill. Mental Health Report (Government document).

Thorburn, M. J., Desai, P., Davidson, L. L. (1992) Categories, classes and criteria in childhood disability – Experience from a survey in Jamaica. Disability & Rehabilitation, 14, 122-132.

Wong, M. S., Bundy, D. A., Golden, M. H. (1988) Quantitative assessment of geophagous behaviour as a potential source of exposure to geohelminth infection. Transactions of the Royal Society of Tropical Medicine & Hygiene, 82, 621-625.

Japan

GENERAL INFORMATION

Japan is a country with an approximate area of 378 thousand sq. km. (UNO, 2001). The country has many mountainous islands. Its population is 127.799 million, and the sex ratio (men per hundred women) is 96 (UNO, 2004). The proportion of population under the age of 15 years is 14% (UNO, 2004), and the proportion of population above the age of 60 years is 24% (WHO, 2004). The literacy rate is 99% for men and 99% for women (UNESCO/MoH, 2004).

The country is a high income group country (based on World Bank 2004 criteria). The proportion of health budget to GDP is 8%. The per capita total expenditure on health is 2131 international $, and the per capita government expenditure on health is 1660 international $ (WHO, 2004).

The main language(s) used in the country is (are) Japanese. The largest ethnic group(s) is (are) Japanese. The largest religious group(s) is (are) Shinto and Buddhist.

The life expectancy at birth is 78.4 years for males and 85.3 years for females (WHO, 2004). The healthy life expectancy at birth is 72 years for males and 78 years for females (WHO, 2004).

EPIDEMIOLOGY

There is substantial epidemiological data on mental illnesses in Japan in internationally accessible literature. No attempt was made to include this information here.

MENTAL HEALTH RESOURCES

Mental Health Policy A mental health policy is present. The policy was initially formulated in 1950.

The components of the policy are advocacy, promotion, prevention, treatment and rehabilitation.

Substance Abuse Policy A substance abuse policy is present. The policy was initially formulated in 1953.

National Mental Health Programme A national mental health programme is present. The programme was formulated in 1950. In 1995, the Government announced the Plan for People with Disabilities – a 7-year Strategy for Normalization.

National Therapeutic Drug Policy/Essential List of Drugs A national therapeutic drug policy/essential list of drugs is absent.

Mental Health Legislation The Mental Health Law was enacted in 1950 and is reviewed every 5 years. It was modified to the Mental Health and Welfare Law of 1995, wherein it provided the legal basis to perform adequate treatment (including voluntary treatment) and prevent abuse and supported the adoption of community care. The most recent amendment of 2000 emphasized that community-based programmes were eligible for public funds and exempted the family of a patient with mental disorder from responsibility for damages caused by the patient to self or others during the course of treatment.

The latest legislation was enacted in 2000.

Mental Health Financing There are budget allocations for mental health.

The country spends 5% of the total health budget on mental health.

The primary sources of mental health financing in descending order are tax based, social insurance, out of pocket expenditure by the patient or family and private insurances.

All residents are insured by the national health care system. Semi-governmental insurance organizations typically cover up to 70% of the cost of services. The remaining 30% is borne by the consumer/family. However, some groups (children, elderly, disabled, those with specific chronic physical and mental illnesses) are exempted from this co-payment. Hospital reimbursement schemes are being changed to favour shorter inpatient stays. The National Government provides for half of the expenditure on community care and the remaining is shared by the prefectural Government, provider agencies and NGOs.

The country has disability benefits for persons with mental disorders.

Mental Health Facilities Mental health is a part of primary health care system. Actual treatment of severe mental disorders is not available at the primary level. Only psychiatric emergency service networks are provided. Various treatments for mental disorders are available in mental hospitals and clinics.

Regular training of primary care professionals is not carried out in the field of mental health.

There are community care facilities for patients with mental disorders. In 1994, the law concerning the activities of community health centres was revised and called the Community Health Care Law. It led to the development of more adequate mental health care in the regional health care system. The Mental Health Welfare Law supports community-based services and deinstitutionalization. However, the majority of beds (89%) are in the private sector, which makes the implementation of the policy somewhat more difficult. However, reform measures are beginning to promote the concepts of deinstitutionalization, disability benefits, differentiation of services, revisions in payment and quality assessment. A number of workshops and group homes have developed. There are about 1250 facilities offering psychiatric day care and night care of which a quarter are detached from psychiatric hospitals.

Psychiatric Beds and Professionals

Total psychiatric beds per 10 000 population	28.4
Psychiatric beds in mental hospitals per 10 000 population	20.6
Psychiatric beds in general hospitals per 10 000 population	7.8
Psychiatric beds in other settings per 10 000 population	0
Number of psychiatrists per 100 000 population	9.4
Number of neurosurgeons per 100 000 population	5
Number of psychiatric nurses per 100 000 population	59
Number of neurologists per 100 000 population	2
Number of psychologists per 100 000 population	7
Number of social workers per 100 000 population	15.7

The Government has decided to reduce 72 000 beds (20% of the existing bed strength) within 10 years. The majority of psychiatric beds are in psychiatric hospitals in the private sector. Only about 0.2% of beds have been allocated to child mental health services. Japan has no specialized legal provision for mentally ill criminal offenders. Acquitted mentally ill offenders are treated in the same way as any other patient with psychiatric disorder according to the laws related to mental health. Convicted offenders with psychiatric illness are treated within the prison system. The discharge of a patient from a psychiatric hospital depends on the assessment of the treating doctor and hospital superintendent and this is reviewed by the Psychiatric Review Board. In 2003, the Diet (parliament) has passed a proposal for setting up forensic wards in public sector hospitals. Physicians, nurses, social workers and occupational therapists are licensed by the Ministry of Health, Labour and Welfare, and clinical psychologists are licensed by the Japanese Certification Board for Clinical Psychologists under the Ministry of Education, Culture, Sports, Science and Technology. Except for a mandatory 1-day course for extending qualification for an additional 5 years, no other systematic effort is made at refresher training of psychiatrists. There are about 300 child and adolescent psychiatrists in the country.

Non-Governmental Organizations NGOs are involved with mental health in the country. They are mainly involved in advocacy, promotion, prevention, treatment and rehabilitation. NGOs help in community care delivery. Consumer (e.g. National Federation of Psychiatric Survivors and Users in Japan) and family (National federation of families with mentally ill in Japan) groups influence policies.

Information Gathering System There is mental health reporting system in the country.
The country has data collection system or epidemiological study on mental health.

Programmes for Special Population The country has specific programmes for mental health for disaster affected population, elderly and children.
The Health and Medical Service Law for the Aged was promulgated in 1987, and the Ten-year Gold Plan to promote Health Care and Welfare of the Elderly was prepared in 1988. It recommends the development of day care services and specialized outpatient, inpatient and residential care for the elderly including those with dementia. A new 5-year elderly health and welfare promotion campaign (Gold Plan 21) that is focussed on mental health was launched in 2003. As a part of this initiative, the Government and other organizations have launched a 'Zero Physical Restraint Campaign'.

Therapeutic Drugs The following therapeutic drugs are generally available at the primary health care level of the country: carbamazepine, ethosuximide, phenobarbital, phenytoin sodium, sodium valproate, amitriptyline, chlorpromazine, diazepam, fluphenazine, haloperidol, lithium, biperiden, carbidopa, levodopa.
The National Health Insurance designates the availability of drugs.

Other Information Prior to the second world war, Japan had two laws related to mental health, the Confinement and Protection for Lunatics Act (1900) and the Mental Hospital Act (1919). In 1950, the Mental Hygiene Law was passed, which allowed for compulsory institutionalized care for patients with psychiatric disorders. In 1958, a nationwide compulsory health insurance scheme was started and from 1961 onwards the Government restricted the construction of any public hospitals and encouraged private hospitals. Following the killing of two patients in one hospital, the Mental Hygiene Law was revised and was renamed as Mental Health Law (1987). Human rights issues of patients and community care and rehabilitation facilities were stressed upon. Voluntary admission was introduced. The Mental Health and Welfare Law (1995) added the social eligibility criteria for mental disabilities. Community care has not been well funded by the Government and private sectors were encouraged to provide psychiatric care throughout the past decades. Typically the major share of psychiatric care is provided by a mid-size private psychiatric hospital. The average length of inpatient stay is very long. Ambulatory services are provided by a third of the hospitals, and small scale vocational workshops are the most prevalent community care facilities in the country. The public health centres deliver a variety of services in spite of low intensity of service provision. The first patient satisfaction survey in Japanese psychiatric hospitals was conducted in 1997. A nation-wide outcome survey is now planned.

Additional Sources of Information

Asai, K. (2000) Mental Health Japan. Asai Hospital. Japan.

Ito, H. (2000) The present and the future of mental health care in Japan. Epidemiologia e Psychiatria Sociale, 9, 79-83.

Kuno, E., Asukai, N. (2000) Efforts toward building a community-based mental health system in Japan. International Journal of Law and Psychiatry, 23, 361-373.

Nakatani,Y. (2000) Psychiatry and the law in Japan. International Journal of Law and Psychiatry, 23, 589-604.

Ohara, K., Sakuta, T, Ohara, K., et al (1999) Social psychiatry in Japan. International Medical Journal, 6, 83-85.

Tsuchiya, K. J., Takei, N. (2004) Focus on psychiatry in Japan. British Journal of Psychiatry, 184, 88-92.

Jordan

GENERAL INFORMATION

Jordan is a country with an approximate area of 89 thousand sq. km. (UNO, 2001). Its population is 5.613 million, and the sex ratio (men per hundred women) is 108 (UNO, 2004). The proportion of population under the age of 15 years is 37% (UNO, 2004), and the proportion of population above the age of 60 years is 5% (WHO, 2004). The literacy rate is 95.5% for men and 85.9% for women (UNESCO/MoH, 2004).

The country is a lower middle income group country (based on World Bank 2004 criteria). The proportion of health budget to GDP is 9.5%. The per capita total expenditure on health is 412 international $, and the per capita government expenditure on health is 194 international $ (WHO, 2004).

The main language(s) used in the country is (are) Arabic. The largest ethnic group(s) is (are) Arab. The largest religious group(s) is (are) Muslim (nine-tenths).

The life expectancy at birth is 68.6 years for males and 73.3 years for females (WHO, 2004). The healthy life expectancy at birth is 60 years for males and 62 years for females (WHO, 2004).

EPIDEMIOLOGY

Al Jaddou and Malkawi (1997) administered an Arabic version of the General Health Questionnaire (GHQ-28) to 794 primary care patients and found the prevalence of psychiatric morbidity to be 61%. Multiple logistic regression analysis revealed that unemployment and perceived severity of physical illness were positively correlated with psychiatric disorders. Haddad and Malak (2002) interviewed randomly selected cluster samples drawn from medical and engineering colleges (n=650) using the modified Arabic version of the WHO Smoking Questionnaire and the Attitudes towards Smoking Questionnaire. The prevalence of smoking was 28.6% (50.2% among males and 6.5% among females). Smoking commenced after 15 years of age in four-fifths of the cases. Warren et al (2000), who conducted the Global Youth Tobacco Survey, reported that tobacco use in the surveyed age group ranged from 10% to 33% in various countries. Oweis (2001) interviewed about 280 primiparous women with no previous history of psychiatric illness and complicated pregnancy and child birth using a number of standardized and locally validated tools including the Edinburgh Postnatal Depression Scale (EPDS). They found high rate of postpartum depression. The prevalence of postpartum depression was associated with perceived stress of childbirth, having a girl child, years of education and income and giving birth in a public or military hospital (as against a private hospital, which was perceived as less stressful). Shuriquie et al (1999) assessed 201 female nursing students (17- 21 years) with the Arabic version of the Abnormal Eating Attitude Scale. They found abnormal eating attitudes and over-concern with food and body image in 12.4%. Abnormal attitudes were inversely correlated with socioeconomic status. Daradkeh (1989) found that the annual suicide rate during 1985-1990 was 2.1 per 100 000. The peak suicide rate was in the age group 15-34 years. The majority of males who committed suicide were single and either unemployed or unskilled manual workers. Over two-thirds of females who committed suicide were either housewives or students. Nearly two-thirds of the total population that committed suicide had previous psychiatric treatment. Violent methods of suicide were most frequently used. Abu al-Ragheb and Salhab (1989) reported that during the 13-year period (1973-1985) at least 329 deaths in Jordan resulted from poisoning by pesticides (organophosphates: 93.6%) of which 61% were due to self-ingestion. Three fifths of the suicides were committed by subjects in the 15-24 years of age. Significantly fewer parasuicides were reported during Ramadan than the month preceding it and the month that follows Ramadan (Daradkeh, 1992). Kharabsheh et al (2001) reported on a mass psychogenic illness involving more than 800 young people who believed they had suffered from the side-effects of tetanus-diphtheria toxoid vaccine administered at school; 122 of them were admitted to hospital. The media, the children's parents and the medical profession played a role in the escalation of this mass reaction. Janson and Dawani (1994) examined 2528 children aged 0-7 years representing 95% of a catchment area. Almost 7.8% had a disability or a chronic disease. Severe mental retardation was one of the commonest disabilities.

MENTAL HEALTH RESOURCES

Mental Health Policy A mental health policy is absent.
A draft for the mental health policy had been prepared in 1986, but is still to be implemented.

Substance Abuse Policy A substance abuse policy is present. The policy was initially formulated in 2000.

National Mental Health Programme A national mental health programme is present. The programme was formulated in 1994. The national mental health programme aims to integrate mental health into public health and to promote mental health awareness. It also outlines service strategies, training strategies and management and promotion strategies.

National Therapeutic Drug Policy/Essential List of Drugs A national therapeutic drug policy/essential list of drugs is present. It was formulated in 1988.

Mental Health Legislation There is the Chapter 49/50/51 from the Law of Common Health regarding the compulsory admission to psychiatric hospitals.
The latest legislation was enacted in 2003.

Mental Health Financing There are no budget allocations for mental health.
Details about expenditure on mental health are not available.
The primary sources of mental health financing in descending order are tax based and out of pocket expenditure by the patient or family.
The country has disability benefits for persons with mental disorders.

Mental Health Facilities Mental health is a part of primary health care system. Actual treatment of severe mental disorders is available at the primary level. There have been initiatives to train general physicians and nurses on aspects of mental health care. Regular training of primary care professionals is carried out in the field of mental health. In the last two years, about 160 personnel were provided training.
There are no community care facilities for patients with mental disorders. Psychiatrists now cover health centres in 5 regions. Psychological counselling centres have been established in the main schools.

Psychiatric Beds and Professionals

Total psychiatric beds per 10 000 population	1.57
Psychiatric beds in mental hospitals per 10 000 population	1.4
Psychiatric beds in general hospitals per 10 000 population	0.08
Psychiatric beds in other settings per 10 000 population	0.07
Number of psychiatrists per 100 000 population	1
Number of neurosurgeons per 100 000 population	0.2
Number of psychiatric nurses per 100 000 population	2
Number of neurologists per 100 000 population	0.3
Number of psychologists per 100 000 population	0.6
Number of social workers per 100 000 population	2

Prior to 1966, there was only one mental hospital in Bethlehem. After the 1967 war, patients on the East Bank did not have access to the services of the hospital and so a new 60-bed mental hospital was constructed and in 1987 the National Centre for Mental Health was opened. A day care centre and a rehabilitation centre are there. Recently, a 46 bedded centre for treatment of drug abuse was created. Although there are 3000 psychologists and 2000 social workers only a few work in the field of mental health. Many professionals seek vacancies with better salaries in neighbouring countries, while others move to private sectors. Among military psychiatrists, two have a diploma in forensic psychiatry and one in child psychiatry (they were trained in the UK). Clinical psychologists have to obtain a licence from the Ministry to practice.

Non-Governmental Organizations NGOs are involved with mental health in the country. They are mainly involved in promotion and rehabilitation.

Information Gathering System There is mental health reporting system in the country.
The country has data collection system or epidemiological study on mental health.

Programmes for Special Population The country has specific programmes for mental health for elderly and children.
Two geriatric homes with a capacity for 200 elderly individuals are under construction. As a part of the national mental health programme, initiative has been taken to start a school mental health programme.

Therapeutic Drugs The following therapeutic drugs are generally available at the primary health care level of the country: carbamazepine, phenobarbital, phenytoin sodium, sodium valproate, amitriptyline, chlorpromazine, diazepam, fluphenazine, haloperidol, lithium, biperiden.
Sinemet is available instead of carbidopa and levodopa (it combines 25 mg of the former and 250 mg of the latter). The cost per 100 tablets is 0.47 USD.

Other Information

Additional Sources of Information

Abu al-Ragheb, S. Y., Salhab, A. S. (1989) Pesticide mortality. A Jordanian experience. American Journal of Forensic Medicine & Pathology, 10, 221-225.

Al Jaddou, H., Malkawi, A. (1997) Prevalence, recognition and management of mental disorders in primary health care in Northern Jordan. Acta Psychiatrica Scandinavica, 96, 31-35.

Daradkeh, T. K. (1989) Suicide in Jordan 1980-1985. Acta Psychiatrica Scandinavica, 79, 241-244.

Daradkeh, T. K. (1992) Parasuicide during Ramadan in Jordan. Acta Psychiatrica Scandinavica, 86, 253-254.

Haddad, L. G., Malak, M. Z. (2002) Smoking habits and attitudes towards smoking among university students in Jordan. International Journal of Nursing Studies, 39, 793-802.

Janson, S., Dawani, H. (1994) Chronic illness in preschool Jordanian children. Annals of Tropical Paediatrics, 14, 137-144.

Kharabsheh, S., Al-Otoum, H., Clements, J., et al (2001) Mass psychogenic illness following tetanus-diphtheria toxoid vaccination in Jordan. Bulletin of the World Health Organization, 79, 764-770.

Oweis, A. I. (2001) Relationships among the situational variables of perceived stress of the childbirth experience, perceived length and perceived difficulty of labor, selected personal variables, perceived nursing support and postpartum depression in primiparous Jordanian women living in Jordan. Widener University School of Nursing.

Shuriquie, N. (2003) Military psychiatry – a Jordanian experience. Psychiatric Bulletin, 27, 386-388.

Shuriquie, N., Elias, T., Abdulhamid, M. (1999) A study of abnormal eating attitude among Jordanian female college students. Bahrain Medical Bulletin, 21, 88-90.

Takriti A. (2004) Psychiatry in Jordan. International Psychiatry, 5, 9-11.

Warren, C. W., Riley, L., Asma, S., et al (2000) Tobacco use by youth: a surveillance report from the Global Youth Tobacco Survey project. Bulletin of the World Health Organization, 78, 868-876.

Kazakhstan

GENERAL INFORMATION

Kazakhstan is a country with an approximate area of 2725 thousand sq. km. (UNO, 2001). Its population is 15.403 million, and the sex ratio (men per hundred women) is 92 (UNO, 2004). The proportion of population under the age of 15 years is 24% (UNO, 2004), and the proportion of population above the age of 60 years is 12% (WHO, 2004). The literacy rate is 99.7% for men and 99.2% for women (UNESCO/MoH, 2004).

The country is a lower middle income group country (based on World Bank 2004 criteria). The proportion of health budget to GDP is 3.1%. The per capita total expenditure on health is 204 international $, and the per capita government expenditure on health is 123 international $ (WHO, 2004).

The main language(s) used in the country is (are) Kazakh and Russian. The largest ethnic group(s) is (are) Kazakh, and the other ethnic group(s) are (is) Russian. The largest religious group(s) is (are) Muslim, and the other religious group(s) are (is) Russian Orthodox Christian.

The life expectancy at birth is 58.7 years for males and 68.9 years for females (WHO, 2004). The healthy life expectancy at birth is 53 years for males and 59 years for females (WHO, 2004).

EPIDEMIOLOGY

Seisembekov et al (1989) used a questionnaire to assess alcohol use among 1458 students and found that 35.3% used alcohol with 62% having started the use between 15-18 years of age. Alcohol use seemed to be increasing. In a tuberculosis dispensary, Khauadamova et al (1992) found the prevalence of alcohol dependence to be 11.2%. Among patients with active tuberculosis the prevalence was 1.6%. In another sample, Shefer and Nabokova (1989) found that 37.8% of tuberculosis patients were heavy alcohol drinkers and 17.2% suffered from alcohol dependence. Mustafetova and Pogosov (1999) compared cocnar dependence (n=172) and opium dependence (n=302) in a clinic-based study and found that those using cocnar were older (70 years compared to 40 years in opium use), continued use for longer (33 years compared to 5 years in the opium using group) and had lesser criminal activities. Wasserman et al (1998 a, b) reported that suicide rates varied greatly between different regions of the former USSR during 1984-1990. It was 11.8 per 100 000 in Central Asia (Kazakhstan, Kirgizia, Turkmenistan, Uzbekistan and Tajikistan). During 1984-1990, a decline in suicide rates (32% for males and 19% for females) took place in the former Soviet Union. Buckley (1997) conducted a descriptive analysis of suicide rates in post-Soviet Kazakhstan during the period 1990-94 and found a 27% increase in male suicide rates, while the suicide rates in females remained stable. They felt that men were more affected because their identity is grounded in the economic arena and the post-Soviet Kazakhstan is facing hardships in the form of unemployment, inflation and economic uncertainty. Stoliarov et al (1990) examined changes in the rate of suicides in some cities of South Kazakhstan. They found that while positive changes were expected in light of measures aimed at the control of heavy drinking and alcohol dependence, the share of alcoholic intoxication as a cause for suicides remained at the former level. A similar relation between alcohol use and suicide was reported by Petrov et al (1991).

MENTAL HEALTH RESOURCES

Mental Health Policy A mental health policy is present. The policy was initially formulated in 1997.
The components of the policy are advocacy, promotion, prevention, treatment and rehabilitation. Providing social assistance and education is also a component of the mental health policy.

Substance Abuse Policy A substance abuse policy is present. The policy was initially formulated in 1998.

National Mental Health Programme A national mental health programme is absent.

National Therapeutic Drug Policy/Essential List of Drugs A national therapeutic drug policy/essential list of drugs is present. It was formulated in 1998.

Mental Health Legislation The Law of Republic of Kazakhstan on Psychiatric Assistance and Guarantee of Rights of Patients is the most recent legislation on mental health. The law requires the state to establish special production units, shops or sections with easier working conditions for labour therapy, vocational training and employment for persons with mental illness along with mandatory quotas for employment of the mentally ill.
The latest legislation was enacted in 1997.

Mental Health Financing There are budget allocations for mental health.
The country spends 7% of the total health budget on mental health.
The primary sources of mental health financing in descending order are tax based and social insurance.
The country has disability benefits for persons with mental disorders.

Mental Health Facilities Mental health is a part of primary health care system. Actual treatment of severe mental disorders is not available at the primary level.
Regular training of primary care professionals is carried out in the field of mental health.
Details about community care facilities in mental health are not available.

Psychiatric Beds and Professionals

Total psychiatric beds per 10 000 population	6.5
Psychiatric beds in mental hospitals per 10 000 population	5.9
Psychiatric beds in general hospitals per 10 000 population	0.2
Psychiatric beds in other settings per 10 000 population	
Number of psychiatrists per 100 000 population	6
Number of neurosurgeons per 100 000 population	1
Number of psychiatric nurses per 100 000 population	
Number of neurologists per 100 000 population	8
Number of psychologists per 100 000 population	0.1
Number of social workers per 100 000 population	

There are 855 psychiatrists and 526 narcologists. The psychiatric service in the Republic of Kazakhstan is provided through psychiatric hospitals, prophylactic centres and psychiatric departments in general hospitals. In the central regional hospitals, there are outpatient clinics, polyclinics, psychiatric emergency clinics. There are also day hospitals and workshops for treatment and social rehabilitation.

Non-Governmental Organizations NGOs are not involved with mental health in the country.

Information Gathering System There is mental health reporting system in the country.
The country has data collection system or epidemiological study on mental health. According to the National Statistics Agency data are being collected on mental disorders.

Programmes for Special Population Details about any special programmes in mental health are not available.
There are 20 centres for preventive psychiatry, and 60 doctors work in this area.

Therapeutic Drugs The following therapeutic drugs are generally available at the primary health care level of the country: carbamazepine, phenobarbital, sodium valproate, amitriptyline, chlorpromazine, diazepam, fluphenazine, haloperidol, lithium.

Other Information

Additional Sources of Information

Buckley, C. (1997) Suicide in post-Soviet Kazakhstan: role stress, age and gender. Central Asian Survey, 16, 45-52.

Khauadamova, G. T., Bekmuratov, E. B., Kabeliuk, V. N., et al (1992) Characteristics of the course of newly diagnosed tuberculosis among socially maladapted persons. Problemy Tuberkuleza, 39-41.

Mustafetova, P. K, Pogosov, A. V. (1999) Clinical features of cocnar addiction. Zhurnal Nevrologii i Psikhiatrii Imeni S.S. Korsakova, 99, 25-28.

Petrov, P. P., Borokhov, D. Z., Kul'zhanov, M. K., et al (1991) Suicidal behavior as a socio-hygienic problem. Sovetskoe Zdravookhranenie, 27-31.

Seisembekov, T. Z., Umbetalina, N. S., Satov, I. T. (1989) Several aspects of alcohol use among students. Sovetskoe Zdravookhranenie, 36-40.

Shefer, L. B., Nabokova, I. P. (1989) Socio-hygienic aspects of the contingents of adult patients with pulmonary tuberculosis. Problemy Tuberkuleza, 17-20.

Stoliarov, A. V., Borokhov, A. D., Zhamanbaev, E. K., et al (1990) Alcohol as a provoking factor of suicidal behavior. Zhurnal Nevropatologii i Psikhiatrii Imeni S-S-Korsakova, 90, 55-58.

Wasserman, D., Varnik, A., Dankowicz, M. (1998a) Regional differences in the distribution of suicide in the former Soviet Union during perestroika, 1984-1990. Acta Psychiatrica Scandinavica, Supplement 394, 5-12.

Wasserman, D., Varnik, A., Eklund, G. (1998b) Female suicides and alcohol consumption during perestroika in the former USSR. Acta Psychiatrica Scandinavica, Supplementum 394, 26-33.

Kenya

GENERAL INFORMATION

Kenya is a country with an approximate area of 580 thousand sq. km. (UNO, 2001). Its population is 32.42 million, and the sex ratio (men per hundred women) is 98 (UNO, 2004). The proportion of population under the age of 15 years is 41% (UNO, 2004), and the proportion of population above the age of 60 years is 4% (WHO, 2004). The literacy rate is 90% for men and 78.5% for women (UNESCO/MoH, 2004).

The country is a low income group country (based on World Bank 2004 criteria). The proportion of health budget to GDP is 7.8%. The per capita total expenditure on health is 114 international $, and the per capita government expenditure on health is 24 international $ (WHO, 2004).

The main language(s) used in the country is (are) English (official) and Swahili (national). The largest ethnic group(s) is (are) African (Kikuyu, Luhya, Luo, Kalenjin and Kamba tribes are most populous), and the other ethnic group(s) are (is) Asian and European. The largest religious group(s) is (are) Christian (more than three-fourths), and the other religious group(s) are (is) Muslim, Hindu and indigenous groups.

The life expectancy at birth is 49.8 years for males and 51.9 years for females (WHO, 2004). The healthy life expectancy at birth is 44 years for males and 45 years for females (WHO, 2004).

EPIDEMIOLOGY

Ndetei and Muhangi (1979) studied 140 rural medical walk-in-clinic patients and found that 20% suffered from psychiatric illnesses, especially depression and anxiety. Sebit (1996) assessed 186 patients attending primary care facilities using the Self Rating Questionnaire (SRQ), the Clinical Interview Schedule/Revised (CIS-R) and the WHO Audit Instrument for Alcohol abuse. The diagnosis of a psychiatric disorder was made according to DSM-III-R criteria. The overall prevalence rate of psychiatric disorder was only 0.43% with an incidence of 0.43 per 1000 persons. In a cross-sectional survey involving 15 324 household heads who reported on a population of 68 487 people in a district. Some (1994) found that there was at least one person who regularly used drugs in 44.3% of the households. The prevalence of regular drug use was 6.4% for alcohol, 2.7% for cigarette smoking, 0.6% for marijuana and 0.2% for non-prescribed medicines. Significant social, financial, occupational/academic, legal, health and injury related complications were noted. Odek-Ogunde and Pande-Leak (1999) assessed 558 undergraduates with a questionnaire on drug use. The lifetime prevalence of commonly used substances was tobacco (54.7%), alcohol (84.2%), cannabis (19.7%) and inhalants (7.2%). The lifetime prevalence of hard drugs (heroin, cocaine, mandrax, amphetamines and LSD) was low (< 5%). Substance use was commoner in males. Rates for regular use (> 20 days/month) were high for tobacco (24.7%) and alcohol (11.5%). More than half of the subjects started using drugs at upper primary and secondary levels but nearly one fifth started substance use in lower primary school. Kuria (1996) interviewed 547 urban and 405 rural students with the WHO youth survey questionnaire. Alcohol was the most commonly abused drug (15% and 14% in urban and rural schools, respectively). Tobacco, cannabis and inhalants followed in that order. Male students abused drugs more often than female students. 'Hard' drugs were used more often in the rural schools. Ayaya et al (2001) found features of tobacco dependence in 37.6% of street children (n=191) who also frequently used other drugs. Saunders et al (1993) evaluated 1888 subjects in 6 countries. After non-drinkers and known alcoholics had been excluded, 18% of subjects had a hazardous level of alcohol intake and 23% had experienced at least one alcohol-related problem in the previous year. Intercountry variations were noted. Omolo and Dhadphale (1987) found a high prevalence of Khat chewing among patients attending a primary health clinic (n=100). Dhadphale et al (1989) used a two-stage screening procedure to diagnose depression according to ICD-9 descriptions in a primary care sample of 881 patients. The prevalence of depressive disorders was 9.2%, with about a third having moderate to severe depression. Maj et al (1994) conducted a multi-country (including Kenya) WHO Neuropsychiatric AIDS Study. The mean global score on the Montgomery-Asberg Depression Rating Scale was significantly higher in symptomatic seropositive individuals than in matched seronegative controls in all centres. Sebit (1995) reported similar results in a study done in Kenya and Zaire (n=408). Maj (1996) also reported that in contexts where social rejection of HIV-seropositive subjects was harsh, symptomatic stages of HIV infection were associated with a greater prevalence of syndromal depression. Weisz et al (1993) interviewed parents of 11-15 year old children living in different societies – Embu in Kenya, Thai, African-American and Caucasian-American. Caucasian-Americans were rated particularly high on under-controlled problems (e.g. arguing, disobedient at home, cruel to others). Embu children were rated particularly high on over-controlled problems (e.g. fears, feels guilty, somatic concerns), largely because of the numerous somatic problems reported. Geissler et al (1998) identified geophagy in 73% of 285 school children. The prevalence decreased with age until age 15 and then stabilized for girls till age 18 but continued to decrease for boys.

MENTAL HEALTH RESOURCES

Mental Health Policy A mental health policy is absent.

In 1982, Kenya adopted mental health as the ninth essential element of its primary health care provision.

Substance Abuse Policy A substance abuse policy is absent.

National Mental Health Programme A national mental health programme is present. The programme was formulated in 1996. The main emphasis is on decentralization of mental health services, integration into general health care provision and establishment of community mental health services. Multidisciplinary and intersectoral collaboration are a central feature. The implementation of this programme has been slow due to inadequate resources, especially human resources.

National Therapeutic Drug Policy/Essential List of Drugs A national therapeutic drug policy/essential list of drugs is present. It was formulated in 1994.

Mental Health Legislation There is a Mental Health Act. The new act of 1989, provides for voluntary and involuntary treatment of people with mental illness and creates a regulatory board to oversee its implementation (The Act was implemented in May 1991). The latest legislation was enacted in 1989.

Mental Health Financing There are budget allocations for mental health.
The country spends 0.01% of the total health budget on mental health.
The primary sources of mental health financing in descending order are tax based, out of pocket expenditure by the patient or family, private insurances and social insurance.
The National Hospital Insurance Fund is a contributory fund for people in employment. It mainly covers bed charges. About 4.8% of Kenyans have health insurance, but the insurance does not cover mental illness. The Ministry of Health is working on a broader national social health insurance scheme.
The country does not have disability benefits for persons with mental disorders.

Mental Health Facilities Mental health is a part of primary health care system. Actual treatment of severe mental disorders is not available at the primary level.
Regular training of primary care professionals is not carried out in the field of mental health. Health care guidelines for primary health care workers are being developed. Only limited training facilities for training are available. However, a system of referral and back-referral exists and some outreach services have been established. More than 70 traditional health practitioners have been identified and are currently being trained in mental health to improve their intervention skills.
There are no community care facilities for patients with mental disorders.

Psychiatric Beds and Professionals

Total psychiatric beds per 10 000 population	0.4
Psychiatric beds in mental hospitals per 10 000 population	0.3
Psychiatric beds in general hospitals per 10 000 population	0.05
Psychiatric beds in other settings per 10 000 population	0.02
Number of psychiatrists per 100 000 population	0.2
Number of neurosurgeons per 100 000 population	0.01
Number of psychiatric nurses per 100 000 population	2
Number of neurologists per 100 000 population	0.02
Number of psychologists per 100 000 population	0.01
Number of social workers per 100 000 population	0.2

One-third of the total psychiatrists work in the public sector. Mathari is the national referral and teaching hospital. Most of the patients admitted in this hospital are referred by the criminal justice system for assessment. As a result of the new legislation psychiatric wards were set up in general hospitals. The provincial units are 22-bed units. Seven out of 70 district units have also been set up. Nearly half of the psychiatrists are practicing in Nairobi. The provincial and district psychiatric units are under-staffed. Psychiatric nurses and medical officers are involved in mental health care.

Non-Governmental Organizations NGOs are involved with mental health in the country. They are mainly involved in advocacy and rehabilitation.

Information Gathering System There is no mental health reporting system in the country.
The country has no data collection system or epidemiological study on mental health.
The national tally sheets contain only one section relating to mental disorders. A proposal for the inclusion of 8 categories has been submitted as a part of health sector reforms.

Programmes for Special Population Special clinics for children and adolescents are run.

Therapeutic Drugs The following therapeutic drugs are generally available at the primary health care level of the country: carbamazepine, phenobarbital, phenytoin sodium, amitriptyline, chlorpromazine, diazepam, fluphenazine, haloperidol.

Other Information Initially, Kenya had a system of psychiatric practice that was dependent on traditional practices. The first western style system developed in 1912 when a smallpox unit was transformed into a centre where 'mad' people used to be locked up. Today, Mathare Hospital is the mental health referral and training centre. The Government is in the process of legislating to regulate the practice of traditional practitioners and incorporate it into the health sector.

Additional Sources of Information

Ayaya, S. O., Esamai, F. O. (2001) Health problems of street children in Eldoret, Kenya. East African Medical Journal,78, 624-629.

Dadphale, M., Cooper, G., Cartwright-Taylor, L. (1989) Prevalence and presentation of depressive illness in a primary health care setting in Kenya. American Journal of Psychiatry, 146, 659-661.

Geissler, P. W., Mwaniki, D. L., Thiong'o, F., et al (1998) Geophagy, iron status and anaemia among primary school children in Western Kenya. Tropical Medicine & International Health, 3, 529-534.

Kiima, D. M., Njenga, F. G., Okonji, M. O., et al. (2004) Kenya mental health profile. International review of Psychiatry, 16, 48-53.

Kuria, M. W. (1996) Drug abuse among urban as compared to rural secondary schools students in Kenya: a short communication. East African Medical Journal, 73, 339.

Maj, M. (1996) Depressive syndromes and symptoms in subjects with human immunodeficiency virus (HIV) infection. British Journal of Psychiatry, Supplement, 30, 117-122.

Maj, M., Janssen, R., Starace, F., et al (1994) WHO Neuropsychiatric AIDS study, cross-sectional phase I. Study design and psychiatric findings. Archives of General Psychiatry, 51, 39-49.

Ndetei, D. M. (1980). Psychiatry in Kenya: Yesterday, Today and Tomorrow. Acta Psychiatrica Scandinavica, 62, 201-211.

Ndetei, D. M., Muhangi, J. (1979) The prevalence and clinical presentation of psychiatric illness in a rural setting in Kenya. British Journal of Psychiatry, 135, 269-272.

Njenga, F. (2002) Focus on psychiatry in East Africa. British Journal of Psychiatry, 181, 354-359.

Odek-Ogunde, M., Pande-Leak, D. (1999) Prevalence of substance use among students in a Kenyan university: a preliminary report. East African Medical Journal, 76, 301-306.

Omolo, O. E., Dhadphale, M. (1987) Prevalence of khat chewers among primary health clinic attenders in Kenya. Acta Psychiatrica Scandinavica, 75, 318-320.

Saunders, J. B., Aasland, O. G., Amundsen, A., et al (1993) Alcohol consumption and related problems among primary health care patients: WHO collaborative project on early detection of persons with harmful alcohol consumption--I. Addiction, 88, 349-362. Sebit, M. B. (1995) Neuropsychiatric HIV-1 infection study: in Kenya and Zaire cross-sectional phase I and II. Central African Journal of Medicine, 41, 315-322.

Sebit, M. B. (1996) Prevalence of psychiatric disorders in general practice in Nairobi. East African Medical Journal, 73, 631-633.

Siringi, S. (2001). Doctors in Kenya call for fair mental health policy. Lancet, 357, 1273.

Some, E. S. (1994) Misuse of drugs: perceptions of household heads in Kisumu district, Kenya. East African Medical Journal, 71, 93-97.

Weisz, J. R., Sigman, M., Weiss, B., et al (1993) Parent reports of behavioral and emotional problems among children in Kenya, Thailand, and the United States. Child Development, 64, 98-109.

Kiribati

GENERAL INFORMATION

Kiribati is a country with an approximate area of 0.73 thousand sq. km. (UNO, 2001). The country consists of more than 30 islands, two-thirds of which are inhabited. Its population is 0.077 million, and the sex ratio (men per hundred women) is 98 (UNO, 2004). The proportion of population above the age of 60 years is 7% (WHO, 2004).
The country is a lower middle income group country (based on World Bank 2004 criteria). The proportion of health budget to GDP is 8.6%. The per capita total expenditure on health is 143 international $, and the per capita government expenditure on health is 141 international $ (WHO, 2004).
The main language(s) used in the country is (are) English. The largest ethnic group(s) is (are) Micronesian. The largest religious group(s) is (are) Roman Catholic, and the other religious group(s) are (is) Protestant.
The life expectancy at birth is 61.8 years for males and 66.7 years for females (WHO, 2004). The healthy life expectancy at birth is 52 years for males and 56 years for females (WHO, 2004).

EPIDEMIOLOGY

There is a paucity of epidemiological data on mental illnesses in Kiribati in internationally accessible literature.

MENTAL HEALTH RESOURCES

Mental Health Policy A mental health policy is present. The policy was initially formulated in 1999.
The components of the policy are advocacy, promotion, prevention, treatment and rehabilitation.

Substance Abuse Policy A substance abuse policy is absent.

National Mental Health Programme A national mental health programme is present. The programme was formulated in 1999.

National Therapeutic Drug Policy/Essential List of Drugs A national therapeutic drug policy/essential list of drugs is present. It was formulated in 1997.

Mental Health Legislation There is no mental health legislation. Some issues related to mental health are covered in other legislations.
Details about the year of enactment of the mental health legislation are not available.

Mental Health Financing There are no budget allocations for mental health.
The country spends 1.6% of the total health budget on mental health.
The primary source of mental health financing is tax based.
The country does not have disability benefits for persons with mental disorders. There are no social benefits.

Mental Health Facilities Mental health is a part of primary health care system. Actual treatment of severe mental disorders is not available at the primary level.
Regular training of primary care professionals is not carried out in the field of mental health.
There are no community care facilities for patients with mental disorders.

Psychiatric Beds and Professionals

Total psychiatric beds per 10 000 population	7.3
Psychiatric beds in mental hospitals per 10 000 population	7.3
Psychiatric beds in general hospitals per 10 000 population	0
Psychiatric beds in other settings per 10 000 population	0
Number of psychiatrists per 100 000 population	1
Number of neurosurgeons per 100 000 population	0
Number of psychiatric nurses per 100 000 population	0
Number of neurologists per 100 000 population	0
Number of psychologists per 100 000 population	0
Number of social workers per 100 000 population	0

Non-Governmental Organizations NGOs are not involved with mental health in the country.

Information Gathering System There is mental health reporting system in the country. Details can be obtained from the Health Information and Statistics Centre of the Ministry of Health.
The country has no data collection system or epidemiological study on mental health.

Programmes for Special Population There are no special services available.

Therapeutic Drugs The following therapeutic drugs are generally available at the primary health care level of the country: carbamazepine, phenobarbital, phenytoin sodium, amitriptyline, chlorpromazine, diazepam, fluphenazine, haloperidol, lithium, carbidopa, levodopa.

Other Information

Additional Sources of Information

Mental Health Annex 1 (Government document).

Kuwait

GENERAL INFORMATION

Kuwait is a country with an approximate area of 18 thousand sq. km. (UNO, 2001). Its population is 2.595 million, and the sex ratio (men per hundred women) is 151 (UNO, 2004). The proportion of population under the age of 15 years is 26% (UNO, 2004), and the proportion of population above the age of 60 years is 3% (WHO, 2004). The literacy rate is 84.7% for men and 81% for women (UNESCO/MoH, 2004).
The country is a high income group country (based on World Bank 2004 criteria). The proportion of health budget to GDP is 3.9%. The per capita total expenditure on health is 612 international $, and the per capita government expenditure on health is 482 international $ (WHO, 2004).
The main language(s) used in the country is (are) Arabic. The largest ethnic group(s) is (are) Kuwaiti, and the other ethnic group(s) are (is) other Arab. The largest religious group(s) is (are) Muslim (five-sixths).
The life expectancy at birth is 75.4 years for males and 77.7 years for females (WHO, 2004). The healthy life expectancy at birth is 67 years for males and 67 years for females (WHO, 2004).

EPIDEMIOLOGY

There is substantial epidemiological data on mental illnesses in Kuwait in internationally accessible literature. No attempt was made to include this information here.

MENTAL HEALTH RESOURCES

Mental Health Policy A mental health policy is present. The policy was initially formulated in 1957.
The components of the policy are advocacy, promotion, prevention, treatment and rehabilitation.

Substance Abuse Policy A substance abuse policy is present. The policy was initially formulated in 1983.

National Mental Health Programme A national mental health programme is present. The programme was formulated in 1997.

National Therapeutic Drug Policy/Essential List of Drugs A national therapeutic drug policy/essential list of drugs is present. It was formulated in 1980.

Mental Health Legislation There is no written legislation. However, efforts had been made to formalize a legislation, though it has not been successful.
Details about the year of enactment of the mental health legislation are not available.

Mental Health Financing There are budget allocations for mental health.
Details about expenditure on mental health are not available.
The primary sources of mental health financing in descending order are social insurance, private insurances and out of pocket expenditure by the patient or family.
The country has disability benefits for persons with mental disorders. Treatment is provided by the Government and social benefits by the Ministry of Social Affairs.

Mental Health Facilities Mental health is a part of primary health care system. Actual treatment of severe mental disorders is available at the primary level. Primary care is provided by the family doctor. Facilities should be developed further.
Regular training of primary care professionals is carried out in the field of mental health. In the last two years, about 40 personnel were provided training. Primary care physicians and family physicians are attached to specialist mental health services for a 4 and 8 weeks period, respectively.
There are community care facilities for patients with mental disorders. Community care is provided through district and general hospitals and family doctors. Community care facilities are not well developed. However, there are 2 day care centres which cater to more than 30 clients and one half-way house that caters to 30 clients.

Psychiatric Beds and Professionals

Total psychiatric beds per 10 000 population	3.4
Psychiatric beds in mental hospitals per 10 000 population	3.4
Psychiatric beds in general hospitals per 10 000 population	0
Psychiatric beds in other settings per 10 000 population	0
Number of psychiatrists per 100 000 population	3.1
Number of neurosurgeons per 100 000 population	
Number of psychiatric nurses per 100 000 population	22.5
Number of neurologists per 100 000 population	
Number of psychologists per 100 000 population	1.4
Number of social workers per 100 000 population	0.4

There are 19 occupational therapists. There is a plan to increase the beds strength in mental hospital from the current level of 3.4 per 10 000 to 4.58 per 10 000 population in 2005. Some beds have been earmarked for the management of drug abusers (260), geriatric and forensic patients. There is a specialized unit for treating PTSD patients. Although there are more than 1000 psychologists and social workers, only a few work in the field of mental health. Thirty-one of them are employed by the psychiatric hospital which serves as the main psychiatric set-up for Kuwait.

Non-Governmental Organizations NGOs are involved with mental health in the country. They are mainly involved in advocacy, promotion, prevention, treatment and rehabilitation.

Information Gathering System There is mental health reporting system in the country. Only data from the psychiatric hospital is available.
The country has data collection system or epidemiological study on mental health.

Programmes for Special Population The country has specific programmes for mental health for disaster affected population, elderly and children.

Therapeutic Drugs The following therapeutic drugs are generally available at the primary health care level of the country: carbamazepine, ethosuximide, phenobarbital, phenytoin sodium, sodium valproate, amitriptyline, chlorpromazine, diazepam, fluphenazine, haloperidol, lithium, biperiden, carbidopa, levodopa.

Other Information

Additional Sources of Information

Bale, R. (2000) A project to develop quality improvements in the Kuwait mental health service. Journal of Psychiatric Practice, 24, 112-12.

Kyrgyzstan

GENERAL INFORMATION

Kyrgyzstan is a country with an approximate area of 199 thousand sq. km. (UNO, 2001). Its population is 5.208 million, and the sex ratio (men per hundred women) is 96 (UNO, 2004). The proportion of population under the age of 15 years is 31% (UNO, 2004), and the proportion of population above the age of 60 years is 9% (WHO, 2004). The literacy rate is 99% for men and 96% for women (UNESCO/MoH, 2004).
The country is a low income group country (based on World Bank 2004 criteria). The proportion of health budget to GDP is 4%. The per capita total expenditure on health is 108 international $, and the per capita government expenditure on health is 53 international $ (WHO, 2004).
The main language(s) used in the country is (are) Kyrgyz and Russian. The largest ethnic group(s) is (are) Kyrgyz, and the other ethnic group(s) are (is) Russian. The largest religious group(s) is (are) Muslim (three-fourths), and the other religious group(s) are (is) Russian Orthodox Christian.
The life expectancy at birth is 60.4 years for males and 68.9 years for females (WHO, 2004). The healthy life expectancy at birth is 52 years for males and 58 years for females (WHO, 2004).

EPIDEMIOLOGY

There is a paucity of epidemiological data on mental illnesses in Kyrgyzstan in internationally accessible literature. Some commentaries on childhood disabilities (Ul'ianova & Khokhnova, 1977) and alcohol dependence (Urakov & Ismailov, 1975) are available. Zharikov et al (1973) studied the association of age and sex on schizophrenia.

MENTAL HEALTH RESOURCES

Mental Health Policy A mental health policy is present. The policy was initially formulated in 2000.
The components of the policy are advocacy, promotion, prevention, treatment and rehabilitation. Restructuring of the system is also a part of the mental health policy.

Substance Abuse Policy A substance abuse policy is present. The policy was initially formulated in 1998.

National Mental Health Programme A national mental health programme is present. The programme was formulated in 2000.

National Therapeutic Drug Policy/Essential List of Drugs A national therapeutic drug policy/essential list of drugs is present. It was formulated in 1996.

Mental Health Legislation The Law on Psychiatric Assistance and Human Rights.
The latest legislation was enacted in 1999.

Mental Health Financing There are budget allocations for mental health.
The country spends 7.9% of the total health budget on mental health.
The primary source of mental health financing is tax based.
The country has disability benefits for persons with mental disorders.

Mental Health Facilities Mental health is a part of primary health care system. Actual treatment of severe mental disorders is not available at the primary level.
Regular training of primary care professionals is carried out in the field of mental health. In the last two years, about 350 personnel were provided training.
There are no community care facilities for patients with mental disorders.

Psychiatric Beds and Professionals

Total psychiatric beds per 10 000 population	6.25
Psychiatric beds in mental hospitals per 10 000 population	5.62
Psychiatric beds in general hospitals per 10 000 population	0.63
Psychiatric beds in other settings per 10 000 population	0
Number of psychiatrists per 100 000 population	4.5
Number of neurosurgeons per 100 000 population	0.77
Number of psychiatric nurses per 100 000 population	13.7
Number of neurologists per 100 000 population	8
Number of psychologists per 100 000 population	0.4
Number of social workers per 100 000 population	

Non-Governmental Organizations NGOs are involved with mental health in the country. They are mainly involved in advocacy and rehabilitation. A non-governmental organization, 'Awakening', was established with the purpose of uniting families and friends of the mentally ill. The main goal of the organization is the improvement of the standard of living of mentally ill people and their social rehabilitation.

Information Gathering System There is mental health reporting system in the country.
The country has data collection system or epidemiological study on mental health. There is a service data collection system.

Programmes for Special Population A programme for medical care of children with donor support was started.

Therapeutic Drugs The following therapeutic drugs are generally available at the primary health care level of the country: carbamazepine, phenobarbital, sodium valproate, amitriptyline, chlorpromazine, diazepam, fluphenazine, haloperidol.

Other Information

Additional Sources of Information

Toktosunov, E. (2001) Self-help union in the Kyrgyz Republic. Mental Health Reforms, 6, 2-3.

Ul'ianova, L. A., Khokhlova, G. A. (1977) Complex ambulatory balneoclimatic treatment of neurasthenia at the Sochi health resort. Voprosy Kurortologii, Fizioterapii i Lechebnoi Fizicheskoi Kultury, 38-40.

Urakov, I., Ismailov, B. (1975) Problems of alcoholism and the tasks of public health authorities. Zdravookhranenie Kirgizii, 3-6.

Zharikov, N. M., Liberman, I. I., Shmaonova, L. M., et al (1973) Evaluation of the role of sex and age factors in the formation of schizophrenia (according to epidemiological study data). Zhurnal Nevropatologii i Psikhiatrii Imeni S-S-Korsakova, 73, 551-559.

Lao People's Democratic Republic

GENERAL INFORMATION

Lao People's Democratic Republic is a country with an approximate area of 237 thousand sq. km. (UNO, 2001). Its population is 5.787 million, and the sex ratio (men per hundred women) is 100 (UNO, 2004). The proportion of population under the age of 15 years is 41% (UNO, 2004), and the proportion of population above the age of 60 years is 6% (WHO, 2004). The literacy rate is 77.4% for men and 55.5% for women (UNESCO/MoH, 2004).

The country is a low income group country (based on World Bank 2004 criteria). The proportion of health budget to GDP is 3.1%. The per capita total expenditure on health is 51 international $, and the per capita government expenditure on health is 29 international $ (WHO, 2004).

The main language(s) used in the country is (are) Lao. The largest ethnic group(s) is (are) Lao Lourm, and the other ethnic group(s) are (is) Lao Theung and Lao Soung. The largest religious group(s) is (are) Buddhist (three-fifths), and the other religious group(s) are (is) indigenous groups.

The life expectancy at birth is 54.1 years for males and 56.2 years for females (WHO, 2004). The healthy life expectancy at birth is 47 years for males and 47 years for females (WHO, 2004).

EPIDEMIOLOGY

The Opium Survey was conducted across 11 provinces of northern Laos. The average prevalence rate of dependence was almost 3% in those above 15 years of age. Opium dependence was associated with age (age group 41-50 years and 61-70 years) and gender (male) (UNODC and LCDC, 2004). Choulamany (2000) showed that the use of Amphetamine-Type-Stimulants (ATS) had increased since the mid 1980s. Lifetime prevalence of drug use among school population ranged from 5.5% to 17.5% in different regions. ATS use was associated with gender (male), age (15-19 years), socioeconomic status (higher), presence of psychopathology related to methamphetamine use and deterioration in neurocognitive performance. Westermeyer (1976) noted that initially heroin use mostly occurred among indigenous Asian addicts, who had gradually switched from opium to heroin. Following the passage of an anti-opium law, a new group of indigenous addicts emerged: young, single, unemployed males in urban areas whose first narcotic drug was heroin. Gradually, American expatriates also started to use heroin. Westermeyer (1979) estimated opioid dependence rates in 10 communities (representing eight ethnic groups and three provinces). In six rural communities, data were obtained by a house-to-house survey and in four urban communities by opium den registration. Communities raising opium poppy as a cash crop had highest crude rates of dependence (7.0-9.8%). Those involved in opium commerce had intermediate rates (4.1-5.5%). Where neither opium production nor commerce was present the communities had the lowest rates of dependence (1.8-2.3%). Westermeyer (1977) showed that drug use was affected by availability in another study that compared opium use among two cultures in Laos, the Hmong (who have easy access to opium) and the Lao (who have a more difficult access). The Hmong's open availability appeared to favour the following: a greater proportion of female addicts; younger age of opiate usage and addiction; use of the more intoxicating route of administration; earlier onset of problems related to addiction; and shorter duration of addiction before seeking treatment. Westermeyer (1988) reported that much diversity occurred among the various ethnic groups with regard to male-female use of drugs and alcohol. Social changes were reflected in choice of substance made by younger and older people (e.g. cigarettes vs. pipes or cigars, heroin vs. opium, manufactured vs. village-produced alcohol). Westermeyer and Peng (1977) compared 51 heroin dependent patients with 51 matched opium dependent patients. Heroin dependent patients were more often from an urban background, had more frequent daily doses of drug, spent considerably more money for their drug, required higher initial methadone doses for detoxification and showed earlier worsening of condition leading to an earlier treatment contact. Westermeyer (1978a) compared a sample of drug dependent patients of Lao origin with expatriate Asian dependent patients living in Laos. Lao and expatriate addicts show marked similarity in their sociodemographic profiles and patterns of narcotic use. Some differences in their recent use of narcotic drugs appear related to the greater cash income of the expatriate Asians and their greater access to heroin. Treated prevalence figures in the year 2003 and 2004 suggest that neurosis (one-fourth of all cases), Schizophrenia (one-sixth), Epilepsy (one-sixth), Substance abuse (one-tenth) mainly ATS and depression (one-fifteenth) were common (Mental Health Unit, 2004). Westermeyer (1978b) found that subjects with psychosis had reduced longevity as compared to the general population and those with organic psychosis had a greater mortality than those with functional psychosis. Hempel et al (2000) found similarities between patients of Amok and those of sudden mass assault by a single individual. Both groups showed social isolation, loss, depression, anger, pathological narcissism and paranoia. According to a survey conducted by Handicap International and NCRM (1999) in 370 villages in 7 districts (n=400 000) the rate of handicap was 0.8%. Intellectual handicap was the 4th leading cause of disability (10% of all cases) and psychological problems were ranked 6th (7% of all cases), multiple handicaps represented 6% and epilepsy 4% of all disabilities.

MENTAL HEALTH RESOURCES

Mental Health Policy A mental health policy is absent.

Substance Abuse Policy A substance abuse policy is present. The policy was initially formulated in 2003. The Lao National Commission for Drug Control and Supervision (LCDC) launched national drug demand reduction strategies in January 2003, including the following components: prevention, treatment and rehabilitation of drug abuse/drug abusers. It emphasized the need for reliable data collection and drug information systems and the understanding of geographical distribution (e.g. urban versus rural areas), type of risk groups and main categories of substances abused.

National Mental Health Programme A national mental health programme is absent.

National Therapeutic Drug Policy/Essential List of Drugs A national therapeutic drug policy/essential list of drugs is present. It was formulated in 1997.

Mental Health Legislation The article 18 in the penal code mentions that persons suffering from mental disorders are not responsible for committing damages. The code of penal procedure dated on 23/11/1989 gives more details on the process. In most cases, conciliation is obtained either by village leaders or the police before the offences reach the tribunal. It there is a suspicion of mental disorder, the police will lead an investigation and refer the person to the hospital for diagnostic evaluation before sending a report to the tribunal. However, psychiatric evaluation is only available in the capital. Civil damages are to be paid by the family who is considered as responsible. If there is a need to look after the mentally disturbed, the head of the village might be requested to arrange this. Mental illness is not considered as a reason for divorce.
Details about the year of enactment of the mental health legislation are not available.

Mental Health Financing There are no budget allocations for mental health.
Details about expenditure on mental health are not available.
The primary sources of mental health financing in descending order are out of pocket expenditure by the patient or family and tax based.
Nearly all medication have to be bought by the patient's family.
The country has disability benefits for persons with mental disorders.

Mental Health Facilities Mental health is not a part of primary health care system. Actual treatment of severe mental disorders is not available at the primary level.
Regular training of primary care professionals is not carried out in the field of mental health. Two provincial hospitals provide limited mental health care on an outpatient basis because of the availability of two general practitioners who received on-the-job training at the mental health unit of the Mahosot hospital.
There are no community care facilities for patients with mental disorders.

Psychiatric Beds and Professionals

Total psychiatric beds per 10 000 population	0.07
Psychiatric beds in mental hospitals per 10 000 population	0
Psychiatric beds in general hospitals per 10 000 population	0.07
Psychiatric beds in other settings per 10 000 population	0
Number of psychiatrists per 100 000 population	0.03
Number of neurosurgeons per 100 000 population	0.07
Number of psychiatric nurses per 100 000 population	0
Number of neurologists per 100 000 population	0.02
Number of psychologists per 100 000 population	0
Number of social workers per 100 000 population	0

There are two full fledged psychiatric units, one in a general hospital setting and one in the military setting. The mental health unit at Mahosot hospital has 9 general nurses, 2 psychiatrists, 1 neurologist and 4 general practitioners. While the military hospital is staffed with 13 general nurses and 4 general practitioners. All psychiatrists and neurologists were trained in Europe.

Non-Governmental Organizations NGOs are involved with mental health in the country. They are mainly involved in advocacy, promotion, prevention, treatment and rehabilitation. NGOs focus on the management of substance use issues. Monks have participated in TV and radio programmes on health promotion and prevention of drug abuse. In 2002, they sponsored youth gatherings in temples as part of a national campaign on drug abuse. Save the Children/UK and UNICEF provide some child mental health services. Handicap International provide free access to care for people suffering from epilepsy and mental handicap/retardation in some sites in collaboration with the mental health unit. However, these services are mainly accessible to those living in and around the Capital.

Information Gathering System There is mental health reporting system in the country. Reporting system on mental health is still in a preliminary stage of development and is mainly based on daily data register of out and inpatients seeking treatment at the mental health unit, Mahosot Hospital. This unit sends monthly data to the Department of Planning and Statistics of the Ministry of Health.

The country has no data collection system or epidemiological study on mental health. A mental health situation analysis (Didier & Choulmany, 2002) was carried out using in-depth interviews, with medical professionals and key informants including village leaders, teachers, monks or healers, focus groups and case reports. Lao folk diagnosis of mental problems covered 32 types. Spiritual causes were perceived as being predominant, followed by genetic and biological causes. Karma was referred as well as a cause. People suffering from mental health problems had had several ways of seeking help or services, e.g. modern medicines, moral support, traditional medicine, religious treatment and magical string and traditional souls calling ceremony. Major mental illnesses were also discussed.

Programmes for Special Population Details about any special mental health programmes are not available.

Detoxification centres are available in the community where opium dependent patients are detoxified using tincture of opium, mainly in the northern parts of the country. The cost of a 15 day detoxification, including medication and food for the opium addict, was found to be around US$ 25 per addict. This does not include logistics costs for Government staff and villagers. (Kham Noan Hsam: Community Based Treatment and Rehabilitation as part of Drug Demand Reduction in on-going UNODC projects in the Northern Provinces of the Lao PDR, 2002). However, there is no rehabilitation programme.

Therapeutic Drugs The following therapeutic drugs are generally available at the primary health care level of the country: phenobarbital, diazepam.

The 4th revision was made in 2004.

J–M

Other Information

Additional Sources of Information

Choulamany, C. (2000, 2001) 'Drug abuse among youth in Lao PDR'.

Choulamany, C., et al. (July 2003) 'Evaluating the treatment of ATS abuse in the Mental Health Unit, Mahosot Hospital'.

Bertrand, D., Choulamany, C. (December 2002) 'Mental health situation analysis in Lao PDR'.

Einfield, S. (1999) Child psychiatry in Laos. Australasian Psychiatry, 7, 189-191.

Government document (2000) République Démocratique Populaire LAO. Paix, Indépendence, Démocratie, Unité, Prosperité.

Hempel, A. G., Levine, R. E., Meloy, J. R., et al (2000) A cross-cultural review of sudden mass assault by a single individual in the oriental and occidental cultures. Journal of Forensic Sciences, 45, 582-588.

Kham Noan Hsam: Community Based Treatment and Rehabilitation as part of Drug Demand Reduction in on-going UNODC Projects in the Northern Provinces of the Lao PDR, 2002.

LCDC and UNODC (2003) 'National drug demand reduction strategies'.

Mental Health Unit (October 2004) 'Statistics on new mental health cases seeking treatment at the Mental Health Unit, from 2000 – 2004'.

Service de Santé Mentale (Government document).

UNODC and LCDC (July 2004) 'Laos Opium Survey 2004'.

Westermeyer, J. (1976) The pro-heroin effects of anti-opium laws in Asia. Archives of General Psychiatry, 33, 1135-1139.

Westermeyer, J. (1977) Narcotic addiction in two Asian cultures: a comparison and analysis. Drug & Alcohol Dependence, 2, 273-285.

Westermeyer, J. (1977) Opium and heroin addicts in Laos. I. A comparative study. Journal of Nervous & Mental Disease, 164, 346-350.

Westermeyer, J. (1978a) Indigenous and expatriate addicts in Laos: a comparison. Culture, Medicine & Psychiatry, 2, 139-150.

Westermeyer, J. (1978b) Mortality and psychosis in a peasant society. Journal of Nervous & Mental Disease, 166, 769-774.

Westermeyer, J. (1979) Influence of opium availability on addiction rates in Laos. American Journal of Epidemiology, 109, 550-562.

Westermeyer, J. (1988) Sex differences in drug and alcohol use among ethnic groups in Laos, 1965-1975. American Journal of Drug & Alcohol Abuse, 14, 443-461.

Westermeyer, J., Peng, G. (1977) Opium and heroin addicts in Laos. II. A study of matched pairs. Journal of Nervous & Mental Disease, 164, 351-354.

Latvia

GENERAL INFORMATION

Latvia is a country with an approximate area of 65 thousand sq. km. (UNO, 2001). Its population is 2.286 million, and the sex ratio (men per hundred women) is 85 (UNO, 2004). The proportion of population under the age of 15 years is 15% (UNO, 2004), and the proportion of population above the age of 60 years is 22% (WHO, 2004). The literacy rate is 99.8% for men and 99.7% for women (UNESCO/MoH, 2004).

The country is a higher middle income group country (based on World Bank 2004 criteria). The proportion of health budget to GDP is 6.4%. The per capita total expenditure on health is 509 international $, and the per capita government expenditure on health is 267 international $ (WHO, 2004).

The main language(s) used in the country is (are) Latvian. The largest ethnic group(s) is (are) Latvian, and the other ethnic group(s) are (is) Russian. The largest religious group(s) is (are) Evangelical Lutheran.

The life expectancy at birth is 64.6 years for males and 75.8 years for females (WHO, 2004). The healthy life expectancy at birth is 58 years for males and 68 years for females (WHO, 2004).

EPIDEMIOLOGY

Wasserman et al (1998 a) reported that suicide rates in the former USSR during 1984-1990 varied greatly between different regions, from 3.5 cases per 100 000 inhabitants in the Caucasus (Georgia, Azerbaijan and Armenia) to 28.0 in the Baltic region (Latvia, Lithuania and Estonia). This pattern was observed for both men and women, with suicide rates for men ranging from 4.9 in the Caucasian region to 45.9 in the Baltics, and suicide rates for women ranging from 2.1 in the Caucasus to 2.3 in the Baltics. During 1984-90, a decline in suicide rates of 32% for males and 19% for females took place in the former Soviet Union (Wasserman et al, 1998b). During 1968-84, the mean value of male suicide rates per 100 000 males and females in Latvia was 52.5 and 14.3, respectively. Suicide rates fell across all the Republics of the USSR during Perestroika. In Latvia, the male suicide rate reduced by 26.6% in the period 1986-90 compared to 1968-84. Female suicide rates were relatively stable and the male-female ratio reduced from 3.7 in 1968-84 to 3.1 in 1986-90 (Varnik et al, 1994). Rancans et al (2001a) found that there were rapid swings of suicide rates during 1980-98, driven by changes in male suicide rates which reached a maximum of 72 per 100 000 population in 1993. The sudden drop in gross domestic product, the rapid increase in first-time alcohol psychosis and the percentage of people unemployed did not correspond strictly with the dynamics of suicide rates. Rancans et al (2001b) found that the overall rate of suicide attempts in a city was 149 per 100 000. The male to female ratio for persons aged 15 years or more was 1:0.9. The highest figures were for females aged 15-24 and men aged 25-34. Females used poisonings in 75% of cases. Males used more violent methods (60%) like cutting, and suicide was associated with alcohol use in men. In a sample of 1412 Latvian liquidators drawn from the State Latvian Chernobyl Clean-up Workers Registry, Viel et al (1997) found greater psychosomatic distress in those exposed to work for longer periods of time in hazardous work areas.

MENTAL HEALTH RESOURCES

Mental Health Policy A mental health policy is present. The policy was initially formulated in 2004.
The components of the policy are advocacy, promotion, prevention, treatment and rehabilitation. The work on the basic document for state mental health has started.

Substance Abuse Policy A substance abuse policy is present. The policy was initially formulated in 2004. Details about the drug policy can be obtained from the Latvia Drug Control and Drug Abuse Prevention Masterplan (1999-2003). The Alcohol use control programme (2004-2008) has been initiated.

National Mental Health Programme A national mental health programme is present. The programme was formulated in 2004. The adopted State Health Care Programme also includes the Psychiatric Aid Strategy and an underlying action plan (national mental health programme) with financial sources and evaluation activities.

National Therapeutic Drug Policy/Essential List of Drugs A national therapeutic drug policy/essential list of drugs is present. It was formulated in 1996.

Mental Health Legislation The most recent legislation on mental health is the Medical Law. In 1999, the new Latvian Criminal Law introduced the concept of diminished responsibility; however, the law was drafted without consultation with mental health professionals.
The latest legislation was enacted in 1997.

Mental Health Financing There are budget allocations for mental health.
The country spends 6.3% of the total health budget on mental health.
The primary sources of mental health financing in descending order are tax based, social insurance, private insurances and out of pocket expenditure by the patient or family.

There are state budget allocations for mental health services through the State Compulsory Health Insurance Agency. The social security system is responsible for severely mentally ill and handicapped children and adolescents until the age of 18 years, covering expenses for medication, shelter and rehabilitation.
The country has disability benefits for persons with mental disorders.

Mental Health Facilities Mental health is a part of primary health care system. Actual treatment of severe mental disorders is available at the primary level. The psychiatrist at the local level promote networking and support services and support local primary health care specialists. Treatment of moderately severe and severe mental disorders is done by psychiatrists.
Regular training of primary care professionals is carried out in the field of mental health. In the last two years, about 160 personnel were provided training. There are training programmes for family doctors and general physicians. Training is provided through seminars, workshops and conferences as well as through general programmes and diplomas. Latvia has a community of well-trained mental health professionals who are committed to the welfare of people with mental illness. Since independence, many staff have received training in psychotherapy and other techniques which were not used before.
There are community care facilities for patients with mental disorders. The state plans and coordinates activities, ensures psychiatric aid with the highly specialized services and ensures academic training. Regional services include inpatient facilities, day hospitals and ambulatory models. The local aid and support services are divided into treatment oriented aid and medical rehabilitation and support services. Rehabilitation is provided through employment centres and psychosocial rehabilitation houses.

Psychiatric Beds and Professionals

Total psychiatric beds per 10 000 population	13.8
Psychiatric beds in mental hospitals per 10 000 population	13.5
Psychiatric beds in general hospitals per 10 000 population	0.3
Psychiatric beds in other settings per 10 000 population	0
Number of psychiatrists per 100 000 population	10
Number of neurosurgeons per 100 000 population	2
Number of psychiatric nurses per 100 000 population	40
Number of neurologists per 100 000 population	10
Number of psychologists per 100 000 population	2
Number of social workers per 100 000 population	0.5

The system remains centred on large under-funded mental hospitals and nursing homes; large institutions consume most of the available mental health budget, while community care is under funded. The process of deinstitutionalization, however, has begun, and a 25% reduction in the number of beds in psychiatric hospitals has been achieved. Almost 160 beds are allotted to child and adolescent psychiatry. The trend in psychiatric institutions in Latvia is now towards the establishment of multidisciplinary teamwork – a process which is still in its infancy. Multidisciplinary teamwork is available in some hospitals. Generally, the multidisciplinary team in Latvia consists of: a nurse, nursing assistant, psychologist, psychiatrist, rehabilitation specialist and social worker. Occupational therapists help the patient develop and improve their functioning, while observing changes in the patient's state, analysing the results of therapy, as well as assessing the level of current functioning and gradually increasing the complexity of exercises. Rehabilitation specialists help the patients to acquire skills such as drawing, painting, pottery and flower arranging. Additional training or refresher courses of mental health professionals is being organized with help from Denmark, Norway, Sweden, Germany and the Netherlands. The country has almost 30 child and adolescent psychiatrists.

Non-Governmental Organizations NGOs are involved with mental health in the country. They are mainly involved in advocacy. NGOs are involved in running alternative mental health services. The Soros Foundation supports many projects. Self-help groups have also developed.

Information Gathering System There is mental health reporting system in the country.
The country has data collection system or epidemiological study on mental health. There are accounting information systems, reports and registers from which data can be collected.

Programmes for Special Population The country has specific programmes for mental health for disaster affected population, indigenous population, elderly and children.
A programme directed at suicide prevention that incorporates psychotherapeutic support groups and telephone hotlines has been organized in collaboration with the Soros Foundation. The World Bank is supporting a project on mental health promotion and prevention of mental disorders. Child and adolescent psychiatric services are restricted to cities. A few youth centres for handicapped adolescents have been started.

Therapeutic Drugs The following therapeutic drugs are generally available at the primary health care level of the country: carbamazepine, ethosuximide, phenobarbital, sodium valproate, amitriptyline, chlorpromazine, diazepam, fluphenazine, haloperidol, lithium, carbidopa, levodopa.
Cyclodol is available instead of biperiden (commonest strength: 2 mg, cost for 100 tablets: 1.62 USD)

Other Information The Psychiatry Aid Strategy of Latvia has certain priorities: patients with serious mental disorders, mentally ill offenders, children and teenagers, young schizophrenics, patients with comorbidity and elderly. The policy project Improving of Citizens' Mental Health Status is based on WHO World Health Report 2001.

Additional Sources of Information

Fedosejeva, R., Girgensons, R. (2000) The mentally ill in prison: developments in Latvia. Lancet, 356 (suppl. 1), 47.

Kishuro, A. (1999) Child and adolescent psychiatry in Latvia. In: H. Remschmidt, H. van Engeland (Eds). Child and Adolescent Psychiatry in Europe. Historical Developments, Current Situation, Future Perspectives. Darmstadt, Steinkopff. pp197-204.

National Drug Control and Drug Abuse Combat Coordination Committee and UNDCP (1999). Latvia Drug Control and Drug Abuse Prevention Masterplan for the Period 1999 – 2003.

Rancans, E., Alka, I., Renberg, E. S., et al (2001b) Suicide attempts and serious suicide threats in the city of Riga and resulting contacts with medical services. Nordic Journal of Psychiatry, 55, 279-286.

Rancans, E., Salander, Renberg E., et al (2001a) Major demographic, social and economic factors associated to suicide rates in Latvia 1980-98. Acta Psychiatrica Scandinavica, 103, 275-281.

Varnik, A., Wasserman, D., Eklund, G. (1994) Suicides in the Baltic countries, 1968-90. Scandinavian Journal of Social Medicine, 22, 166-169.

Viel, J. F., Curbakova, E., Dzerve, B., et al (1997) Risk factors for long-term mental and psychosomatic distress in Latvian Chernobyl liquidators. Environmental Health Perspectives, 105, 1539-1544.

Wasserman, D., Varnik, A., Dankowicz, M. (1998a) Regional differences in the distribution of suicide in the former Soviet Union during perestroika, 1984-1990. Acta Psychiatrica Scandinavica, Supplement 394, 5-12.

Wasserman, D., Varnik, A., Eklund, G. (1998b) Female suicides and alcohol consumption during perestroika in the former USSR. Acta Psychiatrica Scandinavica, Supplement 394, 26-33.

Lebanon

GENERAL INFORMATION

Lebanon is a country with an approximate area of 10 thousand sq. km. (UNO, 2001). Its population is 3.708 million, and the sex ratio (men per hundred women) is 96 (UNO, 2004). The proportion of population under the age of 15 years is 28% (UNO, 2004), and the proportion of population above the age of 60 years is 9% (WHO, 2004). The literacy rate is 92.1% for men and 80.3% for women (UNESCO/MoH, 2004).

The country is a higher middle income group country (based on World Bank 2004 criteria). The proportion of health budget to GDP is 12.2%. The per capita total expenditure on health is 673 international $, and the per capita government expenditure on health is 189 international $ (WHO, 2004).

The main language(s) used in the country is (are) Arabic. The largest ethnic group(s) is (are) Arab. The largest religious group(s) is (are) Muslim (two-thirds), and the other religious group(s) are (is) Christian (almost one third) and Druz.

The life expectancy at birth is 67.6 years for males and 72 years for females (WHO, 2004). The healthy life expectancy at birth is 59 years for males and 62 years for females (WHO, 2004).

EPIDEMIOLOGY

Weissman et al (1996, 1997) conducted a study in 10 countries including Lebanon to estimate the rates and patterns of major depression, bipolar disorder and panic disorder based on cross-national epidemiologic surveys (n=40 000). The lifetime rates for major depression ranged from 1.5% in Taiwan to 19% in Beirut. The annual rates ranged from 0.8% in Taiwan to 5.8% in New Zealand. The mean age at onset showed less variation, and the rates of major depression were higher for women than men at all sites. Major depression was also associated with increased risk for comorbidity with substance abuse and anxiety disorders at all sites. The lifetime rates of bipolar disorder were more consistent across countries (0.3% in Taiwan to 1.5% in New Zealand). The sex ratios were nearly equal and the age at first onset was on an average 6 years earlier than the onset of major depression. The lifetime prevalence rates for panic disorder ranged from 0.4% in Taiwan to 2.9% in Italy. The mean age at first onset was usually in early to middle adulthood, and females were affected more than males. Panic disorder was associated with an increased risk of agoraphobia and major depression in all countries. Karam et al (2000) conducted a study on a stratified cluster sample of 1851 students from two major universities using the Diagnostic Interview Schedule (DIS) and DSM-III criteria. They found that the prevalence of alcohol, nicotine, tranquilizer and heroin use was 49.4%, 18.3%, 10.2% and 0.4%, respectively. Alcohol abuse was present in 2.1% and alcohol dependence in 2.4%. Abuse and dependence of other substances besides nicotine and alcohol ranged between 0.1 to 0.8%. Naja et al (2000) found that in a randomly selected community sample of 1000 people, the prevalence of benzodiazepine use during the past month was 9.6%, with half being dependent on the drug. Current use was associated with age greater than 45 years, female gender, cigarette smoking and recent life events. Karam et al (1998) interviewed randomly selected 658 subjects, aged 18-65 years, from four Lebanese communities with the Arabic version of the DIS (DSM-III-R criteria) and the War Events Questionnaire. The lifetime prevalence of major depression across the four communities varied from 16.3 to 41.9%. Level of exposure to war and a history of pre-war depression predicted the development of depression during war. Chaaya et al (2002) interviewed about 400 postpartum women at two points in time, 24 hours and 3-5 months after delivery. During the latter visit, subjects were screened using the Edinburgh Postnatal Depression Scale. The overall prevalence of postpartum depression was 21%, but it was significantly lower in urban (16%) compared to the rural (26%) area. Lack of social support and prenatal and lifetime depression, stressful life events, vaginal delivery, poor education, unemployment and chronic health problems were significantly related to postpartum depression. El Khoury et al (1999) used the DIS to interview a group of women (n=150) at two points in time of pregnancy, the first on the second post-delivery day and the second, one year later. The prevalence of major depression was 31.3% during lifetime, 10% during pregnancy and 10.9% during one year follow-up. Lifetime depression was associated with the number of children in the household. Depression during pregnancy was inversely related to economic and educational level. Weissman et al (1999) assessed over 40 000 subjects in 9 countries including Lebanon, using the DIS. The lifetime prevalence of suicide ideation ranged from 2.1% (Lebanon) to 18.5% (New Zealand) and for suicide attempts from 0.7% (Lebanon) to 5.9% (Puerto Rico). Women had a 2-3 fold higher rate of suicide attempts than men in most countries. Suicide ideation and attempts were associated with being divorced/separated. Chiementi et al (1989) used a questionnaire to interview mothers of more than 1000 three to nine year old children. Children who had experienced death of a family member, forced displacement of family or destruction of home or had witnessed death were about 1.7 times more likely to exhibit nervous, regressive, aggressive and depressive behaviour than those who had not experienced trauma. Macksoud and Aber (1996) interviewed 224 Lebanese children (10-16 years old) and found that PTSD varied according to the number and level of stressful exposure. Various types of war traumas were differentially related to PTSD, mental health symptoms and adaptational outcomes.

MENTAL HEALTH RESOURCES

Mental Health Policy A mental health policy is absent.

Substance Abuse Policy A substance abuse policy is absent.

National Mental Health Programme A national mental health programme is present. The programme was formulated in 1987. Though the national mental health programme had been initiated in 1987, its progress has not been satisfactory due to the war.

National Therapeutic Drug Policy/Essential List of Drugs A national therapeutic drug policy/essential list of drugs is present. It was formulated in 1987.

Mental Health Legislation Details about the mental health legislation are not available.

Mental Health Financing There are no budget allocations for mental health.
Details about expenditure on mental health are not available.
The primary sources of mental health financing in descending order are tax based, out of pocket expenditure by the patient or family and social insurance.
Lebanon depends mainly on the private sector for the provision of health services. The Ministry of Health has contracts with the private sector and needy patients receive free treatment.
The country does not have disability benefits for persons with mental disorders. There is no disability funding for mental health.

Mental Health Facilities Mental health is a part of primary health care system. Actual treatment of severe mental disorders is not available at the primary level. In order to improve mental health services the Government is shifting from comprehensive care to areas of importance. The two areas of importance have been ambulatory mental health service within the primary care centres and a psychogeriatric care system within a comprehensive geriatric service with emphasis on a community-oriented programme.
Regular training of primary care professionals is not carried out in the field of mental health. A training programme was supposed to have started in 2001. General practitioners and general nurses receive 2-3 months training. Training is also under way on psychogeriatric issues.
There are no community care facilities for patients with mental disorders.

Psychiatric Beds and Professionals

Total psychiatric beds per 10 000 population	7.5
Psychiatric beds in mental hospitals per 10 000 population	7.4
Psychiatric beds in general hospitals per 10 000 population	0.1
Psychiatric beds in other settings per 10 000 population	
Number of psychiatrists per 100 000 population	2
Number of neurosurgeons per 100 000 population	1
Number of psychiatric nurses per 100 000 population	5.3
Number of neurologists per 100 000 population	3
Number of psychologists per 100 000 population	0.6
Number of social workers per 100 000 population	1.5

The figures for personnel are approximations. The number of psychologists working in mental health is around 10% of the total number of psychologists. There is only one psychiatric hospital run by the nuns. This centre also runs schools, medical clinics and hospice centres. All psychiatrists have private clinics.

Non-Governmental Organizations NGOs are involved with mental health in the country. They are mainly involved in prevention, treatment and rehabilitation.

Information Gathering System There is mental health reporting system in the country.
The country has no data collection system or epidemiological study on mental health.

Programmes for Special Population The country has specific programmes for mental health for children.
A comprehensive system of care has been developed for management of some child psychiatric disorders like attention-deficit/ hyperactivity disorder.

Therapeutic Drugs The following therapeutic drugs are generally available at the primary health care level of the country: carbamazepine, phenobarbital, phenytoin sodium, sodium valproate, amitriptyline, chlorpromazine, diazepam, fluphenazine, haloperidol, lithium, biperiden, carbidopa, levodopa.
All drugs (including second and third generation anti-psychotics, anti-depressants, anti-convulsants and non-conventional medication) can be prescribed by primary care physicians and are available free of cost for poor patients through Ministry of Health.

Other Information

Additional Sources of Information

Aboujaoude, E. (1982) The psychiatric hospital of the cross: a sane asylum in the Middle East. American Journal of Psychiatry, 159, 1982.

Chaaya, M., Campbell, O. M., El Kak, F., et al (2002) Postpartum depression: prevalence and determinants in Lebanon. Archives of Women's Mental Health, 5, 65-72.

Chimienti, G., Nasr, J. A., Khalifeh, I. (1989) Children's reactions to war-related stress. Affective symptoms and behaviour problems. Social Psychiatry & Psychiatric Epidemiology, 24, 282-287.

El Khoury, N., Karam, E. G., Melhem, N. M. (1999) Depression and pregnancy. Journal Médical Libanais, 47, 169-174.

Fayyad, J. A., Jahshan, C. S., Karam, E. G. (2001) Systems development of child mental health services in developing countries. Child & Adolescent Psychiatric Clinics of North America, 10, 745-762.

Karam, E. G., Howard, D. B., Karam, A. N., et al (1998) Major depression and external stressors: The Lebanon Wars. European Archives of Psychiatry & Clinical Neuroscience, 248, 225-230.

Karam, E., Melhema, N., Mansour, C., et al (2000) Use and abuse of licit and illicit substances: prevalence and risk factors among students in Lebanon. European Addiction Research, 6, 189-197.

Macksoud, M. S., Aber, J. L. (1996) The war experiences and psychosocial development of children in Lebanon. Child Development, 67, 70-88.

Mohit, A. (2001). Mental health and psychiatry in the Middle East: historical development. Eastern Mediterranean Health Journal, 7, 336-347.

Naja, W. J., Pelissolo, A., Haddad, R. S., et al (2000) A general population survey on patterns of benzodiazepine use and dependence in Lebanon. Acta Psychiatrica Scandinavica, 102, 429-431.

Weissman, M. M., Bland, R. C., Canino, G. J., et al (1996) Cross-national epidemiology of major depression and bipolar disorder. JAMA, 276, 293-299.

Weissman, M. M., Bland, R. C., Canino, G. J., et al (1997) The cross-national epidemiology of panic disorder. Archives of General Psychiatry, 54, 305-309.

Weissman, M. M., Bland, R. C., Canino, G. J., et al (1999) Prevalence of suicide ideation and suicide attempts in nine countries. Psychological Medicine, 29, 9-17.

Lesotho

GENERAL INFORMATION

Lesotho is a country with an approximate area of 30 thousand sq. km. (UNO, 2001). Its population is 1.8 million, and the sex ratio (men per hundred women) is 87 (UNO, 2004). The proportion of population under the age of 15 years is 39% (UNO, 2004), and the proportion of population above the age of 60 years is 7% (WHO, 2004). The literacy rate is 73.7% for men and 90.3% for women (UNESCO/MoH, 2004).

The country is a low income group country (based on World Bank 2004 criteria). The proportion of health budget to GDP is 5.5%. The per capita total expenditure on health is 101 international $, and the per capita government expenditure on health is 80 international $ (WHO, 2004).

The main language(s) used in the country is (are) English and Sesotho. The largest ethnic group(s) is (are) Sesotho. The largest religious group(s) is (are) Christian.

The life expectancy at birth is 32.9 years for males and 38.2 years for females (WHO, 2004). The healthy life expectancy at birth is 30 years for males and 33 years for females (WHO, 2004).

EPIDEMIOLOGY

In a small community based study done in 2001, that involved all adults in a small lowland town, depression (10%) and anxiety (8%) were found to be common. The female to male ratio was 3:1. These rates were deemed similar to levels observed in the neighbouring country – South Africa (Makara, 2004). Hollifield et al (1990) interviewed adults in a village to determine the community prevalence of major depression, panic disorder and generalized anxiety disorder using the Diagnostic Interview Schedule. There was a significantly higher prevalence of all three diagnoses in Lesotho as compared with the United States. Women were at an increased risk for these disorders, although statistical significance was not demonstrated for depression. In an inpatient sample (year 2002), the point prevalence (n= 376) of mental disorders was as follows: 29% had cannabis related mental disorders, 20.2 % had psychotic disorders, 17% had schizophrenia, 9% had organic mental disorders, 7.2% had bipolar mood disorders 6.4% had depression and 6.1% had alcohol related disorders. A similar audit of outpatients (year 2003) showed that about one-third of patients had epilepsy related diagnosis and 17% had depression. Depression was five times more common in women in comparison to men. Schizophrenia (14.6%) and alcohol and drug related mental disorders (9.3%) were also common (Makara, 2004). Hollifield et al (1994) conducted a study in the outpatient clinic of a general hospital to assess depression, generalized anxiety and panic disorder using a translated version of the Diagnostic Interview Schedule and DSM-III-R criteria. Out of the 126 randomly selected out-patients the researchers found that 23% had depression, 24% had panic disorder and 29% had GAD. Forty-six (36%) had either depression or panic disorder, with thirteen having concurrent illness. Patients with depression and/or panic disorder presented with a significantly higher number of physical symptoms and a higher percentage of symptoms that were pain or autonomic nervous system related than patients with no disorder ever. As part of a larger baseline survey of community health status, Siegfried et al (2001) randomly sampled households in 29 villages. Consenting adults (n=348) participated in a face-to-face interview about alcohol use, which included the CAGE. Blood was taken from participants for CDT determination.53% of men (37/69) and 19% of women (53/279) reported drinking alcohol. 36% of men and 9% of women were found to have hazardous patterns of drinking as per predefined criteria. Hazardous drinkers were significantly more likely to be male and older. Using hazardous drinking as the standard, CAGE (score >=2) had a positive predictive value of 75% for men and 62% for women. CDT values also showed high specificity. Meursing and Morojele (1989) conducted a study to ascertain degree of alcohol consumption and attitudes and knowledge of alcohol use among 1133 high school students aged 11-22 years. They primarily used a questionnaire but additional information was obtained by means of classroom discussion and detailed interviews. About half of the students (54% of the boys and 42% of the girls) had drunk alcohol at some point in their lives. Drinking was found to be related to age, sex, drinking of friends, family income and drinking in the family.

MENTAL HEALTH RESOURCES

Mental Health Policy A mental health policy is absent.
The mental health policy is in the draft stage. It is likely to be adopted in 2005.

Substance Abuse Policy A substance abuse policy is absent. The substance abuse policy is also in the draft stage.

National Mental Health Programme A national mental health programme is present. The programme was formulated in 1964.

National Therapeutic Drug Policy/Essential List of Drugs A national therapeutic drug policy/essential list of drugs is absent.

Mental Health Legislation There is the Mental Health Law No. 7. It is being updated.
The latest legislation was enacted in 1964.

Mental Health Financing There are budget allocations for mental health.
The country spends 7% of the total health budget on mental health.
The primary source of mental health financing is tax based.
The country has disability benefits for persons with mental disorders. Psychosocial assessment is done and needy patients are being financially supported. However, this is in some areas only.

Mental Health Facilities Mental health is a part of primary health care system. Actual treatment of severe mental disorders is available at the primary level. The primary level care is provided through health centre/clinics where mental health services are integrated into the general health care and are carried out by general nurses with support and supervision from psychiatric nurses from local hospitals. Regular training of primary care professionals is carried out in the field of mental health. There is a continuous medical education programme for mental health workers at secondary care level (psychiatric nurses and medical officers). Community health workers are trained in four project areas and in future this will be extended to other areas.
There are community care facilities for patients with mental disorders. Community care is available through health posts where integrated services are carried out by community health workers. Support is also provided by mobile units comprising of psychiatric nurses and by resident social workers.

Psychiatric Beds and Professionals

Total psychiatric beds per 10 000 population	0.8
Psychiatric beds in mental hospitals per 10 000 population	0.3
Psychiatric beds in general hospitals per 10 000 population	0.5
Psychiatric beds in other settings per 10 000 population	0
Number of psychiatrists per 100 000 population	0.05
Number of neurosurgeons per 100 000 population	0
Number of psychiatric nurses per 100 000 population	0.2
Number of neurologists per 100 000 population	0
Number of psychologists per 100 000 population	0.09
Number of social workers per 100 000 population	1.2

Mohlomi Hospital is the national main referral hospital with 60 beds. Services are delivered by a multi-disciplinary team consisting of 1 psychiatrist, 2 psychologists, 3 social workers, 3 occupational therapists and 20 psychiatric nurses. Secondary level care is available though 9 Treatment and Observation Units attached to General Districts Hospital and is provided by psychiatric nurses. There is only one psychiatrist for the whole country but psychiatric nurses receive in-services training (workshops) once a year in order to effectively manage patients.

Non-Governmental Organizations NGOs are involved with mental health in the country. They are mainly involved in advocacy, promotion, prevention, treatment and rehabilitation. The Christian Health of Lesotho (CHAL), the main partner in health service provision is also involved in all mental health care services including promotion, curative and rehabilitative services.

Information Gathering System There is mental health reporting system in the country. Mental health statistics are integrated in the Health Management Systems collected daily and reported monthly for compilation and analysis. Annual Statistics are published regularly together with other statistics generated by the Ministry of Health and Social Welfare.
The country has data collection system or epidemiological study on mental health. Service data collection is present.

Programmes for Special Population A proposal supported by the African Development Bank Project for specialized services for children, elderly and forensic patients has been developed. These services will be initiated in the year 2005.
Two Drug and Alcohol Rehabilitation Centres based in the city of Maseru offer services for clients with problems related to substance abuse.

Therapeutic Drugs The following therapeutic drugs are generally available at the primary health care level of the country: phenobarbital, phenytoin sodium, amitriptyline, chlorpromazine, diazepam.
The therapeutic drug policy is in the draft stage. Anti-psychotics and anti-epileptics are given free to the indoor and outdoor patients. Carbamazepine, ethosuximide, fluphenazine, haloperidol, lithium and biperiden are available at the secondary level of care and sodium valproate is available at the tertiary level. All of the above mentioned drugs are in the drug list.

Other Information The Government of Lesotho adopted the strategy of primary health care in 1979. The country is divided into 18 Health Service Areas based on catchment areas of 18 hospitals that supervise 165 satellite health centres. The health centres in turn supervise Village Health Workers at community level. Almost half of the health facilities are owned by the Christian Health Association of Lesotho (CHAL). The complimentary services delivered by CHAL and the Government covers almost 80% of the population (i.e. almost 80% of the population lives within 2 hours walking distance form a static health facility). A resident Fly Doctors Service covers inaccessible mountain areas.

Additional Sources of Information

Hollifield, M., Katon, W., Morojele, N. (1994) Anxiety and depression in an outpatient clinic in Lesotho, Africa. International Journal of Psychiatry in Medicine, 24, 179-188.

Hollifield, M., Katon, W., Spain, D., et al (1990) Anxiety and depression in a village in Lesotho, Africa: a comparison with the United States. British Journal of Psychiatry, 156, 343-350.

Makara, M. (2004). Information on Lesotho Mental Health Profile. (Personal Communication)

Meursing, K., Morojele, N. (1989) Use of alcohol among high school students in Lesotho. British Journal of Addiction, 84, 1337-1342.

Siegfried, N., Parry, C. D. H., Morojele, N. K., et al (2001) Profile of drinking behaviour and comparison of self-report with the CAGE questionnaire and carbohydrate-deficient transferring in a rural Lesotho community. Alcohol & Alcoholism, 36, 243-248.

Liberia

GENERAL INFORMATION

Liberia is a country with an approximate area of 111 thousand sq. km. (UNO, 2001). Its population is 3.487 million, and the sex ratio (men per hundred women) is 100 (UNO, 2004). The proportion of population under the age of 15 years is 47% (UNO, 2004), and the proportion of population above the age of 60 years is 4% (WHO, 2004). The literacy rate is 72.3% for men and 39.3% for women (UNESCO/MoH, 2004).
The country is a low income group country (based on World Bank 2004 criteria). The proportion of health budget to GDP is 4.3%. The per capita total expenditure on health is 127 international $, and the per capita government expenditure on health is 97 international $ (WHO, 2004).
The main language(s) used in the country is (are) English. The largest ethnic group(s) is (are) African. The largest religious group(s) is (are) Christian (four-fifths), and the other religious group(s) are (is) Muslim (one-sixth).
The life expectancy at birth is 40.1 years for males and 43.7 years for females (WHO, 2004). The healthy life expectancy at birth is 34 years for males and 37 years for females (WHO, 2004).

EPIDEMIOLOGY

There is a paucity of epidemiological data on mental illnesses in Liberia in internationally accessible literature. Swiss et al (1998) assessed a random sample of 205 women and girls between the ages of 15 and 70 years (88% participation rate). And found that 49% of them reported experiencing at least 1 act of physical or sexual violence by a soldier or fighter. 15% had been raped, subjected to attempted rape, or sexually coerced. Women who were accused of belonging to a particular ethnic group or fighting faction or who were forced to cook for a soldier or fighter were at increased risk for physical and sexual violence. Young women (those younger than 25 years) were more likely than women 25 years or older to report experiencing attempted rape and sexual coercion.

MENTAL HEALTH RESOURCES

Mental Health Policy A mental health policy is absent.
From September 2004, an emergency mental health strategy is being developed in collaboration between MOH and WHO.

Substance Abuse Policy A substance abuse policy is absent. An emergency substance abuse strategy has been integrated in an overall emergency mental health strategy being developed in collaboration between the Ministry of Health and WHO.

National Mental Health Programme A national mental health programme is absent.

National Therapeutic Drug Policy/Essential List of Drugs A national therapeutic drug policy/essential list of drugs is present. It was formulated in 1970.

Mental Health Legislation The Public Health Act refers to mental health. There is no mental health legislation as such.
The latest legislation was enacted in 1970.

Mental Health Financing There are no budget allocations for mental health.
Details about expenditure on mental health are not available.
The primary source of mental health financing is out of pocket expenditure by the patient or family.
There are no budget allocations for mental health within MOH. Funds were earlier allocated within the Regional University Hospital (JFK) to a psychiatric hospital, but the hospital was destroyed in 1990.
The country does not have disability benefits for persons with mental disorders.

Mental Health Facilities Mental health is not a part of primary health care system. Actual treatment of severe mental disorders is not available at the primary level.
Regular training of primary care professionals is not carried out in the field of mental health.
There are no community care facilities for patients with mental disorders. A few facilities offer layman counselling and shelter, but these services do not cater to the needs of the severely mentally ill.

Psychiatric Beds and Professionals

Total psychiatric beds per 10 000 population	0.08
Psychiatric beds in mental hospitals per 10 000 population	0.08
Psychiatric beds in general hospitals per 10 000 population	0
Psychiatric beds in other settings per 10 000 population	0
Number of psychiatrists per 100 000 population	0.03
Number of neurosurgeons per 100 000 population	0
Number of psychiatric nurses per 100 000 population	0.03
Number of neurologists per 100 000 population	0
Number of psychologists per 100 000 population	0
Number of social workers per 100 000 population	0

There is only one psychiatrist and one psychiatric nurse in the country. No mental health services are currently available in the country as the psychiatric hospital was destroyed during the war. Under the emergency programme, a 25-bedded public hospital is reopening in Monrovia in Fall 2004 along with limited outpatient functions. These will constitute the only clinical mental health services in the country. Mental health is integrated in pre-graduate training of nurses and doctors, but due to the war and the lack of clinical services, the training is sporadic and mainly theoretical. Special training programmes for mental health are not present. The emergency programme plans restarting of in-service training and has restarted training of medical students.

Non-Governmental Organizations NGOs are involved with mental health in the country. They are mainly involved in advocacy and prevention. One NGO is involved in reconstruction of emergency mental health services. A few other international NGOs are mainly involved in psychosocial and trauma work. A few local NGOs provide services for substance misuse.

Information Gathering System There is no mental health reporting system in the country.
The country has no data collection system or epidemiological study on mental health. There is a strong need, but no current resources, for a national survey on needs and resources in mental health and substance abuse.

Programmes for Special Population There are no services for special population groups.

Therapeutic Drugs The following therapeutic drugs are generally available at the primary health care level of the country: phenobarbital, phenytoin sodium, amitriptyline, chlorpromazine, diazepam, haloperidol.
The listed therapeutic drugs are generally not available at the primary health care level. The list and prices are based on pharmacy prices in the capital. Prices vary significantly (minimum and maximum prices from survey 2004 is shown). Benzhexol (5 mg) is used as anti-parkinsonian drugs.

Other Information There is an urgent need for needs assessment as because of the civil war mental health problems have increased. Technical help is needed.
The years of war have had a significant effect on the deterioration of the health system in general with an expected shift also in the population in need of mental health care. Besides patients with classic mental health problems, there are now also serious war/conflict related mental health problems including substance abuse, while resources (funds and professional staff) for assistance are few or non-existent. There are no systematic or recent Needs and Resource Assessment of Mental Health and Substance abuse. In fall 2004, nearly all mental health services were closed due to lack of resources (funds and staff). Traditional and religious healing is common in the communities. The Ministry of Health has appointed a focal point for Mental Health in September 2004. Funding for the Mental Health emergency programme is urgently needed.

Additional Sources of Information

Jense, S. B., Harris, L. (2004) Mental health in Liberia: a 2-year emergency intervention plan report: WHO Liberia.

Swiss, S., Jennings, P. J., Aryee, G. V., et al (1998) Violence against women during the Liberian civil conflict. JAMA, 279, 625-629.

Libyan Arab Jamahiriya

GENERAL INFORMATION

Libyan Arab Jamahiriya is a country with an approximate area of 1760 thousand sq. km. (UNO, 2001). Its population is 5.659 million, and the sex ratio (men per hundred women) is 107 (UNO, 2004). The proportion of population under the age of 15 years is 30% (UNO, 2004), and the proportion of population above the age of 60 years is 6% (WHO, 2004). The literacy rate is 91.8% for men and 70.7% for women (UNESCO/MoH, 2004).

The country is a higher middle income group country (based on World Bank 2004 criteria). The proportion of health budget to GDP is 2.9%. The per capita total expenditure on health is 239 international $, and the per capita government expenditure on health is 134 international $ (WHO, 2004).

The main language(s) used in the country is (are) Arabic, Italian and English. The largest ethnic group(s) is (are) Berber and Arab. The largest religious group(s) is (are) Muslim.

The life expectancy at birth is 70.4 years for males and 75.5 years for females (WHO, 2004). The healthy life expectancy at birth is 62 years for males and 65 years for females (WHO, 2004).

EPIDEMIOLOGY

There is a paucity of epidemiological data on mental illnesses in Libyan Arab Jamahariya in internationally accessible literature. Avasthi et al (1991) conducted a study on 1009 psychiatric in-patients. Using ICD-9 descriptions, they found schizophrenic psychosis in 39%, affective psychosis in 17%, neurotic disorders in 12%, organic psychosis in 8% and acute psychosis in 7%. Neurotic depression was the commonest type of neurotic disorder, and anti-social personality was the commonest among personality disorders. Pu et al (1986) did a sociodemographic study on 100 patients suffering from hysteria in one particular area. Verma (1990) conducted a cytogenetic analysis of cases of Down syndrome and found the prevalence to be 1 in 516 live births. 82% of the mothers of cases of Down syndrome were over 30 years of age as compared to 36% of the mothers of controls. Cytogenetically 96% of the cases were that of trisomy 21.

MENTAL HEALTH RESOURCES

Mental Health Policy A mental health policy is absent.
In Libya, the mental health policy is part of the general health policy.

Substance Abuse Policy A substance abuse policy is absent.

National Mental Health Programme A national mental health programme is present. The programme was formulated in 1988. The national mental health programme was put forward with the objective of providing essential mental health care for all in all spheres of life, like work, family, community and national growth.

National Therapeutic Drug Policy/Essential List of Drugs Details about the national therapeutic drug policy/essential list of drugs are not available.

Mental Health Legislation A ministerial resolution No. 654 in 1975 regulates the treatment of mentally ill in mental hospitals. It requires to be revised. There is a national committee looking into the aspect of a new legislation.
The latest legislation was enacted in 1975.

Mental Health Financing There are no budget allocations for mental health.
Details about expenditure on mental health are not available.
Details about sources of financing are not available.
The country has disability benefits for persons with mental disorders. A monthly stipend of 90 Libyan Dinars is provided to the mentally disabled.

Mental Health Facilities Mental health is a part of primary health care system. Actual treatment of severe mental disorders is available at the primary level.
Regular training of primary care professionals is carried out in the field of mental health. Psychiatric services are integrated in the primary care system. Training programmes for social workers, primary care physicians and clinical psychologists are components of the mental health programme. However, the facilities are poor and manuals for doctors and workers are not available.
There are community care facilities for patients with mental disorders.

Psychiatric Beds and Professionals

Total psychiatric beds per 10 000 population	1
Psychiatric beds in mental hospitals per 10 000 population	1
Psychiatric beds in general hospitals per 10 000 population	0
Psychiatric beds in other settings per 10 000 population	0
Number of psychiatrists per 100 000 population	0.18
Number of neurosurgeons per 100 000 population	0.18
Number of psychiatric nurses per 100 000 population	0.5
Number of neurologists per 100 000 population	0.15
Number of psychologists per 100 000 population	5
Number of social workers per 100 000 population	1.5

Most of psychologists are social psychologists. There are beds for the mentally retarded (500), elderly (130), drug abusers (50) and children, besides the beds mentioned. Patients with drug abuse are admitted only once. There is an acute shortage of occupational therapists.

Non-Governmental Organizations Details about NGO facilities in mental health are not available.

Information Gathering System Details about mental health reporting systems are not available.
Details about data collection system or epidemiological study on mental health are not available.
Hospital data collection is done.

Programmes for Special Population The country has specific programmes for mental health for elderly and children.
There are services for children and elderly and also forensic psychiatry services.

Therapeutic Drugs The following therapeutic drugs are generally available at the primary health care level of the country: unknown.

Other Information

Additional Sources of Information

Avasthi, A., Khan, M. K., Elroey, A. M. (1991) Inpatient sociodemographic and diagnostic study from a psychiatric hospital in Libya. International Journal of Social Psychiatry, 37, 267-279.

Pu, T., Mohamed, E., Imam, K., et al (1986) One hundred cases of hysteria in eastern Libya. A socio-demographic study. British Journal of Psychiatry, 148, 606-609.

Verma, I. C., Mathews, A. R., Faquih, A., et al (1990) Cytogenetic analysis of Down syndrome in Libya. Indian Journal of Pediatrics, 57, 245-248.

Lithuania

GENERAL INFORMATION

Lithuania is a country with an approximate area of 65 thousand sq. km. (UNO, 2001). Its population is 3.422 million, and the sex ratio (men per hundred women) is 87 (UNO, 2004). The proportion of population under the age of 15 years is 18% (UNO, 2004), and the proportion of population above the age of 60 years is 20% (WHO, 2004). The literacy rate is 99.6% for men and 99.6% for women (UNESCO/MoH, 2004).
The country is a higher middle income group country (based on World Bank 2004 criteria). The proportion of health budget to GDP is 6%. The per capita total expenditure on health is 478 international $, and the per capita government expenditure on health is 337 international $ (WHO, 2004).
The main language(s) used in the country is (are) Lithuanian. The largest ethnic group(s) is (are) Lithuanian, and the other ethnic group(s) are (is) Russian and Polish. The largest religious group(s) is (are) Roman Catholic (five-sixths).
The life expectancy at birth is 66.2 years for males and 77.6 years for females (WHO, 2004). The healthy life expectancy at birth is 59 years for males and 68 years for females (WHO, 2004).

EPIDEMIOLOGY

Data from treatment services records show that about 4.6% of the total population sought treatment in mental health services (2.6% for mental disorders and 2% for drug use disorders). A pressing problem is the spread of drug use disorders. In 1994, there were only 26.1 clients per 100 000 and their number increased to 135.2 per 100 000 in 2003. Moreover, 11.5% of them were juveniles. In treatment samples, considerable increase was also noted of patients with affective disorders and Alzheimer disease, likely due to improved access to services and better recognition (Gaizauskiene et al, 2003; Davidoniene, 2004; State Mental Health Centre, 2004). Gailiene et al (1995) used national archive data to study suicide trends in Lithuania in 1924-39 and 1962-93. In pre-war independent Lithuania (1924-39), the suicide rate was 5-10 per 100 000 citizens. During the Soviet period, it gradually increased to 35.8 per 100 000 in 1984. During the period of perestroika, the suicide rate diminished (25.1 per 100 000 in 1986). In 1993, the rate had again increased to 42/100 000 because of economic hardships (Varnik et al, 1994) and has remained extremely high – 42.1 per 100 000 population in 2003. The rate was higher among the elderly (Davidoniene, 2004). Between 1968-84 the male suicide rate rose gradually from 33.0 to 61.3 and the female rate from 8.0 to 13.1; the average male and female suicide rates per 100 000 population for this period were 51.7 and 10.4, respectively. The mean male suicide rate dropped by 14.4% in 1986-90 compared to 1968-84, though the female suicide rate remained stable, and the male-female ratio was accordingly lower in 1986-90 (4.2) than in 1968-84 (5.0) (Varnik et al, 1994). Currently, very high suicide rates are seen among males (up to 77.2 per 100 000) and rural population (62.8 per 100 000) (Davidoniene, 2004). Kalediene (1999) also found that between 1970-95, age-standardized suicide rates had almost doubled in Lithuania. There was an increase in suicides in birth cohorts of males from 1910 to 1950, and in cohorts born after 1965. In females, an increase was observed in all successive birth years from 1905 to 1925 and after 1970. The period effect in males and the cohort effect in females were dominant. Suicide rates in the former USSR during 1984-90 varied greatly between different regions, from 3.5 cases per 100 000 inhabitants in the Caucasus (Georgia, Azerbaijan and Armenia) to 28.0 in the Baltic region (Latvia, Lithuania and Estonia). The same pattern was observed for both men and women, with suicide rates for men ranging from 4.9 in the Caucasian region to 45.9 in the Baltics, and suicide rates for women ranging from 2.1 in the Caucasus to 2.3 in the Baltics. During 1984-90, a decline in suicide rates of 32% for males and 19% for females took place in the former Soviet Union (Varnik & Wasserman, 1992; Wasserman et al, 1998 a, b). It was shown that the time of year, solar activity and geomagnetic activity were related to the monthly death distribution, especially regarding death from IHD and suicide. Age and gender differences were apparent in the relationship between death distribution and physical environmental factors (Stoupel et al, 2002). Ramanauskiene et al (2002) interviewed more than 5000 adolescents in three regions and found that prevalence of depressive symptoms varied from 47.9% and 58.8% and the suicidal ideas varied from 13.2% and 15.4%. Girls attempted suicide more often. Ribakoviene (2002), compared girls who attempted suicide and an age and locality matched control group of schoolgirls. Suicide attempters demonstrated significantly more internalized behaviour especially depression, somatic complaints, aggression and delinquency. Ribakoviene and Puras (2002) found that compared to healthy adolescent girls, girls with suicide attempts were more often from families that were broken, conflictual or financially strained. They also reported a greater frequency of abuse, conduct symptoms (truancy, arguments, delinquency) and poor academic performance. Puras (1987) estimated that severe mental retardation occurred in 0.3% of children aged 4-13 years. There were a higher number of males among the cases with undifferentiated forms.

MENTAL HEALTH RESOURCES

Mental Health Policy A mental health policy is present. The policy was initially formulated in 1993.
The components of the policy are advocacy, promotion, prevention, treatment and rehabilitation.

Substance Abuse Policy A substance abuse policy is present. The policy was initially formulated in 1999. There are different policies on substance abuse, including the Goverment Commission on Drug Control (1995), the State Alcohol Control Programme (1999) and the National Drug Control and Drug Use Prevention Programme (1999).

National Mental Health Programme A national mental health programme is present. The programme was formulated in 1999. Details are available from the website: www.vpsc.lt. The National Programme for Prevention of Mental Disorders (1999) has the following main goals: to stabilize the morbidity of mental disorders, to reduce the rate of suicide, to develop an effective system of rehabilitation and reintegration into society of persons with mental disabilities, to develop a network of municipal mental health centres, to provide for adequate human resources, to develop a system of monitoring suicides and mental disorders and to develop intersectoral cooperation in the field of mental health. Lithuania has a national strategy for suicide prevention and a draft national programme for the same.

National Therapeutic Drug Policy/Essential List of Drugs A national therapeutic drug policy/essential list of drugs is present. It was formulated in 1995.
Details can be obtained from the State Medicines Control Agency at the Ministry of Health of the country (www.vvkt.lt).

Mental Health Legislation The Law on Mental Health was passed in 1995. There is also a law on substance dependence – Law of the Control of Narcotic and Psychotropic Substances (1998). Under the Mental Health Act, each municipality has to establish a mental health centre for outpatient care. A psychiatrist, a child and adolescent psychiatrist, a psychologist and a social worker are included in the list of obligatory team members. Currently, there are 59 centres throughout the country, and it is estimated that there should be about 100 in the near future. An increasing number of municipal mental health centres are effectively cooperating with local social services, schools and other services. Consumer rights are assured in the Civil Code, the Patient's Rights and Compensation Harm to Health Law and the Mental Health Care Law.
The latest legislation was enacted in 1995.

Mental Health Financing There are budget allocations for mental health.
The country spends 7% of the total health budget on mental health.
The primary source of mental health financing is social insurance.
The national health insurance system allocates a certain amount of money per inhabitant for primary mental health care. After active lobbying, the amount of money allocated per inhabitant for municipal mental health rose from the equivalent of $0.7 in 1997 to $2.8 in 1999. Of the insurance funds, 49%, 37% and 14% are directed towards inpatient services, psychotropic drugs and outpatient services, respectively. There exist three levels of prescription coverage to outpatients with specified diagnoses: 100%, 80% and 50%. The 100% coverage is applied to the treatment of schizophrenia and schizoaffective disorder (including new generation neuroleptic like amisulpride, clozapine, olanzapine, risperidone, and quetepine). The 80% coverage is stipulated for the remaining psychotic disorders, moderate/severe depression (including anti-depressants of the new generation) and dementia. The 50% cover applies to organic psychoses. The insurance does not pay for the services of non-medical professionals (psychologists, speech therapists, social workers) and for day care. A recent proposal suggests the need for mixed funding (from health insurance and from budget) for mental health services. Drug abuse centres and mental health programmes of specific sectors (defence, interior affairs, education) are covered by the state budget and long term care institutions are financed through social welfare budget. A lot of progress has been made in the field of drug and alcohol abuse prevention – now officially recognized as integrated into Lithuanian public health provision, since it is attracting the maximum amount of funding given to prevention programmes. Private health insurance and accumulative funds systems are currently not in place.
The country has disability benefits for persons with mental disorders. Severe mental illness leading to global disturbance of functioning is considered for disability benefits.

Mental Health Facilities Mental health is a part of primary health care system. Actual treatment of severe mental disorders is not available at the primary level. Severe mental disorders are treated at secondary and tertiary psychiatric care levels.
Regular training of primary care professionals is carried out in the field of mental health. In the last two years, about 287 personnel were provided training. General physicians have been trained.
There are community care facilities for patients with mental disorders. Starting in 1998-1999, an increasing number of projects (supported by the Soros Foundation, state budget programmes and other sources) directed towards community-based services for mentally ill people have been developed. Currently, there are 64 mental health centres with multidisciplinary teams consisting of psychiatrists (adult, child and dependences), nurses, social workers and psychologists. Social service agency and various NGOs also provide care for the mentally ill in the community. Many new schools and day care centres have been opened for moderately or severely mentally retarded children and young adults who would have been institutionalized in the earlier system.

Psychiatric Beds and Professionals

Total psychiatric beds per 10 000 population	10
Psychiatric beds in mental hospitals per 10 000 population	8.6
Psychiatric beds in general hospitals per 10 000 population	1.1
Psychiatric beds in other settings per 10 000 population	0.3
Number of psychiatrists per 100 000 population	15

Number of neurosurgeons per 100 000 population	2
Number of psychiatric nurses per 100 000 population	36
Number of neurologists per 100 000 population	14
Number of psychologists per 100 000 population	5
Number of social workers per 100 000 population	

The process of deinstitutionalization was started with persons affected by mental retardation due to active efforts of Viltis, a voluntary organization of parents of mentally challenged individuals. About 200 beds for alcohol and drug abusers, 130 beds for child and adolescent mental health care and 110 beds for forensic services are available. Most of mental health professionals are still working in mental hospitals. About 50 psychiatrists provide child and adolescent services.

Non-Governmental Organizations NGOs are involved with mental health in the country. They are mainly involved in advocacy, promotion and rehabilitation. Viltis is an organization formed by parents of children with mental handicaps. It has been able to bring about great changes in mental health care in Lithuania. It is now gradually beginning to function as a reform model for the surrounding countries.

Information Gathering System There is mental health reporting system in the country. Data are collected from mental health care institutions and state mental health centres and included in the annual report.
The country has data collection system or epidemiological study on mental health. Only data from the state mental health centre on morbidity and sickness with mental disorders and suicides are available.

Programmes for Special Population The whole population of Lithuania is provided with mental health care. Emergency mental health care is provided for every person including tourists.
Programmes dealing with prevention of suicide, juvenile delinquency, child abuse, violence and drug and alcohol abuse have been launched. Three large institutions under the Ministry of Social Welfare and a large network of special schools (more than 40 throughout Lithuania) cater to the needs of mentally challenged children.

Therapeutic Drugs The following therapeutic drugs are generally available at the primary health care level of the country: carbamazepine, ethosuximide, phenobarbital, phenytoin sodium, sodium valproate, amitriptyline, chlorpromazine, diazepam, fluphenazine, haloperidol, lithium, biperiden, levodopa.
A special list of medicines is compensated by the Sickness Funds.

Other Information The joint efforts of professionals, non-governmental organizations, politicians, mass media, and the general public has led to a new level of awareness about the burden of mental disorders on society and effective ways of their prevention.

Additional Sources of Information

Davidoniene, O. (2004) Mental health care reform in Lithuania: the main trends (Personal Communication).

Gailiene, D., Domanskiene, V., Keturakis, V. (1995) Suicide in Lithuania. Archives of Suicide Research, 1, 149-158.

Kalediene, R. (1999) Time trends in suicide mortality in Lithuania. Acta Psychiatrica Scandinavica, 99, 419-422.

Kishuro, A. (1999) Child and adolescent psychiatry in Latvia. In: H. Remschmidt, H. van Engeland (Eds). Child and Adolescent Psychiatry in Europe. Historical Developments, Current Situation, Future Perspectives. Darmstadt, Steinkopff. pp 197-204.

Lithuanian Ministry for Health and Lithuanian Health Information Centre (1998). Health Statistics of Lithuania.

Polubinskaya, S.V. (2000) Reform in Psychiatry in Post-Soviet Countries. Acta Psychiatrica Scandanavia, 101 (suppl. 399), 106-108.

Puras, D. K. (1987) Severe mental retardation in an urban child population. Zhurnal Nevropatologii i Psikhiatrii Imeni S-S-Korsakova, 87, 389-392.

Ramanauskiene, T., Matulioniene, V., Martinkiene, V. (2002) Depression and suicidal risk of the adolescents (comparative analysis in the cities of Klaipeda, Kaunas and Siauliai). Medicina (Kaunas), 38, 393-397.

Ribakoviene, V. (2002) Externalizing and internalizing problems of adolescent suicide attempters. Medicina (Kaunas), 38, 398-404.

Ribakoviene, V., Puras, D. (2002) Relationships between social factors and suicidal attempts of adolescent girls. Medicina (Kaunas), 38, 379-386.

Stoupel, E., Israelevich, P., Petrauskiene, J., et al (2002) Cosmic rays activity and monthly number of deaths: a correlative study. Journal of Basic & Clinical Physiology & Pharmacology, 13, 23-32.

Timmermans, H. (1998) Projects in progress. Mental Health Reforms, 3, 18.

Varnik, A., Wasserman, D. (1992) Suicides in the former Soviet republics. Acta Psychiatrica Scandinavica, 86, 76-78.

Varnik, A., Wasserman, D., Eklund, G. (1994) Suicides in the Baltic countries, 1968-90. Scandinavian Journal of Social Medicine, 22, 166-169.

Wasserman, D., Varnik, A., Dankowicz, M. (1998a) Regional differences in the distribution of suicide in the former Soviet Union during perestroika, 1984-1990. Acta Psychiatrica Scandinavica, Supplement 394, 5-12.

Wasserman, D., Varnik, A., Eklund, G. (1998b) Female suicides and alcohol consumption during perestroika in the former USSR. Acta Psychiatrica Scandinavica, Supplement 394, 26-33.

Gaizauskiene, A., et al (2003) Health Statistics of Lithuania 2003, Lithuanian Health Information Centre: www.lsic.lt

State Mental Health Centre (2004) Statistical data of State Mental Health Centre: www.vpsc.lt

Luxembourg

GENERAL INFORMATION

Luxembourg is a country with an approximate area of 3 thousand sq. km. (UNO, 2001). Its population is 0.459 million, and the sex ratio (men per hundred women) is 97 (UNO, 2004). The proportion of population under the age of 15 years is 19% (UNO, 2004), and the proportion of population above the age of 60 years is 18% (WHO, 2004). The literacy rate is 99% for men and 99% for women (UNESCO/MoH, 2004).
The country is a high income group country (based on World Bank 2004 criteria). The proportion of health budget to GDP is 6%. The per capita total expenditure on health is 2905 international $, and the per capita government expenditure on health is 2611 international $ (WHO, 2004).
The main language(s) used in the country is (are) Luxembourgish, German and French. The largest ethnic group(s) is (are) Celtic. The largest religious group(s) is (are) Roman Catholic.
The life expectancy at birth is 75.7 years for males and 81.7 years for females (WHO, 2004). The healthy life expectancy at birth is 69 years for males and 74 years for females (WHO, 2004).

EPIDEMIOLOGY

There is substantial epidemiological data on mental illnesses in Luxembourg in internationally accessible literature. No attempt was made to include this information here.

MENTAL HEALTH RESOURCES

Mental Health Policy A mental health policy is present. The policy was initially formulated in 1991.
The components of the policy are prevention, treatment and rehabilitation.

Substance Abuse Policy A substance abuse policy is present. The policy was initially formulated in 1995. It consists of a drug substitution programme, syringe distribution, books and special locations for drug abusers.

National Mental Health Programme A national mental health programme is present. The programme was formulated in 1991. The document was prepared after consultation with WHO and a large representative panel of concerned professionals, institutions and NGOs.

National Therapeutic Drug Policy/Essential List of Drugs A national therapeutic drug policy/essential list of drugs is present. It was formulated in 1992.

Mental Health Legislation The law on compulsory admission of persons with mental disorders is the latest legislation on mental health.
The latest legislation was enacted in 2000.

Mental Health Financing There are budget allocations for mental health.
The country spends 13.4% of the total health budget on mental health.
The primary sources of mental health financing in descending order are social insurance, tax based, private insurances and out of pocket expenditure by the patient or family.
The country has disability benefits for persons with mental disorders. Similar benefits as per physical illnesses are provided.

Mental Health Facilities Mental health is a part of primary health care system. Actual treatment of severe mental disorders is available at the primary level.
Regular training of primary care professionals is carried out in the field of mental health.
There are community care facilities for patients with mental disorders. During the 1990s, the evolution of services was constant. Different day-centres and sheltered living and work places offered all aspects of community mental health care. Gradually de-institutionalization has become more advanced.

Psychiatric Beds and Professionals

Total psychiatric beds per 10 000 population	10.5
Psychiatric beds in mental hospitals per 10 000 population	7.5
Psychiatric beds in general hospitals per 10 000 population	3
Psychiatric beds in other settings per 10 000 population	0
Number of psychiatrists per 100 000 population	12
Number of neurosurgeons per 100 000 population	0.9
Number of psychiatric nurses per 100 000 population	35
Number of neurologists per 100 000 population	4
Number of psychologists per 100 000 population	28
Number of social workers per 100 000 population	35

Over the last three decades, almost a three-fourth reduction in number of psychiatry beds has been achieved. In addition, a significant proportion of currently available beds are in the general hospital sector. Mental health services are easily accessible, e.g. in schools through governmental or non-governmental (financed by public authorities) agencies. During the last one and a half decade, staff working in community psychiatric care increased tenfold.

Non-Governmental Organizations NGOs are involved with mental health in the country. They are mainly involved in advocacy, promotion, prevention and treatment.

Information Gathering System There is mental health reporting system in the country. There is an annual report of the Ministry of Health.
The country has data collection system or epidemiological study on mental health. Data collection is done by the Ministry of Health and the 'Union Des Caisses De Maladie'.

Programmes for Special Population The country has specific programmes for mental health for refugees, disaster affected population, indigenous population, elderly and children.
Support networks are available for young people as well as adults suffering from, or in danger of, developing mental health problems.

Therapeutic Drugs The following therapeutic drugs are generally available at the primary health care level of the country: carbamazepine, ethosuximide, phenobarbital, phenytoin sodium, sodium valproate, amitriptyline, diazepam, fluphenazine, haloperidol, lithium, biperiden, carbidopa, levodopa.
All drugs are reimbursed either partly or wholly. Chlorpromazine is not available in the market since last year.

Other Information At the end of the 1980s, the authorities became conscious that there was an urgent need to modernize mental health care. The Ministry of Health appointed the Central Institute for Mental Health of Mannheim (Germany) to examine the situation in Luxembourg and make recommendations for organizational models of psychiatric care. The research work was done all over the country and was published in 1993 as Mental Health Care in Luxembourg, Current State and Recommendations for Future Development. The recommendations referred to results of international research and evaluation studies on psychiatric care, as well as to reliably reported experience in different European countries. Having full regard to the needs of psychiatric patients, this part of the study was submitted to a group of WHO experts, who gave an international dimension to the work. This helped the local decision-makers to propose optimal solutions, regardless of the pressure from local interest groups. These proposals were designed in collaboration with the national health authorities to serve as guidelines for the future development of psychiatric care in Luxembourg. This described the principles, guidelines, and priorities, as well as a timetable to implement the recommendations, depending on the available financial resources.

Additional Sources of Information

Memorial – Offical Journal of Luxemborg. (2000) Amendment to Legislation Concerning the Placement of the Mentally Ill and the Application of Criminal Law to the Mentally Ill, Memorial A, nr. 95, September 7, 2000.

Ministry of Health (2000) Annual Report. March 2001.

Origer, A. (2000) Annual National Report on the Drug Situation. European Monitoring Centre for Drugs and Drug Addiction.

Rössler, W., Salize, H. J., Häfner, H. (1993) Gemeindepsychiatrie Grundlagen und Leitlinien – Planungsstudie Luxemborg. Verlag Integrative Psychiatrie.

Madagascar

GENERAL INFORMATION

Madagascar is a country with an approximate area of 587 thousand sq. km. (UNO, 2001). Its population is 17.901 million, and the sex ratio (men per hundred women) is 99 (UNO, 2004). The proportion of population under the age of 15 years is 44% (UNO, 2004), and the proportion of population above the age of 60 years is 5% (WHO, 2004). The literacy rate is 73.6% for men and 59.7% for women (UNESCO/MoH, 2004).

The country is a low income group country (based on World Bank 2004 criteria). The proportion of health budget to GDP is 2%. The per capita total expenditure on health is 20 international $, and the per capita government expenditure on health is 13 international $ (WHO, 2004).

The main language(s) used in the country is (are) Malagasy and French. The largest ethnic group(s) is (are) Merina and Betsileo, and the other ethnic group(s) are (is) Betsimisaraka, Bara, Tsimihety, Sakalava, etc. The largest religious group(s) is (are) indigenous groups, and the other religious group(s) are (is) Christian, Muslim and sects like Jesosy Mamonjy.

The life expectancy at birth is 54.4 years for males and 58.4 years for females (WHO, 2004). The healthy life expectancy at birth is 47 years for males and 50 years for females (WHO, 2004).

EPIDEMIOLOGY

There is a paucity of epidemiological data on mental illnesses in Madagascar in internationally accessible literature. A national survey carried out in 2003 showed that disabilities were diagnosed in 8% of the population. One-fifth of the disabled people had mental (intellectual) deficiencies and 2.3% had mental illness (psychic deficiencies) (MoH, 2004). Ratsifandrihamanana and Terrnova (1961) analysed 92 cases of delirium in a mental hospital and compared the symptoms with those seen in European patients.

MENTAL HEALTH RESOURCES

Mental Health Policy A mental health policy is present. The policy was initially formulated in 2000.
The components of the policy are advocacy, promotion, prevention, treatment and rehabilitation.

Substance Abuse Policy A substance abuse policy is absent.

National Mental Health Programme A national mental health programme is present. The programme was formulated in 2000.

National Therapeutic Drug Policy/Essential List of Drugs A national therapeutic drug policy/essential list of drugs is present. It was formulated in 2000.

Mental Health Legislation The mental health law dates back to the 19th century.
The latest legislation was enacted in 1838.

Mental Health Financing There are budget allocations for mental health.
The country spends 0.82% of the total health budget on mental health.
The primary sources of mental health financing in descending order are tax based, out of pocket expenditure by the patient or family, social insurance and private insurances.
The country has disability benefits for persons with mental disorders. Persons suffering from mental illness can avail 6-12 months of leave.

Mental Health Facilities Mental health is a part of primary health care system. Actual treatment of severe mental disorders is available at the primary level. Mental health is being integrated into districts.
Regular training of primary care professionals is carried out in the field of mental health. Training models and tools are being worked out.
There are no community care facilities for patients with mental disorders.

Psychiatric Beds and Professionals

Total psychiatric beds per 10 000 population	0.17
Psychiatric beds in mental hospitals per 10 000 population	0.08
Psychiatric beds in general hospitals per 10 000 population	0.08
Psychiatric beds in other settings per 10 000 population	0.01
Number of psychiatrists per 100 000 population	0.08
Number of neurosurgeons per 100 000 population	0.013
Number of psychiatric nurses per 100 000 population	0.3
Number of neurologists per 100 000 population	0.08
Number of psychologists per 100 000 population	0.03
Number of social workers per 100 000 population	0.02

Non-Governmental Organizations NGOs are involved with mental health in the country. They are mainly involved in advocacy, promotion, prevention, treatment and rehabilitation.

Information Gathering System There is mental health reporting system in the country.
The country has no data collection system or epidemiological study on mental health. A documentation centre is being planned.

Programmes for Special Population The country has specific programmes for mental health for children.
There are also programmes for workers in the enterprise having alcohol abuse problems and programmes on epilepsy.

Therapeutic Drugs The following therapeutic drugs are generally available at the primary health care level of the country: carbamazepine, phenobarbital, sodium valproate, chlorpromazine, diazepam, haloperidol.

Other Information

Additional Sources of Information

Ministry of Health (Coordination des Soins aux Personnes Handicapéees [Center for the Treatment of Handicapped Persons]) 2004.

Ratsifandrihamanana, B., Terranova, R. (1967) Social psychiatric therapy in a mental hospital at Madagascar. Diseases of the Nervous System, 28, 398-401.

Malawi

GENERAL INFORMATION

Malawi is a country with an approximate area of 118 thousand sq. km. (UNO, 2001). Its population is 12.337 million, and the sex ratio (men per hundred women) is 98 (UNO, 2004). The proportion of population under the age of 15 years is 47% (UNO, 2004), and the proportion of population above the age of 60 years is 5% (WHO, 2004). The literacy rate is 75.5% for men and 48.7% for women (UNESCO/MoH, 2004).

The country is a low income group country (based on World Bank 2004 criteria). The proportion of health budget to GDP is 7.8%. The per capita total expenditure on health is 39 international $, and the per capita government expenditure on health is 14 international $ (WHO, 2004).

The main language(s) used in the country is (are) English and Chichewa. The largest ethnic group(s) is (are) Chewa, and the other ethnic group(s) are (is) Nyanja, Tumbuko and Yao. The largest religious group(s) is (are) Christian, and the other religious group(s) are (is) Muslim.

The life expectancy at birth is 39.8 years for males and 40.6 years for females (WHO, 2004). The healthy life expectancy at birth is 35 years for males and 35 years for females (WHO, 2004).

EPIDEMIOLOGY

There is a paucity of epidemiological data on mental illnesses in Malawi in internationally accessible literature. Carr et al (1994) compared characteristics of patients abusing marijuana with those of matched psychiatric patients and found that the abusers of marijuana (chamba) were more likely to be living in areas that grew chamba, less likely to be raised by natural parents and more likely to be educated. MacLachlan et al (1998) conducted focus groups to elicit responses from 44 male and 10 female psychiatric patients about their perceptions of marijuana (chamba) use in Malawi. Peltzer (1998) compared PTSD symptomatology among torture survivors from Malawi and refugees from Sudan in Uganda and found that among Africans somatic numbing was more common than psychic numbing as outlined in DSM-IV criteria. Simukonda and Rappsilber (1989) found high levels of anxiety among a group of male nursing students. They felt stressed about role differences between nurses and other male health workers.

MENTAL HEALTH RESOURCES

Mental Health Policy A mental health policy is present. The policy was initially formulated in 2002.

The components of the policy are advocacy, promotion, prevention, treatment and rehabilitation. Provision of comprehensive and accessible mental health care services is the main goal of the policy. It hopes to do so through the inclusion of mental health in the National Health Plan and integration of mental health in primary health care. Human resource development is also a component of the policy.

Substance Abuse Policy A substance abuse policy is absent.

National Mental Health Programme A national mental health programme is present. The programme was formulated in 1999.

National Therapeutic Drug Policy/Essential List of Drugs A national therapeutic drug policy/essential list of drugs is present. It was formulated in 1995.

Mental Health Legislation The Mental Treatment Act was amended in 1968. Currently, the Act is being reviewed.
The latest legislation was enacted in 1959.

Mental Health Financing There are budget allocations for mental health.
The country spends 2% of the total health budget on mental health.
The primary sources of mental health financing in descending order are tax based and grants.
The country does not have disability benefits for persons with mental disorders. Mental disorders are not considered a disability.

Mental Health Facilities Mental health is a part of primary health care system. Actual treatment of severe mental disorders is available at the primary level.

Regular training of primary care professionals is carried out in the field of mental health. In the last two years, about 1000 personnel were provided training. In medical undergraduate training, students are encouraged to consider how they may address mental health issues through the many and varied roles which doctors in resource poor countries must fulfil (administrator, trainer, primary health care doctor, and hospital physician). Training of general health workers in mental health issues is planned in 3 regions.

There are community care facilities for patients with mental disorders. Currently, the district mental health care provides community mental health services throughout the country. These centres are staffed by psychiatric nurses. Plans are under way to provide for monitoring and supervisory visits to all districts.

Psychiatric Beds and Professionals

Total psychiatric beds per 10 000 population	0.37
Psychiatric beds in mental hospitals per 10 000 population	
Psychiatric beds in general hospitals per 10 000 population	
Psychiatric beds in other settings per 10 000 population	
Number of psychiatrists per 100 000 population	0
Number of neurosurgeons per 100 000 population	0
Number of psychiatric nurses per 100 000 population	2.5
Number of neurologists per 100 000 population	0
Number of psychologists per 100 000 population	0
Number of social workers per 100 000 population	0

There is one occupational therapist and 2 psychiatric clinical officers. Mental health services are now provided at central level, Zomba Mental Hospital, district hospitals and non-governmental hospitals and also at the health centre level, though the latter is not fully developed. Although, there are only few mental health professionals available in the country, general duty doctors are not deployed to the mental health services area. About 300 psychiatric nurses have been trained and posted in district health centres. Management guidelines and protocols are being developed.

Non-Governmental Organizations NGOs are involved with mental health in the country. They are mainly involved in advocacy, promotion, prevention, treatment and rehabilitation.

Information Gathering System There is mental health reporting system in the country.
The country has no data collection system or epidemiological study on mental health.

Programmes for Special Population The country has specific programmes for mental health for minorities, refugees and disaster affected population.

Therapeutic Drugs The following therapeutic drugs are generally available at the primary health care level of the country: carbamazepine, phenobarbital, phenytoin sodium, amitriptyline, chlorpromazine, diazepam, fluphenazine, haloperidol, lithium. Procyclidine is available.

Other Information

Additional Sources of Information

Carr, S., Ager, A., Nyando, C., et al (1994) A comparison of chamba (marijuana) abusers and general psychiatric admissions in Malawi. Social Science & Medicine, 39, 401-406.

Herzig, H. (2003) Teaching psychiatry in poor countries: priorities and needs. A description of how mental health is taught to medical students in Malawi, Central Africa. Education for Health, 16, 32-39.

MacLachlan, M., Nyirenda, T., Nyando, C. (1995) Attributions for admission to Zomba Mental Hospital: implications for the development of mental health services in Malawi. International Journal of Psychiatry, 41, 79-87.

MacLachlan, M., Page, R. C., Robinson, G. L., et al (1998) Patients' perceptions of chamba (marijuana) use in Malawi. Substance Use & Misuse, 33, 1367-1373.

Peltzer, K. (1998) Ethnocultural construction of posttraumatic stress symptoms in African contexts. Journal of Psychology in Africa, 1, 17-30.

Simukonda, F. S., Rappsilber, C. (1989) Anxiety in male nursing students at Kamuzu College of Nursing. Nurse Education Today, 9, 180-185.

Malaysia

GENERAL INFORMATION

Malaysia is a country with an approximate area of 330 thousand sq. km. (UNO, 2001). Its population is 24.876 million, and the sex ratio (men per hundred women) is 103 (UNO, 2004). The proportion of population under the age of 15 years is 33% (UNO, 2004), and the proportion of population above the age of 60 years is 7% (WHO, 2004). The literacy rate is 91.4% for men and 83.4% for women (UNESCO/MoH, 2004).

The country is a higher middle income group country (based on World Bank 2004 criteria). The proportion of health budget to GDP is 3.8%. The per capita total expenditure on health is 345 international $, and the per capita government expenditure on health is 185 international $ (WHO, 2004).

The main language(s) used in the country is (are) Malay, Chinese, Tamil and English. The largest ethnic group(s) is (are) Malay and other indigenous groups, and the other ethnic group(s) are (is) Chinese and Indian. The largest religious group(s) is (are) Muslim, and the other religious group(s) are (is) Buddhist and Hindu.

The life expectancy at birth is 69.6 years for males and 74.7 years for females (WHO, 2004). The healthy life expectancy at birth is 62 years for males and 65 years for females (WHO, 2004).

EPIDEMIOLOGY

The Ministry of Health (1996) conducted the National Health & Morbidity Survey on 30 114 respondents aged 16 years and above using General Health Questionnaire (GHQ-10). The adjusted prevalence of mental disorders was 10.7%. Prevalence of mental disorders was associated with gender (female), age (under 25 years and over 65 years), ethnicity (Indian), marital status (widowed, divorced), employment (unemployed, agricultural and production workers), income (low), physical illness (asthma, cancer and diabetes) and disability (physical, hearing and speech). The National Working Group (Ministry of Health, 2001) study on promotion of mental health conducted on a sample of 5651 adults and 2075 children using the General Health Questionnaire (GHQ-28) showed the prevalence of mental health problems to be 18.8%. Ramli et al (1991) carried out a 2-stage survey for psychiatric morbidity in a rural area, and found the point prevalence of all psychiatric disorders to be 9.7%. Neurotic disorders (6.15%), especially neurotic depression (3.31%) was common, particularly in women. Maniam (1994) used the 30-item version of the General Health Questionnaire (cut-off score of 6/7) to assess psychiatric morbidity in 206 patients attending an urban general practice. The corrected prevalence estimate of psychiatric morbidity was 29.9%. Though no significant difference was observed in sex or age distribution, Malays had higher scores than Chinese. Navaratnam and Foong (1989) did a trend analysis on data from the national drug abuse monitoring system and found that there was a significant increase in incidence and prevalence (from .084% to .75%) of drug dependence in Malaysia in the period 1970-86. Gan (1995) reported that 59.5% of 472 rural women interviewed by them chewed tobacco and women with less education were more likely to do so. In a sample of 1000 elderly men, Chen (1987) reported that nearly 20% smoked 15 or more cigarettes a day and 40% indicated that their families complained about their alcohol intake. Navaratnam et al (1979) surveyed a representative sample of 12-16 year olds in three different areas (n >16 000) and found that 10.5% (males 11.9% and females 8.6%) used drugs. Drug use was highest among 12-year old children (13.5%) and the common drugs used were sedatives (5.5%), tranquillizers (4.5%), stimulants (3.9%), heroin (3.6%), other opioids (3.9%), hallucinogens (3.1%) and cannabis (2.7%). About a quarter of the students had tried four or more drugs and had rapidly progressed to heroin use. Grace et al (2001) administered the Edinburgh Post-Natal Depression Scale (EPNDS) and the Bradford Somatisation Inventory (BSI) to 154 consecutive mothers who came for a post-natal check up at 6-weeks and found the rate of post natal depression to be 3.9%. The prevalence among Indians (8.5%), Malays (3.0%) and Chinese (0%) was significantly different. Maniam (1995) reported that the corrected suicide rate was between 8-13 per 100 000 population. Nadesan (1999) reviewed all autopsies in a hospital over 3 years and found that 48.8% of the suicides were committed by those of Indian origin, 38.1% by those of Chinese origin and 3.6% by Malays. The commonest age group was between 20-40 years, and poisoning and hanging were the usual methods of committing suicide. Maniam (1988) reviewed records of 95 cases of suicide and 134 cases of parasuicide in a district. Nearly four-fifths of those committing or attempting suicides were Indians. About 94% of suicides and 66% of parasuicides involved ingestion of agricultural poisons. Habil et al (1992) reviewed the records of 306 in-patients with suicide attempts. Suicidal behaviour was more common in young, females, social class IV and V (45%) and persons of Indian origin. Poisoning was the commonest method used. Adjustment disorder was diagnosed in 58.5% of the patients. Cheah et al (1997) conducted a two-phase study involving 589 children aged 10-12 years and found that the prevalence of emotional/behavioural deviance based on parent interview to be 40% in a rural school, 30.2% in an agricultural resettlement school and 32.3% in the urban school. On the teachers' interview, the prevalence of deviance was 40% in the rural school, 10.8% in the agricultural resettlement school and 8.9% in the urban school. In the rural school, significantly higher prevalence of deviance was found among boys. However, Kasmini et al (1993) found a rate of only 6.1% for psychiatric morbidity in a sample of 507 rural children, aged 1-15 years, when they applied the WHO Research Questionnaire for Children (RQC) for initial screening and a semi structured interview at the second stage. Boo et al (1989) examined records of 34 495 live-births delivered in a maternity hospital and found the rate of Down syndrome to be 1044 per 1000 live-births.

MENTAL HEALTH RESOURCES

Mental Health Policy A mental health policy is present. The policy was initially formulated in 1998.
The components of the policy are advocacy, promotion, prevention, treatment and rehabilitation. Accessibility and equity, continuity and integration, community participation, community care, quality of services and multi sectoral collaboration are the major components of the policy. The National Mental Health Framework was formulated in July 2002 as a blue print of strategic planning and implementation for the delivery of mental health services and activities in hospital, primary health care and community based settings. The frame work also set standards and guidelines for the services.

Substance Abuse Policy A substance abuse policy is present. The policy was initially formulated in 1997.

National Mental Health Programme A national mental health programme is present. The programme was formulated in 1998.

National Therapeutic Drug Policy/Essential List of Drugs A national therapeutic drug policy/essential list of drugs is present. It was formulated in 1983.

Mental Health Legislation Mental Health laws are governed by the Mental Health Ordinance (1952) and the Laws of North Borneo. The new Mental Health Act (2001) provides the framework for care, treatment (including community treatment), control, protection and rehabilitation of people with mental disorders. The regulations for the Act were formulated in 2004 and awaiting approval. The regulations specify the specific standards for psychiatric facilities, personnel, rights of the patients, etc.
The latest legislation was enacted in 1952.

Mental Health Financing There are budget allocations for mental health.
The country spends 1.5% of the total health budget on mental health.
The primary sources of mental health financing in descending order are tax based, out of pocket expenditure by the patient or family, private insurances and social insurance.
The country does not have disability benefits for persons with mental disorders. Efforts have been made to categorize the severe mentally ill as a Disabled Person with the aim to improve the quality of life for the severe mentally ill and their integration into mainstream of society. A proposal paper was formulated and awaiting cabinet approval.

Mental Health Facilities Mental health is a part of primary health care system. Actual treatment of severe mental disorders is available at the primary level. Mental Health is integrated into the primary health care system since 1998. In 2003, 733 (i.e. 85%) primary health care clinics were providing treatment for the mentally ill and 25 of these clinics were also providing psychosocial rehabilitation services. Defaulter tracing, family education and treatment in the home are also provided. Mental health has been incorporated in the Adolescent and Elderly Health Services provided in the primary health care. Guidelines and Standard Operating Procedures for implementation of mental health services in the primary health care level have been developed to facilitate the primary health care service providers to carry out their respective programmes and activities. The psychiatric clinics in the District Hospitals are run by medical officers supervised by visiting psychiatrists and also visiting psychiatrists providing services for more difficult cases and consultation. The visiting psychiatrists also provides on the job training as well as continuous medical education (CME) to the medical officers.
Regular training of primary care professionals is carried out in the field of mental health. In the last two years, about 1505 personnel were provided training. Training for the primary health care personnel are carried out regularly based on modular training, in-service and continuous medical training (CME) at national, state and local level. In-service training and continuous medical training (CME) are also been carried out by the psychiatric departments.
There are community care facilities for patients with mental disorders. There has been an emphasis for community based mental health care by the psychiatric departments since 1998. Home based services are being developed and provided at various levels by the psychiatric departments. These include home based care for the acutely ill in 6 districts and assertive follow-up in most districts with psychiatric departments. Families' involvement has been a key feature for management of the mentally ill in Malaysia. In 2002, initiatives to formalize and develop the Family Support Group (FSG) started in Johor Baharu District and till the end of 2004, about 16 FSGs have been formed through the country with a total of 1084 carers. Training for the FSGs was carried out using a module developed in 2002.

Psychiatric Beds and Professionals

Total psychiatric beds per 10 000 population	2.7
Psychiatric beds in mental hospitals per 10 000 population	2.4
Psychiatric beds in general hospitals per 10 000 population	0.3
Psychiatric beds in other settings per 10 000 population	0
Number of psychiatrists per 100 000 population	0.6
Number of neurosurgeons per 100 000 population	0.06
Number of psychiatric nurses per 100 000 population	0.5
Number of neurologists per 100 000 population	0.05
Number of psychologists per 100 000 population	0.05
Number of social workers per 100 000 population	0.2

There are 148 occupational therapists and 295 medical assistants. There are 4 mental institutions, 32 hospitals (27 under Ministry of Health, 3 University Hospitals and 1 Army Hospital) with psychiatric wards (each with 20 – 120 beds). Two of the 4 mental hospitals have over 1500 beds, each. Private nursing homes (nearly 70 at present) are currently licensed by the local authority. However, they will now have to seek legal permission under the 2001 mental health act. About one third of psychiatrists are in full or part-time private practice. Half of these private practitioners are in Kuala Lumpur, but most cities have private psychiatric practice. Most psychiatric units now have occupational therapists working with them. Recently, courses on child psychiatry have started.

Non-Governmental Organizations NGOs are involved with mental health in the country. They are mainly involved in advocacy, promotion, prevention, treatment and rehabilitation. At least 19 NGOs work in the area of mental health. NGOs provide community care facilities like day care centres besides public education and advocacy. The Government has recognized their influential role and a nominal amount of funding is available to some NGOs. They are also involved in planning and policy making. A National Council on Mental Health was formed in 1998 to ensure wide community participation on policy issues. The Befrienders operate a 24-hour telephone as well as face-to-face counselling service in many cities. Other NGOs care for abused children and women or provide marital counselling services.

Information Gathering System There is mental health reporting system in the country. The Ministry of Health has an Information Documentation System (IDS), where data on activities from the hospital and health care systems are collected and collated. Reporting on diseases (including mental disorders) are based on ICD-9.
The country has data collection system or epidemiological study on mental health.

Programmes for Special Population The country has specific programmes for mental health for elderly and children.
Training modules and manuals have been developed for training of psychiatrists, paediatricians, family medicine specialists and primary health care staff in child and adolescent mental health. Mental health promotion has been identified as a key strategy for improving the mental health status of the population through improving coping skills, lifestyle and increasing mental health literacy. Towards this end, the Ministry of Health launched the Healthy Life Style Campaign in 2000. The campaign targeted children, adolescents, working adults, parents and elderly. The activities were implemented through a national level training for trainers for all state facilitators, who conducted training for district facilitators, who were responsible for carrying out activities at the grass root level. Other mental health promotion activities include public forums, health talks and exhibitions. There are more than 30 governmental treatment and rehabilitation centres for drug abusers. Each can house over 300 patients for up to 18 months. A public education programme and a school education programme on drug abuse have been conducted over the past few years. Methadone is not routinely available and there is no needle exchange programme. But these centres provide training in work skills and aftercare for 5 years. A national anti-drug association PEMADAM (NGO) does valuable work in public education, prevention and aftercare. There are also a number of privately run treatment and rehabilitation centres for substance abuse. A few Alcoholic Anonymous and other counselling groups have also come up. Forensic psychiatry care is mainly provided through psychiatric hospitals. Two forensic psychiatrists work in the general hospital setting.

Therapeutic Drugs The following therapeutic drugs are generally available at the primary health care level of the country: carbamazepine, phenobarbital, phenytoin sodium, sodium valproate, amitriptyline, chlorpromazine, diazepam, fluphenazine, haloperidol, lithium, carbidopa, levodopa.

Other Information

Additional Sources of Information

Boo, N. Y., Hoe, T. S., Lye, M. S., et al (1989) Maternal age-specific incidence of Down's syndrome in Malaysian neonates. Journal of the Singapore Paediatric Society, 31, 138-142.

Cheah, Y. C., Kadir, A. B., Jeyarajah, S. (1997) Prevalence of emotional and behavioural problems in Johor Bahru District school children--comparing three geographical areas. Medical Journal of Malaysia, 52, 124-133.

Chen, P. C. (1987) Psychosocial factors and the health of the elderly Malaysian. Annals of the Academy of Medicine, Singapore, 16, 110-114.

Deva, M. P. (2004) Malaysia mental health country profile. International Review of Psychiatry, 16, 167-176.

Gan, C.Y. (1995) Smokeless tobacco use among rural Kadazan women in Sabah, Malaysia. Southeast Asian Journal of Tropical Medicine & Public Health, 26, 291-296

Government document (1998) National Tobacco Control Programme.

Government document (1998) National Alcohol Control Programme.

Government document (1952) The Mental Disorders Ordinance.

Grace, J., Lee, K. K., Ballard, C., et al (2001) The relationship between post-natal depression, somatization and behaviour in Malaysian women. Transcultural Psychiatry, 38, 27-34.

Habil, M. H., Ganesvaran, T., Agnes, L. S. (1992) Attempted suicide in Kuala Lumpur. Asia-Pacific Journal of Public Health, 6, 5-7.

Kasmini, K., Kyaw, O., Krishnaswamy, S., et al (1993) A prevalence survey of mental disorders among children in a rural Malaysian village. Acta Psychiatrica Scandinavica, 87, 253-257.

Maniam, T. (1988) Suicide and parasuicide in a hill resort in Malaysia. British Journal of Psychiatry, 153, 222-225.

Maniam, T. (1994) Psychiatric morbidity in an urban general practice. Medical Journal of Malaysia, 49, 242-246.

Maniam, T. (1995) Suicide and undetermined violent deaths in Malaysia, 1966-1990: evidence for the misclassification of suicide statistics. Asia-Pacific Journal of Public Health, 8, 181-185.

Ministry of Health (1998) National Mental Health Policy. Health Education Division, Ministry of Health Malaysia.

Ministry of Health (1998) Community Health Programme, Plan of Action. Division of Family Health Development, Ministry of Health.

Nadesan, K. (1999) Pattern of suicide: a review of autopsies conducted at the University Hospital, Kuala Lumpur. Malaysian Journal of Pathology, 21, 95-99.

Navaratnam, V., Aun, L. B., Spencer, C. P. (1979) Extent and patterns of drug abuse among children in Malaysia. Bulletin on Narcotics, 31, 59-68.

Navaratnam, V. Foong, K. (1989) An epidemiological assessment of drug dependence in Malaysia--a trend analysis. Medical Journal of Malaysia, 44, 92-103.

Ministry of Health (1996) The National Health & Morbidity Survey.

Ministry of Health (2001) The National Working Group Study on Promotion of Mental Health.

Ramli H., Kasmini K., Hassan S., et al (1991).

Maldives

GENERAL INFORMATION

Maldives is a country with an approximate area of 0.3 thousand sq. km. (UNO, 2001). The country includes nearly 1200 coral islands. Its population is 0.328 million, and the sex ratio (men per hundred women) is 105 (UNO, 2004). The proportion of population under the age of 15 years is 42% (UNO, 2004), and the proportion of population above the age of 60 years is 5% (WHO, 2004). The literacy rate is 97.3% for men and 97.2% for women (UNESCO/MoH, 2004).
The country is a lower middle income group country (based on World Bank 2004 criteria). The proportion of health budget to GDP is 6.7%. The per capita total expenditure on health is 263 international $, and the per capita government expenditure on health is 220 international $ (WHO, 2004).
The main language(s) used in the country is (are) Dhivehi. The largest ethnic group(s) is (are) Sinhalese, and the other ethnic group(s) are (is) Dravidian, Arab and African. The largest religious group(s) is (are) Muslim.
The life expectancy at birth is 66.5 years for males and 65.6 years for females (WHO, 2004). The healthy life expectancy at birth is 59 years for males and 57 years for females (WHO, 2004).

EPIDEMIOLOGY

There is a paucity of epidemiological data on mental illnesses in Maldives in internationally accessible literature.

MENTAL HEALTH RESOURCES

Mental Health Policy A mental health policy is absent.

Substance Abuse Policy A substance abuse policy is present. The policy was initially formulated in 1977.

National Mental Health Programme A national mental health programme is absent.

National Therapeutic Drug Policy/Essential List of Drugs A national therapeutic drug policy/essential list of drugs is present. Details about the year of formulation are not available.

Mental Health Legislation There is no mental health legislation.
Details about the year of enactment of the mental health legislation are not available.

Mental Health Financing There are no budget allocations for mental health.
Details about expenditure on mental health are not available.
The primary sources of mental health financing in descending order are out of pocket expenditure by the patient or family and grants.
The Government has special budget allocations for provision of free medication to mental health patients and provides care and treatment for severe cases at the Home for People with Special Needs. The National Narcotics Control Bureau and the Rehabilitation Centre also have separate budgets allocated for their function.
The country has disability benefits for persons with mental disorders.

Mental Health Facilities Mental health is not a part of primary health care system. Actual treatment of severe mental disorders is not available at the primary level.
Regular training of primary care professionals is carried out in the field of mental health. Training is integrated in the community health workers training programme. The Government plans to make comprehensive mental health services available at the central level. At the regional level, services are provided by visiting psychiatrists. At the atoll and island levels, trained community health workers and nurses provide basic psychiatric services. Home-based care of psychiatric cases will be given priority over institutional treatment. Emphasis will also be given to the prevention of mental illness and the promotion of mental health and well-being through awareness programmes.
There are no community care facilities for patients with mental disorders.

Psychiatric Beds and Professionals

Total psychiatric beds per 10 000 population	
Psychiatric beds in mental hospitals per 10 000 population	
Psychiatric beds in general hospitals per 10 000 population	
Psychiatric beds in other settings per 10 000 population	
Number of psychiatrists per 100 000 population	0.36
Number of neurosurgeons per 100 000 population	0.36
Number of psychiatric nurses per 100 000 population	0
Number of neurologists per 100 000 population	0
Number of psychologists per 100 000 population	1.2
Number of social workers per 100 000 population	0

Most of the personnel work in the capital and in tertiary centres. The psychiatrists visits other islands whenever needed.

Non-Governmental Organizations NGOs are involved with mental health in the country. They are mainly involved in treatment and rehabilitation. One NGO is involved in providing care and support to patients with severe mental illnesses and special needs. Two other NGOs are involved in providing counselling for drug users.

Information Gathering System There is mental health reporting system in the country. A national registry that covers mental disorders is maintained at the Ministry of Gender, Family Development and Social Security. Similarly, a register is maintained at the National Narcotics Control Bureau.
The country has no data collection system or epidemiological study on mental health. However, a prevalence study on mental disorders using the Self-Reporting Questionnaire (SRQ) developed by WHO is under way (in 2004).

Programmes for Special Population There are no programmes for any special population.

Therapeutic Drugs The following therapeutic drugs are generally available at the primary health care level of the country: carbamazepine, phenobarbital, phenytoin sodium, sodium valproate, amitriptyline, chlorpromazine, diazepam, fluphenazine, haloperidol, lithium, carbidopa, levodopa.

Other Information

Additional Sources of Information

Government of Maldives. Health Master Plan. http://www.health.gov.mv/hmp/plan1.htm.

Mali

GENERAL INFORMATION

Mali is a country with an approximate area of 1240 thousand sq. km. (UNO, 2001). Its population is 13.408 million, and the sex ratio (men per hundred women) is 98 (UNO, 2004). The proportion of population under the age of 15 years is 49% (UNO, 2004), and the proportion of population above the age of 60 years is 4% (WHO, 2004). The literacy rate is 26.7% for men and 11.9% for women (UNESCO/MoH, 2004).

The country is a low income group country (based on World Bank 2004 criteria). The proportion of health budget to GDP is 4.3%. The per capita total expenditure on health is 30 international $, and the per capita government expenditure on health is 12 international $ (WHO, 2004).

The main language(s) used in the country is (are) French. The largest ethnic group(s) is (are) Dogon, and the other ethnic group(s) are (is) Voltaic and Touareg. The largest religious group(s) is (are) Muslim.

The life expectancy at birth is 43.9 years for males and 45.7 years for females (WHO, 2004). The healthy life expectancy at birth is 38 years for males and 38 years for females (WHO, 2004).

EPIDEMIOLOGY

Carta et al (1997, 1999) conducted a two-level community study to estimate the prevalence of mental disorders with the help of the Questionnaire pour le Dépistage en Santé Mentale (QDSM), a 23-item screening questionnaire derived from the Self-Reporting Questionnaire (SRQ). In the first phase of the study, 466 randomly selected subjects from the major tribes were evaluated by means of the QDSM. In the second phase, all subjects who were 'positive' at the screening, as well as a sample who were 'negative' were examined by means of a semistructured interview. The estimated prevalence of psychiatric cases was 6.4%. A significant risk was associated with age and education. The common somatic diseases associated with psychiatric disorders were genitourinary tract disorders, tuberculosis and cardiac disorders. True et al (2001) assessed 42 mother-infant (10-12.5 months) pairs from a rural setting. The distribution of the Strange Situation classifications was 67% secure, 0% avoidant, 8% resistant and 25% disorganized. Infant attachment security was significantly related to the quality of observed mother-infant communication. Mothers of disorganized infants had significantly higher ratings of frightened or frightening behaviours.

MENTAL HEALTH RESOURCES

Mental Health Policy A mental health policy is present. The policy was initially formulated in 1983.
The components of the policy are treatment and rehabilitation. Decentralization is a component of the policy.

Substance Abuse Policy A substance abuse policy is present. The policy was initially formulated in 1983.

National Mental Health Programme A national mental health programme is present. The programme was formulated in 1983.

National Therapeutic Drug Policy/Essential List of Drugs A national therapeutic drug policy/essential list of drugs is present. It was formulated in 1985.

Mental Health Legislation The 1938 decree of Gouverneur Général de l'AOF concerning the mentally alienated and the French legislation of 1838 were replaced by the new legislation.
The latest legislation was enacted in 1990.

Mental Health Financing There are budget allocations for mental health.
The country spends 0.02% of the total health budget on mental health.
The primary sources of mental health financing in descending order are out of pocket expenditure by the patient or family, tax based, social insurance and private insurances.
The country does not have disability benefits for persons with mental disorders.

Mental Health Facilities Mental health is a part of primary health care system. Actual treatment of severe mental disorders is available at the primary level.
Regular training of primary care professionals is carried out in the field of mental health. In the last two years, about 48 personnel were provided training.
There are community care facilities for patients with mental disorders.

Psychiatric Beds and Professionals

Total psychiatric beds per 10 000 population	0.2
Psychiatric beds in mental hospitals per 10 000 population	0
Psychiatric beds in general hospitals per 10 000 population	0.1
Psychiatric beds in other settings per 10 000 population	0.05
Number of psychiatrists per 100 000 population	0.06
Number of neurosurgeons per 100 000 population	0.01
Number of psychiatric nurses per 100 000 population	0.15
Number of neurologists per 100 000 population	0.02
Number of psychologists per 100 000 population	0.02
Number of social workers per 100 000 population	0.01

The number of personnel are insufficient.

Non-Governmental Organizations NGOs are involved with mental health in the country. They are mainly involved in advocacy, promotion, prevention, treatment and rehabilitation.

Information Gathering System There is mental health reporting system in the country. Mental disorders are classified under 'other disorders'.
The country has no data collection system or epidemiological study on mental health.

Programmes for Special Population There are no programmes for special population.

Therapeutic Drugs The following therapeutic drugs are generally available at the primary health care level of the country: carbamazepine, phenobarbital, phenytoin sodium, sodium valproate, amitriptyline, chlorpromazine, diazepam, fluphenazine, haloperidol, levodopa.
Trihexiphenydyl is used. Availability of drugs is inadequate.

Other Information

Additional Sources of Information

Carta, M. G., Coppo, P., Carpiniello, B., et al (1997) Mental disorders and health care seeking in Bandiagara: a community survey in the Dogon Plateau. Social Psychiatry & Psychiatric Epidemiology, 32, 222-229.

Carta, M. G., Coppo, P., Reda, M. A., et al (1999) Psychopathology in the Dogon Plateau: an assessment using the QDSM and principal components analysis. Social Psychiatry & Psychiatric Epidemiology, 34, 282-285.

Koumare, B. et al. (1992) Psychopathologie Africaine, 14, 287.

True, M. M., Pisani, L., Oumar, F. (2001) Infant-mother attachment among the Dogon of Mali. Child Development, 72, 1451-1466.

J–M

Malta

GENERAL INFORMATION

Malta is a country with an approximate area of 0.32 thousand sq. km. (UNO, 2001). The country consists of five islands. Its population is 0.396 million, and the sex ratio (men per hundred women) is 98 (UNO, 2004). The proportion of population under the age of 15 years is 19% (UNO, 2004), and the proportion of population above the age of 60 years is 18% (WHO, 2004). The literacy rate is 91.8% for men and 93.4% for women (UNESCO/MoH, 2004).

The country is a high income group country (based on World Bank 2004 criteria). The proportion of health budget to GDP is 8.8%. The per capita total expenditure on health is 813 international $, and the per capita government expenditure on health is 557 international $ (WHO, 2004).

The main language(s) used in the country is (are) Maltese and English. The largest religious group(s) is (are) Roman Catholic.

The life expectancy at birth is 76.1 years for males and 81.2 years for females (WHO, 2004). The healthy life expectancy at birth is 70 years for males and 73 years for females (WHO, 2004).

EPIDEMIOLOGY

Baron et al (2001) interviewed carers at 13 residential homes using a semistructured questionnaire (n=309) about children and adolescents below the age of 16 years. They found behavioural problems in 20.7% and developmental delay (global or specific) in 23.3% of the subjects. Maslowski (1987, 1988) compared the cultural factors and symptomatology of schizophrenia among patients from Poland (n=120), Malta (n=80) and Libya (n=97). Differences were observed in symptomatology and prognosis. Savona-Ventura et al (2001) reported that domestic abuse was common in Mediterranean communities and that abused women were more likely to smoke cigarettes during pregnancy than their counterparts.

MENTAL HEALTH RESOURCES

Mental Health Policy A mental health policy is present. The policy was initially formulated in 1994.

The components of the policy are advocacy, promotion, prevention, treatment and rehabilitation. The policy strives to create healthy environments in family, school, workplace and community and also aims to offer a range of appropriate services to empower people to cope better with mental health issues, thus maximizing their productive and social life.

Substance Abuse Policy A substance abuse policy is present. Details about the year of formulation are not available. The substance abuse policy is under review.

National Mental Health Programme A national mental health programme is present. Details about the year of formulation of the programme are not available.

The national mental health programme is entitled 'National Community Mental Health Strategy'.

National Therapeutic Drug Policy/Essential List of Drugs A national therapeutic drug policy/essential list of drugs is present. It was formulated in 1983.

Mental Health Legislation The Mental Health Act was enacted in 1981 and amended in 1983. Currently, it is under review. A draft of the new Mental Health Act was prepared by the Mental Health Commission in 1999.

The latest legislation was enacted in 1981.

Mental Health Financing There are budget allocations for mental health.

The country spends 10% of the total health budget on mental health.

The primary sources of mental health financing in descending order are tax based, out of pocket expenditure by the patient or family and social insurance.

Residents receive comprehensive care, funded from general taxation. Those determined by means-testing to have a 'low income' and those suffering from chronic conditions (e.g. schizophrenia) are entitled to free drug treatment on an outpatient basis.

The country has disability benefits for persons with mental disorders. Persons suffering from severe mental subnormality or those with certain neurological disorders like epilepsy are entitled to means-related disability benefit, and those suffering from chronic schizophrenia, drug abuse or resident in a therapeutic community are entitled to a means-related social assistance benefit.

Mental Health Facilities Mental health is a part of primary health care system. Actual treatment of severe mental disorders is available at the primary level. The approach is to move out of an institutional system to a community set-up. Many patients are either followed up on an out-patient basis in the state system or by a psychiatrist or general physician in private.

Regular training of primary care professionals is carried out in the field of mental health.

There are community care facilities for patients with mental disorders. Community services are in the form of day centres, sheltered homes, long stay hostels, respite centres and independent living.

Psychiatric Beds and Professionals

Total psychiatric beds per 10 000 population	18.9
Psychiatric beds in mental hospitals per 10 000 population	18.86
Psychiatric beds in general hospitals per 10 000 population	0.04
Psychiatric beds in other settings per 10 000 population	0
Number of psychiatrists per 100 000 population	4
Number of neurosurgeons per 100 000 population	0.8
Number of psychiatric nurses per 100 000 population	102
Number of neurologists per 100 000 population	1
Number of psychologists per 100 000 population	2.6
Number of social workers per 100 000 population	3.1

There are 12 occupational therapists. There is a specialist registration system. The main psychiatric hospital still adheres to old custodial care approach with old management facilities and ineffective human resources management. There are hardly any specialized care units. The main psychiatric hospital focuses on personalized, holistic healing both of which are implemented in a multi-disciplinary 'team' approach. New infrastructures have been introduced into hospitals in order to enhance accountability for resource utilization and performance. Beds have been earmarked for elderly, children and adolescents, those with learning disabilities and forensic patients. Malta has a relatively high numbers of psychiatric beds per 1000 population in comparison to other European countries. However, acute inpatient options are limited. Formal training in psychiatry leading on to full qualification as a psychiatrist is partially provided in Malta and hence doctors must finalize their formal training abroad. Specialists are registered. There is a lack of trained personnel and a multi-disciplinary approach is lacking. Over the past three years, a large portion of resources have been utilized to train staff and management in modern psychiatric care.

Non-Governmental Organizations NGOs are involved with mental health in the country. They are mainly involved in advocacy, promotion and rehabilitation.

Information Gathering System There is no mental health reporting system in the country.
The country has no data collection system or epidemiological study on mental health.

Programmes for Special Population There are no programmes for special populations.
Provision for substance misuse falls under the Ministry of Family and Social Solidarity. Most of the substance misuse services are provided by a Government-funded autonomous agency, the National Agency against Drug and Alcohol Abuse (Sedqa). The services principally employ a multi-disciplinary
approach and provide a range of treatment modalities, including outpatient and inpatient detoxification, community-based one-to-one as well as group psychosocial interventions, family therapy facilities and longer-term residential rehabilitation facilities. Other community-based provision includes prevention programmes and a parental skills programme. Acute provision for substance misuse, however, falls under the Department of Psychiatry within the main psychiatric hospital. A non-governmental organization, Caritas, works alongside the National Agency; its main roles are prevention and community-based rehabilitation. The Department of Psychiatry also provides for psychiatric care within the criminal justice system.

Therapeutic Drugs The following therapeutic drugs are generally available at the primary health care level of the country: carbamazepine, ethosuximide, phenobarbital, phenytoin sodium, sodium valproate, amitriptyline, chlorpromazine, diazepam, haloperidol, lithium, carbidopa, levodopa.
The essential list of drugs is updated regularly. All drugs are dispensed free. The Division of Health uses a locally-produced National Formulary which includes all drugs available under the Maltese NHS and this was derived from the WHO list. Prior approval of the Minister or Director General is required before introducing a new drug. On an outpatient basis, drugs are dispensed free of charge or on a means-test, or if a client is suffering from an illness scheduled under the Social Security Act.

Other Information

Additional Sources of Information

Baron, A. M., Baron, Y. M., Spencer, N. J. (2001) The care and health needs of children in residential care in the Maltese Islands. Child: Care, Health & Development, 27, 251-262.

Galea, S., Mifsud, J. (2004) The mental health care system in Malta. International Psychiatry, 5, 11-13.

Maslowski, J. (1987) Cross cultural study of productive phenomenology of schizophrenia. Bulletin of the Institute of Maritime & Tropical Medicine in Gdynia, 38, 126-132.

Maslowski, J. (1988) Cultural factors and symptoms of schizophrenia, a comparative study in Malta and Poland. Bulletin of the Institute of Maritime & Tropical Medicine in Gdynia, 39, 253-264.

Ministry for Home Affairs and Social Development, Department of Health Policy and Planning. (1994). National Policy on Mental Health Service.

Savona-Ventura, C., Savona-Ventura, M., Drengsted-Nielsen, S., et al (2001) Domestic abuse in a central Mediterranean pregnant population. European Journal of Obstetrics, Gynecology, & Reproductive Biology, 98, 3-8.

Marshall Islands

GENERAL INFORMATION

Marshall Islands is a country with an approximate area of 0.18 thousand sq. km. (UNO, 2001). The country consists of two archipelagic island chains of about 30 atolls and more than 1000 islands. Its population is 0.057 million, and the sex ratio (men per hundred women) is 105 (UNO, 2004). The proportion of population under the age of 15 years is 42% (UNO, 2004), and the proportion of population above the age of 60 years is 7% (WHO, 2004). The literacy rate is 100% for men and 88% for women (UNESCO/MoH, 2004).

The country is a lower middle income group country (based on World Bank 2004 criteria). The proportion of health budget to GDP is 9.8%. The per capita total expenditure on health is 343 international $, and the per capita government expenditure on health is 222 international $ (WHO, 2004).

The main language(s) used in the country is (are) Marshallese and English. The largest ethnic group(s) is (are) Micronesian. The largest religious group(s) is (are) Christian.

The life expectancy at birth is 61.1 years for males and 64.6 years for females (WHO, 2004). The healthy life expectancy at birth is 54 years for males and 56 years for females (WHO, 2004).

EPIDEMIOLOGY

There is a paucity of epidemiological data on mental illnesses in Marshall Islands in internationally accessible literature. Dodd (1980) found that depression and alcohol abuse were common conditions encountered in a medical facility.

MENTAL HEALTH RESOURCES

Mental Health Policy A mental health policy is absent.

Substance Abuse Policy Details about the substance abuse policy are not available.

National Mental Health Programme A national mental health programme is present. The programme was formulated in 1982.

National Therapeutic Drug Policy/Essential List of Drugs A national therapeutic drug policy/essential list of drugs is absent.

Mental Health Legislation There are National Mental Health Planning Council By-Laws.
The latest legislation was enacted in 1997.

Mental Health Financing There are budget allocations for mental health.
The country spends 0.4% of the total health budget on mental health.
The primary source of mental health financing is tax based.
The country has disability benefits for persons with mental disorders.

Mental Health Facilities Mental health is a part of primary health care system. Actual treatment of severe mental disorders is available at the primary level. The Ministry of Health and Environment offers mental health programmes under the auspices of Bureau of Primary Health Care, but all medical supplies and drugs are for curative health care.

Regular training of primary care professionals is carried out in the field of mental health. There have been some workshops and training programmes, namely The Crisis Prevention and Intervention Training, Partners in Mental Health Performance Outcome Workshop, etc.

There are community care facilities for patients with mental disorders. Usually a community-based system of care is provided. Outreach prevention and treatment programmes are provided to communities around the country.

Psychiatric Beds and Professionals

Total psychiatric beds per 10 000 population	0
Psychiatric beds in mental hospitals per 10 000 population	0
Psychiatric beds in general hospitals per 10 000 population	0
Psychiatric beds in other settings per 10 000 population	0
Number of psychiatrists per 100 000 population	0
Number of neurosurgeons per 100 000 population	0
Number of psychiatric nurses per 100 000 population	0
Number of neurologists per 100 000 population	0
Number of psychologists per 100 000 population	1
Number of social workers per 100 000 population	3

Only one medical doctor works with the mental health programme. A psychiatrist is going to be recruited.

Non-Governmental Organizations NGOs are involved with mental health in the country. They are mainly involved in promotion, prevention, treatment and rehabilitation.

Information Gathering System There is mental health reporting system in the country. Monthly reports are sent to the office of the Director; annual reports are sent to the office of the Assistant Secretary of the Primary Health Care and the Planning and Statistics Office.

The country has data collection system or epidemiological study on mental health. The Ministry of Health and Environment has collected data from 1992-2000.

Programmes for Special Population The country has specific programmes for mental health for minorities, elderly and children. Mental health programme and community outreach prevention and treatment programmes provide the services.

Therapeutic Drugs The following therapeutic drugs are generally available at the primary health care level of the country: carbamazepine, phenobarbital, phenytoin sodium, amitriptyline, diazepam, fluphenazine, haloperidol, lithium, carbidopa, levodopa. Benztropine 2mg is usually used for akathisia/dystonia.

Other Information The purposes of the National Mental Health Planning Council are: (1) to serve as advocate for chronically mentally ill persons; (2) to monitor, review and evaluate not less than once a year, the allocation and adequacy of mental health services with the republic; and (3) to carry out other activities that might be related to the purpose of the council.

Additional Sources of Information

Dodd, L. E. Jr. (1980) A doctor's tour on the Eniwetok atoll. Aviation Space & Environmental Medicine, 51, 720-724.

Government document (1997) By-laws of the RMI Mental Health Planning Council (a Standing Committee of the RMI Health Advisory Board).

Mauritania

GENERAL INFORMATION

Mauritania is a country with an approximate area of 1026 thousand sq. km. (UNO, 2001). Its population is 2.98 million, and the sex ratio (men per hundred women) is 98 (UNO, 2004). The proportion of population under the age of 15 years is 43% (UNO, 2004), and the proportion of population above the age of 60 years is 5% (WHO, 2004). The literacy rate is 51.5% for men and 31.3% for women (UNESCO/MoH, 2004).

The country is a low income group country (based on World Bank 2004 criteria). The proportion of health budget to GDP is 3.6%. The per capita total expenditure on health is 45 international $, and the per capita government expenditure on health is 33 international $ (WHO, 2004).

The main language(s) used in the country is (are) Arabic, Fula, Soninke, Wolof and French. The largest ethnic group(s) is (are) Maur, and the other ethnic group(s) are (is) African. The largest religious group(s) is (are) Muslim.

The life expectancy at birth is 49.8 years for males and 54.5 years for females (WHO, 2004). The healthy life expectancy at birth is 43 years for males and 46 years for females (WHO, 2004).

EPIDEMIOLOGY

There is a paucity of epidemiological data on mental illnesses in Mauritania in internationally accessible literature. According to the National General Survey on Mental Health, 16% of subjects had depressive disorders, 20% had anxiety disorders and 2% had psychoactive substance use disorders (MOH, 2004).

MENTAL HEALTH RESOURCES

Mental Health Policy A mental health policy is absent.

Substance Abuse Policy A substance abuse policy is absent. A decree was issued in November 1990 for the creation of the National Commission against Drugs and Psychotropic Substances.

National Mental Health Programme A national mental health programme is present. The programme was formulated in 1999.

National Therapeutic Drug Policy/Essential List of Drugs A national therapeutic drug policy/essential list of drugs is absent.

Mental Health Legislation The country does not have any mental health legislation. A draft legislation is in preparation.
Details about the year of enactment of the mental health legislation are not available.

Mental Health Financing There are budget allocations for mental health.
The country spends 1% of the total health budget on mental health.
The primary sources of mental health financing in descending order are tax based and out of pocket expenditure by the patient or family.
The country has disability benefits for persons with mental disorders.

Mental Health Facilities Mental health is a part of primary health care system. Actual treatment of severe mental disorders is available at the primary level.
Regular training of primary care professionals is not carried out in the field of mental health. Some training of primary care professionals is carried out in the field of mental health through workshops, seminars etc.
There are community care facilities for patients with mental disorders. Special units for mental health treatment have been developed in the community.

Psychiatric Beds and Professionals

Total psychiatric beds per 10 000 population	0.2
Psychiatric beds in mental hospitals per 10 000 population	0.2
Psychiatric beds in general hospitals per 10 000 population	0
Psychiatric beds in other settings per 10 000 population	0
Number of psychiatrists per 100 000 population	0.08
Number of neurosurgeons per 100 000 population	0
Number of psychiatric nurses per 100 000 population	0
Number of neurologists per 100 000 population	0.6
Number of psychologists per 100 000 population	0.1
Number of social workers per 100 000 population	0.1

Training of specialists in mental health is not adequate.

Non-Governmental Organizations NGOs are involved with mental health in the country. They are mainly involved in advocacy, promotion, treatment and rehabilitation.

Information Gathering System There is mental health reporting system in the country. Only hospital data collection is done. The country has no data collection system or epidemiological study on mental health. A general survey on mental health was conducted. Data are not available as yet.

Programmes for Special Population There are no special services.

Therapeutic Drugs The following therapeutic drugs are generally available at the primary health care level of the country: carbamazepine, phenobarbital, sodium valproate, amitriptyline, chlorpromazine, diazepam, haloperidol.
Trihexiphenidyl (5mg) is present.

Other Information

Additional Sources of Information

Mauritius

GENERAL INFORMATION

Mauritius is a country with an approximate area of 2 thousand sq. km. (UNO, 2001). Its population is 1.233 million, and the sex ratio (men per hundred women) is 99 (UNO, 2004). The proportion of population under the age of 15 years is 25% (UNO, 2004), and the proportion of population above the age of 60 years is 9% (WHO, 2004). The literacy rate is 88.2% for men and 80.5% for women (UNESCO/MoH, 2004).

The country is a higher middle income group country (based on World Bank 2004 criteria). The proportion of health budget to GDP is 3.4%. The per capita total expenditure on health is 323 international $, and the per capita government expenditure on health is 192 international $ (WHO, 2004).

The main language(s) used in the country is (are) English, French and Creole Patois. The largest ethnic group(s) is (are) Indo-Mauritian, and the other ethnic group(s) are (is) Creole. The largest religious group(s) is (are) Hindu (more than half), and the other religious group(s) are (is) Christian and Muslim.

The life expectancy at birth is 68.4 years for males and 75.5 years for females (WHO, 2004). The healthy life expectancy at birth is 60 years for males and 65 years for females (WHO, 2004).

EPIDEMIOLOGY

There is a paucity of epidemiological data on mental illnesses in Mauritius in internationally accessible literature. Reynolds et al (2000) used the Schizotypal Personality Questionnaire in a sample of 1201 subjects and found that the three-factor model (cognitive-perceptual deficits, interpersonal deficits and disorganization) underlies individual differences across widely varying groups. Venables (1996, 1997) found that women's exposure to influenza in pregnancy was associated with an elevation of positive schizotypy scores and electrodermal hyperresponsivity (associated with schizophrenia), whereas exposure to low environmental temperatures was associated with an elevation of anhedonia scores and electrodermal hyporesponsiveness in their offspring.

MENTAL HEALTH RESOURCES

Mental Health Policy A mental health policy is present. The policy was initially formulated in 1983.
The components of the policy are promotion, prevention, treatment and rehabilitation.

Substance Abuse Policy A substance abuse policy is present. The policy was initially formulated in 1996. A Substance Abuse Strategic Plan was formulated in 2004.

National Mental Health Programme A national mental health programme is present. The programme was formulated in 2000.
A Mental Health Decentralization and Integration of Mental Health in Primary Health Plan was prepared in 2002.

National Therapeutic Drug Policy/Essential List of Drugs A national therapeutic drug policy/essential list of drugs is present. It was formulated in 1972.

Mental Health Legislation There is a Mental Health Care Act (act no 24). It repealed the older Lunacy Act. The Act is detailed and has provisions for procedure of admission and discharge of patients, rights of patients, living conditions of the hospitals, legal issues pertaining to courts and ability to stand for trial. There are also provisions for actual treatment issues like person responsible for care, plan of treatment, follow-up, etc. A new Mental Health Care Act is under preparation to cover developments related to community psychiatric services/care.
The latest legislation was enacted in 1998.

Mental Health Financing There are budget allocations for mental health.
The country spends 0.3% of the total health budget on mental health.
The primary sources of mental health financing in descending order are tax based, out of pocket expenditure by the patient or family and private insurances.
The country has disability benefits for persons with mental disorders. Two types of benefits are present: (1) basic invalidity pension for those who have 60% of mental handicap; (2) basic invalidity pension and carer's allowance for those who are non-ambulant, have severe disability and who need constant carer's assistance.

Mental Health Facilities Mental health is a part of primary health care system. Actual treatment of severe mental disorders is available at the primary level. Primary care is provided as an outpatient service and as follow-up after treatment at the main psychiatric hospital.
Regular training of primary care professionals is carried out in the field of mental health.
There are community care facilities for patients with mental disorders. Six centres provide community care facilities.

Psychiatric Beds and Professionals

Total psychiatric beds per 10 000 population	9.5
Psychiatric beds in mental hospitals per 10 000 population	8
Psychiatric beds in general hospitals per 10 000 population	1
Psychiatric beds in other settings per 10 000 population	0.5
Number of psychiatrists per 100 000 population	1
Number of neurosurgeons per 100 000 population	0.5
Number of psychiatric nurses per 100 000 population	5
Number of neurologists per 100 000 population	0.1
Number of psychologists per 100 000 population	1
Number of social workers per 100 000 population	1

There are 5 occupational therapists and 4 assistants.

Non-Governmental Organizations NGOs are involved with mental health in the country. They are mainly involved in rehabilitation.

Information Gathering System There is mental health reporting system in the country. Details about services, morbidity, cause of death are published in the Annual Health Statistics. Some information is available about neurotic disorders and alcohol dependence as per ICD 9 criteria.
The country has data collection system or epidemiological study on mental health. Details are given in the Annual Health Statistics. Hospital and community clinic attendance and discharge are reported under the broad group of 'mental disorders'. An epidemiological survey was carried out in 1997-1998 under the aegis of Ministry of Health/Mauritius Institute of Health and Mauritius Psychiatric Association in collaboration with Ins CCOMS Paris, under the title 'Recherche Epidemiologique Multicentrique: La Santé Mentale en Population Generale. Image et Realite'.
The Republic of Mauritius publishes two separate Annual Health Statistics from its two islands of Mauritius and Rodrigues.

Programmes for Special Population The country has specific programmes for mental health for elderly and children.

Therapeutic Drugs The following therapeutic drugs are generally available at the primary health care level of the country: carbamazepine, ethosuximide, phenobarbital, phenytoin sodium, sodium valproate, amitriptyline, chlorpromazine, diazepam, fluphenazine, haloperidol, lithium, biperiden, carbidopa, levodopa.
Other anti-cholinergics (benzhexol, orphenadrine and procyclidine) and newer anti-psychotics (olanzapine, risperidone) and antidepressants (paroxetine) are also available. All the drugs are strictly controlled and dispensed against prescriptions. The prices are Government controlled. Other drugs are available from private pharmacies.

Other Information

Additional Sources of Information

Government Gazette of Mauritius (1998) Legal Supplement – Mental Health Care Act of 1998.

Ministry of Health (2000) Health Statistics Annual. Ministry of Health and Quality of Life. Island of Mauritius.

Ministry of Health (2000) Health Statistics Annual. Ministry of Health and Quality of Life. Island of Rodrigues.

Reynolds, C. A., Raine, A., Mellingen, K., et al (2000) Three-factor model of schizotypal personality: invariance across culture, gender, religious affiliation, family adversity, and psychopathology. Schizophrenia Bulletin, 26, 603-618.

Venables, P. H. (1996) Schizotypy and maternal exposure to influenza and to cold temperature: the Mauritius study. Journal of Abnormal Psychology, 105, 53-60.

Venables, P. H. (1997) Maternal exposure to influenza and cold in pregnancy and electrodermal activity in offspring: the Mauritius Study. Psychophysiology, 34, 427-435.

Mexico

GENERAL INFORMATION

Mexico is a country with an approximate area of 1958 thousand sq. km. (UNO, 2001). Its population is 104.931 million, and the sex ratio (men per hundred women) is 96 (UNO, 2004). The proportion of population under the age of 15 years is 32% (UNO, 2004), and the proportion of population above the age of 60 years is 7% (WHO, 2004). The literacy rate is 92.6% for men and 88.7% for women (UNESCO/MoH, 2004).

The country is a higher middle income group country (based on World Bank 2004 criteria). The proportion of health budget to GDP is 6.1%. The per capita total expenditure on health is 544 international $, and the per capita government expenditure on health is 241 international $ (WHO, 2004).

The main language(s) used in the country is (are) Spanish. The largest ethnic group(s) is (are) Mestizo (three-fourths), and the other ethnic group(s) are (is) Native American. The largest religious group(s) is (are) Roman Catholic (nine-tenths).

The life expectancy at birth is 71.7 years for males and 76.9 years for females (WHO, 2004). The healthy life expectancy at birth is 63 years for males and 68 years for females (WHO, 2004).

EPIDEMIOLOGY

Caraveo-Anduaga et al (1997, 1999) assessed 1932 adults using a modified version of the Composite International Diagnostic Interview (CIDI). The prevalence of any disorder according to ICD-10 was 28.7% (commonest disorders were alcohol use disorders and depressive disorders). Comorbidity was present in 33% of cases (commonest comorbid conditions were anxiety disorders). The lifetime and 12-month prevalence of depression was 7.9% and 4.5%, respectively. The 1-year incidence of depression was 1.3%. Lifetime prevalence of dysthymia was 4.4 %, with a female-male ratio of 2:1. Based on the same study, Caraveo-Anduaga and Colmenares (2000) reported that the lifetime prevalence of various phobic disorders ranged from 2.1% to 2.8%. Most phobic disorders were more frequent in women. De Snyder and Diaz-Perez (1999) assessed 945 rural adults using the Fresno version of the Composite International Diagnostic Interview and ICD 10. The lifetime prevalence of depression, dysthymia and nervios, respectively were 6.2% (women 9.1% and men 2.9%), 3.4% (women 5.2% and men 1.4%) and 15.4% (women 20.8% and men 9.5%). Caraveo-Anduaga and Bermudez (2002) assessed 1734 adults with a modified version of CIDI (DSM-III-R criteria) as a part of the International Consortium of Psychiatric Epidemiology (ICPE) study. Psychiatric disorders were more common among women while substance use disorders were more common in men. Depressive disorders (major depression and dysthymia) were two times more frequent in women (10% and 1.8%) than in men (5.5% and 0.9%); while mania was more frequent in men (2.1%) than in women (0.9%). Agoraphobia, social and simple phobias also predominated in women (5.1%, 2.9% and 3.4% women vs. 2.9%, 1.6% and 2.3% men). Alcohol use disorders were 8.6 times more common than any other substance use disorder, with life time prevalence estimates of 18.6% for alcohol abuse and 7.5% for alcohol dependence. Vega et al (2002) reported the results of the ICPE study on substance use. Using CIDI, the lifetime prevalence rates of use of alcohol (>11 times), marijuana (>4 times) and other drugs were 43.2%, 1.7% and 1.7%, respectively. Tapia-Conyer et al (1990) reported that alcohol dependence was present in 6% (12% of men and <1% of women) and tobacco dependence in 17% of adults. A number of surveys (including national surveys) on drug use among school students and adolescents have been conducted on large samples (500 to 60 000 subjects). Between 22.5%-58.3% reported use of substances in the past month. Drug use by school children/adolescents was found to be associated with gender (male), age (older), socioeconomic status (low) and drug use by peers and family members (e.g. Berenzon et al, 1996; Rojas, 1998). Moreno et al (1999) found depression in 35% of 246 elderly subjects (above 65 years) who were assessed with the General Health Questionnaire. Depression was associated with gender (female), marital status (widowed/divorced), socio-economic status (low), education (poor) and unemployment. Pando-Moreno et al (2001) found sleep disorders (as per DSM-IV) in 33.3% of elders living in the community. Borges et al (1996) analysed death certificates and census data, and found that the rate of suicide increased between 1970 (1.1 per 100 000) and 1994 (2.9 per 100 000), particularly among males and in young (below 19 years) and old (above 65 years) people. The highest suicide rate was in elderly males. Hijar et al (1996) reviewed the mortality database and found that suicides accounted for a greater proportion of deaths in 1993 in comparison to 1979. The main methods of committing suicide were hanging, use of firearms and explosives and poisoning. Mondragon et al (1998) reported that use of different methodologies and samples yielded variable rates of suicide attempts and suicidal ideation (highest rates were 10% and 40.7%, respectively). Borges et al (2000) assessed 1094 adult patients in a general hospital. The lifetime prevalence of suicide attempts was 6.1%. Suicide attempts were associated with gender (female), marital status, age, depressed mood, hopelessness, alcohol use and psychopathology. Gonzalez-Forteza et al (2001) assessed 996 adolescents and found that the rate of sexual abuse, depression and suicide attempts in girls was 7%, 15% and 11%, respectively, and among boys 2%, 14% and 4%, respectively. Sexual abuse and depression were associated with suicide attempts. In a study on 4157 adolescents, Swanson et al (1992) reported that 39.4% had depression (Center for Epidemiologic Studies' Depression Scale score >16) and 11.6% reported current suicidal ideation. Caraveo et al (1995) validated the Reporting Questionnaire for Children (RQC) during the National Mental Health Survey – 1988. Studies in children (sample size >1000) using the parent administered RQC showed that between 13.4% and 20.7% of children had mental disorders (Caraveo et al, 1995; Rico et al, 1998). Rate of mental disorders in children was associated with gender (male), age (above 7 years), birth order (>3) and family type (single parent family) (Rico et al, 1998).

MENTAL HEALTH RESOURCES

Mental Health Policy A mental health policy is present. The policy was initially formulated in 1983.
The components of the policy are promotion, prevention, treatment and rehabilitation. It was revised in 2001 by a process that involved politicians, mental health professionals, NGOs, public servants and consumers. Between 25 to 50% of its original content was put into practice. A psychiatric reform will be launched following the model of Miguel Hidalgo. The National Council of Mental Health was established in 2004. The model contemplates the creation of structures based on the respect of the rights of the users and on provision of integrated medical/psychiatric care with quality and warmth. The model emphasizes community care in the form of preventive services (offered through health centres, health centres with mental health modules, mental health community centres and mental health integrated centres), short-term hospitalization (in psychiatric units in general hospitals, acute wards of psychiatric hospitals and new hospital structures (villas) being created) and social reintegration (half way houses, community housing, independent flats, residences for the elderly, sheltered workshops, mixed cooperatives, social clubs, etc.). Presently, this model is being implemented in 3 federal entities: Tamaulipas, Hidalgo and State of Mexico.

Substance Abuse Policy A substance abuse policy is present. The policy was initially formulated in 2000. It has a specific budget for its implementation and 25 to 50% of its content has been implemented. The law on substance abuse currently in use was formulated in 1983. The National Council of Addictions was established in 1984 and upgraded to the level of Commission in 2000. It has the function of setting the policies and strategies on addiction, as well as setting up the National Programme against Addiction.

National Mental Health Programme A national mental health programme is present. The programme was formulated in 2001. The reform programme of the health sector 2001-2006 includes the establishment and implementation of the national mental health programme. The 2000-01 programme included the New Model of Care in Mental Health, which proposed broader options including health centres, community centres, half-way houses, community residences, etc. It also took into account the patient's rights and focused on their social reinsertion. The programme implementation for the years 2001-2006 includes the prevention and control of depression, schizophrenia, epilepsy, dementia and attention deficit disorder. It has been implemented to the extent of 10 to 25% by local, regional and national authorities. Its main components are strategy of services reform, promotion and prevention, integration of mental health services in primary care and development of specialized services. The various provinces/regions have different mental health programmes currently in place.

National Therapeutic Drug Policy/Essential List of Drugs A national therapeutic drug policy/essential list of drugs is present. It was formulated in 1970.

Mental Health Legislation The most recent legislation in the area was a chapter about mental health in the general health legislation. It was revised in 2000. Regular funds are available for its implementation and it has been implemented to the extent of 75% to 90%. Promotion, prevention, users' rights, involuntary treatment, mental health services regulation, human rights and advocacy are some of its components. However, it lacks regulations on housing for mentally ill people. Under its provisions, about 50% of total admissions for treatment are involuntary.
The latest legislation was enacted in 1983.

Mental Health Financing There are budget allocations for mental health.
The country spends 1% of the total health budget on mental health.
The primary sources of mental health financing in descending order are tax based, out of pocket expenditure by the patient or family, social insurance and private insurances.
The amount spent on mental health is assigned exclusively to the mental health services and the seven units depending on it. The psychiatric units of the decentralized institutions have their own budgets. In addition, there are two systems of social security (IMSS and ISSSTE) and Ministry of Health supports those who do not have social security.
The country has disability benefits for persons with mental disorders. Disability benefits are included in the New Law of the Mexican Institute of Social Security (IMSS) and the Law of the Institute of State Workers Security and Social Services (ISSSTE). Benefits are available for severe disorders, but the process of documenting the disability is complicated and often difficult to obtain. Further, disability benefits are available only for those covered by social security (less than 10% of the population).

Mental Health Facilities Mental health is a part of primary health care system. Actual treatment of severe mental disorders is available at the primary level. Human resources are limited and cannot fulfil the demands of mental health. Less than 25 % of the population is covered by this kind of service and they are usually provided by primary health care doctors. Treatment for severe disorders is limited at the primary care level. A system of referral is in place.
Regular training of primary care professionals is carried out in the field of mental health. There is a major movement towards decentralization that is likely to lead to educational programmes for the health staff, close contact with the communities and the inclusion of mental health programmes and activities at primary health care services.
There are community care facilities for patients with mental disorders. The community based care system is mainly provided through outpatient clinics and includes prevention and promotion interventions, residential facilities and vocational training.

Psychiatric Beds and Professionals

Total psychiatric beds per 10 000 population	0.667
Psychiatric beds in mental hospitals per 10 000 population	0.51
Psychiatric beds in general hospitals per 10 000 population	0.051
Psychiatric beds in other settings per 10 000 population	
Number of psychiatrists per 100 000 population	2.7
Number of neurosurgeons per 100 000 population	1.5
Number of psychiatric nurses per 100 000 population	0.1
Number of neurologists per 100 000 population	1.2
Number of psychologists per 100 000 population	
Number of social workers per 100 000 population	0.2

There are 2920 other mental health workers. There are 45 629 psychologists working under the Department of Health and related Ministries. Most public specialist mental health services are in big cities. There are few private psychiatric hospitals but recently services for drug abuse patients have increased. 28% of these beds are occupied by long stay patients. Only about 33% of psychiatrists work in public institutions.

Non-Governmental Organizations NGOs are involved with mental health in the country. They are mainly involved in advocacy, promotion, prevention, treatment and rehabilitation. Joint collaboration, as well as counselling in the implementation of the New Model of Mental Health Care is done with the NGOs. They participate in psychosocial and pharmacological interventions related to women, children, drug addition, domestic violence and consumers. It is estimated that they are responsible for 25% of the promotion, prevention and advocacy activities that are carried out in Mexico.

Information Gathering System There is mental health reporting system in the country. Mental disorders of discharged hospital patients are reported in the annual statistics of the Health Ministry. ICD 10 is used for recording purposes.
The country has data collection system or epidemiological study on mental health. The 'Dirección General de Estatística e Informática' is in charge of the data collection system for mental disorders. Data collection is done only for part of the health system (public institutions).

Programmes for Special Population The country has specific programmes for mental health for refugees, disaster affected population, indigenous population, elderly and children. There are facilities for victims of domestic violence.
Also, there are programmes for women, children in vulnerable situation and domestic violence. They have the participation of national organizations.

Therapeutic Drugs The following therapeutic drugs are generally available at the primary health care level of the country: carbamazepine, phenobarbital, phenytoin sodium, sodium valproate, amitriptyline, chlorpromazine, diazepam, fluphenazine, haloperidol, lithium, biperiden, carbidopa, levodopa.
The national therapeutic drugs policy was revised in 2000. All the drugs are in the essential list and hence should be available always, but that is not so, especially in the rural areas. Some prices are subsided in some regions.

Other Information There are two essential developments in mental health services. First, the establishment in 1997 of the Mental Health Services, formerly the Mental Health Coordination, as a decentralized institution, in order to set up, organize, supervise and evaluate the development of activities related to health care services, as well as improving psychiatric and mental health services in the country. Second, the setting up and implementation of the New Model of Mental Health Care, which is the beginning of the restructuring of the mental health care services system in Mexico.

Additional Sources of Information

Benassini, O. (1997) Atencion en salud mental regionalizacion y reorientacion en el marco de la descentralizacion de servicios de la salud en Mexico. Salud Mental, 20, 48-53.

Benassini, O. (2001) La atencion psiquiatrica en Mexico hacia el silgo XXI. Salud Mental, 24, 62-73.

Berenzon, S., Medina-Mora, M. E., Carreno, S., et al (1996) The use and abuse of psychoactive substances among Mexican high school students. Salud Mental, 19, 44-52.

Borges, G., Rosovsky, H., Gomez, C., et al (1996) Epidemiology of suicide in Mexico, 1970-1984. Salud Publica de Mexico, 38, 197-206.

Borges, G., Saltijeral, M. T., Bimbela, A., et al (2000) Suicide attempts in a sample of patients from a general hospital. Archives of Medical Research, 31, 366-372.

Caraveo-Anduaga, J. J., Bermudez, E. C. (2002) Psychiatric disorders and substance abuse in Mexico: Epidemiological perspective. Salud Mental, 25, 9-15.

Caraveo-Anduaga, J. J., Colmenares, E. (2000) Prevalence of phobic anxiety disorders in the adult population of Mexico City. Salud Mental, 23, 10-19.

Caraveo-Anduaga, J. J., Colmenares, E. B., Saldivar, G. J. H. (1999) Psychiatric morbidity in Mexico City: Prevalence and comorbidity during life time. Salud Mental, 22, 62-67.

Caraveo-Anduaga, J. J., Martinez-Velez, N. A., Rivera-Guevara, B. E., et al (1997) Life prevalence of depressive episodes and the use of specialized services. Salud Mental, 20, 15-23.

Caraveo, J., Medina-Mora, M.E., Villatoro, J., et al (1995) Detection of mental health problems in childhood. Salud Publica de Mexico, 37, 446-451.

De Snyder, V. N. S., Diaz-Perez, MaDJ (1999) Affective disorders among the rural population. Salud Mental, 22, 68-74.

Gonzalez-Forteza, C., Ramos, L. L., Vignau Brambila, L. E., et al (2001) Sexual abuse and suicide attempt associated with recent depressive distress and suicide ideation in adolescents. Salud Mental, 24, 16-25.

Hijar, M. M., Rascon, P. RA, Blanco, M. J., et al (1996) Suicide in Mexico. Sexual and geographical characteristics (1979-1993). Salud Mental, 19, 14-21.

Ley General de Salud. Titulo Decimosegundo, Control sanitario de productos y servicios y de su importacion y expotacion chp.6

Ley General de Salud. Titulo Primero, Disposiciones generales.

Ley General de Salud. Titulo Tercero, Prestacion de los servicios de salud.

Ley General de Salud. Titulo Decimoprimero, Programa contra las adicciones.

Ministry of Health (2000) Mental Health Policy.

Mondragon, L., Saltijeral, M. T., Bimbela, A., et al (1998) Suicidal ideation and its relation with hopelessness and drug and alcohol abuse. Salud Mental, 21, 20-27.

Moreno, M. P., Beltran, C. A., Leon Barbosa, J. L. P., et al (1999) Mental health in senior citizens in the metropolitan zone of Guadalajara. Aging-Clinical & Experimental Research, 11, 96-100.

Pando-Moreno, M., Beltran, C. A., Aldrete, M. E., et al (2001) Prevalence of sleep disorders in the elderly. Cadernos de Saude Publica, 17, 63-69.

Rico, H., Magis, C., Guerrero, M. G., et al (1998) Frequency of mental disorders in elementary first grade scholars. Salud Mental, 21, 12-18.

Rojas, E., Medina-Mora, M. E., Villatoro, J., et al (1998) Evolution of drug abuse problems among Mexico City students. Salud Mental, 21, 37-42.

Secretaria de Salud (2000). Para la prevencion, tratamiento y control de las adicciones.

Secretaria de Salud (2000). Chapter 4 Sistemas de Informacion. Sistima de vigilancia epidemiolégica de las adicciones, terminologia y clasificacion, Direccion General de Epidemiologia, Secretaria de Salud, Mexico.

Secretaria de Salud (1995). Para la prestacion de servicios de salud enunidades de atencion integral hospitalaria medico-psiquiatrics.

Secretaria de Salud (1987). Para la Prestacion de servicios de atencion medica en Hospitales Psiquatricos. Secretaria de Salud.

Swanson, J.W., Linskey, A.O., Quintero-Salinas, R., et al (1992) A binational school survey of depressive symptoms, drug use, and suicidal ideation. Journal of the American Academy of Child & Adolescent Psychiatry, 31, 669-678.

Tapia-Conyer, R., Medina-Mora, M.E., Sepulveda, J., et al (1990) The national addictions survey of Mexico. Salud Pública de Mexico, 32, 507-522.

Vega, W. A., Aguilar-Gaxiola, S., Andrade, L., et al (2002) Prevalence and age of onset for drug use in seven international sites: Results from the international consortium of psychiatric epidemiology. Drug & Alcohol Dependence, 68, 285-297.

Micronesia, Federated States of

GENERAL INFORMATION

Micronesia, Federated States of is a country with an approximate area of 0.7 thousand sq. km. (UNO, 2001). The country consists of four major island groups with more than 600 islands. Its population is 0.111 million, and the sex ratio (men per hundred women) is 102 (UNO, 2004). The proportion of population under the age of 15 years is 38% (UNO, 2004), and the proportion of population above the age of 60 years is 5% (WHO, 2004). The literacy rate is 91% for men and 88% for women (UNESCO/MoH, 2004). The country is a lower middle income group country (based on World Bank 2004 criteria). The proportion of health budget to GDP is 7.8%. The per capita total expenditure on health is 319 international $, and the per capita government expenditure on health is 230 international $ (WHO, 2004).

The main language(s) used in the country is (are) English and Micronesian languages (e.g. Chuukese, Pohnpeian, Yapese, Kosraean). The largest ethnic group(s) is (are) Micronesian (Chuukese/Mortlockese, Yapese, Outer Island Yapese, Pohnpeian and Kosraean), and the other ethnic group(s) are (is) Chinese, Caucasian and Filipino. The largest religious group(s) is (are) Roman Catholic (more than half of the population), and the other religious group(s) are (is) Protestant (about two-fifths).

The life expectancy at birth is 64.9 years for males and 68.1 years for females (WHO, 2004). The healthy life expectancy at birth is 57 years for males and 58 years for females (WHO, 2004).

EPIDEMIOLOGY

Waldo (1999) studied schizophrenia in one island of Micronesia and found 22 patients giving a prevalence rate of 6.8/1000 and a male to female ratio of 6.3:1. Although the profile was similar to that found in western societies, the majority of the patients were episodically mute, especially when untreated or inadequately treated. Rubinstein (1983) reported that suicide rates had increased substantially in Micronesia among the post-war cohort, especially among the young adults. The authors inferred that gradual dissolution of social cohesiveness due to break-up of village and communal lineage-houses was the reason for such an increase. Allan and Hunter (1985) commented on regional variations in rates of occurrence of disorders, manifestation of symptoms, demographic characteristics and referral patterns and their relationship to social and cultural factors.

MENTAL HEALTH RESOURCES

Mental Health Policy A mental health policy is present. The policy was initially formulated in 1986.
The components of the policy are advocacy, promotion, prevention and treatment.

Substance Abuse Policy A substance abuse policy is present. The policy was initially formulated in 1989.

National Mental Health Programme A national mental health programme is present. The programme was formulated in 1989.

National Therapeutic Drug Policy/Essential List of Drugs A national therapeutic drug policy/essential list of drugs is present. It was formulated in 1991.

Mental Health Legislation Details about existing mental health legislation are not available. However, there is a tobacco law. All four states of Micronesia have passed the law making it illegal to sell tobacco to minors. This was formulated in 1994.
Details about the year of enactment of the mental health legislation are not available.

Mental Health Financing There are budget allocations for mental health.
The country spends 7.3% of the total health budget on mental health.
The primary sources of mental health financing in descending order are grants, social insurance, out of pocket expenditure by the patient or family and tax based.
A small amount ($14 000.00) is allotted to purchase medication for the mental health patients each year.
The country has disability benefits for persons with mental disorders. Mentally ill children of a state/federation employee are provided with a small benefit of $50 if the parent dies.

Mental Health Facilities Mental health is a part of primary health care system. Actual treatment of severe mental disorders is available at the primary level.
Regular training of primary care professionals is carried out in the field of mental health. In the last two years, about 21 personnel were provided training. The Hawaii State Hospital is the primary site for teaching clinical psychiatry to the Pacific Basin Medical Officer Training Program. Transcultural issues are discussed.
There are community care facilities for patients with mental disorders. CMHS supports the activities on mental health issues.

Psychiatric Beds and Professionals

Total psychiatric beds per 10 000 population	0.7
Psychiatric beds in mental hospitals per 10 000 population	0
Psychiatric beds in general hospitals per 10 000 population	0.7
Psychiatric beds in other settings per 10 000 population	0
Number of psychiatrists per 100 000 population	0
Number of neurosurgeons per 100 000 population	0
Number of psychiatric nurses per 100 000 population	0
Number of neurologists per 100 000 population	0
Number of psychologists per 100 000 population	0
Number of social workers per 100 000 population	4

There is 1 occupational therapist, 4 hospital administrators, 5 medical assistants, 12 medical officers and 4 other kind of staff. The Government is considering the deployment of social workers as counsellors.

Non-Governmental Organizations NGOs are involved with mental health in the country. They are mainly involved in advocacy, promotion, prevention and rehabilitation.

Information Gathering System There is mental health reporting system in the country. Quarterly and annual reports are made. The country has data collection system or epidemiological study on mental health. There is a mental health information system. This uses EPI and epidemiological surveillance system called MHIS.

Programmes for Special Population The country has specific programmes for mental health for minorities, disaster affected population, indigenous population, elderly and children. The whole population is composed of minorities and indigenous people (as per SAMHSA definitions).

Therapeutic Drugs The following therapeutic drugs are generally available at the primary health care level of the country: carbamazepine, phenobarbital, phenytoin sodium, amitriptyline, chlorpromazine, diazepam, fluphenazine, haloperidol, lithium.

Other Information Outreach service is hindered by the distances between the islands. The field trip ship runs about once every three months. Small planes can fly only to one island (once a week) with an airfield. Motor boats are used to extend the services.

Additional Sources of Information

Allan, A. T., Hunter, E. M. (1985) Cross-cultural psychiatry in Micronesia: the consultant's view. International Journal of Social Psychiatry, 31, 59-66.

Bernstein, D., Young, D. M. (1996) Shrinking the Western Pacific: psychiatric training for medical students from Micronesia. Hawaii Medical Journal, 55, 70-71.

Government document (1994) Third Pohnpei Legislature, Fourteenth Special Session.

Rubinstein, D. H. (1983) Epidemic suicide among Micronesian adolescents. Social Science & Medicine, 17, 657-665.

Rubenstein, D. H. (1992) Suicide in Micronesia and Samoa: a critique of explanations. Pacific Studies, 15, 51-75.

Waldo, M. C. (1999) Schizophrenia in Kosrae, Micronesia: prevalence, gender ratios, and clinical symptomatology. Schizophrenia Research, 35, 175-181.

J–M

Monaco

GENERAL INFORMATION

Monaco is a country with an approximate area of 0.002 thousand sq. km. (UNO, 2001). Its population is 0.032 million, and the sex ratio (men per hundred women) is 94 (UNO, 2004). The proportion of population under the age of 15 years is 13% (UNO, 2004), and the proportion of population above the age of 60 years is 20% (WHO, 2004).

The country is a high income group country (based on World Bank 2004 criteria). The proportion of health budget to GDP is 7.6%. The per capita total expenditure on health is 2016 international $, and the per capita government expenditure on health is 1131 international $ (WHO, 2004).

The main language(s) used in the country is (are) French. The largest ethnic group(s) is (are) French. The largest religious group(s) is (are) Monegasque Christian, and the other religious group(s) are (is) Roman Catholic.

The life expectancy at birth is 77.8 years for males and 84.5 years for females (WHO, 2004). The healthy life expectancy at birth is 71 years for males and 75 years for females (WHO, 2004).

EPIDEMIOLOGY

There is substantial epidemiological data on mental illnesses in Monaco in internationally accessible literature. No attempt was made to include this information here.

MENTAL HEALTH RESOURCES

Mental Health Policy A mental health policy is present. Details about the year of formulation are not available.

Substance Abuse Policy A substance abuse policy is present. The policy was initially formulated in 1995.

National Mental Health Programme A national mental health programme is present. Details about the year of formulation of the programme are not available.

National Therapeutic Drug Policy/Essential List of Drugs A national therapeutic drug policy/essential list of drugs is absent.

Mental Health Legislation The Law No 1039 of 1981 concerning the placement and protection of the mentally ill.
The latest legislation was enacted in 1981.

Mental Health Financing There are budget allocations for mental health.
Details about expenditure on mental health are not available.
The primary source of mental health financing is social insurance.
The country has disability benefits for persons with mental disorders.

Mental Health Facilities Mental health is a part of primary health care system. Actual treatment of severe mental disorders is available at the primary level.
Details about training facilities are not available.
There are no community care facilities for patients with mental disorders.

Psychiatric Beds and Professionals

Total psychiatric beds per 10 000 population	17.27
Psychiatric beds in mental hospitals per 10 000 population	0
Psychiatric beds in general hospitals per 10 000 population	17.27
Psychiatric beds in other settings per 10 000 population	0
Number of psychiatrists per 100 000 population	28.5
Number of neurosurgeons per 100 000 population	0
Number of psychiatric nurses per 100 000 population	
Number of neurologists per 100 000 population	6
Number of psychologists per 100 000 population	33
Number of social workers per 100 000 population	81

Non-Governmental Organizations NGOs are not involved with mental health in the country.

Information Gathering System There is mental health reporting system in the country.
The country has no data collection system or epidemiological study on mental health.

Programmes for Special Population The country has specific programmes for mental health for elderly.

Therapeutic Drugs The following therapeutic drugs are generally available at the primary health care level of the country: carbamazepine, ethosuximide, phenobarbital, sodium valproate, amitriptyline, chlorpromazine, diazepam, fluphenazine, lithium, biperiden, carbidopa, levodopa.
Phenytoin and Haloperidol are only for hospitals.

Other Information

Additional Sources of Information

Usuelles, L. (1993) Law Number 1039 Concerning the Placement and Protection of Mentally Ill.

Mongolia

GENERAL INFORMATION

Mongolia is a country with an approximate area of 1567 thousand sq. km. (UNO, 2001). Its population is 2.63 million, and the sex ratio (men per hundred women) is 100 (UNO, 2004). The proportion of population under the age of 15 years is 31% (UNO, 2004), and the proportion of population above the age of 60 years is 6% (WHO, 2004). The literacy rate is 98% for men and 97.5% for women (UNESCO/MoH, 2004).

The country is a low income group country (based on World Bank 2004 criteria). The proportion of health budget to GDP is 6.4%. The per capita total expenditure on health is 122 international $, and the per capita government expenditure on health is 88 international $ (WHO, 2004).

The main language(s) used in the country is (are) Mongolian. The largest ethnic group(s) is (are) Mongolian (Khalkh Mongol, four-fifths of the population), and the other ethnic group(s) are (is) Kazakh, Tuvin, Uzbek, Russian and Chinese. The largest religious group(s) is (are) Buddhist.

The life expectancy at birth is 60.1 years for males and 65.9 years for females (WHO, 2004). The healthy life expectancy at birth is 53 years for males and 58 years for females (WHO, 2004).

EPIDEMIOLOGY

There is a paucity of epidemiological data on mental illnesses in Mongolia in internationally accessible literature. Dorjjadamba (1970) reported that historical cultural background, geographical environment and custom of ethnic groups were closely related to mental health including the rate, type and presentation of mental disorders. According to the results of epidemiological survey conducted in 1976-1984, the prevalence of major mental disorder ranged from 1.0% to 2.4% in different regions (Tsetsegdary, 2004). A study conducted in 2002-2003 showed a three-fold increase in rate of suicide over a decade (1992-2002), with figures for 2002 being 36 cases per 100 000 people. The prevalence of schizophrenia was 0.1% (Tsetsegdary, 2004).

MENTAL HEALTH RESOURCES

Mental Health Policy A mental health policy is absent.

But the State Policy on Public Health adopted by the Parliament in 2001 included some statements on mental health.

Substance Abuse Policy A substance abuse policy is absent. The State Policy on Public Health adopted by the Parliament in 2001 also included some statements on substance abuse policy. There are laws on fighting against harm related to alcohol (1994 & 2000), tobacco (1993/under revision) and a Law on Control of Tracking in Narcotic Drugs and Psychotropic Substances (2002). There is also the National Programme on Prevention of Narcotics and Drug Abuse (2000) and Alcohol Prevention and Control (2003).

National Mental Health Programme A national mental health programme is present. The programme was formulated in 2002. The programme emphasized mental health promotion, community mental health care, accessibility to care and intersectoral collaboration.

National Therapeutic Drug Policy/Essential List of Drugs A national therapeutic drug policy/essential list of drugs is present. It was formulated in 1996.

Mental Health Legislation The Law of Mongolia on Mental Health emphasized mental health promotion, community mental health care, accessibility to care, rights of mentally ill persons and their legal representatives, forced hospitalization, provision of security and social welfare assistance for mentally ill persons and intersectoral collaboration.

The latest legislation was enacted in 2000.

Mental Health Financing There are budget allocations for mental health.

The country spends 5% of the total health budget on mental health.

The primary sources of mental health financing in descending order are tax based and social insurance.

Nearly 90% of total budget allocated from the State for the treatment, rehabilitation and social care of people with mental disorders is spent to cover hospital expenditures and for providing inpatient and outpatient mental health care. Three-fourths of the population is covered by health insurance.

The country has disability benefits for persons with mental disorders. Disability benefits are provided according to the Law on Social Welfare adopted in 1998.

Mental Health Facilities Mental health is a part of primary health care system. Actual treatment of severe mental disorders is not available at the primary level.

Regular training of primary care professionals is carried out in the field of mental health. In the last two years, about 350 personnel were provided training. WHO has assisted in the training of trainers, and translated training materials are available. Every province was covered. Almost 45% of general physicians and 3% of primary health workers have been trained. An evaluation of this programme has been carried out in 1999. Training on management of mental health issues during disasters was provided to family doctors, social welfare workers, Red Cross personnel, police and local administrators in provinces affected by dzud (winter natural disaster).

There are community care facilities for patients with mental disorders. In the community drugs are provided free of cost, psychosocial rehabilitation welfare service towards children with mental retardation is also present. There are seven day care centres and about 12 residential (tent based) programmes that carry out occupational rehabilitation. There is a plan to start a sheltered workshop in the community.

Psychiatric Beds and Professionals

Total psychiatric beds per 10 000 population	2.4
Psychiatric beds in mental hospitals per 10 000 population	1.7
Psychiatric beds in general hospitals per 10 000 population	0.7
Psychiatric beds in other settings per 10 000 population	0
Number of psychiatrists per 100 000 population	3.3
Number of neurosurgeons per 100 000 population	0.4
Number of psychiatric nurses per 100 000 population	4.4
Number of neurologists per 100 000 population	7
Number of psychologists per 100 000 population	6
Number of social workers per 100 000 population	3

Psychologists and social workers are trained by state pedagogical institutes and work in social welfare organizations. There are 21 general hospital psychiatric units with 5 to 15 beds, each. Some beds in the psychiatry hospitals are earmarked for children. Forensic psychiatric services are available at the State Psychiatric hospital at Ulaanbbtar. About 50 beds for voluntary and 160 beds for involuntary (Under the Ministry of Justice) treatment of alcohol misuse are available. Designated psychiatrists have 4-6 months of on the job training in psychiatry in their internship. Postgraduate psychiatric education includes residential training (1-2 years), Master's degree course (2 years), Refresher training course (2-3 month), PhD (3 years) and Scientific degree – Dr. Sc. Med. The Health Law of 1998 includes provisions related to the licensing of medical practitioners and the accreditation of health institutions.

Non-Governmental Organizations NGOs are involved with mental health in the country. They are mainly involved in advocacy, promotion and rehabilitation. The WHO initiated the formation of the Mongolian Mental Health Association (with psychiatrists, volunteers and representatives from other NGOs as members), which is active in promoting mental health public education and community care and rehabilitation. American, Belgian and Dutch NGOs and the Asian Development Bank have helped with equipment, funds and training of primary health care staff.

Information Gathering System There is mental health reporting system in the country. Details are available from the Health Statistics office of Directorate Medical Service under the Ministry of Health, and Statistics Unit of Mental Health and Narcology Center.
The country has data collection system or epidemiological study on mental health. It was established with the support of WHO. A mental health database has been established with the help of WHO.

Programmes for Special Population The country has specific programmes for mental health for minorities, disaster affected population, elderly and children. There are Government programmes on elderly and adolescent health and on disaster management. The Ministry of Health and the Ministry of Education, Culture and Science are introducing the concept of life skills education at the secondary school level. Teachers, school doctors and social workers are being trained to implement a school mental health programme. Telephone counselling services for adolescents have been set up in two provinces and three districts of Ulaanbaatar with the aid of WHO. A school for the intellectually disabled has been set up at the State Psychiatric Hospital with the help of the ADRA (the Adventist Development Relief Agency). UNICEF is providing psychosocial support to children in areas affected by dzud (winter natural disaster) in 4 provinces. A network of sobering stations function under the charge of the Ministry of the Interior (Police).

Therapeutic Drugs The following therapeutic drugs are generally available at the primary health care level of the country: carbamazepine, phenobarbital, amitriptyline, chlorpromazine, diazepam, haloperidol, lithium, carbidopa, levodopa.
The fourth revision was made in 2000. Information on availability of drugs is from the Mongolian Government drug supply company 'Mongol Em Impex'and Drug Information Center of the Directorate Medical Service, Ministry of Health.

Other Information Ensuring adequate health services throughout a sparsely populated (1.5 inhabitants per sq. km.) terrain with extremes in climate is a challenging task to the health system, particularly because one-fifth of the populace leads a nomadic life.

Additional Sources of Information

Byambasuren S. (2000) Community based mental health service. Advanced training materials for family doctors. Ulaanbaatar, 3, 291.

Byambasuren, S., Tsetsegdary, G. (2004) Mental health in Mongolia. International Psychiatry, (in press).

Byambasuren, S., Erdenebayar, L., Tsetsegdary, G., et al (2003) Epidemiology of suicides among population in Ulaanbaatar city. Mongolian Medical Science, 3, 40-44.

Dorjjadamba, S. (1970) Some problems of epidemiology of neuromental derangements in Mongolian People's Republic. Sante Publique, 249-254.

Health Sector Review (1999) Mongolia, 1-2.

Human Development Report of Mongolia, 2003.

Khishigsuren, Z., Gantsetseg, T., Byambasuren, S. et al (2004) Epidemiology of schizophrenia in Ulaanbaatar, Mongolia. Mongolian Medical Science, 1, 39-42.

Morocco

GENERAL INFORMATION

Morocco is a country with an approximate area of 447 thousand sq. km. (UNO, 2001). Its population is 31.064 million, and the sex ratio (men per hundred women) is 100 (UNO, 2004). The proportion of population under the age of 15 years is 31% (UNO, 2004), and the proportion of population above the age of 60 years is 7% (WHO, 2004). The literacy rate is 63.3% for men and 38.3% for women (UNESCO/MoH, 2004).

The country is a lower middle income group country (based on World Bank 2004 criteria). The proportion of health budget to GDP is 5.1%. The per capita total expenditure on health is 199 international $, and the per capita government expenditure on health is 78 international $ (WHO, 2004).

The main language(s) used in the country is (are) Arabic. The largest ethnic group(s) is (are) Arab, and the other ethnic group(s) are (is) Berber. The largest religious group(s) is (are) Muslim.

The life expectancy at birth is 68.8 years for males and 72.8 years for females (WHO, 2004). The healthy life expectancy at birth is 60 years for males and 61 years for females (WHO, 2004).

EPIDEMIOLOGY

A WHO assisted study on prevalence of mental disorders has been conducted on representative samples (n=6000) from many regions of the country using the Mini International Neuropsychiatry Interview (MINI), and the results are being compiled. Data is regularly collected from public psychiatric institutions. In 2002, among outpatients (n=1 504 508), 34% had schizophrenia, 25.1% had mood disorders, 16.7% had neuroses and 1.8% had alcohol and drug use disorders. Among inpatients (n=15 398) 65.2% had schizophrenia, 11.9% had mood disorders, 2.5% had neuroses and 5.1% had alcohol and drug use disorders (Ministry of Health, 2004). Kadri et al (2002) used DSM-IV criteria to assess sexual dysfunction in a representative sample of the population of women aged 20 and older in one city (n=728). The 6-month prevalence was 26.6% with dysfunctions of sexual arousal as the commonest disorder. Age, financial dependency, number of children and sexual harassment were positively associated with presence of sexual disorder. Ghazal et al (2001) evaluated a randomly selected and representative sample of students attending six secondary schools (n=1887) and a second group composed of students of the French secondary school (n=157). Subjects completed a sociodemographic questionnaire and the Bulimic Investigatory Test of Edinburgh (BITE). In the first group, 15.3% of subjects took at least one substance, 12.7% were dependent on tobacco and 5.7% consumed alcohol occasionally. Almost a sixth of students reported a familial history of disturbed eating behaviour. The overall prevalence of bulimia in this group was 0.8% (1.2% in female and 0.1% in male subjects). The mean age of bulimic subjects was 18.6 years. In the group from the French school, the prevalence of bulimia was 1.9% in the whole sample (3.4% among girls and no case among boys). Bulimic subjects did not differ from the non bulimic subjects with regard to sociodemographic characteristics. Kadri et al (2000) assessed 100 adult males for two consecutive years over a 6-week period during Ramadan with clinical interviews, visual analog scales and the Hamilton Anxiety Scale. Smokers were significantly more irritable than non-smokers before the beginning of Ramadan. An increase in irritability was noted in both groups during Ramadan, but irritability increased more in smokers than in non-smokers. Taoudi Benchekroun et al (1999) reported that during Ramadan the sleep chronotype as evaluated by the Horne and Ostberg scale changed significantly with an increase of the evening type and a decrease in the morning type. Daytime sleepiness as evaluated by the Epworth Sleepiness Scale was significantly increased.

MENTAL HEALTH RESOURCES

Mental Health Policy A mental health policy is present. The policy was initially formulated in 1972.

The components of the policy are promotion, prevention, treatment and rehabilitation. Decentralization is also a component of the policy. Since 1972, the mental health policy has been reviewed several times with the help of the ' Moroccan Society of Psychiatry'. The legislation on mental health, which was formulated in 1959 by 'Dahir', is the highest legislation form in the country.

Substance Abuse Policy A substance abuse policy is present. The policy was initially formulated in 1972.

National Mental Health Programme A national mental health programme is present. The programme was formulated in 1973. The mental health programme has been revised in 1992 and 1995. The programme was formulated according to the 'Dahir'. The programme has been reviewed several times.

National Therapeutic Drug Policy/Essential List of Drugs A national therapeutic drug policy/essential list of drugs is present. It was formulated in 1972.

The list is revised each year. The last review was in 2000. New as well as old drugs (neuroleptics, anti-depressants, mood-regulators) are on the list.

Mental Health Legislation The Dahir 1-58-295 relating to the prevention of mental illnesses and protection of the patients is the latest mental health legislation. Though it is old, its articles are well formulated and were examined by WHO experts in 1998. Reviews may be done in the future. The main aim is to guarantee the medical characteristics of mental institutions by entrusting them with the prime mission of treating the sick while protecting their rights and their property during their period of illness. The Law created the Central Service for Mental Health and Degenerative Diseases and the Mental Health Committee, organized mental institutions and other psychiatric set-ups and specified different manners of patient admission and discharge among its many other laws, as well as the modalities of protection of the sick and of its material owns.

The latest legislation was enacted in 1959.

Mental Health Financing There are budget allocations for mental health.
Details about expenditure on mental health are not available.
The primary sources of mental health financing in descending order are tax based, social insurance, out of pocket expenditure by the patient or family and private insurances.
Each state has its own budget line specified for equipment and investment work in hospitals at regional levels.
The country has disability benefits for persons with mental disorders. Those who become handicapped or lose their autonomy benefit from the system in the form of paid sick leave plus disability card if the disability is definite. Common diseases are supported like other illnesses.

Mental Health Facilities Mental health is a part of primary health care system. Actual treatment of severe mental disorders is available at the primary level. Outpatient clinics are integrated to some extent into the primary health care system. Two hundred health centres spread over the country offer mental health services within primary health care.
Regular training of primary care professionals is carried out in the field of mental health. Training on primary mental health care is integrated in basic academic courses of general physicians, in faculties of medicine and in the institutes of health works (Instituts de Formation en Carrières de Santé: IFCS).
There are community care facilities for patients with mental disorders. The community programme includes the family which plays an important role in the therapeutic programme.

Psychiatric Beds and Professionals

Total psychiatric beds per 10 000 population	0.783
Psychiatric beds in mental hospitals per 10 000 population	0.52
Psychiatric beds in general hospitals per 10 000 population	0.17
Psychiatric beds in other settings per 10 000 population	0.1
Number of psychiatrists per 100 000 population	0.4
Number of neurosurgeons per 100 000 population	0.12
Number of psychiatric nurses per 100 000 population	2.2
Number of neurologists per 100 000 population	0.3
Number of psychologists per 100 000 population	0.03
Number of social workers per 100 000 population	0.007

The condition is unsatisfactory, especially in public sector; e.g. occupational therapy is provided by psychiatrists, nurses and social workers.

Non-Governmental Organizations NGOs are involved with mental health in the country. They are mainly involved in advocacy, promotion, prevention, treatment and rehabilitation.

Information Gathering System There is mental health reporting system in the country.
The country has data collection system or epidemiological study on mental health. Several specific studies were conducted by the main psychiatric university centers like Ibn Rochd (Casablanca) and Ar-Razi (Rabat-Salé). An exhaustive list of studies and results is available from the Ministry of Health.

Programmes for Special Population The country has specific programmes for mental health for children.

Therapeutic Drugs The following therapeutic drugs are generally available at the primary health care level of the country: carbamazepine, phenobarbital, phenytoin sodium, sodium valproate, amitriptyline, chlorpromazine, diazepam, fluphenazine, haloperidol, lithium, levodopa.
Other drugs are available in the primary health centres.

Other Information There has been a psychiatric tradition in Morocco since the Middle ages – 'The Moristanes' (health care places for the mentally ill) were psychiatric hospital precursors of public sector. Then, two Psychiatric University Centres came up in Salé in the 1960s and in Casblanca in the 1970s. Recently, two university centers were created in Marrakesh and in Fès. According to mental health policy of the Ministry of Health, several mental health services are being created each year in the general hospitals. The goal is to have sectorized coverage of mental needs of the population in the entire country.

Additional Sources of Information

Des organismes charges de la prevention et du traitment des maladies mentales et de la protection des malades mentaux (Government document).

Ghazal, N., Agoub, M., Moussaoui, D., et al (2001) Prevalence of bulimia nervosa among secondary school students in Casablanca. Encephale, 27, 338-342.

Kadri, N., Tilane, A., El Batal, M., et al (2000) Irritability during the month of Ramadan. Psychosomatic Medicine, 62, 280-285.

Kadri, N., McHichi Alami, K. H., McHakra Tahiri, S. (2002) Sexual dysfunction in women: population based epidemiological study. Archives of Women's Mental Health, 5, 59-63.

Moussaoui, D. (2002) Creating a department of psychiatry in a developing country. World Psychiatry, 1, 57-58.

Taoudi Benchekroun, M., Roky, R., Toufiq, J., et al (1999) Epidemiological study: chronotype and daytime sleepiness before and during Ramadan. Therapie, 54, 567-572.

Mozambique

GENERAL INFORMATION

Mozambique is a country with an approximate area of 802 thousand sq. km. (UNO, 2001). Its population is 19.183 million, and the sex ratio (men per hundred women) is 93 (UNO, 2004). The proportion of population under the age of 15 years is 44% (UNO, 2004), and the proportion of population above the age of 60 years is 5% (WHO, 2004). The literacy rate is 62.3% for men and 31.4% for women (UNESCO/MoH, 2004).

The country is a low income group country (based on World Bank 2004 criteria). The proportion of health budget to GDP is 5.9%. The per capita total expenditure on health is 47 international $, and the per capita government expenditure on health is 32 international $ (WHO, 2004).

The main language(s) used in the country is (are) Portuguese (official), Emakua, Xichangana and Elomwé. The largest ethnic group(s) is (are) African. The largest religious group(s) is (are) Roman Catholic, and the other religious group(s) are (is) Muslim and indigenous groups.

The life expectancy at birth is 41.2 years for males and 43.9 years for females (WHO, 2004). The healthy life expectancy at birth is 36 years for males and 38 years for females (WHO, 2004).

EPIDEMIOLOGY

There is a paucity of epidemiological data on mental illnesses in Mozambique in internationally accessible literature. In 2003, the Ministry of Health conducted a mental health community study in an urban and a rural district. The prevalence of psychoses, mental retardation and epilepsy in the urban area were 1.5%, 1.1% and 1.3%, while the prevalence of these disorders in the rural area were 5%, 1.8% and 3.9%, respectively. Rural-urban differences were highly significant (MoH, 2002-2003). Granja et al (2002) conducted a retrospective hospital-based study on deaths from injuries among pregnant/postpartum women (n=27) and found that suicide was the cause in one-third of cases.

MENTAL HEALTH RESOURCES

Mental Health Policy A mental health policy is absent.

The final draft is now ready and is awaiting approval.

Substance Abuse Policy A substance abuse policy is present. The policy was initially formulated in 1997. The policy is to be reviewed every two years.

National Mental Health Programme A national mental health programme is present. The programme was formulated in 1990. The draft National Mental Health Strategic Plan is likely to be approved in 2004.

National Therapeutic Drug Policy/Essential List of Drugs A national therapeutic drug policy/essential list of drugs is present. It was formulated in 1999.

Mental Health Legislation Specific legislation on mental health is not available. However, Law No 1/99 (formulated in 1999) controls and regulates access of youngsters to the night clubs as well as projection of certain videos and also controls the sale of alcohol and tobacco.

Details about the year of enactment of the mental health legislation are not available.

Mental Health Financing There are budget allocations for mental health.

Details about expenditure on mental health are not available.

The primary source of mental health financing is tax based.

The state budget as well as funds from different partners are allocated to the health sector as a whole and re-distributed through different programmes. The specific amount for mental health is determined according the national yearly plans and priorities, which often vary.

The country has disability benefits for persons with mental disorders. Disability benefits are provided for persons with chronic mental disorders, such as epilepsy and psychosis by the National Institute of Social Welfare. Patients with chronic mental illness are also given a discount on their medical prescription.

Mental Health Facilities Mental health is a part of primary health care system. Actual treatment of severe mental disorders is not available at the primary level. Few health centres have outpatient facilities.

Regular training of primary care professionals is not carried out in the field of mental health. Seminars are organized from time to time to train health workers in mental health.

There are community care facilities for patients with mental disorders. Few such centres exist.

Psychiatric Beds and Professionals

Total psychiatric beds per 10 000 population	0.23
Psychiatric beds in mental hospitals per 10 000 population	0.2
Psychiatric beds in general hospitals per 10 000 population	0.04
Psychiatric beds in other settings per 10 000 population	0.01
Number of psychiatrists per 100 000 population	0.04
Number of neurosurgeons per 100 000 population	0.01
Number of psychiatric nurses per 100 000 population	0.01
Number of neurologists per 100 000 population	0.01
Number of psychologists per 100 000 population	0.05
Number of social workers per 100 000 population	0.01

Each province has at least 2 mental health professionals. Since May 2004, three newly trained Mozambican psychiatrists have joined the workforce; the remaining 7 are foreigners. Twenty-seven psychiatric technicians are now working in the health system. It is expected that by September 2005 the number will increase to 58 (31 technicians are under training). There is one psychiatric hospital in the country located in Maputo City, the nation's capital, with a bed capacity of 260. The second psychiatric hospital located in the northern province of Nampula was closed as it did not offer minimal conditions for service delivery, and a Mental Health Community Centre was opened in its place. Service delivery (outpatient and inpatient care) primarily occurs at the provincial hospital level. Admissions are also made in general medicine wards, where approximately 3 to 5 beds are allocated to mental health.

Non-Governmental Organizations NGOs are involved with mental health in the country. They are mainly involved in promotion, prevention and rehabilitation. Some NGOs focus on rehabilitation of drug abusers.

Information Gathering System There is mental health reporting system in the country. New indicators for mental health reporting system in the country have been approved; they are introduced in the General Health Information System.
The country has data collection system or epidemiological study on mental health. Data collecting systems are being tested, statistical information on patients are being collected.

Programmes for Special Population A school for mentally challenged children exists. Efforts are now being made to mainstream the education of such children.

Therapeutic Drugs The following therapeutic drugs are generally available at the primary health care level of the country: carbamazepine, phenobarbital, phenytoin sodium, sodium valproate, amitriptyline, chlorpromazine, diazepam, fluphenazine, haloperidol, biperiden, levodopa.
The essential drug list is under revision. Inclusion of newer (more effective) drugs has been proposed. The final list and new policy might be approved in early 2005.

Other Information WHO has undertaken a project in Cuamba district to integrate mental health into general health care at the primary level. Special emphasis is given to psychosocial support in collaboration with traditional healers. WHO has also assisted the Ministry of Health in drafting a mental health policy and updating the mental health programme. This programme would also be used in building the capacity of mental health professionals to provide community-based care.

Additional Sources of Information

Essential Drug List. (Government document).

Granja, A. C., Zacarias, E., Bergstrom, S. (2002) Violent deaths: the hidden face of maternal mortality. BJOG: an International Journal of Obstetrics & Gynaecology, 109, 5-8.

Ministry of Health (2002-3) Community Mental Health Study – A Household Key Informant Survey in Rural and Urban Mozambique. Mental Health Program, Department of Community Health-National Health Directory. Mozambique.

WHO (2002) Working with countries: mental health policy and service development projects. WHO. Geneva. WHO/MSD/MPS/02.1

Myanmar

GENERAL INFORMATION

Myanmar is a country with an approximate area of 677 thousand sq. km. (UNO, 2001). Its population is 50.101 million, and the sex ratio (men per hundred women) is 98 (UNO, 2004). The proportion of population under the age of 15 years is 32% (UNO, 2004), and the proportion of population above the age of 60 years is 7% (WHO, 2004). The literacy rate is 89.2% for men and 81.4% for women (UNESCO/MoH, 2004).
The country is a low income group country (based on World Bank 2004 criteria). The proportion of health budget to GDP is 2.1%. The per capita total expenditure on health is 26 international $, and the per capita government expenditure on health is 5 international $ (WHO, 2004).
The main language(s) used in the country is (are) Burmese. The largest ethnic group(s) is (are) Kachin, and the other ethnic group(s) are (is) Kayah, Kayin, Chin, Mon, Bamar, Rakhine and Shan. The largest religious group(s) is (are) Buddhist (nine-tenths), and the other religious group(s) are (is) Christian, Muslim, Hindu and indigenous groups.
The life expectancy at birth is 56.2 years for males and 61.8 years for females (WHO, 2004). The healthy life expectancy at birth is 50 years for males and 54 years for females (WHO, 2004).

EPIDEMIOLOGY

A community survey done in an urban area (n=915) showed that 8.6% of the population had psychiatric morbidity (Tin Nyunt Pu et al, 1976). Another survey in a sub-urban area (459 households were covered) revealed psychiatric morbidity in 5.6% of residents, with the prevalence of psychoses being 0.05%, mental retardation 0.4% and epilepsy 0.4% (Thane Htay Pe et al, 1982). A recent survey in an urban area (861 households, n=5106) showed that 8.6% of the population had mental disorders, with the prevalence rate of psychoses being 0.6%, epilepsy 0.4%, mental retardation (moderate and severe) 0.5%, alcohol use disorders 2.3% (7% in males over 18 years of age) and dementia (moderate and severe) in about 2.5% of those over 65 years of age. A similar survey in a rural area (225 households, n=1000) showed that 7.7% of the population had mental disorders, with the prevalence rate of psychoses being 0.6%, epilepsy 0.2%, mental retardation (moderate and severe) 0.1%, alcohol use disorders 2.3% (7% in males over 18 years of age) and dementia (moderate and severe) in about 3.5% of those over 65 years of age (Win Aung Myint et al, 2004).

MENTAL HEALTH RESOURCES

Mental Health Policy A mental health policy is present. The policy was initially formulated in 1990.
The components of the policy are advocacy, promotion, prevention, treatment and rehabilitation. Community integration is also a component of the mental health policy.

Substance Abuse Policy A substance abuse policy is present. The policy was initially formulated in 1993. The Narcotic Drug and Psychotropic Substances Law aims to prevent the danger of narcotic drugs and psychotropic substances, to implement the provisions of the UN Convention Against Illicit Traffic in Narcotic Drugs and Psychotropic Substances, to carry out more effective measures for imparting knowledge and education on the danger of these substances and for medical treatment and rehabilitation of drug users, to impose more effective penalties for offenders and to cooperate with state parties and other international organizations in respect of the prevention of the danger of narcotic drugs and psychotropic substances.

National Mental Health Programme A national mental health programme is present. The programme was formulated in 1990.

National Therapeutic Drug Policy/Essential List of Drugs A national therapeutic drug policy/essential list of drugs is present. It was formulated in 1992.

Mental Health Legislation There is a Lunacy Act from 1912. A mental health act had been proposed in 1994.
The latest legislation was enacted in 1912.

Mental Health Financing There are budget allocations for mental health.
The country spends 1.3% of the total health budget on mental health.
The primary source of mental health financing is tax based.
The country has disability benefits for persons with mental disorders. Any Government employee who is mentally ill and has a poor prospect of recovery is recommended for invalidation.

Mental Health Facilities Mental health is a part of primary health care system. Actual treatment of severe mental disorders is not available at the primary level. Consultant psychiatrists are posted in different states and divisions and patients are referred to them. Regular training of primary care professionals is carried out in the field of mental health. In the last two years, about 2000 personnel were provided training. Consultants train medical officers and primary care workers about mental health illnesses and means of treating them.
There are community care facilities for patients with mental disorders.

Psychiatric Beds and Professionals

Total psychiatric beds per 10 000 population	0.55
Psychiatric beds in mental hospitals per 10 000 population	0.33
Psychiatric beds in general hospitals per 10 000 population	0.11
Psychiatric beds in other settings per 10 000 population	0.11
Number of psychiatrists per 100 000 population	0.2
Number of neurosurgeons per 100 000 population	0.02
Number of psychiatric nurses per 100 000 population	0.6
Number of neurologists per 100 000 population	0.02
Number of psychologists per 100 000 population	0.01
Number of social workers per 100 000 population	0.3

There are two occupational therapists and medical assistants.

Non-Governmental Organizations NGOs are involved with mental health in the country. They are mainly involved in promotion, prevention and rehabilitation. In line with the National Health Policy, NGOs such as Myanmar Maternal and Child Welfare Association and Myanmar Red Cross Society also take a share of service provision. Their role is becoming more important as the needs of collaborative actions for health become more prominent.

Information Gathering System There is mental health reporting system in the country. Mental illnesses are included in health management information system.
The country has data collection system or epidemiological study on mental health. Necessary training and educational material was given to primary care workers for data collection.

Programmes for Special Population The country has specific programmes for mental health for minorities, disaster affected population, indigenous population, elderly and children. Child Guidance Clinics and Geriatric Care Clinics are conducted twice a week.

Therapeutic Drugs The following therapeutic drugs are generally available at the primary health care level of the country: carbamazepine, phenobarbital, sodium valproate, amitriptyline, chlorpromazine, diazepam, fluphenazine, haloperidol.

Other Information

Additional Sources of Information

Health in Myanmar (2001) Excerpt of Health Management Information System Mental Health Project.

Thane Htay Pe et al (1982) Psychiatric Prevalence study at Seinpan Myaing Ward Mayangon Twonship.

The State Law and Order Restoration Council (1993) Narcotic Drugs and Psychotropic Substances Law.

Tin Nyunt Pu et al (1976) Psychiatric prevalence survey at Lllegu area. Unpublished paper.

Win Aung Myint, Zaw Sein Lwin, Tin Oo et al (2004) Prevalence study of common mental disorders in Daw Pone Township, Yangon Civision, Union of Myanmar.

Namibia

GENERAL INFORMATION

Namibia is a country with an approximate area of 824 thousand sq. km. (UNO, 2001). Its population is 2.011 million, and the sex ratio (men per hundred women) is 96 (UNO, 2004). The proportion of population under the age of 15 years is 43% (UNO, 2004), and the proportion of population above the age of 60 years is 6% (WHO, 2004). The literacy rate is 83.8% for men and 82.8% for women (UNESCO/MoH, 2004).

The country is a lower middle income group country (based on World Bank 2004 criteria). The proportion of health budget to GDP is 7%. The per capita total expenditure on health is 342 international $, and the per capita government expenditure on health is 232 international $ (WHO, 2004).

The main language(s) used in the country is (are) Afrikaans, German and English. The largest ethnic group(s) is (are) African (Ovambo, Kavango, Herero, Damara, Nama, Afrikaners), and the other ethnic group(s) are (is) Asian (descent). The largest religious group(s) is (are) indigenous groups, and the other religious group(s) are (is) Christian.

The life expectancy at birth is 48.1 years for males and 50.5 years for females (WHO, 2004). The healthy life expectancy at birth is 43 years for males and 44 years for females (WHO, 2004).

EPIDEMIOLOGY

There is a paucity of epidemiological data on mental illnesses in Namibia in internationally accessible literature.

MENTAL HEALTH RESOURCES

Mental Health Policy A mental health policy is absent.

The final draft of the mental health policy is ready and has been submitted for approval.

Substance Abuse Policy A substance abuse policy is absent. The final draft of the substance abuse policy is ready and has been submitted for approval.

National Mental Health Programme A national mental health programme is absent.

The mental health programme was drafted with assistance of WHO. It will be presented to the Primary Health Care Management Committee for final inputs and then it will be forwarded for approval.

N–R

National Therapeutic Drug Policy/Essential List of Drugs A national therapeutic drug policy/essential list of drugs is present. It was formulated in 1995.

Mental Health Legislation Mental health services are provided under the South African Mental Health Act no. 18 of 1973. This is in spite of the fact that the South African Mental Health Act has been updated in South Africa. Namibia is therefore using an outdated legislation. A new Bill is in the early stages of development. This is an essential element of reform that is needed as part of the implementation of the Mental Health Policy.

The latest legislation was enacted in 1973.

Mental Health Financing There are no budget allocations for mental health.

Details about expenditure on mental health are not available.

The primary sources of mental health financing in descending order are tax based, grants, out of pocket expenditure by the patient or family and private insurances.

Namibia has no cost recovery mechanisms in place. As a result of this, incomes generated by health services through user fees, insurance recovery and donations are deposited in the general revenue of the Government. The Ministry of Health is currently exploring possibilities regarding retaining a portion of the collected fees. Mental health is under the primary health care programme and there is no special budget for mental health. The budget is allocated according to the annual mental health activities.

The country has disability benefits for persons with mental disorders. If a person is classified as chronically mentally ill then the application is forwarded to the social services for disability grant.

Mental Health Facilities Mental health is a part of primary health care system. Actual treatment of severe mental disorders is not available at the primary level. Treatment is generally available at the hospital level, but follow-up of discharged psychiatric patients is done in all health care facilities.

Regular training of primary care professionals is not carried out in the field of mental health. There is a proposal to train more mental health nurses and social workers. Community psychiatric nurses based in state hospitals also run satellite psychiatric clinics. However, such services are not available in the interior. Nurses cannot prescribe medication, for which they have to consult medical officers or psychiatrists. The psychiatric unit in the country's capital also plans to identify medical officers with interest in psychiatry and provide them with one-week intensive training followed by on-site basic psychiatry training. Traditional healers are also being encouraged to undertake training, and depot anti-psychotics are provided to them for managing psychotic disorders. The Namibia University has no medical school. The general nursing training includes a component of psychiatric nursing.

There are community care facilities for patients with mental disorders. Only follow-up of discharged psychiatric patients is done in the community.

Psychiatric Beds and Professionals

Total psychiatric beds per 10 000 population	1.5
Psychiatric beds in mental hospitals per 10 000 population	1.5
Psychiatric beds in general hospitals per 10 000 population	0
Psychiatric beds in other settings per 10 000 population	0
Number of psychiatrists per 100 000 population	0.2
Number of neurosurgeons per 100 000 population	0
Number of psychiatric nurses per 100 000 population	0
Number of neurologists per 100 000 population	0
Number of psychologists per 100 000 population	6
Number of social workers per 100 000 population	6

The above mentioned psychologists and social workers work in the public sector. Two occupational therapists are working in Windhoek Mental Health Care Centre. A relatively broad range of mental health services are currently available only at tertiary care centres (Windhoek Mental Health Care Centre with 112 beds and Oshakati Psychiatric Unit with 80 beds). Emergency mental health services are also provided at the district hospitals as part of general wards (which do not have specialist mental health staff). All general hospitals are expected to have at least one or two rooms for severely psychotic patients. Follow-up and a limited range of psychotropic medications are available at some health care centres and clinics. Ninety-nine beds at the Windhoek Mental Health Care Centre are earmarked for forensic psychiatry services. At present, the referral system is not well established. The responsible doctors follow referral guidelines sent out to all regions for mentally ill patients for at least 72 hours. However, health professionals at these levels find it hard to adhere to these guidelines due to their limited training and experience in mental health areas. Even the specialized mental health centres lack the full complement of mental health professionals in terms of specialization and numbers. Recently, one registered nurse from Windhoek psychiatric centre completed her degree in psychiatric nursing with the financial support from Finland. A major portion of psychiatric care in primary and secondary care settings is provided by nurses and social workers, due to lack of trained psychiatrists. Private practitioners also provide mental health services (10 psychologists, 3 psychiatrists), but these services are limited to those who can afford them. Traditional healers also play a considerable role, however, the number of those mentally ill individuals seeking the services in this sector is unknown.

Non-Governmental Organizations NGOs are involved with mental health in the country. They are mainly involved in advocacy, promotion, prevention and rehabilitation. In the capital city, the German Evangelic Lutheran Church provides one accommodation facility for psychiatric patients who do not have a family to take care of them.

Information Gathering System There is mental health reporting system in the country. The Health Information System was revised in 2000, and new system was introduced in 2001. The analyses are based on the records of outpatients who attended clinics, health centres and hospital outpatient departments. Information on inpatients is also available. The facility based information contains data on all public health sectors and services including mission health care facilities. Mental illnesses are audited if they are among the first ten common disorders.
The country has data collection system or epidemiological study on mental health. Disorders are classified according to ICD 10 criteria.

Programmes for Special Population The country has specific programmes for mental health for children.
The Windhoek Mental Health Care Centre provides outpatient and inpatient services for children.

Therapeutic Drugs The following therapeutic drugs are generally available at the primary health care level of the country: carbamazepine, phenobarbital, phenytoin sodium, sodium, valproate, amitriptyline, chlorpromazine, diazepam, fluphenazine, haloperidol, lithium, biperiden, carbidopa, levodopa.
A Namibian Essential Medicines List (NEMLIST) has been formulated. These drugs are frequently not made available because of a lack of review mechanisms and lack of staff skills.

Other Information

Additional Sources of Information

Feinstein, A. (2002). Psychiatry in post-apartheid Namibia: a troubled legacy. Psychiatric Bulletin, 26, 310-312.

Nauru

GENERAL INFORMATION

Nauru is a country with an approximate area of 0.02 thousand sq. km. (UNO, 2001). Its population is 0.01 million, and the sex ratio (men per hundred women) is 105 (UNO, 2004). The proportion of population under the age of 15 years is 42% (UNO, 2004), and the proportion of population above the age of 60 years is 7% (WHO, 2004).

The country is a high income group country (based on World Bank 2004 criteria). The proportion of health budget to GDP is 7.5%. The per capita total expenditure on health is 1015 international $, and the per capita government expenditure on health is 900 international $ (WHO, 2004).

The main language(s) used in the country is (are) Nauruan. The largest ethnic group(s) is (are) Nauruan Islander, and the other ethnic group(s) are (is) Chinese and European. The largest religious group(s) is (are) Protestant (more than half), and the other religious group(s) are (is) Roman Catholic, Confucian and Taoist.

The life expectancy at birth is 59.7 years for males and 66.5 years for females (WHO, 2004). The healthy life expectancy at birth is 53 years for males and 58 years for females (WHO, 2004).

EPIDEMIOLOGY

There is a paucity of epidemiological data on mental illnesses in Nauru in internationally accessible literature.

MENTAL HEALTH RESOURCES

Mental Health Policy A mental health policy is absent.

Substance Abuse Policy A substance abuse policy is absent.

National Mental Health Programme A national mental health programme is absent.

National Therapeutic Drug Policy/Essential List of Drugs A national therapeutic drug policy/essential list of drugs is present. It was formulated in 1997.

Mental Health Legislation The Mentally Disordered Persons Ordinance is the latest legislation.
The latest legislation was enacted in 1963.

N–R

Mental Health Financing There are no budget allocations for mental health.
Details about expenditure on mental health are not available.
The primary source of mental health financing is tax based.
The country does not have disability benefits for persons with mental disorders. Mental illness is not considered a disability.

Mental Health Facilities Mental health is not a part of primary health care system. Actual treatment of severe mental disorders is not available at the primary level.
Regular training of primary care professionals is not carried out in the field of mental health.
There are community care facilities for patients with mental disorders. Community services are very limited. Care facilities for children with mental disabilities have been set up with the cooperation of the Government and parents of these children. Mentally ill persons are easily absorbed into the community.

Psychiatric Beds and Professionals

Total psychiatric beds per 10 000 population	0
Psychiatric beds in mental hospitals per 10 000 population	0
Psychiatric beds in general hospitals per 10 000 population	0
Psychiatric beds in other settings per 10 000 population	0
Number of psychiatrists per 100 000 population	0
Number of neurosurgeons per 100 000 population	0
Number of psychiatric nurses per 100 000 population	0
Number of neurologists per 100 000 population	0
Number of psychologists per 100 000 population	0
Number of social workers per 100 000 population	0

There are no mental health personnel in the country. There are no specified beds for psychiatry.

Non-Governmental Organizations NGOs are involved with mental health in the country. They are mainly involved in treatment. The International Organization for Migration (IOM) has appointed a psychiatrist for asylum seekers living in camps in Nauru. The psychiatrist also provides assessment and management to referred Nauruan patients.

Information Gathering System There is no mental health reporting system in the country.
The country has no data collection system or epidemiological study on mental health.

Programmes for Special Population There are no special services available.

Therapeutic Drugs The following therapeutic drugs are generally available at the primary health care level of the country: carbamazepine, phenobarbital, phenytoin sodium, sodium valproate, amitriptyline, chlorpromazine, diazepam, fluphenazine, haloperidol, carbidopa, levodopa.
Other drugs like nortriptyline and midazolam are also available.

Other Information Suicide rates are on the increase in these islands and there is a need for mental health personnel.

Additional Sources of Information

Nepal

GENERAL INFORMATION

Nepal is a country with an approximate area of 147 thousand sq. km. (UNO, 2001). Its population is 25.724 million, and the sex ratio (men per hundred women) is 104 (UNO, 2004). The proportion of population under the age of 15 years is 40% (UNO, 2004), and the proportion of population above the age of 60 years is 6% (WHO, 2004). The literacy rate is 61.6% for men and 26.4% for women (UNESCO/MoH, 2004).

The country is a low income group country (based on World Bank 2004 criteria). The proportion of health budget to GDP is 5.2%. The per capita total expenditure on health is 63 international $, and the per capita government expenditure on health is 19 international $ (WHO, 2004).

The main language(s) used in the country is (are) Nepali. The largest ethnic group(s) is (are) indigenous Nepalese, and the other ethnic group(s) are (is) Indo-Nepalese and Tibeto-Nepalese. The largest religious group(s) is (are) Hindu, and the other religious group(s) are (is) Buddhist, Muslim and Christian.

The life expectancy at birth is 59.9 years for males and 60.2 years for females (WHO, 2004). The healthy life expectancy at birth is 52 years for males and 51 years for females (WHO, 2004).

EPIDEMIOLOGY

Wright et al (1989) interviewed patients attending a primary care center for psychiatric illnesses using the Self-Reporting Questionnaire. Psychiatric morbidity was detected in one-quarter of all patients screened; more women were affected. Sharma (1975) examined 226 subjects with cannabis abuse and an equal number of matched (age, sex, education) normal controls. Compared with the controls, the cannabis users had a poor work record, poor social and family relationships, a lack of interest in sex and a general loss of initiative and efficiency. Regmi et al (2002) screened 100 women 2-3 months post-delivery and 40 control women using the Edinburgh Postpartum Depression Scale (EPDS). All those who screened positive for depression and 20% of the negatives also underwent a structured interview to assess depression by DSM-IV criteria. Predictive errors were minimized by using an EPDS score 13 to define depression. Using this threshold, there was no difference in depression prevalence between postpartum women (12%) and the control group (12.5%). Van Ommeren et al (2001) used standardized tools to interview 418 tortured Bhutanese refugees and 392 non-tortured Bhutanese refugees. Tortured refugees were more likely to report 12-month ICD-10 posttraumatic stress disorder, persistent somatoform pain disorder and dissociative (amnesia and conversion) disorders. In addition, tortured refugees were more likely to report lifetime posttraumatic stress disorder, persistent somatoform pain disorder, affective disorder, generalized anxiety disorder and dissociative (amnesia and conversion) disorders. Tortured women, compared with tortured men, were more likely to report lifetime generalized anxiety disorder, persistent somatoform pain disorder, affective disorder and dissociative (amnesia and conversion) disorders. Shrestha et al (1998) did a case-control study on a random sample of 526 tortured Bhutanese refugees and an equal number of non-tortured refugees matched for age and sex. The tortured refugees, as a group, suffered more DSM-III-R PTSD symptoms and had higher Hopkins Symptom Checklist-25 (HSCL-25) anxiety and depression scores and more musculoskeletal system- and respiratory system-related complaints than the non-tortured refugees. Buddhists were less likely to be depressed or anxious, and males were less likely to experience anxiety. Van Ommeren et al (2002) found that the number of PTSD symptoms, independent of depression and anxiety, predicted both number of reported somatic complaints and number of organ systems involving such complaints. Emmelkamp et al (2002) evaluated 315 Bhutanese refugees and found that the total number of coping strategies was correlated with anxiety and depression. Negative coping, in contrast to positive coping, was related to all symptom outcome measures. Received social support was more strongly related to symptoms than perceived social support. The findings from the first sample were replicated in the second sample of 57 Nepalese torture victims. In a case-control study that involved 68 cases and 66 controls in a Bhutanese refugee camp, Van Ommeren et al (2001) found that recent loss, early loss, childhood trauma and pulse-rate were predictors of case status during an epidemic of medically unexplained illness consisting of somatoform symptoms, acute anxiety and dissociation (which included visual and auditory hallucinatory experiences in 60% and 28% of cases, respectively). Karki et al (2001) found that 86.5% of patients (n=37) attending the emergency ward with severe organophosphorus poisoning (OPP) had consumed it with the intent of committing suicide.

MENTAL HEALTH RESOURCES

Mental Health Policy A mental health policy is present. The policy was initially formulated in 1997.

The components of the policy are advocacy, promotion, prevention, treatment and rehabilitation. The mental health policy is a part of the general health policy. Psychiatrists, psychologists, psychiatric nurses, lawyers and civil servants were involved in its development. The policy aims to provide minimum mental health care facilities for all by the end of the current National Five-Year Plan by integrating mental health services into the general health services of the country, develop human resource facilities in mental health, protect the fundamental rights of the mentally ill, improve awareness about mental illness and promote better mental health in the community.

Substance Abuse Policy A substance abuse policy is present. The policy was initially formulated in 1994.

National Mental Health Programme A national mental health programme is absent.

It is in accordance with the national mental health policy of the country.

National Therapeutic Drug Policy/Essential List of Drugs A national therapeutic drug policy/essential list of drugs is present. It was formulated in 1986.
Supply of 5 essential psychotropics has been ensured in the lowest level of the health delivery system of the country.

Mental Health Legislation Under the Civil Law there are some sections having legal provisions concerning insanity. A separate mental health legislation, that protects the basic human rights of the mentally ill, has been drafted and is now awaiting the approval of the parliament.
The latest legislation was enacted in 1964.

Mental Health Financing There are budget allocations for mental health.
The country spends 0.08% of the total health budget on mental health.
The primary sources of mental health financing in descending order are out of pocket expenditure by the patient or family, tax based and grants.
The Government and NGOs like the World Health Organization, United Mission to Nepal etc. are important funders of mental health care services. Despite this, the family of the mentally ill has to spend around 25 000 Nepalese rupees per year (USD 320) as direct services costs.
The country has disability benefits for persons with mental disorders. Chronic mental illness has been classified as one of the mental disabilities and these patients have equal rights as other disabilities according to the Disability Act.

Mental Health Facilities Details about mental health facilities at the primary care level are not available. Mental health is not an integral part of primary health care, but treatment of severe mental health disorders are available in ten districts where community health programmes with the support of NGOs are going on.
Regular training of primary care professionals is not carried out in the field of mental health. Primary care physicians and health workers are trained in mental health. Subsequent refresher training and supervision by psychiatrists has been attempted in some regions. A system of referral has been established. Local faith healers have been involved in the referral network. Successful integration of mental health care in primary health care has already occurred in 7 out of 75 districts.
There are no community care facilities for patients with mental disorders.

Psychiatric Beds and Professionals

Total psychiatric beds per 10 000 population	0.08
Psychiatric beds in mental hospitals per 10 000 population	0.02
Psychiatric beds in general hospitals per 10 000 population	0.02
Psychiatric beds in other settings per 10 000 population	0.04
Number of psychiatrists per 100 000 population	0.12
Number of neurosurgeons per 100 000 population	0.04
Number of psychiatric nurses per 100 000 population	0.08
Number of neurologists per 100 000 population	0.08
Number of psychologists per 100 000 population	0.08
Number of social workers per 100 000 population	0.04

At least 40 beds (10 in the governmental and 30 in the private sector) are earmarked for drug dependence treatment. All mental health professionals are stationed in urban and semi-urban areas.

Non-Governmental Organizations NGOs are involved with mental health in the country. They are mainly involved in advocacy, promotion, prevention, treatment and rehabilitation. Apart from usual services, NGOs run mental health services for homeless psychotic patients and refugees and day care centres for drug users.

Information Gathering System There is mental health reporting system in the country. A morbidity form is available for outpatients and is filled by primary health centres.
The country has data collection system or epidemiological study on mental health.

Programmes for Special Population The country has specific programmes for mental health for refugees.
Orientation programmes have been organized for school teachers. Special clinics for children, psychosexual disorders, headache and drug abuse treatment are available at a few centres.

Therapeutic Drugs The following therapeutic drugs are generally available at the primary health care level of the country: carbamazepine, phenobarbital, phenytoin sodium, amitriptyline, chlorpromazine, diazepam.
The drugs listed above are in the essential drug list for health posts and sub-health posts. More psychotropic drugs are available in the district and primary health care level.

Other Information A national level Non-communicable Disease Prevention and Control Committee has been formed in the Ministry of Health. Eight non-communicable diseases (including mental disorder) have been prioritized. An overall national focal point for non-communicable diseases and a coordinator for each of the eight non-communicable diseases have been identified and a national Non-communicable Diseases Policy and strategies have been formulated. Activities for each of the eight non-communicable diseases are being planned.

Additional Sources of Information

DoHS (1998-99) Annual Report – National Health Policy.

Emmelkamp, J., Komproe, I. H., Van Ommeren, M., et al (2002) The relation between coping, social support and psychological and somatic symptoms among torture survivors in Nepal. Psychological Medicine, 32, 1465-1470.

Essential Drug List and National Formulary (Government document).

Karki, P., Hansdak, S. G., Bhandari, S., et al (2001) A clinico-epidemiological study of organophosphorus poisoning at a rural-based teaching hospital in eastern Nepal. Tropical Doctor, 31, 32-34.

Ministry of Health (1995) National Mental Health Policy.

Regmi, S., Sligl, W., Carter, D., et al (2002) A controlled study of postpartum depression among Nepalese women: validation of the Edinburgh Postpartum Depression Scale in Kathmandu. Tropical Medicine & International Health, 7, 378-382.

Regmi, S. K., Pokharel, A., Ojha, S. P. (2004) Nepal mental health country profile. International Review of Psychiatry, 16, 142-149.

Sharma, B. P. (1975) Cannabis and its users in Nepal. British Journal of Psychiatry, 127, 550-552.

Shrestha, N. M., Sharma, B., Van Ommeren, M., et al (1998) Impact of torture on refugees displaced within the developing world: symptomatology among Bhutanese refugees in Nepal. JAMA, 280, 443-448.

Tausig, M., Subedi, S. (1997) The modern mental health system in Nepal: organizational persistence in the absence of legitimating myths. Social Science & Medicine, 45, 441-447.

Van Ommeren, M., de Jong, J. T., Sharma, B., et al (2001) Psychiatric disorders among tortured Bhutanese refugees in Nepal. Archives of General Psychiatry, 58, 475-482.

Van Ommeren, M., Sharma, B., Komproe, I., et al (2001) Trauma and loss as determinants of medically unexplained epidemic illness in a Bhutanese refugee camp. Psychological Medicine, 31, 1259-1267.

Van Ommeren, M., Sharma, B., Sharma, G. K., et al (2002) The relationship between somatic and PTSD symptoms among Bhutanese refugee torture survivors: examination of comorbidity with anxiety and depression. Journal of Traumatic Stress, 15, 415-421.

Wright, C., Nepal, M. K., Bruce-Jones, W. D. (1989) Mental health patients in primary health care services in Nepal. Asia-Pacific Journal of Public Health, 3, 224-230.

Netherlands*

GENERAL INFORMATION

Netherlands is a country with an approximate area of 42 thousand sq. km. (UNO, 2001). Its population is 16.227 million, and the sex ratio (men per hundred women) is 99 (UNO, 2004). The proportion of population under the age of 15 years is 18% (UNO, 2004), and the proportion of population above the age of 60 years is 18% (WHO, 2004). The literacy rate is 99% for men and 99% for women (UNESCO/MoH, 2004).

The country is a high income group country (based on World Bank 2004 criteria). The proportion of health budget to GDP is 8.9%. The per capita total expenditure on health is 2612 international $, and the per capita government expenditure on health is 1654 international $ (WHO, 2004).

The main language(s) used in the country is (are) Dutch. The largest ethnic group(s) is (are) Dutch. The largest religious group(s) is (are) Roman Catholic, and the other religious group(s) are (is) Protestant.

The life expectancy at birth is 76 years for males and 81.1 years for females (WHO, 2004). The healthy life expectancy at birth is 70 years for males and 73 years for females (WHO, 2004).

EPIDEMIOLOGY

There is substantial epidemiological data on mental illnesses in Netherlands in internationally accessible literature. No attempt was made to include this information here.

MENTAL HEALTH RESOURCES

Mental Health Policy A mental health policy is present. The policy was initially formulated in 1999.

The components of the policy are advocacy, promotion, prevention, treatment and rehabilitation. The Government has developed a policy (National Mental Health Plan) to create a mental health care sector that has the following characteristics: the care provided is demand-driven, i.e. tailored to the care needs of the individual client and his or her specific social or cultural characteristics. It comes about through consultation with the client, is easily accessible and consists of both medical and psychiatric treatment and social assistance; the provision of care is organized effectively in accordance with a clear profile from 'light and general to heavy and specialized'; disorders that can be treated in the short term and by general means are dealt with in the locally organized first echelon of mental health care by the general practitioner, the health care psychologist and the social worker; disorders that are beyond the capacities of the first echelon are referred to the regionally organized specialist mental health care centres, which are preferably located in or near the general hospital. These regional centres offer a complete range of facilities (prevention, diagnosis, crisis care, outpatient and short-term inpatient treatment, resocialization and sheltered accommodation); super-specialist help is provided at the supra-regional or national level in the university hospitals and in a number of designated mental health care institutions. The Government had set up a broadly-based committee to advise on an active public mental health policy. This committee was to report at the end of the year 2001. Details can be obtained from the document 'Mental Health Care Policy Document'.

Substance Abuse Policy A substance abuse policy is present. The policy was initially formulated in 1995. In order to manage the drug problem in an effective way, there is a Netherlands National Drug Monitor which assesses the different situation both nationally and internationally and advises on policies. The drug policy distinguishes between drugs which present an unacceptable risk and those like cannabis which are less harmful. The policy is to limit the risks to individuals and socially integrate the patients. The policy is focussed more towards harm-reduction than towards total abstinence.

National Mental Health Programme A national mental health programme is present. The programme was formulated in 1999. The Dutch Government issued an integral policy document on mental health care. It describes the ideal mental health care sector and how to reach (or to come close to) that ideal. Its principles include: demand-driven care, effectively and transparent organized care, deinstitutionalization, further development of the locally organized first echelon of mental health care, a logically configured professional structure, using methods that have been scientifically validated and coherent and integrated services for patients in which mental health care providers work closely with other care sectors, social sectors and local authorities.

National Therapeutic Drug Policy/Essential List of Drugs A national therapeutic drug policy/essential list of drugs is present. Details about the year of formulation are not available.

Mental Health Legislation The specialist mental health care sector, like the care for the handicapped and (in part) the nursing care sector, is managed on the basis of three related pieces of legislation: The Exceptional Medical Expenses Act (entitlements/accreditation), The Hospital Provision Act (planning and building), The Health Care Charges Act (charges). During the past few years, several acts have come into being to strengthen the position of clients in health care, such as: The Medical Treatment Contract Act, which stipulates that a care plan must be drawn up with the consent of the patient; The Client's Right of Complaint Act; The individual Health Care Professional Act, which regulates the duties and responsibilities of care providers; The Psychiatric Hospitals Act, which protects patients' rights in cases of committal and compulsory treatment. The Psychiatric Hospitals Act (1994) has recently been evaluated. Input from patients and family organizations has helped to identify a number of problem areas relating to the limited options for the compulsory treatment of patients who have no insight into their illness, as well as patients' need for more opportunities for autonomy by means of self-binding undertakings. Also, it has become evident that there is need for compulsory outpatient

N–R

treatment. Therefore, it is planned that The Psychiatric Hospitals Act will be changed in the coming years. Forensic psychiatry plays an important role in the care and treatment of prisoners with mental disorders. There are number of legislation related to forensic psychiatry, namely, the Penal Law (TBS), Psychiatric Hospital (Special Admissions) Act and certain articles of the Penitentiary Principles. Prisoners requiring treatment are treated at maximum security hospitals, forensic psychiatry hospitals and psychiatric hospitals for the mentally retarded delinquents. The level of care is high. Besides this, there are forensic psychiatry services in each district, psycho-medical teams, specific care departments, forensic observation and guidance departments, individual guidance departments, special care departments and addiction guidance departments.
The latest legislation was enacted in 1994.

Mental Health Financing There are budget allocations for mental health.
The country spends 7% of the total health budget on mental health.
The primary sources of mental health financing in descending order are social insurance, out of pocket expenditure by the patient or family and private insurances.
Since 1989, mental health care has been financed through the Exceptional Medical Expenses Act except for outpatient substance use care which is mainly paid for via the Welfare Act. Almost 73% of the mental health budget is spent on mental hospitals, 19% on ambulatory care, 6% on general hospitals and the remaining on sheltered living. About 75% is spent on mental health care of the adult and elderly, 15% on children and adolescents, 7% on substance use care and 5% on forensic care. After 1 year the patients in inpatient treatment, psychotherapy or sheltered care have to pay a part of their expenses besides the funding from the Exceptional Medical Expenses Act.
The country has disability benefits for persons with mental disorders. About 300 000 people are receiving benefits for mental disorders.

Mental Health Facilities Mental health is a part of primary health care system. Actual treatment of severe mental disorders is available at the primary level. It is the Dutch policy to strengthen the primary care in the treatment of mental disorders. The majority of patients with mental disorders initially contact their primary carers which include the general practitioner, social worker or psychologist.
Regular training of primary care professionals is carried out in the field of mental health.
There are community care facilities for patients with mental disorders. Until the 1970s, the mental health care system had developed along private and religious lines. The Dutch Association for Community Mental Health Care was established in 1972 and the Government intention to develop community care was proclaimed in 1974. The first Regional Institute for Community Mental Health Care (RIAGG) was established in 1982. As a result of the moves towards care in the community and the changing wishes of patients, the mental health care sector, the other care sectors, social organizations and local authorities are increasingly becoming involved and reliant on one another in the areas of housing, jobs, education and participation. Former psychiatric patients can call on a wide range of social provisions: the regular care sector, social pensions, sheltered accommodation facilities, crisis centres, etc. Most of the alternatives to hospital are in the private non-profit sector. Large scale experiments have also been carried out for replacing inpatient care with day care and assertive home treatment.

Psychiatric Beds and Professionals

Total psychiatric beds per 10 000 population	18.7
Psychiatric beds in mental hospitals per 10 000 population	15.4
Psychiatric beds in general hospitals per 10 000 population	1
Psychiatric beds in other settings per 10 000 population	2.3
Number of psychiatrists per 100 000 population	9
Number of neurosurgeons per 100 000 population	1
Number of psychiatric nurses per 100 000 population	99
Number of neurologists per 100 000 population	3.7
Number of psychologists per 100 000 population	28
Number of social workers per 100 000 population	176

There are other professionals as occupational therapists (177), creative art therapists (856), psychomotor therapists (743), social pedagogical workers (2855), activity supporters (1546), spiritual workers (146), other medical doctors (607) and a large number of other personnel. In the Netherlands, the first effort to reduce traditional inpatient care was not deinstitutionalization but strengthening outpatient care. The substitution policy was successful to an extent that inpatient care was reduced and outpatient and other community-based care increased. Intensive community based care was increased almost 5 times more than hospital-based care was reduced. There are at present 3 times as many professionals involved in inpatient care as in community care.

Non-Governmental Organizations NGOs are involved with mental health in the country. They are mainly involved in advocacy, promotion and rehabilitation. In 1964, Pandora was founded with the purpose to normalize the image of psychiatric patients and help in rehabilitation. This was followed by the League of Clients in 1971, whose primary objectives were advocacy and empowerment. A post called the Independent Patient Confidential Counsellor was forged to look into the negative experiences of the patient during hospitalization. Client councils were initially formed in hospitals but later also developed among the RIAGGs. The National Foundation for Patient Council was formed in 1981. A number of self-help groups started to function since the 1980s and family groups since the 1990s.

Information Gathering System There is mental health reporting system in the country.
The country has data collection system or epidemiological study on mental health.

Programmes for Special Population The country has specific programmes for mental health for minorities, refugees, disaster affected population, indigenous population, elderly and children. The facilities for child and adolescent care are divided into the clinics for child and adolescent psychiatry, the child protection agencies and the child care system.
There are care circuits and programmes for children, elderly and adults with specific disorders. In these there are tailor made programmes for treatment of specific disorders including those related to forensic psychiatry. There are facilities for both sheltered care and short term care.

Therapeutic Drugs The following therapeutic drugs are generally available at the primary health care level of the country: unknown.

Other Information Mental health care in its present form dates back to the 1970s and 1980s when the regional Institutes for outpatient mental health care and facilities for sheltered care and part-time treatment were added. Other facilities like semi-residential care, inpatient care and care circuits are present. Dutch mental health care is facing three major challenges. In the first place, epidemiological research and the statistics on trends in the use of care services point towards a steep rise in demand, particularly for outpatient care. The mental health care sector must respond to this appropriately. In the second place, the nature of the demand for care is changing: many people with chronic psychiatric problems want to be given the opportunity to remain part of the community. This means the further transformation of residential care into outpatient care. A third matter of concern is that the mental health care sector has to establish a much more explicit presence in regard to a number of social problems. Examples include incapacity for work as a result of mental problems, the problems surrounding the 'neglected' and 'degenerate', as well as the mental health problems of prisons, abuse, loneliness and poor living conditions. Details can be obtained about the mental health care facilities from the 'Fact Sheet Mental Health care' published in August 2000. According to the EPSILON Group study, most of the care provided to patients suffering from schizophrenia is on site with some services at the patient's home or other places like police stations and hospital emergencies.
* The verification of this country profile is still being awaited from the Ministry of Health of the Netherlands.

Additional Sources of Information

Becker T., Hullsmann, S., Knudsen, H. C. et al & the EPSILON Group (2002) Provision of services for people with schizophrenia in five European regions. Journal of Social Psychiatry and Psychiatric Epidemiology, 37, 465-474.

Ministry of Foreign Affairs, Ministry of Health Welfare and Sport, Ministry of Justice and Ministry of the Interior (1995) Drug Policy in the Netherlands: Continuity and Change.

Ministry of Health Welfare and Sport (2000) Psychiatric Hospitals (Compulsory Admissions Act).

Ministry of Health Welfare and Sport in conjunction with the Timbros Institute (Netherlands Institute of Mental Health and Addiction) (2000) Fact Sheet – Major Challenges to Dutch Mental Health Care.

Ministry of Health Welfare and Sport (1999) Mental Health Care Policy Document.

Ministry of Health Welfare and Sport (1999) Drug Policy in the Netherlands.

Ministry of Health Welfare and Sport (1997) Drug Policy in the Netherlands.

Pijl, Y. J., Kluiter, H., Wiersma, D. (2000) Change in Dutch mental health care: an evaluation. Social Psychiatry and Psychiatric Epidemiology, 35, 402-407.

Schene, A. H., Faber, A. M. E. (2001) Mental health care reform in the Netherlands. Acta Psychiatrica Scandinavica, 104 (suppl. 410), 74-81.

Van Marle, H. (2000) Forensic psychiatric services in Netherlands. International Journal of Law and Psychiatry, 23, 515-531.

N–R

New Zealand

GENERAL INFORMATION

New Zealand is a country with an approximate area of 271 thousand sq. km. (UNO, 2001). The country consists of two main islands and a number of small outlying scattered islands. Its population is 3.905 million, and the sex ratio (men per hundred women) is 97 (UNO, 2004). The proportion of population under the age of 15 years is 22% (UNO, 2004), and the proportion of population above the age of 60 years is 16% (WHO, 2004). The literacy rate is 99% for men and 99% for women (UNESCO/MoH, 2004). The country is a high income group country (based on World Bank 2004 criteria). The proportion of health budget to GDP is 8.3%. The per capita total expenditure on health is 1724 international $, and the per capita government expenditure on health is 1323 international $ (WHO, 2004).
The main language(s) used in the country is (are) English and Maori. The largest ethnic group(s) is (are) European, and the other ethnic group(s) are (is) Maori. The largest religious group(s) is (are) Christian.
The life expectancy at birth is 76.6 years for males and 81.2 years for females (WHO, 2004). The healthy life expectancy at birth is 70 years for males and 72 years for females (WHO, 2004).

EPIDEMIOLOGY

There is substantial epidemiological data on mental illnesses in New Zealand in internationally accessible literature. No attempt was made to include this information here.

MENTAL HEALTH RESOURCES

Mental Health Policy A mental health policy is present. The policy was initially formulated in 1994.
The components of the policy are advocacy, promotion, prevention, treatment and rehabilitation. Community based care, quality improvement, services for Maori, balancing personal rights with protection of the public, and developing a national drug and alcohol policy are the major issues addressed in the policy (the document 'Looking Forward' outlines the 10-year national mental health strategy). The strategy requires specialized mental health services to be delivered to the 3% of people who are the most severely affected by mental illness and mental health in primary care for the other 17%. A strategy to address Maori mental health issues, 'Te Puawaitanga; Maori Mental Health National Strategic Framework', was published in 2001.

Substance Abuse Policy A substance abuse policy is present. The policy was initially formulated in 1998. The National Drug Policy (1998) emphasizes the need for strong law enforcement (to control the supply of drugs), credible messages about drug-related harm (to reduce demand for drugs) and effective health services (to manage drug problems which do still occur).

N–R

National Mental Health Programme A national mental health programme is present. The programme was formulated in 1997. The Mental Health Commission was established in 1996 to monitor the progress of implementation of the national strategy. In 1997, 'Moving Forward' was released. This document set a national mental health plan for more and better services. In 1998, the Mental Health Commission released the Blueprint for Mental Health Services in New Zealand. It provides a description of the mental health service and workforce developments required for the implementation of the National Mental Health Strategy. It emphasizes appropriate attention to mental health promotion, early intervention services and treatment for moderate and mild mental illness. In June 2000, the five-year mental health workforce plan was completed. Most of the milestones in the national mental health strategy have now been met. A successor strategy, with new milestones for 2006-2010 is being prepared. National mental health standards were developed in 1997 and subsequently revised in 2001. All mental health services must comply with these standards.

National Therapeutic Drug Policy/Essential List of Drugs A national therapeutic drug policy/essential list of drugs is present. Details about the year of formulation are not available.
An organization set up by the Government evaluates drugs considered to be essential for the health services and subsidizes them. Other drugs considered non-essential by the organization have to be paid for in full.

Mental Health Legislation There is a Mental Health (Compulsory Assessment and Treatment) Act of 1992, which was amended in 1999. The Criminal Procedure (Mentally Impaired Persons) Act 2003 regulates forensic issues in conjunction with Part 4 of the Mental Health Act. There is no capacity for diminished responsibility. The Mental Health Commission Act 1998 sets up a Commission to monitor and report on the implementation of the Government's mental health strategy.
The latest legislation was enacted in 1992.

Mental Health Financing There are budget allocations for mental health.
The country spends 11% of the total health budget on mental health.
The primary sources of mental health financing in descending order are tax based, out of pocket expenditure by the patient or family, private insurances and social insurance.
Hospital and community-based mental health services are publicly funded. Since 1999, District Health Boards have taken over the funding role from the erstwhile Health Funding Authority. They provide 70% of the mental health and drug abuse services directly and fund the other 30% of services provided by around 400 NGOs and independent general practitioner associations. Patients pay a proportion of the cost of their drugs and tests. Lower rates are levied for those on benefits. Public sector funding increased by 125%

between the years 1994 and 2003 to support the implementation of the national strategy. The Accident Compensation Corporation funded by employers and employees finances sexual abuse counselling. About 34% of people have private health insurance, but these provide limited mental health cover. Private expenditure on clinical psychological services is primarily out of pocket.
The country has disability benefits for persons with mental disorders. People are eligible for a range of Government funded benefits according to need.

Mental Health Facilities Mental health is a part of primary health care system. Actual treatment of severe mental disorders is available at the primary level. In 2001, a new Primary Health Care Strategy was developed and it led to the establishment of Primary Health Care Organizations (PHOs). The Strategy builds on a population health focus. As part of the implementation of the Strategy, work is under way to better integrate mental health into primary care. Even for those people who have moderate to severe mental illness, their needs are met in primary health care. Some specialist mental health and primary health shared care services operate jointly to manage people with severe mental illness in primary care.
Regular training of primary care professionals is carried out in the field of mental health. To support shared care services, additional training of primary care professionals in managing people with severe mental illness has been undertaken.
There are community care facilities for patients with mental disorders. A broad range of community services are available, for instance, residential care, community support, supported employment, consumer and family networks, education and some home based services. About 6-7% of people estimated to be using mental health services live in supported accommodation. Most of these are provided or funded by Community Housing Limited, with support services provided by DHBs or DHB contracted community providers. Currently, community-based services form around 68% of all mental health services. Increased community-based service delivery is a result of deinstitutionalization and the greater focus in recent years on the recovery based model of mental health as well as increased recognition of the human rights issues.

Psychiatric Beds and Professionals

Total psychiatric beds per 10 000 population	3.8
Psychiatric beds in mental hospitals per 10 000 population	1
Psychiatric beds in general hospitals per 10 000 population	2.8
Psychiatric beds in other settings per 10 000 population	0
Number of psychiatrists per 100 000 population	6.6
Number of neurosurgeons per 100 000 population	0.4
Number of psychiatric nurses per 100 000 population	74
Number of neurologists per 100 000 population	1.23
Number of psychologists per 100 000 population	28
Number of social workers per 100 000 population	

There are 1837 occupational therapists. Specialist mental health services are available for the 3% of people with severe mental illness. As a result of deinstitutionalization, stand-alone psychiatric hospitals have been replaced by mental health units in general hospitals. Inpatient beds have decreased by about one third in the last decade. In the same period, beds in services delivered by the community have more than doubled. There is only one private hospital. About 7% of available beds are earmarked for the elderly. Two-thirds of psychiatrists are based in Christchurch and Auckland. About 15% of psychiatrists and 30.5% of psychologists offering clinical, counselling and psychotherapy services are in private practice. The deployment of mental health professionals in the public mental health services has increased in the last decade (e.g. psychologists by more than 50%), but still a shortage is perceived. Psychologists and psychiatric nurses do not have medication prescribing privileges.

Non-Governmental Organizations NGOs are involved with mental health in the country. They are mainly involved in advocacy, promotion, prevention, treatment and rehabilitation. NGOs also provide residential care facilities. Mental health services run by and for consumers operate throughout the country, and consumer representatives make an invaluable contribution in all policy and service development issues.

Information Gathering System There is mental health reporting system in the country. The centralized information system is known as the Mental Health Information National Collection (MHINC). Details are available from the website:www.nzhis.govt.nz. This provides ongoing information about people accessing mental health treatment and support services in inpatient and community settings, their diagnoses and the services they receive.
The country has no data collection system or epidemiological study on mental health. The development of systems to routinely collect information about client outcomes is in the early stages. A major epidemiology study, as part of the WHO World Mental Health Consortium, to examine the determinants of mental health and to provide information on the prevalence of mental disorders, disability and service utilization is also under way.
The Mental Health Information National Collection (MHINC) provides ongoing information about numbers of adults, children and young people accessing mental health services, their diagnoses and the services they receive. A major epidemiology study that

examines the determinants of mental health and provides information on the prevalence of mental disorders, disability and service utilization is under way.

Programmes for Special Population The country has specific programmes for mental health for minorities, refugees, disaster affected population, indigenous population, elderly and children. In addition, there are specific services for deaf subjects and those with alcohol and substance abuse, as well as forensic and maternal mental health services.
To improve the low mental health status of Maori, as compared with the rest of the population, Kaupapa Maori mental health services have been developed. These services are run by and for Maori, and operate according to Maori perspectives of health and well-being. Similarly, there are services by and for Pacific people living in New Zealand. Mainstream services must also ensure culturally responsive service delivery. The Ministry of Health's Public Health Directorate has developed a national mental health promotion strategy entitled 'Building on Strengths.' The Directorate is also leading a national campaign entitled 'Like Minds, Like Mine: Project to Counter Stigma and Discrimination associated with Mental Illness.' Broadly, the campaign comprises both national and regional components. The national work consists of mass media (including a television and radio advertising campaign), benchmark and tracking surveys on the general public's attitude towards mental illness and collecting information on attitudes, behaviours and policies that are, or could be, discriminatory. In collaboration with the Education sector, two programmes 'Health Promotion in Schools' and 'Mentally Healthy Schools' are available for school use. The Mental Health Directorate has responsibility for managing problem gambling through community services. DHB's have responsibility for developing 'Major Incident and Emergency Plans'.

Therapeutic Drugs The following therapeutic drugs are generally available at the primary health care level of the country: carbamazepine, ethosuximide, phenobarbital, phenytoin sodium, sodium valproate, amitriptyline, chlorpromazine, diazepam, fluphenazine, haloperidol, lithium, biperiden, carbidopa, levodopa.
Though there is no WHO style national drug policy or essential drug list, there is a therapeutic policy and regulation that has all the elements of the WHO policy, and the current regulatory environment meets the WHO definitions. The Government funds pharmaceuticals in New Zealand via a separate agency (PHARMAC) that apply a cost utility approach to selection of medicines to fund. Inherent within the PHARMAC approach is consideration of maintaining a number of medicines in particular therapeutic groups.

Other Information The life expectancy for Maori, the country's indigenous population, is lower than the general population at 69.0 for Maori males and 73.2 for Maori females. The Government has established a broad based approach to social policy. A priority in this initiative is the low mental health status of Maori compared with the rest of New Zealand's population.

Additional Sources of Information

Bale, R. (2002) An experience of New Zealand psychiatry. Psychiatric Bulletin, 26, 192-193.

Brinded, P. M. J. (2000) Forensic psychiatry in New Zealand. International Journal of Law and Psychiatry, 23, 453-465.

Durie, M. (1999) Mental health and Maori development. Austalian and New Zealand Journal of Psychiatry, 33, 5-12.

Joyce, P. E. (2002) Focus on psychiatry in New Zealand. British Journal of Psychiatry, 180, 468-470.

Mental Health Commission (1998) Blueprint for Mental Health Services in New Zealand, How Things Need to Be.

Mental Health Commission (1999) New Zealand's National Mental Health Strategy: Review of Progress 1994-1999. Wellington.

Ministry of Health (1994) Looking Forward, Strategic Directions for the Mental Health Services.

Ministry of Health (1997) Mental Health in New Zealand from a Public Health Perspective. Wellington.

Ministry of Health (1997) Moving Forward, The National Mental Health Plan for More and Better Services.

Ministry of Health (1998) National Drug Policy, A National Drug Policy for New Zealand 1998-2003.

Ministry of Health (2000) Health Expenditure Trends in New Zealand. 1980-1999. Wellington.

Ministry of Health (2000) Social Inequalities in Health-New Zealand. 1999. Wellington.

Ministry of Health (April 2004) Health Expenditure Trends in New Zealand 1990-2002.

Ministry of Health Information Service (2004) Psychologist Workforce in New Zealand 2003.

Wilson, J. (2000) Mental health services in New Zealand. International Journal of Law and Psychiatry, 23, 3-4, 215-228.

Wright, D. (1997) Mental health in New Zealand: positive developments in mental health services in New Zealand, and the role of the Mental Health Commission. Healthcare Review Online, 2, 3.

Statistics New Zealand, 2004.

Stewart, M. W. (2001) Medical psychology in New Zealand. Journal of Clinical Psychology in Medical Settings, 8, 51-59.

Nicaragua

GENERAL INFORMATION

Nicaragua is a country with an approximate area of 130 thousand sq. km. (UNO, 2001). Its population is 5.596 million, and the sex ratio (men per hundred women) is 99 (UNO, 2004). The proportion of population under the age of 15 years is 41% (UNO, 2004), and the proportion of population above the age of 60 years is 5% (WHO, 2004). The literacy rate is 76.8% for men and 76.6% for women (UNESCO/MoH, 2004).

The country is a low income group country (based on World Bank 2004 criteria). The proportion of health budget to GDP is 7.8%. The per capita total expenditure on health is 158 international $, and the per capita government expenditure on health is 77 international $ (WHO, 2004).

The main language(s) used in the country is (are) Spanish. The largest ethnic group(s) is (are) Mestizo (seven-tenths), and the other ethnic group(s) are (is) European and African. The largest religious group(s) is (are) Roman Catholic (five-sixths).

The life expectancy at birth is 67.9 years for males and 72.4 years for females (WHO, 2004). The healthy life expectancy at birth is 60 years for males and 63 years for females (WHO, 2004).

EPIDEMIOLOGY

Penayo (1990) used SRQ-20 as a screening instrument to identify probable psychiatric cases (cut-off score of 9/10) in the general population (n=576) and primary health care (n=781). Confirmation of diagnosis was done through Present State Examination (PSE) assisted interview. Almost 23% of general population and 47% of the primary care subjects were identified as cases. Penayo et al (1992) estimated the prevalence of mental disorders in an area affected by armed conflict. Two-stage cluster sampling was used to select 219 families (n=584). Screening was done with SRQ and confirmation of diagnosis through the Present State Examination. The estimated prevalence rates were: neurosis (7.5%), depression (6.2%), reactive crisis (3.3%), alcoholism (5.8%), organic brain syndrome (3.9%), psychosis (0.5%) and other disorders (0.7%). The estimated overall prevalence of mental disorders in the study population was 27.9%. Disorders were more prevalent among men (30.8%) than women (26.3%). Caldera et al (2001) assessed a sample of 496 adult survivors of a hurricane in 4 primary care centres using the Harvard Trauma Questionnaire (HTQ). Prevalence of PTSD ranged from 9.0% in the worst afflicted area to 4.5% in a less damaged area. PTSD symptoms 6 months after the disaster (HTQ) were significantly associated with the death of a relative, destroyed house, female sex, previous mental health problems and illiteracy. Suicidal thoughts were reported by 8.5% of the sample and it was associated with a history of previous mental health problems and illiteracy. One year after the hurricane, half of those identified as PTSD cases at 6 months retained the diagnosis. Goenjian et al (2001) interviewed 158 adolescents from three differentially exposed cities using a Hurricane Exposure Questionnaire, the Child Posttraumatic Stress Disorder Reaction Index and the Depression Self-Rating Scale 6 months after a hurricane. Severe levels of posttraumatic stress and depressive reactions were found in the two more heavily affected cities and this was proportionate to the level of exposure. Level of impact (city), objective and subjective features and thoughts of revenge accounted for 68% of the variance in severity of posttraumatic stress reaction. Severity of posttraumatic stress reaction, death of a family member and sex accounted for 59% of the variance in severity of depression. Summerfield and Toser (1991) found that 62% of men and 91% of women ex-refugees still living in the war zone met criteria for caseness according to the General Health Questionnaire. Nearly 25% of men and 50% of women merited a diagnosis of posttraumatic stress disorder. Some distress reflected unresolved grief states. Caldera et al (1995) assessed 100 consecutive outpatients with the Structural Clinical Interview for DSM-III Disorders. One fourth of patients had a psychotic disorder where schizophrenia dominated. Among non-psychotic patients, major depression, anxiety and adjustment disorders were most frequent. Personality disorders were common (80%) among non-psychotic patients, with paranoid, obsessive-compulsive, passive-aggressive and masochistic personality disorders being the most frequent. Victims of spousal violence frequently experienced feelings of shame, isolation and entrapment and poor social support (Ellsberg et al, 1999, 2000). Suicide was the leading cause of death in the 15-34 year-old age group and the tenth leading cause of mortality overall in the year 2001. Suicidal behaviour is more common in men than women (2,5:1). The rate for 100 000 inhabitants has ascended of 2.80 in 1992 to 6.74 in 2002. Almost 29% of the parasuicidal behaviour is seen in the population younger than 20 years and more than 50% in those younger than 25 years. In this group women (more than 75%) are overrepresented. Herbicides are often used to attempt suicide (Ministry of Health, 2004).

MENTAL HEALTH RESOURCES

Mental Health Policy A mental health policy is present. The policy was initially formulated in 1975.
The components of the policy are advocacy, promotion, prevention, treatment and rehabilitation. It was revised in 2001 by mental health professionals and public servants. Between 25 to 50 % of its original content was put into practice.

Substance Abuse Policy Details about the substance abuse policy are not available. It was revised in 2002. It has a specific budget for its implementation and has been implemented to the extent of 25 to 50%. Nicaragua also has laws on substance abuse, 'Ley 175 de 1994 – Creación Consejo Nacional Antidrogas', 'Ley 285 Ley antidrogas actualizada' and 'Ley 370 – Ley Creación Instituto contra el Alcoholismo y la Drogadicción'.

National Mental Health Programme A national mental health programme is present. The programme was formulated in 1979. It was revised in 2001. There are no specific funds for its implementation, but it has been implemented to the extent of 25 to 50% by local, regional and national authorities. Its main components are strategy of services reform, promotion and prevention, integration of mental health services in primary care and development of specialized services.

National Therapeutic Drug Policy/Essential List of Drugs A national therapeutic drug policy/essential list of drugs is present. It was formulated in 1999.

Mental Health Legislation The most recent legislation is from 2001 and was revised in 2002. There are no regular funds for its implementation but it has been implemented to the extent of 25 to 50%. It focuses on promotion and prevention and regulation of mental health services, but there is no reference to human rights of patients. Other laws related with mental health are the Handicap Law (Law 202), the Anti-Drug Law (Law 285), the Law on Creation of the Institute Against Alcoholism and the Drug Addiction and the Pharmacy Law.
The latest legislation was enacted in 2001.

Mental Health Financing There are budget allocations for mental health.
The country spends 1% of the total health budget on mental health.
The primary sources of mental health financing in descending order are out of pocket expenditure by the patient or family, tax based, social insurance and private insurances.
The country has disability benefits for persons with mental disorders. Disability benefits are available only to those covered by social security. The health department has to assess a patient every 3 years.

Mental Health Facilities Mental health is a part of primary health care system. Actual treatment of severe mental disorders is available at the primary level. Less than 25 % of the population is covered by this kind of service. Mental health care is provided by primary health care physicians.
Regular training of primary care professionals is not carried out in the field of mental health.
There are community care facilities for patients with mental disorders. The system of community care for the mentally ill includes preventive/promotion interventions, home interventions, family interventions, residential facilities, vocational training; employment programs; however, all of them are available for less than 25% of the population. Community care teams are often multidisciplinary (general clinicians, nurses, social workers), but they are understaffed.

Psychiatric Beds and Professionals

Total psychiatric beds per 10 000 population	0.34
Psychiatric beds in mental hospitals per 10 000 population	0.32
Psychiatric beds in general hospitals per 10 000 population	
Psychiatric beds in other settings per 10 000 population	0.02
Number of psychiatrists per 100 000 population	0.64
Number of neurosurgeons per 100 000 population	0.01
Number of psychiatric nurses per 100 000 population	0.045
Number of neurologists per 100 000 population	0.4
Number of psychologists per 100 000 population	1.45
Number of social workers per 100 000 population	0.71

In addition, there are 10 general nurses, 74 assistants and a 1 pedagogue. Almost half of the psychiatrist work in the private set-up. No attempts have been made to close mental hospitals. However, only 10% of beds are occupied by long-stay patients. There are facilities to assess the quality of care at secondary and tertiary level. The ministerial resolution 31- 93 encourages attendance of psychiatric patients in general hospitals. About 15 general hospitals provide mental health care. There is significant geographic variation of mental health services with 96% of centres providing mental health care being along the Pacific Coast. More than 50% of mental health professionals are employed in public institutions.

Non-Governmental Organizations NGOs are involved with mental health in the country. They are mainly involved in advocacy, promotion, prevention, treatment and rehabilitation. These organizations participate in mental health activities related to women, children, domestic violence and consumers.

Information Gathering System There is mental health reporting system in the country. They use ICD-10 codes. Besides psychiatric diagnoses, other mental health components reported are family violence, homicides, suicides, drug abuse and dependence. Epidemiological assessments of mental disorders are performed.
The country has data collection system or epidemiological study on mental health. The department in charge of service data collection system is the 'Dirección General de Sistemas de Información' of the Ministry of Health. Data is collected only in hospitals and some primary health care centers where mental health services are available. Cases registered in the system of registration of

the MINSA in 2002 showed that out of the 33 583 outpatients applying for mental health care (0.07% of all registrants) only 69% had diagnosable conditions. Sleep related disorders (22%), anxiety states (42%), psychoses (27%), and alcohol dependence (2.9%) were common (Ministry of Health, 2004)

Programmes for Special Population The country has specific programmes for mental health for disaster affected population, indigenous population and children.
Also, there are programmes for women, children in vulnerable situation, and victims of domestic violence.

Therapeutic Drugs The following therapeutic drugs are generally available at the primary health care level of the country: carbamazepine, ethosuximide, phenobarbital, phenytoin sodium, sodium valproate, amitriptyline, chlorpromazine, diazepam, haloperidol, lithium, biperiden, carbidopa, levodopa.
The essential drug list was created in 1979 and revised in 2001. Availability of these medications is erratic. They are free of charge for chronic patients and at the primary care level.

Other Information

Additional Sources of Information

Asioli, F., Kraudy, E., Liberati, A., et al (1987) Organization of services and pattern of psychiatric care in Nicaragua: result of a survey in 1986. Acta Psychiatrica Scandinavica, 76, 545-51.

Byng, R. (1993) Primary mental health care in Nicaragua. Social Science and Medicine, 36, 625-29.

Caldera, T., Kullgren, G., Penayo, U., et al (1995) Is treatment in groups a useful alternative for psychiatry in low-income countries? An evaluation of a psychiatric outpatient unit in Nicaragua. Acta Psychiatrica Scandinavica, 92, 386-391.

Caldera, T., Palma, L., Penayo, U., et al (2001) Psychological impact of the hurricane Mitch in Nicaragua in a one-year perspective. Social Psychiatry & Psychiatric Epidemiology, 36, 108-114.

Ellsberg, M. C., Pena, R., Herrera, A., et al (1999) Wife abuse among women of childbearing age in Nicaragua. American Journal of Public Health, 89, 241-244.

Ellsberg, M., Pena, R., Herrera, A., et al (2000) Candies in hell: women's experiences of violence in Nicaragua. Social Science & Medicine, 51, 1595-1610.

Goenjian, A. K., Molina, L., Steinberg, A. M., et al (2001) Posttraumatic stress and depressive reactions among Nicaraguan adolescents after hurricane Mitch. American Journal of Psychiatry, 158, 788-794.

Penayo, U., Caldera, T., Jacobsson, L., et al (1992) Prevalence of mental disorders in adults in Subtiava, Leon, Nicaragua. Boletin de la Oficina Sanitaria Panamericana, 113, 137-149.

Penayo, U., Kullgren, G., Caldera, T. (1990) Mental disorders among primary health care patients in Nicaragua. Acta Psychiatrica Scandinavica, 82, 82-85.

Summerfield, D., Toser, L. (1991) 'Low intensity' war and mental trauma in Nicaragua: a study in a rural community. Medicine & War, 7, 84-99.

Niger

GENERAL INFORMATION

Niger is a country with an approximate area of 1267 thousand sq. km. (UNO, 2001). Its population is 12.415 million, and the sex ratio (men per hundred women) is 102 (UNO, 2004). The proportion of population under the age of 15 years is 50% (UNO, 2004), and the proportion of population above the age of 60 years is 3% (WHO, 2004). The literacy rate is 25.1% for men and 9.3% for women (UNESCO/MoH, 2004).

The country is a low income group country (based on World Bank 2004 criteria). The proportion of health budget to GDP is 3.7%. The per capita total expenditure on health is 22 international $, and the per capita government expenditure on health is 9 international $ (WHO, 2004).

The main language(s) used in the country is (are) French, Kanuri, Arabe, Gourmantche, Toubou and Boudouma. The largest ethnic group(s) is (are) Hausa, and the other ethnic group(s) are (is) Djerma, Fula and Tuareg. The largest religious group(s) is (are) Muslim (four-fifths), and the other religious group(s) are (is) Roman Catholic.

The life expectancy at birth is 42.6 years for males and 42.7 years for females (WHO, 2004). The healthy life expectancy at birth is 36 years for males and 35 years for females (WHO, 2004).

EPIDEMIOLOGY

There is a paucity of epidemiological data on mental illnesses in Niger in internationally accessible literature.

MENTAL HEALTH RESOURCES

Mental Health Policy A mental health policy is present. The policy was initially formulated in 1993.
The components of the policy are promotion, prevention and treatment.

Substance Abuse Policy A substance abuse policy is present. The policy was initially formulated in 1997.

National Mental Health Programme A national mental health programme is present. The programme was formulated in 2001. A new mental health programme was adopted in 2001. A national action plan in mental health is being formulated, in which activities in primary health care and mental health would be included and this would be adopted soon.

National Therapeutic Drug Policy/Essential List of Drugs A national therapeutic drug policy/essential list of drugs is present. It was formulated in 1995.

N–R

Mental Health Legislation The current legislation on mental health is the decree which created psychiatric services in western French Africa. A process to formulate new mental health legislation is under way. A draft of this legislation was expected before December 2001.
The latest legislation was enacted in 1928.

Mental Health Financing There are no budget allocations for mental health.
Details about expenditure on mental health are not available.
The primary sources of mental health financing in descending order are tax based, out of pocket expenditure by the patient or family, social insurance and private insurances.
The country does not have disability benefits for persons with mental disorders.

Mental Health Facilities Mental health is not a part of primary health care system. Actual treatment of severe mental disorders is not available at the primary level.
Regular training of primary care professionals is not carried out in the field of mental health.
There are community care facilities for patients with mental disorders. Traditional medicine is the only form of community treatment.

Psychiatric Beds and Professionals

Total psychiatric beds per 10 000 population	0.2
Psychiatric beds in mental hospitals per 10 000 population	0
Psychiatric beds in general hospitals per 10 000 population	0.2
Psychiatric beds in other settings per 10 000 population	0
Number of psychiatrists per 100 000 population	0.04
Number of neurosurgeons per 100 000 population	0.01
Number of psychiatric nurses per 100 000 population	0.04
Number of neurologists per 100 000 population	0.01
Number of psychologists per 100 000 population	0.03
Number of social workers per 100 000 population	0.05

Non-Governmental Organizations NGOs are involved with mental health in the country. They are mainly involved in advocacy, promotion, prevention and rehabilitation.

Information Gathering System There is mental health reporting system in the country. Mental disorders are included in 'other disorders' category.
The country has no data collection system or epidemiological study on mental health.

Programmes for Special Population There are no special mental health programmes for any specific population.

Therapeutic Drugs The following therapeutic drugs are generally available at the primary health care level of the country: phenobarbital, chlorpromazine, diazepam, haloperidol.

Other Information

Additional Sources of Information

Nigeria

GENERAL INFORMATION

Nigeria is a country with an approximate area of 924 thousand sq. km. (UNO, 2001). Its population is 127.117 million, and the sex ratio (men per hundred women) is 102 (UNO, 2004). The proportion of population under the age of 15 years is 44% (UNO, 2004), and the proportion of population above the age of 60 years is 5% (WHO, 2004). The literacy rate is 74.4% for men and 59.4% for women (UNESCO/MoH, 2004).

The country is a low income group country (based on World Bank 2004 criteria). The proportion of health budget to GDP is 3.4%. The per capita total expenditure on health is 31 international $, and the per capita government expenditure on health is 7 international $ (WHO, 2004).

The main language(s) used in the country is (are) English, Hausa, Yoruba, Igbo and Pidgin English. The largest ethnic group(s) is (are) Hausa and Fulani in the north, Yoruba in the southwest and Igbo in the southeast., and the other ethnic group(s) are (is) Efik/Ibibio, Tiv, Ijaw, Kanuri, Nupe, Edo and Idoma. The largest religious group(s) is (are) Muslim and Christian, and the other religious group(s) are (is) indigenous groups.

The life expectancy at birth is 48 years for males and 49.6 years for females (WHO, 2004). The healthy life expectancy at birth is 41 years for males and 42 years for females (WHO, 2004).

EPIDEMIOLOGY

Leighton et al (1963) conducted a cross-cultural study in which they found that subjects in Yorubaland, Nigeria had more mental symptoms especially those related to the organic domain but fewer cases of mental disorders in comparison to those in the Stirling County in North America. More men in the former setting and more women in the latter setting had mental disorders. Gureje et al (1992a) assessed 787 primary care patients using the Yoruba translation of the General Health Questionnaire (GHQ–12) and Composite International Diagnostic Interview (CIDI) in a two stage design. A weighted prevalence for specific DSM-III-R disorders was 27.8%. Abiodun (1993) assessed 272 primary care patients using a two-stage procedure with GHQ-12 and the Present State Examination Schedule (PSE). The prevalence of psychiatric disorder was 21.3%. Depressive neurosis (51.7%) and anxiety neurosis (36.3%) were common. Psychiatric morbidity was associated with age (older), gender (female) and marital status (widowed, separated or divorced). Gureje (2002) assessed 704 primary care patients with GHQ-28, a structured diagnostic interview and a disability assessment schedule, at 2 time points one year apart. About 10% met the ICD-10 criteria for any disorder and 25% met GHQ caseness criterion. Being a case on the GHQ at baseline (but not on ICD-10) was associated with disability at 12-month follow-up. Uwakwe (2000) assessed 164 rural community subjects aged above 60 years using the Self-Reporting Questionnaire and the Geriatric Mental State Schedule. Psychiatric diagnoses as per ICD-10 Research Criteria were recorded in 23.1% of the subjects, with depression constituting 79% of all diagnoses. Hendrie et al (2001) and Ogunniyi et al (2000) examined two elderly (65+ years) community-dwelling populations in USA (n=2147 African Americans) and Nigeria (n=2459) following a two stage procedure. The age-standardized annual incidence rates were significantly lower among the Nigerians (Dementia: 1.4%, Alzheimer's disease: 1.2%) compared to the African Americans (Dementia: 3.2%, Alzheimer's disease: 2.5%). The overall age-adjusted prevalence rates of dementia and Alzheimer's disease in Ibadan (2.3% and 1.4%, respectively) were also lower than the respective values (8.2% and 6.2%) obtained for African Americans. In Nigeria, dementia was associated with old age and female gender. The frequencies of the vascular risk factors were lower in Nigerians. In the same sample, Perkins et al (2002) found that dementia was associated with increased mortality at both sites (Ibadan RR = 2.83, Indianapolis RR = 2.05). Obot (1990) conducted a household survey (n=1271) and found that 22.6% of adults smoked regularly. Abiodun et al (1994) examined 1041 secondary school students using a 117-item WHO self-report substance-use questionnaire. Use of salicylates (56.2%), stimulants (21.6%), alcohol (12.0%) and cigarettes (4.4%) was common. Adelekan and Ndom (1997) evaluated more than 1800 secondary school students with the same instrument at two time points 5 years apart. On the whole, substance use was less frequent in the follow-up sample. However, there were significant increases in the current use of cocaine, organic solvents and hallucinogens. Mamman et al (2002) examined 300 women from rural/suburban areas and found that 64% of them used alcohol, with more than half reporting current use. Gureje et al (1992b) administered the GHQ-12, the Alcohol Use Disorders Identification Test (AUDIT) and the Composite International Diagnostic Interview (CIDI) to subjects in an urban primary care clinic. Alcohol abuse or dependence according to DSM-III-R was estimated to be present in 1.7%. The National Expert Committee on Non-Communicable Diseases (1997) reported that 8.9% of adults (n=16 019) smoked cigarettes. Smoking was associated with gender (male), age (25-34 years) and residence (urban). Also more urban males drank alcohol in comparison to rural males. The National HIV/AIDS and Reproductive Health Survey (2003) showed that 12% of adults (n=10 910) had consumed alcoholic beverages regularly in the past 4 weeks and 3% drank daily. Use of psychoactive drugs was reported by 1% of the population. Jablensky et al (1992) reported the findings of the Determinants of Outcome of Severe Mental Disorders (DOSMED) study. They found that schizophrenia had similar presentation and incidence rates across different countries, but a better outcome in developing countries. Aderibigbe et al (1993) examined 162 women during second trimester and 6-8 weeks postpartum using GHQ-28 and PAS. The rate of caseness was 30% at the prenatal assessment and 14% in the postnatal assessment. Marital and family problems were associated with morbidity. Ohaeri and Odejide (1994) evaluated 865 adults from primary care clinics using GHQ-28, the Self-Reporting Questionnaire (SRQ) and the Brief Disability Questionnaire. About 8.2% fulfilled criteria for probable somatoform disorders. Nwosu and Odesanmi (2001) reviewed autopsy records and reported that the rate of completed suicide was 0.4 per 100 000 population with a male to female ratio of 3.6 to 1. The majority of the victims were in the third decade of life and the common methods of committing suicide were consumption of insecticides and use of firearms. Eferakeya (1984) reviewed records of attempted suicides. The incidence of suicide attempt was 7/100 000. The majority of attempters was below 30 years of age and used poisons (88%). Mental illnesses were reported in one-third of the sample. Abiodun (1992) examined 500 rural children aged between 5-15 years and found the prevalence of psychiatric morbidity to be 15%, with emotional and conduct disorders present in two-thirds of these subjects. Children from disrupted families were more likely to suffer from psychiatric morbidity. Adelekan et al (1999) administered the Rutter's A2 scale to parents of 846 primary school children. The criterion of caseness (cut-off of 13) was met by 18.6% (neurotic disorders: 7.3%, anti-social disorders: 8% and undifferentiated disorders: 3.3%) being common. Psychiatric morbidity was associated with gender (boys), physical and emotional problems during pregnancy in mothers, delayed developmental milestones, major illness during childhood, broken homes and attending rural schools. Gureje et al (1994) assessed 227 children (7-14 years) attending a primary care centre with the children's version of the Schedule for Affective Disorders and Schizophrenia. The weighted prevalence of any DSM-III-R disorders was 19.6% (depressive disorders: 6%, anxiety disorders: 4.7% and conduct disorders: 6.1%).

MENTAL HEALTH RESOURCES

Mental Health Policy A mental health policy is present. The policy was initially formulated in 1991.
The components of the policy are advocacy, promotion, prevention, treatment and rehabilitation. Training and research and management information system are also emphasized in the policy.

Substance Abuse Policy A substance abuse policy is present. The policy was initially formulated in 1990. National Drug Law Enforcement Agency Decree No. 48 was amended in 1990.

National Mental Health Programme A national mental health programme is present. The programme was formulated in 1989. It was adopted in 1991.

National Therapeutic Drug Policy/Essential List of Drugs A national therapeutic drug policy/essential list of drugs is present. It was formulated in 1991.
Psychotropics are available and relatively affordable. However, newer formulations are either unavailable or too expensive. For example, a month's supply of risperidone (2mg) would cost more than the minimum monthly wage in the public service.

Mental Health Legislation The existing legislation on mental health dates back to 1916, later adopted as the Lunacy Act CAP 112, Laws of the Federation of Nigeria, 1958. A revised Mental Health Bill is now before the National Assembly (Parliament) for inaction into law. In 2004, it had passed a public hearing stage and adoption by the Senate. It is now before the House of Representatives.
The latest legislation was enacted in 1958.

Mental Health Financing There are budget allocations for mental health.
Details about expenditure on mental health are not available.
The primary sources of mental health financing in descending order are out of pocket expenditure by the patient or family, tax based, grants, social insurance and private insurances.
The country does not have disability benefits for persons with mental disorders.

Mental Health Facilities Mental health is a part of primary health care system. Actual treatment of severe mental disorders is available at the primary level. However, relatively few centres have trained staff and equipment to implement primary health care. Regular training of primary care professionals is carried out in the field of mental health. Each state has a school of Health Technologists for training of primary care professionals including health care workers.
There are community care facilities for patients with mental disorders. Community care is available in a few states. Providers include private medical practitioners, NGOs, especially faith-based organizations, and traditional healers.

Psychiatric Beds and Professionals

Total psychiatric beds per 10 000 population	0.4
Psychiatric beds in mental hospitals per 10 000 population	0.3
Psychiatric beds in general hospitals per 10 000 population	0.04
Psychiatric beds in other settings per 10 000 population	0.01
Number of psychiatrists per 100 000 population	0.09
Number of neurosurgeons per 100 000 population	0.009
Number of psychiatric nurses per 100 000 population	4
Number of neurologists per 100 000 population	0.02
Number of psychologists per 100 000 population	0.02
Number of social workers per 100 000 population	0.02

Many health professionals migrate to industrialized countries leading to a shortage of personnel. Most resources are located in urban centres and predominantly in the southern parts of the country. There is virtually no private practice in the country. Many psychiatrists who have trained in other countries have not returned.

Non-Governmental Organizations NGOs are involved with mental health in the country. They are mainly involved in advocacy, promotion, prevention, treatment and rehabilitation.

Information Gathering System There is mental health reporting system in the country. Mental health morbidity statistics are available in each mental health institution but not always aggregated comprehensively at the national level.
The country has data collection system or epidemiological study on mental health. A national survey of mental health and wellbeing conducted in 2003-2004 to provide information on the size and extent of mental health problems in the country is undergoing analysis.

Programmes for Special Population The country has specific programmes for mental health for refugees, disaster affected population, elderly and children. There is a National Emergency Relief Agency (NEMA) that caters for the needs of refugees and populations affected by disasters. Mental health workers are invited to render necessary assistance, whenever required.
Specific programmes have been developed for substance use disorders.

Therapeutic Drugs The following therapeutic drugs are generally available at the primary health care level of the country: carbamazepine, phenobarbital, phenytoin sodium, amitriptyline, chlorpromazine, diazepam, fluphenazine, haloperidol, biperiden. Benzhexol (5mg) is available.

Other Information Many psychiatric researches have been directed to problems related to the scientific practice and acceptability of psychiatry as a distinct discipline of medicine. These research studies created a positive awareness which led to the establishment of more psychiatry units in the general hospital setting, several specialist psychiatric institutions in the community and psychiatric residency programmes in the country.

Additional Sources of Information

Abiodun, O. A. (1992) Emotional illness in a paediatric population in Nigeria. East African Medical Journal, 69, 557-559.

Abiodun, O. A. (1993) A study of mental morbidity among primary care patients in Nigeria. Comprehensive Psychiatry, 34, 10-13.

Abiodun, O. A., Adelekan, M. L., Ogunremi, O. O., et al (1994) Pattern of substance use amongst secondary school students in Ilorin, northern Nigeria. West African Journal of Medicine, 13, 91-97.

Adamson, T. A. (1998). The productivity and impact of psychiatric research on development of mental health services in Nigeria. West African Medical Journal, 17, 243-247.

Adelekan, M. L., Ndom, R. J. (1997) Trends in prevalence and pattern of substance use among secondary school pupils in Ilorin, Nigeria. West African Journal of Medicine, 16, 157-164.

Adelekan, M. L., Ndom, R. J., Ekpo, M., et al (1999) Epidemiology of childhood behavioural disorders in Ilorin, Nigeria--findings from parental reports. West African Journal of Medicine, 18, 39-48.

Aderibigbe, Y. A., Gureje, O., Omigbodun, O. (1993) Postnatal emotional disorders in Nigerian women. A study of antecedents and associations. British Journal of Psychiatry, 163, 645-650.

Eferakeya A. E. (1984) Drugs and suicide attempts in Benin City, Nigeria. British Journal of Psychiatry, 145, 70-73.

Federal Ministry of Health (1991) The National Mental Health Policy for Nigeria. Federal Ministry of Health, Lagos.

Federal Ministry of Health (1991) The National Mental Health Programme and Action Plan for Nigeria. Federal Ministry of Health, Lagos.

Federal Ministry of Health (2003) Essential Drugs List, Fourth Revision, Federal Ministry of Health, Abuja in collaboration with WHO.

Federal Ministry of Health of Nigeria (2003) National HIV/AIDS and Reproductive Health Survey, 2003. Federal Ministry of Health, Abuja.

Federal Ministry of Health (1997) Non Communicable Diseases in Nigeria: Final Report of a National Survey by the Expert Committee on NCD. Ed OO Akinkugbe. Intec Printers limited, Ibadan.

Gureje, O. (2002) Psychological disorders and symptoms in primary care. Association with disability and service use after 12 months. Social Psychiatry & Psychiatric Epidemiology, 37, 220-224.

Gureje, O. (2003) Psychiatry in Nigeria. International Psychiatry, 2, 10-12.

Gureje, O., Obikoya, B., Ikuesan, B. A. (1992a) Prevalence of specific psychiatric disorders in an urban primary care setting. East African Medical Journal, 69, 282-287.

Gureje, O., Obikoya, B., Ikuesan, B. A. (1992b) Alcohol abuse and dependence in an urban primary care clinic in Nigeria. Drug & Alcohol Dependence, 30, 163-167.

Gureje, O., Omigbodun, O. O., Gater, R., et al (1994) Psychiatric disorders in a paediatric primary care clinic. British Journal of Psychiatry, 165, 527-530.

Hendrie, H. C., Ogunniyi, A., Hall, K. S., et al (2001) Incidence of Dementia and Alzheimer disease in 2 communities: Yoruba residing in Ibadan, Nigeria, and African Americans residing in Indianapolis, Indiana. JAMA, 285, 739-747.

Jablensky, A., Sartorius, N., Ernberg, G., et al (1992) Schizophrenia: manifestations, incidence and course in different cultures. A World Health Organization ten-country study. Psychological Medicine, Monograph Supplement 22, 1-97.

Mamman, L. S., Brieger, W. R., Oshiname, F. O. (2002) Alcohol consumption pattern among women in a rural Yoruba community in Nigeria. Substance Use & Misuse, 37, 579-597.

National Population Commission (1998) 1991 Population Census of the Federal Republic of Nigeria – Analytical Report at the National Level, National Poplation Commission, Lagos, Nigeria

Nwosu, S. O., Odesanmi, W. O. (2001) Pattern of suicides in Ile-Ife, Nigeria. West African Journal of Medicine, 20, 259-262.

Obot, I. S. (1990) The use of tobacco products among Nigerian adults: a general population survey. Drug & Alcohol Dependence, 26, 203-208.

Ogunniyi, A., Baiyewu, O., Gureje, O., et al (2000) Epidemiology of dementia in Nigeria: results from the Indianapolis-Ibadan study. European Journal of Neurology, 7, 485-490.

Ohaeri, J. U., Odejide, O. A. (1994) Somatization symptoms among patients using primary health care facilities in a rural community in Nigeria. American Journal of Psychiatry, 151, 728-731.

Perkins, A. J., Hui, S. L., Ogunniyi, A., et al (2002) Risk of mortality for dementia in a developing country: the Yoruba in Nigeria. International Journal of Geriatric Psychiatry, 17, 566-573.

University College Hospital Ibadan (1998). Essential Drug List.

Uwakwe, R. (2000) The pattern of psychiatric disorders among the aged in a selected community in Nigeria. International Journal of Geriatric Psychiatry, 15, 355-362.

Niue

GENERAL INFORMATION

Niue is a country with an approximate area of 0.26 thousand sq. km. (UNO, 2001). Its population is 0.002 million, and the proportion of population above the age of 60 years is 7% (WHO, 2004).
The country is a high income group country (based on World Bank 2004 criteria). The proportion of health budget to GDP is 7.7%. The per capita total expenditure on health is 1041 international $, and the per capita government expenditure on health is 1010 international $ (WHO, 2004).
The main language(s) used in the country is (are) Niuean and English. The largest ethnic group(s) is (are) Niue.
The life expectancy at birth is 67.6 years for males and 73.3 years for females (WHO, 2004). The healthy life expectancy at birth is 59 years for males and 62 years for females (WHO, 2004).

EPIDEMIOLOGY

There is a paucity of epidemiological data on mental illnesses in Niue in internationally accessible literature.

MENTAL HEALTH RESOURCES

Mental Health Policy A mental health policy is absent.

Substance Abuse Policy A substance abuse policy is absent.

National Mental Health Programme A national mental health programme is absent.

National Therapeutic Drug Policy/Essential List of Drugs A national therapeutic drug policy/essential list of drugs is present. It was formulated in 1998.

Mental Health Legislation There is a Mental Health Act. New Zealand's mental health act is also used in the country.
The latest legislation was enacted in 1969.

Mental Health Financing There are no budget allocations for mental health.
Details about expenditure on mental health are not available.
The primary source of mental health financing is tax based.
The country has disability benefits for persons with mental disorders. There is a Government budget support for disability benefits.

Mental Health Facilities Mental health is not a part of primary health care system. Actual treatment of severe mental disorders is not available at the primary level.
Regular training of primary care professionals is not carried out in the field of mental health.
There are no community care facilities for patients with mental disorders.

Psychiatric Beds and Professionals

Total psychiatric beds per 10 000 population	0
Psychiatric beds in mental hospitals per 10 000 population	0
Psychiatric beds in general hospitals per 10 000 population	0
Psychiatric beds in other settings per 10 000 population	0
Number of psychiatrists per 100 000 population	0
Number of neurosurgeons per 100 000 population	0
Number of psychiatric nurses per 100 000 population	0
Number of neurologists per 100 000 population	0
Number of psychologists per 100 000 population	0
Number of social workers per 100 000 population	0

Non-Governmental Organizations NGOs are not involved with mental health in the country.

Information Gathering System There is mental health reporting system in the country. Mental health reporting is available only as a statistical information.
The country has no data collection system or epidemiological study on mental health.

Programmes for Special Population There are no special services available.

Therapeutic Drugs The following therapeutic drugs are generally available at the primary health care level of the country: carbamazepine, phenobarbital, phenytoin sodium, sodium valproate, amitriptyline, chlorpromazine, diazepam, fluphenazine, haloperidol, carbidopa, levodopa.
The essential list of drugs is revised every 2 years. The most recent revision took place in 2004. It should also be noted that the drugs are dispensed from the hospital pharmacy and not through the primary health care.

Other Information

Additional Sources of Information

Norway

GENERAL INFORMATION

Norway is a country with an approximate area of 324 thousand sq. km. (UNO, 2001). Its population is 4.552 million, and the sex ratio (men per hundred women) is 98 (UNO, 2004). The proportion of population under the age of 15 years is 19% (UNO, 2004), and the proportion of population above the age of 60 years is 20% (WHO, 2004). The literacy rate is 99% for men and 99% for women (UNESCO/MoH, 2004).

The country is a high income group country (based on World Bank 2004 criteria). The proportion of health budget to GDP is 8%. The per capita total expenditure on health is 2920 international $, and the per capita government expenditure on health is 2497 international $ (WHO, 2004).

The main language(s) used in the country is (are) Norwegian. The largest religious group(s) is (are) Evangelical Lutheran, and the other religious group(s) are (is) Muslim, Roman Catholic and Orthodox Christian.

The life expectancy at birth is 76.4 years for males and 81.7 years for females (WHO, 2004). The healthy life expectancy at birth is 70 years for males and 74 years for females (WHO, 2004).

EPIDEMIOLOGY

There is substantial epidemiological data on mental illnesses in Norway in internationally accessible literature. No attempt was made to include this information here.

MENTAL HEALTH RESOURCES

Mental Health Policy A mental health policy is present. The policy was initially formulated in 1997.

The components of the policy are advocacy, promotion, prevention, treatment and rehabilitation. Further information is given in the section on national mental health programme.

Substance Abuse Policy A substance abuse policy is present. The policy was initially formulated in 1991. The national mental health programme puts considerable emphasis on developing well coordinated treatment programmes targeted towards patients suffering from both drug-abuse and severe mental illness.

National Mental Health Programme A national mental health programme is present. The programme was formulated in 1999. The national mental health programme was initiated by a White Paper of 1997 ('Stortingsmelding nr 25 (1996-97) ; Åpenhet og helhet – om psykiske lidelser og tjenestetilbudene') that analysed the then current situation regarding mental health services and the need for developing more user-friendly and decentralized mental health services. The national mental health programme/reform ('St prp nr 63 (1997-98) – Om opptrappingsplan for psykisk helse 1999 – 2006') was adopted by the Norwegian Parliament ('Stortinget') and later extended to apply to the period 1999 to 2008. The mental health programme aims at improving availability, accessibility, quality and organization of mental health services and treatment on all levels. It covers many different aspects and settings including primary health care, the specialized health services, the educational system, social services, occupation and employment, housing, etc. The Programme also focuses on deinstitutionalization, reorganization of specialized mental health services and primary mental health care around decentralized community mental health centers, strengthening of primary health and social care services to people with mental illness, participation of user-/patient organizations in mental health policy planning, educational campaigns to reduce stigma and discrimination towards people with ill mental health. Norway also has other national programmes dealing with mental health issues, such as a suicide prevention programme (started in 1994) and a major programme targeting traumatized individuals.

National Therapeutic Drug Policy/Essential List of Drugs A national therapeutic drug policy/essential list of drugs is present. Details about the year of formulation are not available.

Mental Health Legislation In July 1999, the Norwegian Parliament passed four new acts concerning different aspects of health: The Specialized Health Services Act, The Mental Health Act, The Patients' Rights Act, The Health Personnel Act. These new health acts with their additional provisions were put into practice in January 2001. The mental health act ('Ot prp nr 11[1998-99]: Om lov om etablering og gjennomføring av psykisk helsevern [psykiatriloven]') especially regulates the part of psychiatry that deals with coercion/mandatory treatment. However, the main principle is that psychiatry is to be regulated on the same grounds as other specialized medical disciplines in the Specialized Health Services Act. During the fall 2004/winter 2005 a major evaluation will be undertaken regarding the Mental Health Act and its provisions, based on the experiences Norway has had so far with the law. Also, the Directorate for Health and Social Affairs is currently working on a program where the main objective is reduction and quality assurance regarding use of coercive treatment in psychiatry/mental health services.

The latest legislation was enacted in 1998.

Mental Health Financing There are budget allocations for mental health.

The country spends 0.1% of the total health budget on mental health.

The primary sources of mental health financing in descending order are social insurance, tax based, out of pocket expenditure by the patient or family and private insurances.

The national mental health programme has required extensive economical grants and subsidies to the public health sector from the Government.

The country has disability benefits for persons with mental disorders.

Mental Health Facilities Mental health is a part of primary health care system. Actual treatment of severe mental disorders is available at the primary level. The national mental health programme lays emphasis on the importance of the capability of primary health care services in dealing with persons with mental illnesses and problems and on close collaboration between different services and public entities.
Regular training of primary care professionals is carried out in the field of mental health. In the last two years, about 1600 personnel were provided training.
There are community care facilities for patients with mental disorders. Mental health facilities consist of decentralized community mental health centres and specialized psychiatric hospitals. Many psychiatrists and psychologists with private practices are financially supported from the state, and represent an important part of the overall pool of resources in the fight against mental ill health.

Psychiatric Beds and Professionals

Total psychiatric beds per 10 000 population	12
Psychiatric beds in mental hospitals per 10 000 population	
Psychiatric beds in general hospitals per 10 000 population	
Psychiatric beds in other settings per 10 000 population	
Number of psychiatrists per 100 000 population	20
Number of neurosurgeons per 100 000 population	1
Number of psychiatric nurses per 100 000 population	42
Number of neurologists per 100 000 population	4
Number of psychologists per 100 000 population	68
Number of social workers per 100 000 population	

Non-Governmental Organizations NGOs are involved with mental health in the country. They are mainly involved in advocacy, promotion, prevention, treatment and rehabilitation. Official Norwegian health policy states that user participation is an essential factor if one is going to succeed in the overall improvement of mental health services. As a result, NGOs, including user/patient organizations, are strongly involved with mental health issues in the country.

Information Gathering System There is mental health reporting system in the country. MBDS (Minste Basis Data Sett) is a reporting system that is mandatory in all mental health service facilities. This system also includes a detailed reporting system for psychiatric patients undergoing mandatory/coercive treatment.
The country has data collection system or epidemiological study on mental health. The National Institute for Public Health (Folkehelseinstituttet) gathers epidemiological data, including mental health for the whole country.

Programmes for Special Population The country has specific programmes for mental health for minorities, refugees, disaster affected population, elderly and children. There are services for prisoners.
In addition, there are programmes/projects targeting other special groups/problems (diagnostic, ethnic etc), e.g. severe mental illness and violence, diagnosis and treatment regarding children, adolescents and adults suffering from ADHD, patients with severe mental illness and drug abuse, patients suffering from eating disorders, health and social services for refugees and health services for prisoners/inmates.

Therapeutic Drugs The following therapeutic drugs are generally available at the primary health care level of the country: carbamazepine, ethosuximide, phenobarbital, phenytoin sodium, sodium valproate, amitriptyline, chlorpromazine, diazepam, fluphenazine, haloperidol, lithium, biperiden, carbidopa, levodopa.

Other Information Norway has traditionally emphasized the principle of equal rights and access to well-functioning health and social services for all citizens. This, however, is a challenge due to the country's geographical features and the low population density patterns in the country. A decentralized health service system creates its own problems that must be dealt with. For instance, it is a challenge to recruit qualified personnel to small local clinics in rural areas. Also it is essential to achieve and maintain a well functioning, collaborative and coherent service systems for the benefit of the user/patient.

Additional Sources of Information

Mental Health Services in Norway (2001) Norwegian Ministry of Health and Social Affairs.

Sosial Og Helsedepartementet (1996-1997) Apenhet og Hellet – Om Psykiske Lidelser Og Tjenestetilbudene.

Sosial Og Helsedepartementet (1998-1999) Om Lov Om Etablering Og Gjennnomforing av Pshy Helsevern (Psykiatriloven).

The National Institute of Public Health ('Folkehelseinstituttet'): www.fhi.no

The Norwegian Government's official website with general information on Norway: www.dep.no/odin/engelsk

The Norwegian Ministry of Health's offical website: www.dep.no/hd/engelsk

Oman

GENERAL INFORMATION

Oman is a country with an approximate area of 310 thousand sq. km. (UNO, 2001). Its population is 2.935 million, and the sex ratio (men per hundred women) is 134 (UNO, 2004). The proportion of population under the age of 15 years is 37% (UNO, 2004), and the proportion of population above the age of 60 years is 4% (WHO, 2004). The literacy rate is 82% for men and 65.4% for women (UNESCO/MoH, 2004).

The country is a higher middle income group country (based on World Bank 2004 criteria). The proportion of health budget to GDP is 3%. The per capita total expenditure on health is 343 international $, and the per capita government expenditure on health is 277 international $ (WHO, 2004).

The main language(s) used in the country is (are) Arabic. The largest ethnic group(s) is (are) Arab, and the other ethnic group(s) are (is) Baluchi, South Asian and African. The largest religious group(s) is (are) Muslim.

The life expectancy at birth is 71 years for males and 76.3 years for females (WHO, 2004). The healthy life expectancy at birth is 63 years for males and 65 years for females (WHO, 2004).

EPIDEMIOLOGY

Chand et al (2001) conducted an 8-year retrospective analysis of hospital records of cases with dissociative disorder. These disorders were common, and female predominance was not marked. The most common presentations were dissociative convulsions, dissociative motor and dissociative trance disorders. Zaidan et al (2002) reviewed Accident and Emergency records over a 6-year period and found 123 cases of deliberate self-harm. Most patients with deliberate self-harm were women, students and unemployed. Analgesic (paracetamol) use was the preferred method followed by other non-pharmaceutical chemicals. Al Adawi et al (2002) used the Eating Attitude Test and the Bulimic Investigatory Test to assess eating disorders in Omani teenagers, non-Omani teenagers and Omani adults. On the Eating Attitude Test, 33% of Omani teenagers (29.4% females and 36.4% males) and 9% of non-Omani teenagers (7.5% of males and 10.6% females) showed anorexia-like behaviour. On the Bulimic Investigatory Test, 12.3% of Omani teenagers (13.7% females and 10.9% males) showed a propensity for binge eating or bulimia. Among the non-Omani teenagers, 18.4% showed bulimic tendencies with females outnumbering males. Only 2% of Omani adults showed any problems related to eating behaviours. Kenue et al (1995) assessed 492 children (<15 years of age) and found that 2% had disabilities related to chromosomal abnormality, genetic, perinatal and infectious factors. Down syndrome was present in 31% of children with chromosomal abnormalities.

MENTAL HEALTH RESOURCES

Mental Health Policy A mental health policy is present. The policy was initially formulated in 1992.
The components of the policy are advocacy, promotion, prevention, treatment and rehabilitation.

Substance Abuse Policy A substance abuse policy is present. The policy was initially formulated in 1999. The Royal Decree 17/99, Law on Control of Narcotics and Psychotropics was formulated in 1999. The components of the policy are prevention, treatment, rehabilitation and advocacy.

National Mental Health Programme A national mental health programme is present. The programme was formulated in 1990. The national mental health programme was revised in 1992. It envisages to provide mental health care for all through the primary, secondary and tertiary level, taking into account measures for prevention, treatment, promotion and rehabilitation and keeping in view the culture, family and community. The aim was to involve the whole community along with religious teachers, incorporate programmes for the mentally retarded and substance abusers and train professionals. A review workshop is held every year to assess the progress of the national mental health programme.

National Therapeutic Drug Policy/Essential List of Drugs A national therapeutic drug policy/essential list of drugs is present. It was formulated in 1975.

Mental Health Legislation There is no specific mental health legislation. The provision of mental health care is an essential component of the National Health Policy as contained in the policy statement issued by the Ministry of Health in 1992. The Royal Decree 17/99, Law on Control of Narcotics and Psychotropics was formulated in 1999.
Details about the year of enactment of the mental health legislation are not available.

Mental Health Financing There are budget allocations for mental health.
Details about expenditure on mental health are not available.
The primary sources of mental health financing in descending order are tax based, private insurances and out of pocket expenditure by the patient or family.
Psychiatric services are provided free of charge to most Omani patients.
The country has disability benefits for persons with mental disorders. Disability benefits are provided by the Ministry of Social Affairs to all Omani nationals who have physical or mental disorders.

Mental Health Facilities Mental health is a part of primary health care system. Actual treatment of severe mental disorders is not available at the primary level. Primary care and referral services are available. Patients with severe psychiatric disorders are referred to secondary and tertiary levels and managed at primary level only after they are stabilized.
Regular training of primary care professionals is carried out in the field of mental health. In the last two years, about 250 personnel were provided training. Besides training during residency, there are some training facilities for nursing graduates and some for primary care doctors. The training programme for primary care doctors is held on a regular basis along with regional workshops. The Health Ministry has published a manual for primary health care professionals, which lays down the standard operating policy for primary management of psychiatric problems.
There are community care facilities for patients with mental disorders.

Psychiatric Beds and Professionals

Total psychiatric beds per 10 000 population	0.49
Psychiatric beds in mental hospitals per 10 000 population	0.28
Psychiatric beds in general hospitals per 10 000 population	0.21
Psychiatric beds in other settings per 10 000 population	0
Number of psychiatrists per 100 000 population	1.4
Number of neurosurgeons per 100 000 population	0.4
Number of psychiatric nurses per 100 000 population	5
Number of neurologists per 100 000 population	0.25
Number of psychologists per 100 000 population	0.25
Number of social workers per 100 000 population	0.5

There are 15 other mental health professionals. Besides the central psychiatric hospital near Muscat, there are psychiatrists at the nine regional hospitals, eight of which have four beds for psychiatry. There are also beds allotted to other major hospitals and universities. There is a 15-bed facility for the mentally retarded under the Ministry of Social Affairs with training schools for the handicapped. Some beds are earmarked for female patients.

Non-Governmental Organizations NGOs are involved with mental health in the country. They are mainly involved in advocacy, promotion and rehabilitation.

Information Gathering System There is mental health reporting system in the country.
The country has data collection system or epidemiological study on mental health.

Programmes for Special Population The country has specific programmes for mental health for minorities, elderly and children. There is a school mental health programme that involves participation of administrators, school teachers, school children. The programmes are mainly concentrated in rural areas and they are educated through lectures, debates, essay competitions, posters, etc. School health workers and teachers are given some training in order to pick up certain behavioural problems and learning disorders.

Therapeutic Drugs The following therapeutic drugs are generally available at the primary health care level of the country: carbamazepine, phenobarbital, chlorpromazine, diazepam, haloperidol.
Procyclidine and Maprotiline are available through the primary health care. Other psychotropics, except atypical anti-psychotics, are also available through primary centres if they are prescribed by secondary and tertiary centres.

Other Information

Additional Sources of Information

Al Adawi, S., Dorvlo, A. S., Burke, D. T., et al (2002) Presence and severity of anorexia and bulimia among male and female Omani and non-Omani adolescents. Journal of the American Academy of Child & Adolescent Psychiatry, 41, 1124-1130.

Chand, S. P., Koul, R., Al Hussaini, A. A. (2001) Conversion and dissociative disorders in the Sultanate of Oman. Journal of the American Academy of Child & Adolescent Psychiatry, 40, 869-870.

Kenue, R. K., Raj, A. K., Harris, P. F., et al (1995) Cytogenetic analysis of children suspected of chromosomal abnormalities. Journal of Tropical Pediatrics, 41, 77-80.

Zaidan, Z. A. J., Burke, D. T., Dorvlo, A. S. S., et al (2002) Deliberate self-poisoning in Oman. Tropical Medicine & International Health, 7, 549-556.

Pakistan

GENERAL INFORMATION

Pakistan is a country with an approximate area of 796 thousand sq. km. (UNO, 2001). Its population is 157.315 million, and the sex ratio (men per hundred women) is 105 (UNO, 2004). The proportion of population under the age of 15 years is 41% (UNO, 2004), and the proportion of population above the age of 60 years is 6% (WHO, 2004). The literacy rate is 53.4% for men and 28.5% for women (UNESCO/MoH, 2004).

The country is a low income group country (based on World Bank 2004 criteria). The proportion of health budget to GDP is 3.9%. The per capita total expenditure on health is 85 international $, and the per capita government expenditure on health is 21 international $ (WHO, 2004).

The main language(s) used in the country is (are) Punjabi, Sindhi, Siraiki, Pashtu and Urdu. The largest ethnic group(s) is (are) Punjabi, and the other ethnic group(s) are (is) Sindhi, Siraiki, Pashtun and Muhajir. The largest religious group(s) is (are) Muslim.

The life expectancy at birth is 61.1 years for males and 61.6 years for females (WHO, 2004). The healthy life expectancy at birth is 54 years for males and 52 years for females (WHO, 2004).

EPIDEMIOLOGY

Mumford et al (1996, 1997) used the Bradford Somatic Inventory to screen a general population sample in two rural areas. Further interviews were conducted using ICD-10 research diagnostic criteria. About 46% and 66% of women and 15% and 25% of men suffered from anxiety and depressive disorders. Emotional distress was associated with age, social disadvantage (in both genders), living in unitary households (in women) and lower education (in younger subjects). Ahmad et al (2001) used the Bradford Somatic Inventory (BSI) and Self-Reporting Questionnaire (SRQ) in another rural sample (n=664) and found that 72% of women and 44% of men were suffering from anxiety and depressive disorders. BSI and SRQ scores had negative correlations with socio-economic factors. In contrast, in an urban slum sample only 25% of women and 10% of men had depression and anxiety (Mumford et al, 2000). Emotional distress was associated with age (in both genders), less education (in younger women) and low financial status (in women) as in the previous study, but in the urban setting women living in joint households reported more distress than those living in unitary families. Husain et al (2000) conducted a two-phase survey of a rural general population sample, employing the Personal Health Questionnaire and the Self-Rating Questionnaire for screening (n=259) and the Psychiatric Assessment Schedule and Life Events and Difficulties Schedule for detailed assessment. The adjusted prevalence of depressive disorders was 44.4% (25.5% in males and 57.5% in females). Nearly all cases had lasted longer than 1 year. In comparison to non-cases, the affected individuals were less well educated, had more children and experienced more marked, independent chronic difficulties. Rabbani and Raja (2000) interviewed 260 mothers in an urban squatter settlement with the Aga Khan University Anxiety and Depression Scale (AKUADS) and found probable mental disorder in 28.8%. Psychiatric morbidity was associated with older age group, longer duration of marriage, interpersonal conflicts with husband or in-laws, husband's unemployment, lacking permanent source of income and lack of autonomy in making decisions. Khan and Reza (2000) conducted a 2-year analysis of reports related to suicide in a major newspaper in Pakistan (n= 306 suicides reported from 35 cities). Prevalence of suicide was associated with gender (male), age (under 30 years) and marital status (unmarried for men and married for women). More than half the subjects used organophosphate insecticides. Khalid (2001) analysed the pattern of suicide in a region based on newspaper reports (n=1230 news-items) and found a similar profile. Males adopted more violent methods (61.20%) while females more often ingested chemicals (35.20%). Khan and Reza (1998) reviewed records of 262 female and 185 male suicidal inpatients. Three quarters of the suicidal persons were under the age of 30 years. Compared to men, women were younger and more often married. Benzodiazepines were the commonest drugs used for self-poisoning among both genders, but women used organophosphorus insecticides more often than men. Javed et al (1992) used the Rutter Scale and found emotional and behavioural disorders in 9.3% of children. Yaqoob et al (1995) assessed a stratified sample (n=1303) of urban children from 2 to 24 months of age for serious mental retardation (DQ<50). The incidence per 1000 live births was 22 in the peri-urban slums, 9 in the urban slums, 7 in a village and 4 in an upper middle class group. Down syndrome was the most common cause of severe mental retardation (36%). Durkin et al (1998) conducted a two-stage survey of 2- to 9-year-old children obtained via cluster sampling (n=6365) using the Ten Questions screen for disabilities and structured medical and psychological assessments. Prevalence of mental retardation was 1.9% for serious retardation and 6.5% for mild retardation. Lack of maternal education, perinatal difficulties, neonatal infections, postnatal brain infections and injury and malnourishment were associated with mental retardation. Bashir et al (2002) identified mild mental retardation in 6.2% of children in a community sample of 6-10 year olds by a two stage method using the Ten Questions as a screening tool (n=649 families), psychometric tests (WISC-R and Griffiths) and clinical interviews. The distribution of mild mental retardation was uneven, the prevalence being 1.2% among children from the upper-middle class, 4.8% in the rural setting, 6.1% in urban slums and 10.5% in the poor peri-urban slums. Additional impairments were found in three-quarters of the children with mental retardation, of which speech impairment was the most common.

MENTAL HEALTH RESOURCES

Mental Health Policy A mental health policy is present. The policy was initially formulated in 1997.
The components of the policy are advocacy, promotion, prevention, treatment and rehabilitation. Intersectoral collaboration is also a component of the policy. The mental health policy envisages to train primary care providers, to establish resource centres at teaching hospitals and psychiatric and detoxification centres, to set up monitoring and evaluation systems and to prepare training and teaching modules. Special facilities would be established for mentally handicapped. Crisis intervention and counselling services for special groups of population would be started. Large mental hospitals would be reorganized and upgraded.

Substance Abuse Policy A substance abuse policy is present. The policy was initially formulated in 1997. It includes interventions for both reduction of supply and demand. The policy is being implemented by the Planning Commission of the Government of Pakistan.

National Mental Health Programme A national mental health programme is present. The programme was formulated in 1986. The national mental health programme is a part of the general health policy of the country and is aimed at incorporating mental health in primary care, removing stigma, caring for mental health and substance abuse across the country and maintaining principles of equity and justice in the provision of mental health and substance abuse services. It was fully implemented in 2001. It does not have a specific suicide reduction plan.

National Therapeutic Drug Policy/Essential List of Drugs A national therapeutic drug policy/essential list of drugs is present. It was formulated in 1997.

Mental Health Legislation In February 2001, a new mental health ordinance 2001 was enacted. The new ordinance puts emphasis on promotion of mental health and prevention of mental illness. It provides encouragement to community care and proposes the establishment of powerful federal mental health authority by the Government. It provides protection of the rights of the mentally ill and promotion of the mental health literacy. It also provides the guidelines for the development and establishment of new national standards for the care and the treatment of patients. Informed consent for treatment and investigations can be obtained from the patient or his/her relatives.
The latest legislation was enacted in 2001.

Mental Health Financing There are budget allocations for mental health.
The country spends 0.4% of the total health budget on mental health.
The primary sources of mental health financing in descending order are out of pocket expenditure by the patient or family, tax based, social insurance and private insurances.
The country has disability benefits for persons with mental disorders. Disability benefit is paid to individuals who are not able to work due to mental illness.

Mental Health Facilities Mental health is a part of primary health care system. Actual treatment of severe mental disorders is available at the primary level. The programme has initially started in Punjab, the largest province, in 1985 and is being extended to others over the years. There are many residential and day-care facilities, especially for people with learning disabilities providing social, vocational and educational activities.
Regular training of primary care professionals is carried out in the field of mental health. Training programmes have started in the province of Punjab as a part of in-service training for primary care personnel. Till now, approximately 2000 primary care physicians and 42 000 primary care workers have been trained. Community activists from NGOs (e.g. National Rural Support Programme (NRSP) are also being trained. Though there are training programmes for physicians, nurses and psychologists, there are no such facilities for social workers. Mental health training has been included in the programme of the District Health Development Centres. The Institute of Psychiatry Rawalpindi Medical College was the first WHO collaborating Centre-EMR and is acting as a resource centre at national and regional level for training, services information system and research. Multiple training manuals for primary health care physicians, paramedics, community workers and teachers have been developed. In an additional training package on counselling skills for health professionals, a package for rehabilitation of mentally ill has been developed. People from Sudan, Egypt, Iran, Afghanistan, Yemen, Tunisia, Morocco, Palestine and Nepal have been trained in the Institute of Psychiatry. The National Steering Committee evaluates the quality of care delivery on a regular basis.
There are community care facilities for patients with mental disorders. The community mental health programme was planned in a phased manner. The first phase included collection of data pertaining to demographics, knowledge, attitudes and beliefs about mental health and sensitization of the community towards mental health. The second phase involved training of personnel in mental health. The third phase involved stimulation of community activities through advocacy campaigns using religious leaders and developing a workable referral system. In the final phase, qualitative changes were incorporated in the services and steps were taken to improve the knowledge of the population about mental health. The programmes have been initiated in all provinces but have not been generalized to the whole population. More than 78 junior psychiatrists have been trained in community mental health to act as resource persons in the development of programmes in their areas.

Psychiatric Beds and Professionals

Total psychiatric beds per 10 000 population	0.24
Psychiatric beds in mental hospitals per 10 000 population	0.06
Psychiatric beds in general hospitals per 10 000 population	0.148
Psychiatric beds in other settings per 10 000 population	0.02
Number of psychiatrists per 100 000 population	0.2
Number of neurosurgeons per 100 000 population	0.2
Number of psychiatric nurses per 100 000 population	0.08
Number of neurologists per 100 000 population	0.14
Number of psychologists per 100 000 population	0.2
Number of social workers per 100 000 population	0.4

There are about 2000 other mental health personnel. There are four mental health hospitals in the country. All medical colleges have psychiatric units. Psychiatric units are also present in allied hospitals in both public and private sector. Some psychiatric care facilities are available at the tehsil level. Beds for the treatment of drug abusers are available at most hospital facilities (232 centres). Forensic beds are available at a few centres. There are two child psychiatrists in the country. Mental health professionals are concentrated in big urban centres. Most psychiatrists have private clinics.

Non-Governmental Organizations NGOs are involved with mental health in the country. They are mainly involved in advocacy, promotion, prevention, treatment and rehabilitation. Some of the NGOs like the Fountain House have done exemplary work in order to build the foundation of rehabilitation psychiatry in Pakistan. A concept of agrotherapy for the rural population has evolved. Recently, the organization the 'National Rural Support Programme' decided to include mental health among their activities.

Information Gathering System There is no mental health reporting system in the country. A mental health reporting system has been initiated in the National Health Management Information System.
The country has data collection system or epidemiological study on mental health. An information system for using in tertiary facilities has been developed at the WHO Collaborating Centre at Rawalpindi.
It has been agreed that the HMIS will collect information from primary care centres on depressive illness, substance abuse and epilepsy.

Programmes for Special Population The country has specific programmes for mental health for refugees and children. NGOs are involved in service provision and advocacy for the above groups. Afghan refugees are being provided services by international organizations. There are also facilities for women and victims of torture.
There are some facilities for children in the larger hospitals and regional hospitals, but the most parts of the country have no facilities for child and adolescent psychiatry. There are many residential and day care facilities for people with learning disabilities, especially in big cities. There is a school mental health programme and it aims to develop awareness of mental health among schoolchildren, schoolteachers and the community; to provide essential knowledge about mental health to teachers so that they are able to impart that to the students and are able to recognize and provide some counselling to the students for basic psychological problems. Its positive impact has been evaluated and published in international journals. Mental health issues have been incorporated in the teacher training programme at the national level. Text book boards have been approached for inclusion of mental health topics in school curricula.

Therapeutic Drugs The following therapeutic drugs are generally available at the primary health care level of the country: carbamazepine, phenobarbital, chlorpromazine, diazepam, haloperidol.
Imipramine is supplied instead of amitriptylline. Procyclidine is supplied.

Other Information Active community research has been conducted regarding mental health in the last years which have been published. The innovative community mental health programme included the faith healers. Manpower development at national and international level has been carried out. Print as well as electronic media have been utilized to spread mental health education. Collaboration with schools and NGOs like the National Rural Support Programme has been established. Public educational material on sleep disturbance, anxiety disorder, phobias, drug dependence, depression and psychosis is available. Pakistan is actively involved in developing guidelines for economic analysis of community mental health care programme in low income countries.

Additional Sources of Information

Ahmad, I., Saeed, K., Mubbashar, M. H., et al (2001) Minor psychiatric morbidity and socio-economic factors. Medical Forum Monthly, 12, 5-8.

Bashir, A., Yaqoob, M., Ferngren, H., et al (2002) Prevalence and associated impairments of mild mental retardation in six- to ten-year old children in Pakistan: a prospective study. Acta Paediatrica, 91, 833-837.

Durkin, M. S., Hasan, Z. M., Hasan, K. Z. (1998) Prevalence and correlates of mental retardation among children in Karachi, Pakistan. American Journal of Epidemiology, 147, 281-288.

EMRO Monograph on Mental Health (2000) Institute of Psychiatry and WHO Collaborating centre for Mental Health Research and Training.

Gadit A. A., Khalid N. (2002) State of mental health in Pakistan. Hamdard University.Karachi.

Gater, R., Rehman Ch.U. (2001) Mental health and service developments in the Rawalpindi district of Pakistan. Journal of College of Physicians & Surgeons Pakistan, 11, 210-214.

Husain, N., Creed, F., Tomenson, B. (2000) Depression and social stress in Pakistan. Psychological Medicine, 30, 395-402.

Javed, M. A., Kundi, M. Z., Khan, P. A. (1992) Emotional and behavioural problems among school children in Pakistan. Journal of the Pakistan Medical Association, 42, 181-183.

Karim, S., Saeed, K., Rana, M. H. (2004) Pakistan mental health profile. International Review of Psychiatry, 16, 83-92.

Khalid, N. (2001) Pattern of suicide: causes and methods employed. Medical Forum Monthly, 12, 27-29.

Khan, M. M., Reza, H. (1998) Gender differences in nonfatal suicidal behavior in Pakistan: significance of sociocultural factors. Suicide & Life-Threatening Behavior, 28, 62-68.

Khan, M. M., Reza, H. (2000) The pattern of suicide in Pakistan. Crisis: Journal of Crisis Intervention & Suicide, 21, 31-35.

Mental Health Programme Country Report of Pakistan for Regional Consultation on World Health Report (2000).

Ministry of Health (1998) Report of the Sub-Committee on Health and Substance Abuse. Planning Commission. Government of Pakistan.

Ministry of Health (1997) Mental Health Policy. Ministry of Health Government of Pakistan.

Mubbashar, M. H., Saeed, K. (2002) Developing models of balanced mental health care: the case of Pakistan. World Psychiatry, 1, 100-101.

Mubasshar, M. H. (2003) Development of mental health services in Pakistan. International Psychiatry, 1, 11-13.

Mumford, D. B. (1997) Stress and psychiatric disorder in rural Punjab – A Community survey. British Journal of Psychiatry, 170, 473-78.

Mumford, D. B., Minhas, F. A., Akhtar, I., et al (2000) Stress and psychiatric disorder in urban Rawalpindi. Community survey. British Journal of Psychiatry, 177, 557-562.

Mumford, D. B., Nazir, M., Jilani, F.-U.-M., et al (1996) Stress and psychiatric disorder in the Hindu Kush. A community survey of mountain villages in Chitral, Pakistan. British Journal of Psychiatry, 168, 299-307.

Mumford, D. B., Saeed, K., Ahmad, I., et al (1997) Stress and psychiatric disorder in rural Punjab: a community survey. British Journal of Psychiatry, 170, 473-478.

Rabbani, F., Raja, F. F. (2000) The minds of mothers: maternal mental health in an urban squatter settlement of Karachi. Journal of the Pakistan Medical Association, 50, 306-312.

Yaqoob, M., Bashir, A., Tareen, K., et al (1995) Severe mental retardation in 2 to 24-month-old children in Lahore, Pakistan: a prospective cohort study. Acta Paediatrica, 84, 267-272.

Yousaf, F. (1997) Psychiatry in Pakistan. International Journal of Social Psychiatry, 43, 298-302.

Palau

GENERAL INFORMATION

Palau is a country with an approximate area of 0.46 thousand sq. km. (UNO, 2001). The country consists of about 200 islands. Only eight of the islands are permanently inhabited. Its population is 0.02 million, and the sex ratio (men per hundred women) is 113 (UNO, 2004). The proportion of population above the age of 60 years is 7% (WHO, 2004). The literacy rate is 93% for men and 90% for women (UNESCO/MoH, 2004).

The country is a higher middle income group country (based on World Bank 2004 criteria). The proportion of health budget to GDP is 9.2%. The per capita total expenditure on health is 886 international $, and the per capita government expenditure on health is 816 international $ (WHO, 2004).

The main language(s) used in the country is (are) Palauan and English. The largest ethnic group(s) is (are) Palauan (two-thirds of the population), and the other ethnic group(s) are (is) Asian (Filipino and Chinese, one-fourth). The largest religious group(s) is (are) Roman Catholic (two-fifths), and the other religious group(s) are (is) Protestant (one-third) and Modekngei.

The life expectancy at birth is 66.4 years for males and 70.9 years for females (WHO, 2004). The healthy life expectancy at birth is 59 years for males and 60 years for females (WHO, 2004).

EPIDEMIOLOGY

Jensen and Polloi (1988) conducted a study to assess the prevalence of dementia in people aged 90 years and above (0.2% of total population). They used an adaptation of the Wechsler Logical Memory Test and the Global Deterioration Scale to assess cognitive functions. The prevalence of dementia as determined by clinical assessment was high (25% mild and 42% moderate/severe). This prevalence was lower (44%) as determined by the Global Deterioration Scale. Major physical and mental illnesses were infrequent. But most subjects had at least one chronic illness, the most common being arthritis. Most chewed betel nut but few used alcohol or smoked. Hammond et al (1983) assessed 35 Palauan schizophrenic patients. They found that the sample showed an unusual 4:1 male predominance, a proclivity towards violence and substantial affective symptomatology. Male patients extensively abused alcohol and cannabis. In a field study, Kauders et al (1982) confirmed these findings. Myles-Worsley et al (1999) ascertained 160 strictly defined cases of schizophrenia in a population of 13 750 adults, which yielded a lifetime prevalence of 2% (2.8% in males and 1.2% in females). This greater than 2:1 male-to-female risk ratio for schizophrenia was accompanied by an earlier mean age of onset for males (23.3 years) than for females (27.5 years). The 160 cases belonged to 59 separate families. Eleven families had 5-14 cases representing nearly half of the total cases. When a family was defined to include third-degree relatives, only 11 cases were non-familial. The majority of the ascertained cases could be linked together into extended pedigrees with complex multi-lineal inheritance patterns.

MENTAL HEALTH RESOURCES

Mental Health Policy A mental health policy is absent.
The components of the policy are advocacy, promotion, prevention, treatment and rehabilitation. The executive summary of the Mental Health Plan 2005 outlines programmes for adults, children and technical assistance needs.

Substance Abuse Policy A substance abuse policy is absent.

National Mental Health Programme A national mental health programme is present. The programme was formulated in 1973.

National Therapeutic Drug Policy/Essential List of Drugs A national therapeutic drug policy/essential list of drugs is absent.

Mental Health Legislation There are different legislations in the field of mental health of which RPL 349 amends a previous legislation by adding provisions for non-judicial, involuntary 72-hour detention period for purposes of evaluation, diagnosis and treatment of mental illness and for other purposes.
The latest legislation was enacted in 1991.

Mental Health Financing There are no budget allocations for mental health.
The country spends 2% of the total health budget on mental health.
The primary source of mental health financing is grants.
The country has disability benefits for persons with mental disorders. There is a law now, RPPL 6-25, subsection 5-15 which is entitled 'Palau Severely Disabled Assistance Fund'. It makes small stipends available to persons with disability as set forth in the regulations. Mental illness, depending on severity, is included.

Mental Health Facilities Mental health is a part of primary health care system. Actual treatment of severe mental disorders is available at the primary level.
Regular training of primary care professionals is not carried out in the field of mental health. The Behavioural Health Division provides some training, but a regular system has not evolved. Limited training is also carried out in the area of substance abuse.
There are community care facilities for patients with mental disorders.

Psychiatric Beds and Professionals

Total psychiatric beds per 10 000 population	4.7
Psychiatric beds in mental hospitals per 10 000 population	0
Psychiatric beds in general hospitals per 10 000 population	4.7
Psychiatric beds in other settings per 10 000 population	0
Number of psychiatrists per 100 000 population	5
Number of neurosurgeons per 100 000 population	0
Number of psychiatric nurses per 100 000 population	10
Number of neurologists per 100 000 population	0
Number of psychologists per 100 000 population	0
Number of social workers per 100 000 population	10

Non-Governmental Organizations NGOs are involved with mental health in the country. They are mainly involved in advocacy. The Palau Mental Health Council is involved in monitoring, reviewing and evaluating the allocation and adequacy of services in Palau, besides advocacy, which is its main activity.

Information Gathering System There is mental health reporting system in the country. There are monthly reports to the Ministry. The country has data collection system or epidemiological study on mental health. Data are compiled every month.
Details about patients and service utilization are available from the Behavioural Health Division Report.

Programmes for Special Population Free medicines and counselling are provided to prisoners. A programme for substance abuse exists.

Therapeutic Drugs The following therapeutic drugs are generally available at the primary health care level of the country: carbamazepine, phenobarbital, phenytoin sodium, sodium valproate, amitriptyline, chlorpromazine, diazepam, fluphenazine, haloperidol, lithium.
A national therapeutic drug policy/essential list of drugs is being developed, and in the meantime a formulary is being utilized.

N–R

Other Information

Additional Sources of Information

Government document (2005) Mental Health Plan. Executive Summary.

Hammond, K. W., Kauders, F. R., MacMurray, J. P. (1983) Schizophrenia in Palau: a descriptive study. International Journal of Social Psychiatry, 29, 161-170.

Jensen, G. D., Polloi, A. H. (1998) The very old of Palau: health and mental state. Age & Ageing, 17, 220-226.

Kauders, F. R., MacMurray, J. P., Hammond, K. W. (1982) Male predominance among Palauan schizophrenics. International Journal of Social Psychiatry, 28, 97-102.

Myles-Worsley, M., Coon, H., Tiobech, J., et al (1999) Genetic epidemiological study of schizophrenia in Palau, Micronesia: prevalence and familiality. American Journal of Medical Genetics, 88, 4-10.

Panama

GENERAL INFORMATION

Panama is a country with an approximate area of 76 thousand sq. km. (UNO, 2001). Its population is 3.178 million, and the sex ratio (men per hundred women) is 102 (UNO, 2004). The proportion of population under the age of 15 years is 31% (UNO, 2004), and the proportion of population above the age of 60 years is 8% (WHO, 2004). The literacy rate is 92.9% for men and 91.7% for women (UNESCO/MoH, 2004).

The country is a higher middle income group country (based on World Bank 2004 criteria). The proportion of health budget to GDP is 7%. The per capita total expenditure on health is 458 international $, and the per capita government expenditure on health is 316 international $ (WHO, 2004).

The main language(s) used in the country is (are) Spanish. The largest ethnic group(s) is (are) Mestizo (seven-tenths), and the other ethnic group(s) are (is) Amerindian. The largest religious group(s) is (are) Roman Catholic (five-sixths).

The life expectancy at birth is 72.8 years for males and 78.2 years for females (WHO, 2004). The healthy life expectancy at birth is 64 years for males and 68 years for females (WHO, 2004).

EPIDEMIOLOGY

In 1996, Panama conducted a National Youth Survey on Alcohol and Drug Use on students aged 12-18 years (n= 6477). More males, older students and students in higher grades had used licit and illicit drugs, but male-female differences were small. Public-private school differences and urban-rural trends varied depending on the drug (Gonzales et al, 1999). Delva et al (1999, 2000) estimated clustering of substance use by the Alternating Logistic Regression method. Modest clustering was observed at the school level for tobacco smoking, alcohol consumption, use of inhalants and other drug use. These findings suggested that chances of drug use among school-attending youths increased when another youth in the same school used drugs. They also found opportunities to use drugs and actual drug use to be greater at higher grade levels. Also, the probability of making a transition to use, given an opportunity, was more likely among upper-grade students. Males were more likely to have an opportunity to use marijuana, crack-cocaine and other forms of cocaine, but not more likely than females to make a transition into drug use once an opportunity had occurred to try each drug.

MENTAL HEALTH RESOURCES

Mental Health Policy A mental health policy is present. The policy was initially formulated in 2000.
The components of the policy are advocacy, promotion, prevention, treatment and rehabilitation. The policy was formulated through a process that involved the participation of multiple stakeholder groups including health professionals, other governmental professionals and NGOs of patients and families. Between 50 to 75% of its original content has been implemented.

Substance Abuse Policy A substance abuse policy is present. The policy was initially formulated in 1996. It was revised in 2000. There is a specific budget for its implementation and it has been implemented to the extent of 75 to 90%.

National Mental Health Programme A national mental health programme is present. The programme was formulated in 1972. It was revised in 1996. There is a specific budget for its implementation, but it has been implemented only to the extent of 10 to 25% by local, regional and national authorities. Its main components are strategy of services reform, promotion and prevention, integration of mental health services in primary care and development of specialized services.

National Therapeutic Drug Policy/Essential List of Drugs A national therapeutic drug policy/essential list of drugs is present. It was formulated in 1993.

Mental Health Legislation The law establishing provisions about hospital and community mental health services and promotion of the rights of persons with mental disorders of 1997 was presented to the Legislative Assembly, but is yet to be approved. Details about any previous legislation are not known.
Details about the year of enactment of the mental health legislation are not available.

Mental Health Financing There are no budget allocations for mental health.
Details about expenditure on mental health are not available.
The primary sources of mental health financing in descending order are tax based, social insurance, out of pocket expenditure by the patient or family.
The country has disability benefits for persons with mental disorders. A psychiatrist works at the commission for handicapped persons of the Social Security to look after the disabilities of mentally ill patients.

Mental Health Facilities Mental health is a part of primary health care system. Actual treatment of severe mental disorders is available at the primary level. 50-75% of the population is covered by this kind of service. Mental health care is provided by primary health care doctors, nurses and psychiatrists. A referral system is in place.
Regular training of primary care professionals is not carried out in the field of mental health. Primary care nurses have been trained for management of mental disorders in a programme supported by PAHO/WHO. In an evaluation it was shown that the educational programme had a positive impact on their clinical practice at least in the short term.

There are community care facilities for patients with mental disorders. Some facilities for community care are being developed, e.g. day care centres and hospitals and health promotion centres. The community care system for the mentally ill includes outpatient clinics comprises preventive/promotion interventions, home interventions, family interventions (all the above are available for about half of the intended population), residential facilities, vocational training and employment programmes (these are available for less than 25% of the intended population). Multiple professional disciplines are involved but many teams are understaffed.

Psychiatric Beds and Professionals

Total psychiatric beds per 10 000 population	2.55
Psychiatric beds in mental hospitals per 10 000 population	1.56
Psychiatric beds in general hospitals per 10 000 population	0.99
Psychiatric beds in other settings per 10 000 population	
Number of psychiatrists per 100 000 population	3.7
Number of neurosurgeons per 100 000 population	0.6
Number of psychiatric nurses per 100 000 population	5
Number of neurologists per 100 000 population	0.35
Number of psychologists per 100 000 population	2.6
Number of social workers per 100 000 population	0.07

The figures quoted are only for those working in the Government sector and with the Social Security. 70% of these beds are occupied by long stay patients.

Non-Governmental Organizations NGOs are involved with mental health in the country. They are mainly involved in advocacy, promotion, prevention, treatment and rehabilitation. These organizations participate in mental health activities related to women, children and domestic violence.

Information Gathering System There is no mental health reporting system in the country.
The country has data collection system or epidemiological study on mental health. The 'Departamento de Análisis y Tendencias de Salud' is in charge of the data collection system for mental disorders. Service data collection system is conducted for part of the mental health system (emergencies, regional hospital discharges at national level). In 2001, considering mental health related outpatient consultations (specialized and general) the 3 most frequent psychiatric diagnosis, according to ICD-10 criteria, were anxiety disorders, affective disorders (mainly depression) and mental and behaviour disorders associated with drug use, including alcohol. Patient discharge from both psychiatric and general hospitals in 2000 points out as the most frequent diagnoses bipolar disorders, schizophrenia and drug use associated disorders.

Programmes for Special Population The country has specific programmes for mental health for indigenous population, elderly and children. There is a health section of indigenous people who are making efforts to facilitate inclusion of services for indigenous people.
In addition, there are programmes for women, abused children and victims of domestic violence. A national initiative named 'Know Depression and Face it' was launched in Collaboration with PAHO.

Therapeutic Drugs The following therapeutic drugs are generally available at the primary health care level of the country: carbamazepine, phenobarbital, phenytoin sodium, sodium valproate, amitriptyline, chlorpromazine, diazepam, fluphenazine, haloperidol, lithium, biperiden, carbidopa, levodopa.
The therapeutic drug policy was revised in 2001. The purchasing of general and psychiatric medicines is the responsibility of the Ministry of Health.

Other Information

Additional Sources of Information

Delva, J., Bobashev, G., Gonzalez, G., et al (2000) Clusters of drug involvement in Panama: results from Panama's 1996 National Youth Survey. Drug & Alcohol Dependence, 60, 251-257.

Delva, J., Van Etten, M. L., Gonzalez, G. B., et al (1999) First opportunities to try drugs and the transition to first drug use: evidence from a national school survey in Panama. Substance Use & Misuse, 34, 1451-1467.

Gonzalez, G. B., Cedeno, M. A., Penna, M., et al (1999) Estimated occurrence of tobacco, alcohol, and other drug use among 12- to 18-year-old students in Panama: results of Panama's 1996 National Youth Survey on Alcohol and Drug Use. Pan American Journal of Public Health, 5, 9-16.

Government document (1996) Comision Nacional para el estudio y la prevencion de los delitos relacionados con Droga.

Ministerio de Salud Caja de Seguro Social (1996) Programa nacional de salud mental.

Ministerio de Salud (1996) Plan Nacional de salud mental.

Ministerio de Salud (1993) Formulario nacional de medicamentos esenciales.

Moreno, P., Saravanan, Y., Levav, I., et al. (2003) Evaluation of the PAHO/WHO training program on the detection and treatment of depression for primary care nurses in Panama. Acta Psychiatrica Scandinavica, 108, 61-65.

Papua New Guinea

GENERAL INFORMATION

Papua New Guinea is a country with an approximate area of 463 thousand sq. km. (UNO, 2001). The country consists of the eastern half of the island of New Guinea, and many outlying islands. Its population is 5.836 million, and the sex ratio (men per hundred women) is 106 (UNO, 2004). The proportion of population under the age of 15 years is 41% (UNO, 2004), and the proportion of population above the age of 60 years is 4% (WHO, 2004). The literacy rate is 70.6% for men and 56.8% for women (UNESCO/MoH, 2004).

The country is a low income group country (based on World Bank 2004 criteria). The proportion of health budget to GDP is 4.4%. The per capita total expenditure on health is 144 international $, and the per capita government expenditure on health is 128 international $ (WHO, 2004).

The main language(s) used in the country is (are) English, Tok Pisin and Hiri Motu. The largest ethnic group(s) is (are) Papuan, and the other ethnic group(s) are (is) Melanesian, Micronesian and Polynesian. The largest religious group(s) is (are) Christian (more than half).

The life expectancy at birth is 58.4 years for males and 61.5 years for females (WHO, 2004). The healthy life expectancy at birth is 51 years for males and 52 years for females (WHO, 2004).

EPIDEMIOLOGY

Johnson (1990) administered questionnaires to a cross-section of university students and office workers (n=50). The results showed that both the student and clerical groups were moderately involved in substance abuse. The use of alcohol and cannabis was common. In another study on university students (n=90), Johnson (1998) found that alcohol, tobacco and other drugs were being used frequently. Johnson (1994) reviewed hospital data and noted a rise in alcohol, cannabis and diazepam related health problems, especially among males. Attah Johnson and Mostaghimi (1995) evaluated 132 consecutive adult dermatology outpatients using the Harding Self-Rating Questionnaire (cut-off point of 7) and clinical interview. The common psychiatric diagnoses for the women patients were: anxiety neurosis 16.9% and neurotic depression 56.9%, and for men anxiety neurosis 22.4% and neurotic depression 44.8%. Johnson (1997) found that schizophrenia (49%) was the commonest diagnosis among psychiatric inpatients. Pal (1997) interviewed 64 mentally ill offenders who had committed violent crimes and found schizophrenia in 42.2%, epilepsy in 10.9%, alcohol and cannabis abuse in 32.8% of the subjects and culture-bound syndromes like amok and spirit possession in a few cases. Canetto and Lester (1995) reported that suicide mortality was highest among young adult married females in Papua New Guinea and older single white adult males in the United States. They felt that these differences are due to cultural sanctions in relation to behaviour.

MENTAL HEALTH RESOURCES

Mental Health Policy A mental health policy is present. Details about the year of formulation are not available.
The components of the policy are advocacy, promotion, prevention, treatment and rehabilitation.

Substance Abuse Policy A substance abuse policy is absent.

National Mental Health Programme A national mental health programme is present. The programme was formulated in 1962. There is also a Mental Health and Social Change Program 2001-2010 which has the following priorities: review and update of the Public Health Act; increase staffing and training of psychiatric nurses; establish psychiatric units at all public hospitals; establish four regional referral and supervising units at level 2 hospitals; upgrade Laloki Mental Hospital; improve intersectoral collaboration in forensic psychiatry, domestic violence against women and the control and prevention of substance abuse; improve community knowledge and skills to support community mental health programmes; expand community mental health programmes and improve monitoring and reporting.

National Therapeutic Drug Policy/Essential List of Drugs A national therapeutic drug policy/essential list of drugs is present. It was formulated in 1950.

Mental Health Legislation There is a Public Health Act with certain sections on mental health.
The latest legislation was enacted in 1985.

Mental Health Financing There are budget allocations for mental health.
The country spends 0.7% of the total health budget on mental health.
The primary source of mental health financing is tax based.
The country does not have disability benefits for persons with mental disorders. Mentally ill patients are cared for by their relatives with no support from the Government.

Mental Health Facilities Mental health is not a part of primary health care system. Actual treatment of severe mental disorders is available at the primary level.
Regular training of primary care professionals is carried out in the field of mental health. In seven provinces psychiatric services are provided by psychiatric nurses and in the remaining nine provinces by general physicians or general health workers. Formal training

conducted in 1999 and 2000 with the support of WHO has produced a minimum of one physician in each hospital (total 19) with sufficient skills to handle mental health problems. Outcome evaluation was not done. Training of primary care professionals such as Health Extension Officers is part of their curriculum. Formal training of mental health in primary health care for other workers in districts is also in place.
There are no community care facilities for patients with mental disorders. Community care is provided for known patients on medications prescribed by psychiatrist. Upon discharge of patients from the psychiatric hospital to another province, a member of the staff accompanies the patient to help reintegrate them into their local community and would spend time with the local health worker or psychiatric nurse in an educative role. Discharged patients are followed up at the local centre with advice from staff at the psychiatric hospital. There is a psychosocial rehabilitation centre for about 15 patients. It offers residential and day care facilities. It provides a variety of occupational therapy and social activities for former patients and support groups for families of mentally ill, and the centre carries out public education activities. Training for the staff was provided through the support of WHO. NGOs provide operational support.

Psychiatric Beds and Professionals

Total psychiatric beds per 10 000 population	0.24
Psychiatric beds in mental hospitals per 10 000 population	0.17
Psychiatric beds in general hospitals per 10 000 population	0.07
Psychiatric beds in other settings per 10 000 population	0
Number of psychiatrists per 100 000 population	0.09
Number of neurosurgeons per 100 000 population	0
Number of psychiatric nurses per 100 000 population	1.2
Number of neurologists per 100 000 population	0
Number of psychologists per 100 000 population	0
Number of social workers per 100 000 population	0.04

There is a lack of trained staff. Psychiatric facilities are limited. Since 1999, all hospitals including the 4 regional and 9 provincial hospitals have got psychiatric services. The only psychiatric hospital has 60 beds and some general hospitals have few (up to 10) mental health beds. The country has historically depended on overseas training, principally from Australia, for its professional staff. However, those people continue to work in mental health in the country after overseas training in small (about one-third). A one-year post-basic training course for nurses is now available in the country. A post-graduate training in psychiatry was started and 4 psychiatrists have graduated in 2002. All psychiatrists, except one, are in the capital city.

N–R

Non-Governmental Organizations NGOs are involved with mental health in the country. They are mainly involved in advocacy, promotion, prevention, treatment and rehabilitation. The Center for Domestic Violence provides shelter for women victims and their children.

Information Gathering System There is no mental health reporting system in the country. National Department of Health's forms on reporting have no provision for mental health.
The country has no data collection system or epidemiological study on mental health.

Programmes for Special Population There are services for prisoners and also for other forensic services.
Special programmes for armed forces/ Defence Force of Papau New Guinea are ongoing (2001). Rehabilitation programmes for chronic mental illness are in place. Programmes for school children are ongoing. The correctional institution has an infirmary for psychiatric care of mild mental illnesses in inmates. Those needing more intensive care are transferred to the psychiatric hospital. The Papua New Guinea Narcotics Bureau is engaged in a public awareness campaign, training of administrators and counselling.

Therapeutic Drugs The following therapeutic drugs are generally available at the primary health care level of the country: carbamazepine, phenytoin sodium, sodium valproate, amitriptyline, chlorpromazine, diazepam, haloperidol.
All the drugs are available in primary health care.

Other Information Promoting materials such as posters, video, community awareness tapes are available; street awareness programmes, newspaper articles, radio talk shows are some of the arrays of success funded by the National Department of Health. The country has a radio telephone network, HEALTH NET, which was supplied by the Australian Agency for International Development. It is used to communicate between hospitals and clinics to obtain advice and emergency aid and to disseminate information. It had been underutilized for mental health services but has lately been used to provide training and supervision to the remote population.

Additional Sources of Information

Attah Johnson, F. Y., Mostaghimi, H. (1995) Co-morbidity between dermatologic diseases and psychiatric disorders in Papua New Guinea. International Journal of Dermatology, 34, 244-248.

Canetto, S. S., Lester, D. (1995) Gender and the primary prevention of suicide mortality. Suicide & Life-Threatening Behavior, 25, 58-69.

Johnson, F. Y. (1990) An epidemiological survey of alcohol and drug abuse in the national capital district of Papua New Guinea. Medicine & Law, 9, 797-830.

Johnson, F. Y. (1994) Clinical observations on substance abuse related health problems at the Port Moresby General Hospital, National Capital District, Papua New Guinea. Medicine & Law, 13, 251-262.

Johnson, F.Y. (1997) Ward Six Psychiatric Unit at the Port Moresby General Hospital: a historical review and admission statistics from 1980 to 1989. Papua New Guinea Medical Journal, 40, 79-88.

Johnson, F. Y. (1998) A study of substance abuse on two campuses of University of Papua New Guinea. Medicine & Law, 17, 229-241.

Noble, F. (1997) Long-term psychiatric care in Papua New Guinea. Psychiatric Bulletin, 21, 113-116.

Pal, S. (1997) Mental disorders in abnormal offenders in Papua New Guinea. Medicine & Law, 16, 87-95.

Paraguay

GENERAL INFORMATION

Paraguay is a country with an approximate area of 407 thousand sq. km. (UNO, 2001). Its population is 6.018 million, and the sex ratio (men per hundred women) is 102 (UNO, 2004). The proportion of population under the age of 15 years is 38% (UNO, 2004), and the proportion of population above the age of 60 years is 6% (WHO, 2004). The literacy rate is 94% for men and 91.5% for women (UNESCO/MoH, 2004).

The country is a lower middle income group country (based on World Bank 2004 criteria). The proportion of health budget to GDP is 8%. The per capita total expenditure on health is 332 international $, and the per capita government expenditure on health is 127 international $ (WHO, 2004).

The main language(s) used in the country is (are) Guarani. The largest ethnic group(s) is (are) Mestizo (almost 95%). The largest religious group(s) is (are) Roman Catholic (nine-tenths).

The life expectancy at birth is 68.7 years for males and 74.7 years for females (WHO, 2004). The healthy life expectancy at birth is 60 years for males and 64 years for females (WHO, 2004).

EPIDEMIOLOGY

There is a paucity of epidemiological data on mental illnesses in Paraguay in internationally accessible literature. Miguez et al (1992) administered questionnaires in Spanish and Guarani with acceptable reliability and validity to 2504 individuals selected through a stratified sampling technique. Use of legal substances such as alcohol, tobacco and psychotropic drugs was common. Among illicit substances, inhalants and marijuana use was frequent. Da Costa e Silva and Koifman (1998) analysed the results from prevalence surveys of smoking in 14 Latin American countries and observed that smoking prevalence among men varied from 24.1% (Paraguay) to 66.3% (Dominican Republic) and among women from 5.5% (Paraguay) to 26.6% (Uruguay). By applying point prevalence data to the stage model of the tobacco epidemic in developed countries they concluded that most of Latin American countries were in stage 2, i.e. with a clearly rising prevalence among men, a prevalence for women that is beginning to increase, and mortality attributable to smoking among men still not reflecting peak prevalence. However, Paraguay appeared to be still emerging from stage 1, i.e. with low prevalence rates among men, too. Pages et al (1981) conducted an ethnographic study on mental health issues of the Chiriguanos, a tribe native to Paraguay that has migrated to Bolivia. It is described under the relevant section in Bolivia.

MENTAL HEALTH RESOURCES

Mental Health Policy A mental health policy is present. The policy was initially formulated in 2002.

The components of the policy are advocacy, promotion, prevention, treatment and rehabilitation. It was developed through consultations between mental health professionals, NGOs and consumers. It is in the very beginning of its implementation and there is no regular budget for it.

Substance Abuse Policy A substance abuse policy is absent.

National Mental Health Programme A national mental health programme is present. The programme was formulated in 2002. It is to be implemented by national authorities, but this has not been done yet. There is no specific budget for its implementation. Its main components are strategy of services reform, promotion and prevention, mental health services at primary health care and specialized services.

National Therapeutic Drug Policy/Essential List of Drugs A national therapeutic drug policy/essential list of drugs is present. It was formulated in 2002.

Mental Health Legislation There are no regular funds for its implementation. There is a new code under consideration of the legislature that includes promotion and prevention, human rights, regulation of mental health services, regulation of involuntary treatment, regulation of mental health services, admission and discharge procedures, advocacy and housing. There is la law on substance abuse from 1989.

The latest legislation was enacted in 1980.

Mental Health Financing There are budget allocations for mental health.

The country spends 0.05% of the total health budget on mental health.

Details about sources of financing are not available.

Approximately seven-eighths of the budget is spent on the psychiatric hospital and one-eighth on other services.

The country has disability benefits for persons with mental disorders. According to the law, mental impairment is considered a disability for getting public disability benefits. However, for socio-economical reasons, less than 10% of the eligible persons actually receive the benefits. Psychosis, depression and drug dependence are considered for disability benefits. The evaluation procedure includes several interviews and psycho-diagnostic tests.

Mental Health Facilities Mental health is a part of primary health care system. Actual treatment of severe mental disorders is available at the primary level. Less than 25 % of the population is covered by this kind of service. Mental health care is provided by Primary Health Care doctors and psychiatrists.
Regular training of primary care professionals is not carried out in the field of mental health. The first pilot project was conducted recently.
There are no community care facilities for patients with mental disorders. A pilot project on community care is under way in one health region (number 13).

Psychiatric Beds and Professionals

Total psychiatric beds per 10 000 population	0.731
Psychiatric beds in mental hospitals per 10 000 population	0.614
Psychiatric beds in general hospitals per 10 000 population	0.097
Psychiatric beds in other settings per 10 000 population	
Number of psychiatrists per 100 000 population	1.8
Number of neurosurgeons per 100 000 population	0.2
Number of psychiatric nurses per 100 000 population	0.08
Number of neurologists per 100 000 population	0.3
Number of psychologists per 100 000 population	
Number of social workers per 100 000 population	

About 6 general nurses per 100 000 population are working in the mental health area. On a regular basis, the psychiatric hospitals have approximately 450 inpatients in spite of having 340 beds. About half the beds are occupied by patients staying more than 6 months in hospital.

Non-Governmental Organizations NGOs are involved with mental health in the country. They are mainly involved in promotion and prevention. These organizations participate in mental health activities related to women, children, consumers and domestic violence. Associations of consumers and their families are being organized. There is an organization for the rights of the mentally ill and others for substance users' treatment.

Information Gathering System There is no mental health reporting system in the country.
The country has data collection system or epidemiological study on mental health. The Technical Support for Mental Health is in charge of the data collection system for mental disorders.

Programmes for Special Population The country has specific programmes for mental health for minorities, indigenous population, elderly and children.
There are mental health programmes being run in association with the Ministry of Education, universities and NGOs. At international level, collaborative projects with Argentina (Rio Negro province), Brazil (Ministry of Health), Cuba, Italy (Modena) and PAHO/WHO are being conducted.

Therapeutic Drugs The following therapeutic drugs are generally available at the primary health care level of the country: haloperidol.
There is no essential drug list.

Other Information

Additional Sources of Information

da Costa e Silva, V.L., Koifman, S. (1998) Smoking in Latin America: a major public health problem. Cadernos de Saude Publica, 14 Suppl 3, 99-108.

Miguez, H. A., Pecci, M. C., Carrizosa, A., Jr. et al (1992) Epidemiology of alcohol and drug abuse in Paraguay. Acta Psiquiatrica y Psicologica de America Latina, 38, 19-29.

Pages, Larraya F., Servy, E., Marangunich, L., et al (1981) Migration and mental disorders in the Chiraguano civilization. Acta Psiquiatrica y Psicologica de America Latina, 27, 15-27.

Peru

GENERAL INFORMATION

Peru is a country with an approximate area of 1285 thousand sq. km. (UNO, 2001). Its population is 27.567 million, and the sex ratio (men per hundred women) is 101 (UNO, 2004). The proportion of population under the age of 15 years is 33% (UNO, 2004), and the proportion of population above the age of 60 years is 7% (WHO, 2004). The literacy rate is 91.3% for men and 80.3% for women (UNESCO/MoH, 2004).

The country is a lower middle income group country (based on World Bank 2004 criteria). The proportion of health budget to GDP is 4.7%. The per capita total expenditure on health is 231 international $, and the per capita government expenditure on health is 127 international $ (WHO, 2004).

The main language(s) used in the country is (are) Spanish and Quéchua. The largest ethnic group(s) is (are) Indian and Mestizo. The largest religious group(s) is (are) Roman Catholic (nine-tenths).

The life expectancy at birth is 67.5 years for males and 72 years for females (WHO, 2004). The healthy life expectancy at birth is 60 years for males and 62 years for females (WHO, 2004).

EPIDEMIOLOGY

In an urban community survey, the lifetime prevalence of selected psychiatric disorders according to DSM-III criteria, utilizing the Spanish version of the Diagnostic Interview Schedule (DIS) were: major depressive episode (9.7%), alcohol abuse and dependence (18.6%) and phobia (8.5%) (Hayashi et al, 1985). A later survey using the Spanish version (5.0) of the Mini International Diagnostic Interview (MINI) showed that 37.3% of the urban adult population met the ICD-10 criteria for at least one mental disorder during their lifetime. The most frequent were anxiety disorders (25.3 %) and depressive disorders (19.0%). The lifetime prevalence of depressive episode was 18.2%, generalized anxiety disorder was 9.9%, social phobia was 7.9% and PTSD was 6.0%. The one-year prevalence for alcohol abuse and dependence was 5.3 % (Estudio Epidemiológico Metropolitano en Salud Mental, 2002). Yamamoto et al (1993) studied the prevalence of alcohol use in 815 subjects from the community using a Spanish version of Diagnostic Interview Schedule and DSM-III criteria. The prevalence of alcohol abuse or dependence was higher among the men (34.8%) than among the women (2.5%), but the onset for women was earlier. Alcoholism was strongly associated with antisocial personality disorder and with drug abuse or dependence. The prevalence of alcoholism for the Peruvian men was higher than that for men in the USA, though the women had one of the lowest prevalences reported in literature. Montoya and Chilcoat (1996) estimated that the lifetime prevalence of cocaine or coca paste use was between 0.8%-3% in 5 countries (Bolivia, Colombia, Ecuador, Peru and Venezuela) in a population sample of more than 24 000 subjects. Coca paste or cocaine use was associated with age (middle-age), socioeconomic category (middle-class), gender (males), education (finished high school), income (high) and locality (urban). The most frequent age of first use was 15 to 24 years. Flores Agreda (1986) reported on the prevalence and incidence of drug use in Bolivia, Colombia and Peru. A survey in Peru showed that 37% of secondary school students used drugs and 27% used basic cocaine paste as their first drug. The abuse of basic cocaine paste was spread evenly across urban social classes. The increased drug use ran parallel to an increase in illegal cocaine cultivation in these countries. Gossop et al (1994) evaluated 68 drug users receiving treatment for cocaine problems at treatment centres in Bolivia and Peru. Levels of cocaine consumption were extremely high with a mean level of 16.4 grams. The majority of the users (87%) smoked cocaine in the form of pasta, pitillo or basuco. Severity-of-dependence scale scores were high. Vega-Dienstmaier et al (1999) assessed 321 women in the first postpartum year, 41 nulliparous women and 63 women who were more than 1 year postpartum. The prevalence of major depression in the first postpartum year (5.9%) was significantly lower than its prevalence in women who were more than 1 year postpartum. Depression was higher still in women who were more than 2 years postpartum. The risk factors associated with postpartum depression were obsessive-compulsive disorder, premenstrual dysphoric disorder, previous major depression, maternity blues, young age and lower education level. De Michelena (1993) examined 318 children and teenagers with Down syndrome in specialized educational institutions and a matched (date of birth, sex and maternal age) group of 1196 control individuals that was selected from the birth records of 2 general hospitals of the city. The means of paternal age in the 2 groups were compared, first globally and then by groups of maternal age (<21 years, 21-29 years, 30-34 years, 35-39 years and >39 years). The results obtained in this study gave no evidence that paternal age can be considered a risk factor for the conception of a child with Down syndrome.

MENTAL HEALTH RESOURCES

Mental Health Policy A mental health policy is present. The policy was initially formulated in 1991.

The components of the policy are advocacy, promotion, prevention, treatment and rehabilitation. It was revised in 2001 by civil servants, mental health professionals and NGOs. There are regular funds for its implementation and between 25 to 50% of its original content have been put into practice. At present, some provisions are being developed within the national mental health policy, with the following objectives: to favour development and dissemination of the global health approach by promoting healthy styles and environments and taking care of mental health as a component which is inherent and necessary to the general state of complete health; to ensure access, coverage and quality of intersectoral health services and programmes by developing specific proposals for prevention, care and rehabilitation in accordance with the cultural reality and including equity among all; to improve quality of interventions by revising, evaluating and creating efficient patterns, which include the results of alternative practice and the psychosocial resources of the community; to improve the existing infrastructure in order to increase mental health coverage and contribute to the quality of care; to improve the efficiency of mental health programmes and services by strengthening the process of planning, monitoring and evaluation.

Substance Abuse Policy A substance abuse policy is present. The policy was initially formulated in 1996. It was revised in 2000. There are regular funds for its implementation and between 50 to 75% of its original content has been put into practice. The most recent substance abuse policies are 'Plan Nacional de Prevención y Control de Drogas (1994-2000)', 'Ley de lucha contra el narcotráfico (Decreto Legislativo 824 de 1996)', 'Programa Nacional de Prevención y Rehabilitación (1998-2002)' and 'Estrategia Nacional (de lucha) contra las drogas (2002-2007)'.

National Mental Health Programme A national mental health programme is present. The programme was formulated in 1991. It was revised in 2001. There are no regular funds for its implementation; it has been implemented to the extent of 25 to 50% by local and regional authorities. Its main components are integration of mental health services in primary care and development of specialized services.

National Therapeutic Drug Policy/Essential List of Drugs A national therapeutic drug policy/essential list of drugs is present. It was formulated in 2000.

Mental Health Legislation There is a law (law 27306), which modifies the protection law against domestic violence and this came into force in 2000. It was revised in 2001. This law does not address legal provisions for the protection of the basic human and civil rights of people with mental disorders. There is no comprehensive mental health legislation but the General Health Law, in its article 11, refers to mental health.
The latest legislation was enacted in 2001.

Mental Health Financing There are budget allocations for mental health.
The country spends 2% of the total health budget on mental health.
The primary source of mental health financing is tax based.
The Ministry of Health provides health care for those without any other type of coverage, 73.8% of general population; ESSALUD provides health care for workers with health insurance, covering 21.8% of the general population and the rest is covered by private health services (3.7 %), army health services (1.9 %) and others (3.8 %) (http://corporativo.bibliomed.com.br). Psychiatric hospitals receive 85% of the budget, outpatient care 10%, community care 2% and others 3%.
The country has disability benefits for persons with mental disorders. Public disability benefits are restricted only for those covered by social security (a minority of the population). Less than 10% of the population is entitled for getting benefits.

Mental Health Facilities Mental health is a part of primary health care system. Actual treatment of severe mental disorders is not available at the primary level. Less than 25 % of the population is covered by this kind of service. Mental health care is provided by primary health care physicians. After the initial consultation the patient is referred to a specialized centre.
Regular training of primary care professionals is not carried out in the field of mental health.
There are community care facilities for patients with mental disorders. It does not work as a system. It is intended to strengthen this intervention modality through psychosocial clubs.

Psychiatric Beds and Professionals

Total psychiatric beds per 10 000 population	0.47
Psychiatric beds in mental hospitals per 10 000 population	
Psychiatric beds in general hospitals per 10 000 population	
Psychiatric beds in other settings per 10 000 population	
Number of psychiatrists per 100 000 population	2.06
Number of neurosurgeons per 100 000 population	
Number of psychiatric nurses per 100 000 population	6
Number of neurologists per 100 000 population	
Number of psychologists per 100 000 population	4
Number of social workers per 100 000 population	1

Most of the psychiatric beds and psychiatrists are in Lima. About 70% of the beds are in public institutions. 10% of these beds are occupied by long stay patients. Between 40 to 90% of professionals from various disciplines work in public institutions for mental health.

Non-Governmental Organizations NGOs are involved with mental health in the country. They are mainly involved in advocacy, promotion, prevention, treatment and rehabilitation. These organizations participate in mental health activities related to women, children, domestic violence and consumers.

Information Gathering System There is mental health reporting system in the country. ICD-10 is used for recording purposes. Activities in promotion and prevention are also reported. The report is separated from the rest of health information. The data collection has limitations. The HIS-MIS system does not include most important mental health problems. The mental health programme collects activities information on a parallel system.
The country has data collection system or epidemiological study on mental health. The mental health area from the Ministry of Health is in charge of the data collection system for mental disorders. Service data collection system is conducted for all the mental health system. There is an epidemiological study in progress.

Programmes for Special Population The country has specific programmes for mental health for refugees, disaster affected population, elderly and children. Interventions are carried out in children and adolescent victims of armed violence.
Also, there are special programmes for women and victims of domestic violence.

Therapeutic Drugs The following therapeutic drugs are generally available at the primary health care level of the country: carbamazepine, phenobarbital, phenytoin sodium, amitriptyline, chlorpromazine, diazepam, fluphenazine, lithium, biperiden.

Other Information

Additional Sources of Information

de Michelena, M. I., Burstein, E., Lama, J. R., et al (1993) Paternal age as a risk factor for Down syndrome. American Journal of Medical Genetics, 45, 679-682.

Estudio Epidemiológico Metropolitano en Salud Mental 2002. Anales de Salud Mental, Lima, Perú, 2002. Vol. XVIII, n. 1 y 2.

Flores Agreda, R. (1986) Drug abuse problems in countries of the Andean subregion. Bulletin on Narcotics, 38, 27-36.

Gossop, M., Butron, M., Molla, M., et al (1994) High dose cocaine use in Bolivia and Peru. Bulletin on Narcotics, 46, 25-33.

Hayashi, S., Perales, A., Sogi, C. et al (1985) Prevalencia de vida de trastornos mentales en Independencia (Lima, Peru). Anales de Salud Mental, 1, 206-222.

Montoya, I. D., Chilcoat, H. D., et al (1996) Epidemiology of coca derivatives use in the Andean region: a tale of five countries. Substance Use & Misuse, 31, 1227-1240.

Vega-Dienstmaier, J. M., Mazzotti, G., Stucchi-Portocarrero, S., et al (1999) Prevalence and risk factors for depression in postpartum women. Actas Espanolas de Psiquiatria, 27, 299-303.

Yamamoto, J., Silva, J. A., Sasao, T., et al (1993) Alcoholism in Peru. American Journal of Psychiatry, 150, 1059-1062.

Philippines

GENERAL INFORMATION

Philippines is a country with an approximate area of 300 thousand sq. km. (UNO, 2001). The country is an archipelago of over 7000 islands. Its population is 81.408 million, and the sex ratio (men per hundred women) is 101 (UNO, 2004). The proportion of population under the age of 15 years is 36% (UNO, 2004), and the proportion of population above the age of 60 years is 6% (WHO, 2004). The literacy rate is 92.5% for men and 92.7% for women (UNESCO/MoH, 2004).

The country is a lower middle income group country (based on World Bank 2004 criteria). The proportion of health budget to GDP is 3.3%. The per capita total expenditure on health is 169 international $, and the per capita government expenditure on health is 77 international $ (WHO, 2004).

The main language(s) used in the country is (are) Pilipino and English. The largest ethnic group(s) is (are) Christian Malay. The largest religious group(s) is (are) Roman Catholic (five-sixths).

The life expectancy at birth is 65.1 years for males and 71.7 years for females (WHO, 2004). The healthy life expectancy at birth is 57 years for males and 62 years for females (WHO, 2004).

EPIDEMIOLOGY

Parker and Balza (1977) examined the association between schizophrenia and winter birth in an equatorial region (n=3508). A 15% excess above expectation was found for patients born in the coldest 3-month period of the year (December-February). An excess of births in that period was found in both sexes and in each decade of birth examined. Guiao (1994) examined 200 women from an urban community and found a negative relationship between annual individual income, educational achievement and depression. Ramoso-Jalbuena (1994) conducted a survey on 500 urban women aged 40-50 years and found that climacteric symptoms affected 83% of the respondents, with 79% reporting psychological disorders. Fugita and Crittenden (1990) assessed 966 students from Korea, Philippines, Taiwan and US using the Zung Self-Reported Depressive Symptomatology (SDS) scale. Korean and Philippine students had higher scores than Caucasian Americans. Females had higher SDS scores in all but one group. Howard et al (1999) evaluated 351 tribal and non-tribal disaster victims 6 years after they were displaced following a volcanic eruption. The prevalence rates for PTSD and major depression were 27.6% and 14.0%, respectively. McKelvey and Webb (1997) assessed a group of 101 Vietnamese Amerasians at a transit center in Vietnam and subsequently at a refugee camp in the Philippines with the Hopkins Symptom Checklist-25 and a Camp Comparison Questionnaire. There was a significant decrease in anxiety and depression between the two centers; however, these changes were not related to changes in refugee camp conditions or social support within the camp. McKelvey et al (1993) assessed a cohort of 161 randomly selected Vietnamese youth in Vietnam awaiting placement in the US using the Felsman's 35-item Personal Information Form and the Hopkins Symptom Checklist-25 (HSCL-25). Ninety-five members of the original cohort were re-evaluated at a Philippine refugee center. Those with more pre-migratory risk factors had significantly more total and depressive symptoms in the latter stage. In another study, McKelvey and Webb (1995), found a history of physical and/or sexual abuse in 22% of male and 18% of female Amerasians (n=102). Abused males reported significantly higher levels of psychological distress than non-abused males, while abused and non-abused females did not differ in their levels of psychological distress. Giel et al (1981) assessed 925 children attending primary health care facilities in Sudan, Philippines, India and Columbia through a two stage survey. Rates of behavioural disorders varied between 12% and 29% in the four study areas. In a study on 961 school children, Maxwell (2001) showed that witnessing inter-parental violence was significantly associated with self-reported antisocial and delinquent activities. Williams et al (1986) examined the performance of 911 children with histories of perinatal risk events on a restandardized Philippine (Metro-Manila) version of the Denver Developmental Screening Test (DDST). This study established that the children performed significantly below Philippine norms. Mendez and Adair (1999) evaluated more than 2000 children and found that stunted growth between birth and 2 years was associated with deficits in cognitive ability at 8 and 11 years. Deficits in children's scores were smaller at age 11 years than at age 8 years, suggesting that adverse effects may decline over time.

MENTAL HEALTH RESOURCES

Mental Health Policy A mental health policy is present. The policy was initially formulated in 1990.

The components of the policy are advocacy, promotion, prevention, treatment and rehabilitation. The policy calls for community-based services and services that are integrated with the general health and primary care. It pays special attention to vulnerable groups (e.g. those affected by disasters, women, children, etc.) and overseas Filipino workers.

Substance Abuse Policy A substance abuse policy is present. The policy was initially formulated in 1972. It was amended in 2002.

National Mental Health Programme A national mental health programme is present. The programme was formulated in 1990. The primary objective of the programme is to fully integrate mental health in the nation's health system. Its strategies include: networking, nation-wide democratization of capabilities of mental health facilities, intensification and strengthening the training in psychiatry and mental health, focus on research, advocacy, social mobilization and peripheral development. Currently, efforts are being made to restructure the National Programme for Mental Health to the National Programme for Mental Health and Substance Abuse. The absence of a specific budget makes the implementation of the programme difficult when it is shifted to a lower priority.

National Therapeutic Drug Policy/Essential List of Drugs A national therapeutic drug policy/essential list of drugs is present. It was formulated in 1988.

Mental Health Legislation There is no mental health legislation. The laws that govern the provision of mental health services are contained in various parts of the Administrative and Penal Code promulgated in 1917. The Dangerous Drugs Act (2002) and Tobacco Regulation Act (2003) require that the Department of Health handles demand reduction efforts and accredits physicians to evaluate and manage substance misuse. A certification of mental health is necessary before issuance of a firearms licence, and a certification of being drug free is necessary before the issuance of a driver's licence.
Details about the year of enactment of the mental health legislation are not available.

Mental Health Financing There are budget allocations for mental health.
The country spends 0.02% of the total health budget on mental health.
The primary sources of mental health financing in descending order are tax based, out of pocket expenditure by the patient or family and social insurance.
The new social health insurance programme provides compulsory coverage to the employed sector and voluntary coverage to the self-employed and informal sectors. The indigent sector receives free coverage through financial counterparts in health and other sectors. However, mental health benefit is limited to acute inpatient care.
The country has disability benefits for persons with mental disorders.

Mental Health Facilities Mental health is a part of primary health care system. Actual treatment of severe mental disorders is not available at the primary level.
Regular training of primary care professionals is carried out in the field of mental health. Integration of mental health care in primary care has been achieved in a few demonstration projects. Training modules are available. Under the national mental health programme, trainers training was conducted for critical incident stress debriefing of disaster victims in the Department of Social Welfare and Development. These trainers have since trained other social workers in the field.
There are no community care facilities for patients with mental disorders. One regional hospital has been designated 'collaborating centre for comprehensive mental health'. It will serve as a model for development of comprehensive care including acute psychiatric units and outpatient clinics, home treatment and psychosocial rehabilitation. Family education programmes have been initiated in some areas.

Psychiatric Beds and Professionals

Total psychiatric beds per 10 000 population	0.9
Psychiatric beds in mental hospitals per 10 000 population	0.56
Psychiatric beds in general hospitals per 10 000 population	0.3
Psychiatric beds in other settings per 10 000 population	0.03
Number of psychiatrists per 100 000 population	0.4
Number of neurosurgeons per 100 000 population	0
Number of psychiatric nurses per 100 000 population	0.4
Number of neurologists per 100 000 population	0.2
Number of psychologists per 100 000 population	0.9
Number of social workers per 100 000 population	16

There are 1199 occupational therapists. Three fourths of the beds available for psychiatric care are in the National Centre for Mental Health (NCMH) in the National Capital Region. Regional mental health units have 25-100 functional beds and are present in only 10 regions. These centres provide general psychiatric, consultation-liaison and forensic services. Ten general psychiatric units are also being developed with the aim of eventually phasing out the NMCH. The land on which the National Centre is located is urgently needed for other city programmes. Nearly three-fifths of the psychiatrists practice in the National Capital Region. Post-residency fellowships are available in child, social and consultation-liaison psychiatry. There are now 15 child psychiatrists. Most clinical psychologists work in the private sector. Emigration is a major issue, particularly in the field of nursing. A wave of physicians, both general practitioners and specialists have shifted to nursing in order to apply for vacancies in developed countries where there is an acute need for nurses. This combined with emigration of registered nurses, is causing concern about the future of health care delivery in the country.

Non-Governmental Organizations NGOs are involved with mental health in the country. They are mainly involved in advocacy, promotion, prevention, treatment and rehabilitation. NGOs provide psychosocial rehabilitation services, organize family support groups and carry out public education efforts.

Information Gathering System There is no mental health reporting system in the country.
The country has no data collection system or epidemiological study on mental health.
No nation-wide study on the prevalence of psychiatric disorders has been done.

Programmes for Special Population The country has specific programmes for mental health for minorities, refugees, disaster affected population, indigenous population, elderly and children.
The National Programme for Mental Health in collaboration with the University of the Philippines Psychiatrists Foundation Inc. (UPPFI), an NGO, organized a Mental Health task Force in Disaster, which conceptualizes and implements the psychosocial intervention programme for victims of disasters. The country also has some child protection units. The Department of Health integrates mental health components in its annual advocacy and health promotion efforts especially in its healthy life style theme. Examples of such programmes include those on mental health of children and adolescents and stress in workplace. The Overseas Workers Welfare Assistance (OWWA) of the Department of Labour and Employment has developed a Pre-departure policy consisting of triage for mental disorders and a package on stress (especially cultural stress). It also offers services of physicians and social welfare officers to overseas workers at Consulates. There are policies specifying the need to ascertain a person's mental health before appointment to high positions in the Government or the assumption of specific responsibilities. The Department of Social Welfare and Development has adopted a psychosocial orientation in their training of childcare workers in their various institutions for street children, children victims of abuse and violence and for counsellors in women crisis centres.

Therapeutic Drugs The following therapeutic drugs are generally available at the primary health care level of the country: carbamazepine, phenobarbital, phenytoin sodium, sodium valproate, chlorpromazine, diazepam, fluphenazine, haloperidol, lithium, biperiden, carbidopa, levodopa.

Other Information

Additional Sources of Information

Conde, B. (2004) Philpipines mental health country profile. International Review of Psychiatry, 16, 159-166.

Department of Health (2000) Philippine National Drug Formulary, Essential Drugs List. National Drug Committee, Philippine National Drug Policy Program, Department of Health, 1(5).

Fugita, S. S., Crittenden, K. S. (1990) Towards culture- and population-specific norms for self-reported depressive symptomatology. International Journal of Social Psychiatry, 36, 83-92.

Giel, R., de Arango, M.V., Climent, C.E., et al (1981) Childhood mental disorders in primary health care: results of observations in four developing countries. A report from the WHO collaborative Study on Strategies for Extending Mental Health Care. Pediatrics, 68, 677-683.

Guiao, I. Z. (1994) Predictors of mental health in women of a politically unstable country, the Philippines. Health Care for Women International, 15, 197-211.

Government document (1982) The Dangerous Drugs Act of 1972(RA 6425). Amended by Batas Pambansa blg. 179 and R.A. 7659.

Howard, W. T., Loberiza, F. R., Pfohl, B. M., et al (1999) Initial results, reliability, and validity of a mental health survey of Mount Pinatubo disaster victims. Journal of Nervous & Mental Disease, 187, 661-672.

Maxwell, S. R. (2001) A focus on familial strain: antisocial behavior and delinquency in Filipino society. Sociological Inquiry, 71, 265-292.

McKelvey, R. S., Webb, J. A. (1997) A prospective study of psychological distress related to refugee camp experience. Australian & New Zealand Journal of Psychiatry, 31, 549-554.

McKelvey, R. S., Webb, J. A., Mao, A. R. (1993) Premigratory risk factors in Vietnamese Amerasians. American Journal of Psychiatry, 150, 470-473.

McKelvey, R. S., Webb, J. A. (1995) A pilot study of abuse among Vietnamese Amerasians. Child Abuse & Neglect, 19, 545-553.

Mendez, M. A., Adair, L. S. (1999) Severity and timing of stunting in the first two years of life affect performance on cognitive tests in late childhood. Journal of Nutrition, 129, 1555-1562.

Parker, G., Balza, B. (1977) Season of birth and schizophrenia – an equatorial study. Acta Psychiatrica Scandinavica, 56, 143-146.

Ramoso-Jalbuena, J. (1994) Climacteric Filipino women: a preliminary survey in the Philippines. Maturitas, 19, 183-190.

Tolentino Jr., U. J. L. (2004) The state of mental health in the Philippines. International Psychiatry, 6, 8-11.

Williams, P. D., Williams, A. R., Dial, M. N. (1986) Children at risk: perinatal events, developmental delays and the effects of a developmental stimulation program. International Journal of Nursing Studies, 23, 21-38.

Poland

GENERAL INFORMATION

Poland is a country with an approximate area of 313 thousand sq. km. (UNO, 2001). Its population is 38.551 million, and the sex ratio (men per hundred women) is 94 (UNO, 2004). The proportion of population under the age of 15 years is 17% (UNO, 2004), and the proportion of population above the age of 60 years is 17% (WHO, 2004). The literacy rate is 99.7% for men and 99.7% for women (UNESCO/MoH, 2004).

The country is a higher middle income group country (based on World Bank 2004 criteria). The proportion of health budget to GDP is 6.1%. The per capita total expenditure on health is 629 international $, and the per capita government expenditure on health is 452 international $ (WHO, 2004).

The main language(s) used in the country is (are) Polish. The largest ethnic group(s) is (are) Polish. The largest religious group(s) is (are) Roman Catholic (almost 95%).

The life expectancy at birth is 70.6 years for males and 78.7 years for females (WHO, 2004). The healthy life expectancy at birth is 63 years for males and 68 years for females (WHO, 2004).

EPIDEMIOLOGY

The National Health Interview Survey based on an instrument derived from the General Health Questionnaire (GHQ-12) showed that almost 25% of women and about 18% of men had minor psychiatric morbidity (MPM). MPM was related to marital status (divorced/widowed), unemployment, disability and low education (Kiejna et al, 2001). In a small sample of primary health care patients, an assessment with the Munich-Composite International Diagnostic Interview (M-CIDI) (computer version) revealed that half of subjects had at least one and about a quarter two or more mental disorders. The most common diagnoses were neurotic, stress-related and somatoform disorders (32.9%), substance use disorders (26.5%) and mood disorders (16.5%) (Moscicka et al, 2001). In a two-phase population based study (Mini Mental State Examination followed by diagnostic examination with Cambridge Mental Disorders of the Elderly Examination) on a stratified random sample of 1000 persons, the prevalence of dementia was estimated at 5.7%. Age-specific prevalences in the age-groups 65-69, 70-74, 75-79, 80-84 were 1.9, 5.8, 8.6 and 16.5%, respectively. The rate of vascular dementia (2.7%) was higher than that of the Alzheimer's type (2.3%) (Gabryelewicz et al, 2002). In a study on a large sample of subjects (n=13 023), the point prevalence of dementia was noted to be 10% and the incidence (per year) of Alzheimer's Disease was recorded as 2.6% in those over 65 years of age (Wender et al, 1990). Chodorowski et al (2001) assessed 716 students with the Alcohol Use Disorders Identification Test (AUDIT) and showed that 8.2% were in stage B (comprised) and 10.2% in stage C (dangerous drinking) category. Another study on university students (n=1585) revealed a rate of drug dependence of 1.4% (Chodorowski et al, 2000). A study on 747 schoolgirls (14-16 years) that employed the Eating Attitude Test (EAT-26) revealed a prevalence of 2.3% for sub-clinical eating disorder (Wlodarczyk-Bisaga & Dolan, 1996). Population based suicide statistics suggest that gender (male), age and place of residence are important risk factors of suicides in the elderly age group (Pecyna, 1993). Examination of forensic data on suicide in minors (below 18 years), revealed that the majority (87.5%) were in the age range of 16-18 years (Marek et al, 1976). Polewka et al (2002) reported that the average age of suicide completers was 43.6 years. Completed suicide was associated with male gender (four-fifths), employment (unemployed or pensioner) and mental/alcohol use disorders, while suicide attempts were associated with younger age group, female gender (three-fourths), marital status (divorced), residence (metropolitan), education (elementary/secondary), employment (unemployed or pensioner), mental disorders (depression, personality disorders) and suicide among friends or relatives. Data from regional centres of clinical toxicology showed that 43% of acute poisoning was due to suicide attempts. A mortality rate of 5.4% was observed when forensic data were taken into account (Kamenczak, 1990). A case control study of 323 inpatients with suicidal overdose and 219 patients with accidental overdose showed that the former group had a significantly greater number of people who were divorced/separated, had fewer children, had recently lost their jobs or had financial problems (Goszcz, 1999). Suicide attempts in the elderly was associated with gender (female), age (young old), occupation (retired), marital status (widowed), social isolation and physical disorders. Mental disorders (depression, organic brain disorders and alcohol use disorders) were common in both suicide attempters and suicide completers (Polewka et al, 2002). A comparison of subjects who made repeated suicide attempts and those who had made one attempt showed that the former had a greater proportion of subjects with mental disorders, divorce/separation, elementary education and unemployment/pensioner status (Polewka et al, 2001). Screening of large samples (n>500) of children and adolescents revealed probable depression in 32.8% of first-grade students, 31.7% of adolescents aged 13-14 years and 27.4% of those aged 16-17 years (Bomba, 1987; Bomba & Jaklewicz, 1990). In 490 Polish school districts, the prevalence of mental retardation, major mental retardation (I.Q. from 0 to 49) and Langdon-Down syndrome were 2%, 0.3% and 0.05%, respectively. Major mental retardation was associated with a family history of mental retardation and mental disorders and a history of birth asphyxia (Wald & Stomma, 1968).

MENTAL HEALTH RESOURCES

Mental Health Policy A mental health policy is present. The policy was initially formulated in 1995.
The components of the policy are promotion, prevention, treatment and rehabilitation.

Substance Abuse Policy A substance abuse policy is present. The policy was initially formulated in 1999.

National Mental Health Programme A national mental health programme is present. The programme was formulated in 1995. The three greatest priorities of the national mental health programme are: deinstitutionalization and improvement of the quality of care; development of community-based psychiatry; mental health promotion. Large psychiatric hospitals are to be dismantled or transformed for some other purpose; communal coordinating teams would be created at the level of county areas, consisting of representatives of services providing health care to the mentally disordered. The team would serve also as an advisory body in matters of social policy concerning mental health issues and the needs of psychiatric care (including allotment of financial resources). A programme of postgraduate training for general practitioners is now under development. The monitoring of quality of care in psychiatric facilities is being promoted along with the co-operation of non-governmental organizations. The following activities for mental health promotion are being planned: develop in the community the knowledge and skills needed for an individual's growth and self-actualization, successful coping with stress and environmental demands and gaining better mental health; shape mental health-promoting behaviour and lifestyles; school education; implement programmes aimed at prevention of mental disorders in high-risk groups; organize various forms of service delivery in crisis situations; implement programmes of co-operation within the local communities on mental disorders, mental health promotion, and prevention of substance abuse. It is expected that the National Mental Health Programme will be included into Mental Health Act by the Parliament. Poland has a plan for national action with regard to the prevention of suicides.

National Therapeutic Drug Policy/Essential List of Drugs A national therapeutic drug policy/essential list of drugs is present. It was formulated in 2000.
The list of drugs are prepared on the basis of the Minister of Health Ordinance on the list of drugs which are supplied free of charge or at special low prices for persons suffering from specified diseases. The ordinance is published every year.

Mental Health Legislation The Mental Health Act regulates three major issues: (1) promotion of mental health and the prevention of mental disorders, shaping of appropriate social attitudes towards people with mental disorders and counteracting discrimination; (2) provision of comprehensive and accessible mental health care and assistance for people with mental disorders under the models of community care and social welfare; and (3) protection of the civil rights of people with mental disorders, in particular, definition of the guarantee of the rights of people admitted to and treated in hospitals without consent. The other relevant acts are: The Involuntary Commitment Law, Section 7 of 1986, the Act on Legal Proceedings (1999), the Act on Upbringing in Sobriety and Counteracting Alcoholism of 1998, the Act on Counteracting Drug Abuse of 1997, the Act on Social Assistance of 1990, with subsequent amendments; the Act on Vocational and Social Rehabilitation and Employment of the Disabled of 1997. The Penal Code (1998) has provisions for offenders with mental disorders and has laws to protect the fundamental rights of the victim and perpetrator.
The latest legislation was enacted in 1994.

Mental Health Financing There are no budget allocations for mental health.
Details about expenditure on mental health are not available.
The primary sources of mental health financing in descending order are social insurance and tax based.
The Sickness Fund provides for the bulk of psychiatric services. In 1991, the State Fund for Rehabilitation of Disabled Persons was established. This resulted in organization of occupational therapy workshops.
The country has disability benefits for persons with mental disorders.

Mental Health Facilities Mental health is a part of primary health care system. Actual treatment of severe mental disorders is not available at the primary level.
Regular training of primary care professionals is carried out in the field of mental health. In the last two years, about 3500 personnel were provided training. There are training facilities for primary care doctors.
There are community care facilities for patients with mental disorders. The process of transformation of psychiatric care started in the middle 1970s, but was slow. The counselling system, which is the strong point of Polish psychiatric care, emerged some years before the dismantling of large psychiatric hospitals began. There are outpatient clinics (854 in 2002), day hospitals (221 for 16 160 patients in 2002), mobile community teams (22, mainly in cities), hostels (6 for 158 patients) and sheltered workshops (about 200). Co-ordination teams consisting of representatives of service providers will be created at the level of counties. Article 9 of the mental health act provides for two forms of community-based programmes – a specialist social help services and community self-help houses for persons who are unable to integrate themselves properly into the society due to their illnesses.

Psychiatric Beds and Professionals

Total psychiatric beds per 10 000 population	7.8
Psychiatric beds in mental hospitals per 10 000 population	5.2
Psychiatric beds in general hospitals per 10 000 population	1.2
Psychiatric beds in other settings per 10 000 population	0.6
Number of psychiatrists per 100 000 population	6
Number of neurosurgeons per 100 000 population	
Number of psychiatric nurses per 100 000 population	18.4
Number of neurologists per 100 000 population	8
Number of psychologists per 100 000 population	3.4
Number of social workers per 100 000 population	0.6

The number of substance abuse therapists per 100 000 population is 3.0. Attempts at deinstitutionalization have resulted in a 20% reduction in the number of inpatient beds between 1970 and 1990. However, even now almost a quarter of beds are concentrated in 9 large mental hospitals, which account for 7620 beds. About 19% and 4% of beds are allocated to substance (alcohol and drug) abuse and child and adolescent services, respectively. The social welfare system provides for nursing homes (place for 40 000 clients) for chronically ill patients and for mentally challenged individuals. Currently, about 583 forensic psychiatry beds are available. Psychiatric services are also available in prisons. Such services are usually provided by psychologists in consultation with prison psychiatrists. Child and adolescent psychiatry and psychotherapy are recognized sub-specialities. About 200 psychiatrists and psychologists have forensic psychiatry as their special interest area.

Non-Governmental Organizations NGOs are involved with mental health in the country. They are mainly involved in advocacy, prevention and rehabilitation. A voluntary coalition for mental health was set up in 1993 as a national organization including many self-help and related associations and groups. Substantial part of the social support services is provided by NGOs, some of which are supported by the Government. More than 2005 Alcoholic Anonymous groups, 712 Alanon and 183 Alteen groups have been established.

Information Gathering System There is mental health reporting system in the country.
The country has data collection system or epidemiological study on mental health. There is a Statistical Yearbook on Mental Health Care and Neurological Care published every year.

Programmes for Special Population The country has specific programmes for mental health for elderly and children. There are separate facilities for children and elderly with mental disorders.
Child and adolescent psychiatry has been recognized as a sub-speciality since 1999. The main forms of psychiatric care and delivery of alcohol or drug abuse treatment are outpatient clinics and various forms of intermediate care – day hospitals, mobile community teams, crisis intervention centres, and rehabilitative facilities. Currently, psychiatric institutions in which detention is carried out have been divided into three groups based on their security arrangements. One psychiatric hospital in the country fulfils the criteria for maximum security. Courts decide on detention in psychiatric hospitals, and the National Psychiatric Board for Protective Measures selects the most suitable hospital.

Therapeutic Drugs The following therapeutic drugs are generally available at the primary health care level of the country: carbamazepine, ethosuximide, phenobarbital, phenytoin sodium, sodium valproate, amitriptyline, chlorpromazine, diazepam, fluphenazine, haloperidol, lithium, biperiden, carbidopa, levodopa.
A number of other drugs like cloimipramine, fluoxetine, oxazepam, buspirone, etc. are available. The above mentioned drugs are only the example of fully reimbursed medications. The vast majority of other psychotropic drugs are also available but with patients co-payment, which varies substantially from one drug to the other.

Other Information

Additional Sources of Information

Balicki, M., Leder, S., Piotrowski, A. (2000) Focus on psychiatry in Poland. British Journal of Psychiatry, 177, 377-381.

Bomba, I. (1987) Juvenile depression (epidemiological study). Zhurnal Nevropatologii i Psikhiatrii Imeni S-S-Korsakova, 87, 1501-1503.

Bomba, J., Jaklewicz, H. (1990) Depression in children at the beginning of school education. Prevalence of the phenomenon and its relation to the child's adaptive capacity. Psychiatria Polska, 24, 15-19.

Chodorowski, Z., Anand, J. S., Salamon, M., et al (2001) Evaluation of illicit drug use among students from universities in Gdansk. Przeglad Lekarski, 58, 267-271.

Chodorowski, Z., Sein Anand J., Sein Anand, I., et al (2000) The evaluation of methods of usage of addictive substances among high school students and Gdansk University students. Przeglad Lekarski, 57, 549-552.

Ciszewski, L., Sutula,E.(2000) Psychiatric care for mentally disturbed perpetrators of criminal acts in Poland. International Journal of Law and Psychiatry, 23, 547-554.

Dabrowski, S. (1998) Community specialist social help services as a form of community social support. Psychiatria Polska, 32, 443-451.

Gabryelewicz, T., Parnowski, T., Szafranska, A., et al (2002) The prevalence of dementia in Poland: a population-based, door-to-door survey in an urban community. Archives of Psychiatry & Psychotherapy, 4, 17-26.

Goszcz, H. (1999) Social conditions of suicidal poisonings. Przeglad Lekarski, 56, 422-427.

Instytut Psychiatrii I Neurologi (1995) The Mental Health Act.

Instytut Psychiatrii I Neurologi (1999) Zaklady Psychiatrycznej oraz Neurologicznej Opieki Zdrowotnej – Rocznik Statystyczny 1999. (Statistical Yearbook: Mental Health and Neurological Care Facilities.

Instytut Psychiatrii I Neurologi (2000) Polish Mental Health Act.

Kamenczak, A. (1990) Evaluation of the risk of acute poisoning with chemicals in inhabitants of Krakow in from 1983 to 1987. Folia Medica Cracoviensia, 31, 169-187.

Kiejna, A., Wojtyniak, B., Rymaszewska, J., et al (2001) The prevalence of minor psychiatric morbidity and its correlates in Poland. Archives of Psychiatry & Psychotherapy, 3, 31-43.

Langiewicz, W., Supczyska-Kossobudzka, E. (2000) Psychiatric services in the fifth year of health care reform in Poland. International Psychiatry, 6, 6-8.

Law Gazette of Republic of Poland (2000) List of Psychotropic Drugs Prepared on the Basis of the Minister of Health Ordinance on the List of Drugs which are Supplied Free of Charge or at Special Law Prices for Persons Suffering from Specified Diseases.

Marek, Z., Widacki, J., Zwarysiewicz, W. (1976) Suicides committed by minors. Forensic Science, 7, 103-108.

Ministerstwo Zdrowia (2000) Narodowy Progream Profilaktyki I Rozwiazywania Probemow Alkoholowych. (The National Program on Preventing and Solving Alcohol Problems).

Ministerstwo Zdrowia i Opieki Spolecznej (1999) Karjowy Program: Prezeciwdzialania Narkomanii na lata 1999 – 2001. (The National Program on Preventing Drug Abuse).

Mocicka, A., Makowska, Z., Merecz, D., et al (2001) Mental health status in workers: the results based on the Munich version of the International Composite Diagnostic Interview (M-CIDI). Medycyna Pracy, 52, 329-336.

Panstwowa Agencja Rozwiazywania Problemow Alkoholowych. (1998) Ustawa o Wychowaniu w Trzezwosci i Przeciwdzialaniu Alkoholizmowi i Inne Dokumenty. (The Act on Upbringing in Sobreity and Counteracting Alcoholism).

Pecyna, S. M. (1993) Death of choice in the subpopulation of people aged 60 and more in psycho-epidemiological studies in the years 1978-1991. Polish Population Review, 125-138.

Polewka, A., Groszek, B., Trela, F., et al (2002) The completed and attempted suicide in Krakow: similarities and differences. Przeglad Lekarski, 59, 298-303.

Polewka, A., Pach, J., Zieba, A., et al (2001) A trial for the complex risk assessment of repeated suicide predictors in patients after suicidal poisoning attempts, hospitalized in the Department of Clinical Toxicology CM UJ in Krakow. I. Influence of socio-demographic factors. Przeglad Lekarski, 58, 325-329.

Puzynski St. Program Ochrony Zdrowia Psychicznego (2001) The Mental Health Program (unpublished manuscript).

Puzynski, S., Moskalewicz, J. (2001) Evolution of the mental health care system in Poland. Acta Psychiatrica Scandinavica, 104 (suppl. 410), 69-73.

Puzynski, S., Langiewicz, W., Pietrzykowska, B (2002) The reform of psychiatric care in Poland-2001. Psychiatria Polska, 36, 181-192.

USTAWA (1997) O Przeciwdzialaniu Narkomanii. (The Act on Preventing Drug Abuse).

Wald, I., Stomma, D. (1968) Epidemiology of mental retardation in Poland. Psychiatrie, Neurologie und Medizinische Psychologie – Beihefte, 8-9, 191-198.

Wender, M., Mularczyk, J., Modestowicz, R. (1990) Epidemiology of Alzheimer's disease in the selected region of Wielkopolska (town and commune Steszew). Przeglad. Epidemiologiczny, 44, 215-221.

Wlodarczyk-Bisaga, K., Dolan, B. (1996) A two-stage epidemiological study of abnormal eating attitudes and their prospective risk factors in Polish school-girls. Psychological Medicine, 26, 1021-1032.

Portugal

GENERAL INFORMATION

Portugal is a country with an approximate area of 92 thousand sq. km. (UNO, 2001). Its population is 10.072 million, and the sex ratio (men per hundred women) is 93 (UNO, 2004). The proportion of population under the age of 15 years is 17% (UNO, 2004), and the proportion of population above the age of 60 years is 21% (WHO, 2004). The literacy rate is 93.7% for men and 88.5% for women (UNESCO/MoH, 2004).

The country is a high income group country (based on World Bank 2004 criteria). The proportion of health budget to GDP is 9.2%. The per capita total expenditure on health is 1618 international $, and the per capita government expenditure on health is 1116 international $ (WHO, 2004).

The main language(s) used in the country is (are) Portuguese.

The life expectancy at birth is 73.6 years for males and 80.5 years for females (WHO, 2004). The healthy life expectancy at birth is 67 years for males and 72 years for females (WHO, 2004).

EPIDEMIOLOGY

There is substantial epidemiological data on mental illnesses in Portugal in internationally accessible literature. No attempt was made to include this information here.

MENTAL HEALTH RESOURCES

Mental Health Policy A mental health policy is present. The policy was initially formulated in 1995.

The components of the policy are advocacy, promotion, prevention, treatment and rehabilitation. Mental health and alcohol issues are coordinated by the same department at the Directorate General of Health within the Ministry of Health.

Substance Abuse Policy A substance abuse policy is present. The policy was initially formulated in 1999. The policy has a 5-year duration (1999-2004) (Council of Ministers Resolution 46/99 of 22 April). There is a specific structure within the Ministry of Health for this area. An alcohol policy is also present since 2000.

National Mental Health Programme A national mental health programme is present. The programme was formulated in 1996. A new national mental health plan is being prepared within the context of the National Health Plan 2004-2010. Several other programmes namely for the elderly, children and adolescents, depression, PTSD, alcohol use disorders and drug use disorders are also being prepared. There is a National Network, involving the Ministry of Defence and the Ministry of Health, for PTSD of ex-combatants and a National Network for Alcohol problems is being developed.

National Therapeutic Drug Policy/Essential List of Drugs A national therapeutic drug policy/essential list of drugs is present. It was formulated in 2000.

Mental Health Legislation There is the Mental Health Law 36/98. Other relevant national laws are: Law 35/99 (organization of services), Joint Ruling 407/98 (not specific for mental health) Order 348A/98 (social firms, not specific for mental health), Council of Ministers Resolution 166/2000 (Alcohol Action Plan), Law 281/2003 of (Continuity Care Network) and Joint Ruling 502/2004 (PTSD Network).

The latest legislation was enacted in 1998.

Mental Health Financing There are budget allocations for mental health.

The country spends 2.3% of the total health budget on mental health.

The primary sources of mental health financing in descending order are tax based, social insurance, private insurances and out of pocket expenditure by the patient or family.

The country has disability benefits for persons with mental disorders. Financial incentives were introduced for disabled employees in 1982. More recently, benefits were announced with the Dec.-Law 247/89.

Mental Health Facilities Mental health is a part of primary health care system. Actual treatment of severe mental disorders is available at the primary level. However, major psychiatric illnesses are generally treated in specialized psychiatric set-ups.

Regular training of primary care professionals is carried out in the field of mental health. During their training general practitioners are given theoretical and practical exercises in a mental health setting.

There are community care facilities for patients with mental disorders. Since 1989, community care (vocational training, employment support, day centres and residential support) has been progressively developed through cooperation of health services, social services and NGOs. Since 1998, there has been an integration of social support and continuous health care for people in situations of dependency (physical, mental, social), with mental and psychiatric disorders, for residential and occupational programmes, financed by social security. In 1998, the Ministry of Work and Solidarity defined the framework for recognition and granting of technical and financial support to integration within the context of social employment market as an active employment sponsored by the Institute for Employment and Vocational Training.

Psychiatric Beds and Professionals

Total psychiatric beds per 10 000 population	7.5
Psychiatric beds in mental hospitals per 10 000 population	1.5
Psychiatric beds in general hospitals per 10 000 population	1
Psychiatric beds in other settings per 10 000 population	4.9
Number of psychiatrists per 100 000 population	4.7
Number of neurosurgeons per 100 000 population	1.5
Number of psychiatric nurses per 100 000 population	10.1
Number of neurologists per 100 000 population	3.2
Number of psychologists per 100 000 population	2
Number of social workers per 100 000 population	1.6

Over the last 15 years, a decrease of 40% in bed strength has been achieved.

Non-Governmental Organizations NGOs are involved with mental health in the country. They are mainly involved in advocacy, promotion, prevention, treatment and rehabilitation. NGOs are active in suicide prevention programmes.

Information Gathering System There is mental health reporting system in the country. There is a national participation in European programmes, like 'European Community Health Indicators (ECHI-2)', in order to achieve national health indicators.
The country has data collection system or epidemiological study on mental health. The 3rd National Health Survey contains some information about mental health and the 4th (in preparation) will deeper cover alcohol and mental health. There are three National Psychiatric Census (the latest in 2001). The Directorate General of Health within the Ministry of Health is preparing a national system for mental health information and the first National Morbidity Study.

Programmes for Special Population The country has specific programmes for mental health for disaster affected population, elderly and children. There are services for PTSD. There are separate clinics for child and adolescent psychiatry. For the elderly, there are outpatient clinics, inpatient services, home visit facilities and old people's home.
There are 3 child and adolescent psychiatry departments and 25 services and units (Rede de Referenciação em Psiquiatria e Saúde Mental, Direcção-Geral da Saúde, 2004). In the area of illicit drugs, the country has a nationwide network of 45 C.A.T. (care centers). In addition, there are three regional alcohol abuse treatment centres and 1 centre for psychiatric rehabilitation.

Therapeutic Drugs The following therapeutic drugs are generally available at the primary health care level of the country: carbamazepine, phenobarbital, phenytoin sodium, sodium valproate, amitriptyline, chlorpromazine, diazepam, fluphenazine, haloperidol, lithium, biperiden, carbidopa, levodopa.

Other Information In 2000, there was a ' Resolution of Assembly of Republic' No 76/2000 and a 'Resolution of Council of Ministries' No 166/2000 directed to fighting alcoholism. There was also a law- No 318/2000.
Although suicide rates have been declining in the last few years, there is a regional cluster of suicides in Alentejo and Algarve Regions.

Additional Sources of Information

Directorate General of Health (2004) National Health Plan 2004-2010.
Ministry of Heath (2000) Health Determinants in the European Union: Évora Conference Proceedings.
Ministry of Heath – Directorate General of Health (2002) Health Gains in Portugal.
Ministry of Heath – Directorate General of Health (2004) Statistics elements of Health/2001.

Qatar

GENERAL INFORMATION

Qatar is a country with an approximate area of 11 thousand sq. km. (UNO, 2001). Its population is 0.619 million, and the sex ratio (men per hundred women) is 172 (UNO, 2004). The proportion of population under the age of 15 years is 26% (UNO, 2004), and the proportion of population above the age of 60 years is 3% (WHO, 2004). The literacy rate is 94.9% for men and 82.3% for women (UNESCO/MoH, 2004).

The country is a high income group country (based on World Bank 2004 criteria). The proportion of health budget to GDP is 3.1%. The per capita total expenditure on health is 782 international $, and the per capita government expenditure on health is 574 international $ (WHO, 2004).

The main language(s) used in the country is (are) Arabic and English. The largest ethnic group(s) is (are) Arab, and the other ethnic group(s) are (is) Pakistani, Indian and Iranian. The largest religious group(s) is (are) Muslim (almost 95%).

The life expectancy at birth is 74.8 years for males and 73.8 years for females (WHO, 2004). The healthy life expectancy at birth is 67 years for males and 64 years for females (WHO, 2004).

EPIDEMIOLOGY

There is substantial epidemiological data on mental illnesses in Quatar in internationally accessible literature. No attempt was made to include this information here.

MENTAL HEALTH RESOURCES

Mental Health Policy A mental health policy is present. The policy was initially formulated in 1980.
The components of the policy are advocacy, promotion, prevention, treatment and rehabilitation.

Substance Abuse Policy A substance abuse policy is present. The policy was initially formulated in 1986.

National Mental Health Programme A national mental health programme is present. The programme was formulated in 1990.
The national mental health programme stresses on legislation, family involvement, primary health care and counselling programmes.

National Therapeutic Drug Policy/Essential List of Drugs A national therapeutic drug policy/essential list of drugs is present. It was formulated in 1980.

N–R

Mental Health Legislation Details about the mental health legislation are not available.

Mental Health Financing There are budget allocations for mental health.
The country spends 1% of the total health budget on mental health.
The primary source of mental health financing is tax based.
The country has disability benefits for persons with mental disorders.

Mental Health Facilities Mental health is a part of primary health care system. Actual treatment of severe mental disorders is not available at the primary level. Primary care is provided to a small number of centres. All psychiatric drugs are dispensed except for the controlled ones. Drug abuse patients are referred to the psychiatric clinics and only referrals from the catchment areas are seen. Generally, psychologists attend and handle referrals on-site.

Regular training of primary care professionals is carried out in the field of mental health. In the last two years, about 15 personnel were provided training. Training courses for physicians from primary health care and dermatology are held.

There are community care facilities for patients with mental disorders. A community nursing service was started in 1993 and domiciliary visits for assessments and home management of patients in liaison with their families have started. There are also day-care centres at certain hospitals which impart stress control, assertive training, job training, family education, increase self knowledge, rehabilitate institutionalized chronic patients and carry out family-oriented educational programmes.

Psychiatric Beds and Professionals

Total psychiatric beds per 10 000 population	0.97
Psychiatric beds in mental hospitals per 10 000 population	0.97
Psychiatric beds in general hospitals per 10 000 population	0
Psychiatric beds in other settings per 10 000 population	0
Number of psychiatrists per 100 000 population	3.4
Number of neurosurgeons per 100 000 population	0.8
Number of psychiatric nurses per 100 000 population	10
Number of neurologists per 100 000 population	1
Number of psychologists per 100 000 population	1.2
Number of social workers per 100 000 population	10

There are 3 other mental health professionals of different categories. Beds have been earmarked for women patients and for services related to rehabilitation, mental retardation, special education and psychogeriatrics.

Non-Governmental Organizations NGOs are involved with mental health in the country. They are mainly involved in treatment.

Information Gathering System There is mental health reporting system in the country.
The country has data collection system or epidemiological study on mental health.
A computerized database information system covering all psychiatric clinical services includes modern diagnostic criteria and information on treatment and referral outcomes are possible, but only in the capital city.

Programmes for Special Population The country has specific programmes for mental health for elderly and children.
There are facilities for imparting mental health services to schools. There are also ambulatory child psychiatry facilities.
Psychogeriatric services consist of an inpatient service with follow-up protocol.

Therapeutic Drugs The following therapeutic drugs are generally available at the primary health care level of the country: carbamazepine, ethosuximide, phenobarbital, phenytoin sodium, sodium valproate, amitriptyline, chlorpromazine, diazepam, fluphenazine, haloperidol, lithium, carbidopa, levodopa.

Other Information Qatar's psychiatric service was established in 1971. Almost all hospital services are controlled by the Hamad Medical Corporation, which is a Government corporation.

Additional Sources of Information

El-Islam, M. F. (1995) Psychiatry in Qatar. Psychiatric Bulletin, 19, 779-781.

Republic of Korea

GENERAL INFORMATION

Republic of Korea is a country with an approximate area of 99 thousand sq. km. (UNO, 2001). Its population is 47.95 million, and the sex ratio (men per hundred women) is 101 (UNO, 2004). The proportion of population under the age of 15 years is 20% (UNO, 2004), and the proportion of population above the age of 60 years is 12% (WHO, 2004). The literacy rate is 99.1% for men and 96.4% for women (UNESCO/MoH, 2004).

The country is a high income group country (based on World Bank 2004 criteria). The proportion of health budget to GDP is 6%. The per capita total expenditure on health is 948 international $, and the per capita government expenditure on health is 421 international $ (WHO, 2004).

The main language(s) used in the country is (are) Korean. The largest ethnic group(s) is (are) Korean. The largest religious group(s) is (are) Christian, and the other religious group(s) are (is) Buddhist.

The life expectancy at birth is 71.8 years for males and 79.4 years for females (WHO, 2004). The healthy life expectancy at birth is 65 years for males and 71 years for females (WHO, 2004).

EPIDEMIOLOGY

There is substantial epidemiological data on mental illnesses in the Republic of Korea in internationally accessible literature. No attempt was made to include this information here.

MENTAL HEALTH RESOURCES

Mental Health Policy A mental health policy is present. The policy was initially formulated in 1960.

The components of the policy are advocacy, promotion, prevention, treatment and rehabilitation. The mental health policy of Korea is to decrease long-term hospitalization and to develop and extend the community-based mental health service system. In addition, the mental health policy emphasizes enhancing the priority of mental health, workforce development and developing a comprehensive service system.

Substance Abuse Policy A substance abuse policy is present. The policy was initially formulated in 1970. The substance abuse policy is not only diminishing supply but also diminishing demand of substance by developing prevention programmes on the substance use and abuse.

National Mental Health Programme A national mental health programme is present. The programme was formulated in 1995. The national mental health programme is developing a community mental health service delivery system including national mental hospitals, community mental health centres and community health centres.

National Therapeutic Drug Policy/Essential List of Drugs A national therapeutic drug policy/essential list of drugs is present. It was formulated in 2000.

Most mentally ill patients with medical insurance are able to afford most therapeutic drugs, while the poor people with medical aid have a limited availability to expensive new drugs.

Mental Health Legislation There is a mental health law. It was revised in 2000. The revision allows for legal support to the establishment of social rehabilitative facilities and their role in providing community mental health services. Disability benefits are covered under the Medical Protection Act and the Welfare Law for the Handicapped.

The latest legislation was enacted in 1999.

Mental Health Financing There are no budget allocations for mental health.

The country spends 3% of the total health budget on mental health.

The primary sources of mental health financing in descending order are social insurance, tax based and out of pocket expenditure by the patient or family.

There is a universal public insurance funded by premiums. There is no private health insurance. About 90% of the providers are in the private/non-government sector, whose services are covered through the public health insurance. The Government funds health care for the poor through tax-based funds. Medical insurance covers inpatient, outpatient and day care, while tax-based funds cover nursing home and rehabilitation services.

The country has disability benefits for persons with mental disorders. Since January 2000, mentally ill patients have been made eligible for similar support and rights as other disabled persons.

Mental Health Facilities Mental health is a part of primary health care system. Actual treatment of severe mental disorders is not available at the primary level.

Regular training of primary care professionals is carried out in the field of mental health. In the last two years, about 7565 personnel were provided training. Community mental health nurses have also been trained.

There are community care facilities for patients with mental disorders. Since the formulation of the Mental Health Act in 1995, community care has started to develop. Currently, there are nearly 115 community health centres and 110 rehabilitation centres. Home help service and a visiting nursing programme for mentally ill have been developed by community mental health centres. Vocational rehabilitation programmes including sheltered workshops and supported employment are also coming up with support from the Korea Employment Promotion Agency for the Disabled. Community care is being developed with a catchment area approach. The community health centres are mainly managed by public health centres and nearby university/psychiatric hospitals. Each centre has a part time psychiatrist who acts as the supervisor. The centre provides counselling, home-visit care, treatment, case management, education, rehabilitation and outreach activities. Rehabilitation services are also provided in the private/non-government sphere. Funds for community care are being increased and it is planned that community care capacity would be increased 10-fold over the next decade. At present there is a gap between the inpatient system and the community care system.

Psychiatric Beds and Professionals

Total psychiatric beds per 10 000 population	13.8
Psychiatric beds in mental hospitals per 10 000 population	6.3
Psychiatric beds in general hospitals per 10 000 population	3.8
Psychiatric beds in other settings per 10 000 population	2.7
Number of psychiatrists per 100 000 population	3.5
Number of neurosurgeons per 100 000 population	3.1
Number of psychiatric nurses per 100 000 population	10.1
Number of neurologists per 100 000 population	1.4
Number of psychologists per 100 000 population	0.8
Number of social workers per 100 000 population	2.6

A special 1-year training programme for nurses, social workers and psychologists (certified by the Ministry of Health and Welfare) has been approved under the Mental Health Law to develop an appropriate workforce to implement the National Mental Health Programme.

Non-Governmental Organizations NGOs are involved with mental health in the country. They are mainly involved in advocacy, promotion and rehabilitation. The NGOs played a major advocacy role in the development of the mental health policy. NGOs and family associations work closely together in psychoeducation of families and users and in anti-stigma campaigns.

Information Gathering System There is mental health reporting system in the country.
The country has data collection system or epidemiological study on mental health. The Government is conducting a national epidemiological study to assess the prevalence of mental disorders.

Programmes for Special Population There are no special services.
A nation-wide anti-stigma campaign was launched in 2003 with multi-sectoral participation. A school mental programme has been set up and is run by school nurses trained in detection and counselling. Psychologists have been deployed in universities. Child and adolescent and geriatric care programmes are being developed by community mental health centres.

Therapeutic Drugs The following therapeutic drugs are generally available at the primary health care level of the country: carbamazepine, ethosuximide, phenobarbital, phenytoin sodium, sodium valproate, amitriptyline, chlorpromazine, diazepam, haloperidol, lithium, biperiden, carbidopa, levodopa.

Other Information Since the enactment of the Mental Health Act, many private mental asylums have been changed into mental hospitals. Different psychosocial programmes have been developed for rehabilitation, open wards are slowly developing in mental hospitals and unrecognized 'houses of prayer' have been closed. Custodial care in mental hospitals is still present as is prolonged inappropriate stay of patients in mental hospitals, primarily due to lack of adequate staff to care for the patients in the community. Between 1970 and 1983, families began to be replaced by unauthorized facilities as primary care givers. As a result of increasing human rights problems, the Government began to take an active interest in their care of the mentally ill. This initially led to an increase in the number of mental hospitals and their beds. It was only after the formulation of the Mental Health Act of 1995, that community care and disability benefits began to develop. However, the length of inpatient stay is still very long and there is still a huge amount of stigma against mental disorders and patients. This is being addressed gradually through advocacy campaigns.

Additional Sources of Information

Regional Office for the Western Pacific (2001) Country report on mental health – Republic of Korea.
Suh, G.-H. (2004) Mental health care in South Korea. International Psychiatry, (in press).

Republic of Moldova

GENERAL INFORMATION

Republic of Moldova is a country with an approximate area of 34 thousand sq. km. (UNO, 2001). Its population is 4.263 million, and the sex ratio (men per hundred women) is 92 (UNO, 2004). The proportion of population under the age of 15 years is 20% (UNO, 2004), and the proportion of population above the age of 60 years is 14% (WHO, 2004). The literacy rate is 99.6% for men and 98.6% for women (UNESCO/MoH, 2004).

The country is a low income group country (based on World Bank 2004 criteria). The proportion of health budget to GDP is 5.7%. The per capita total expenditure on health is 112 international $, and the per capita government expenditure on health is 56 international $ (WHO, 2004).

The main language(s) used in the country is (are) Moldovan. The largest ethnic group(s) is (are) Moldavian and Romanian, and the other ethnic group(s) are (is) Ukrainian, Bulgarian, Gaguzian and Russian. The largest religious group(s) is (are) Eastern Orthodox Christian.

The life expectancy at birth is 64 years for males and 71.6 years for females (WHO, 2004). The healthy life expectancy at birth is 57 years for males and 62 years for females (WHO, 2004).

EPIDEMIOLOGY

There is a paucity of epidemiological data on mental illnesses in Republic of Moldova in internationally accessible literature. Wasserman et al (1998) found that the suicide rates in the former USSR during 1984-90 varied greatly between different regions. It was 18.1 per 100 000 in Moldova. In quantitative analyses Wasserman and Varnik (1998) showed that mortality data were reliable for Moldova.

MENTAL HEALTH RESOURCES

Mental Health Policy A mental health policy is present. The policy was initially formulated in 2000.
The components of the policy are advocacy, promotion, prevention, treatment and rehabilitation.

Substance Abuse Policy A substance abuse policy is present. The policy was initially formulated in 2000.

National Mental Health Programme A national mental health programme is absent.

National Therapeutic Drug Policy/Essential List of Drugs A national therapeutic drug policy/essential list of drugs is present. It was formulated in 1997.

Mental Health Legislation In 1998, a programme to improve the psychiatric service was adopted, with emphasis on the rights and interests of persons suffering from mental disorders. This experience showed that it was necessary to pay more attention to the judicial rights of individuals receiving psychiatric help and to formulate appropriate criteria for compulsory admission. In 1998, the Law Concerning Psychiatric Assistance and Guarantees of the Citizen's Rights was adopted. Since January 1999, the project of developing humane mental health care in Moldova through professional training for psychiatric nurses and doctors in multidisciplinary teamwork have been in the process of implementation.
The latest legislation was enacted in 1998.

Mental Health Financing There are budget allocations for mental health.
The country spends 6.5% of the total health budget on mental health.
The primary source of mental health financing is tax based.
The budget is allocated by the National Company of Compulsory Medical Insurance. Both outpatient and inpatient treatment of mentally ill patients is free. Mental health services are financed from both Government and local authority budgets.
The country has disability benefits for persons with mental disorders.

Mental Health Facilities Mental health is a part of primary health care system. Actual treatment of severe mental disorders is not available at the primary level.
Regular training of primary care professionals is carried out in the field of mental health.
There are no community care facilities for patients with mental disorders. Since 1999, the project 'Developing humane mental health care in Moldova through professional training for psychiatric nurses and doctors in multidisciplinary teamwork' has been implemented with the support of the Geneva Initiative in Psychiatry. The number of places in day hospitals is also increasing.

Psychiatric Beds and Professionals

Total psychiatric beds per 10 000 population	6.7
Psychiatric beds in mental hospitals per 10 000 population	5.9
Psychiatric beds in general hospitals per 10 000 population	0.8
Psychiatric beds in other settings per 10 000 population	0.1
Number of psychiatrists per 100 000 population	9
Number of neurosurgeons per 100 000 population	1
Number of psychiatric nurses per 100 000 population	30.5
Number of neurologists per 100 000 population	9
Number of psychologists per 100 000 population	0.7
Number of social workers per 100 000 population	0.5

There are 3 psychiatric hospitals. Outpatient psychiatric care is provided by two psycho-neurological clinics and three departments within general clinics. The first stage of help is given in villages and districts in rural medical ambulatory sectors or in psychiatric clinics at district polyclinics. At the second stage, outpatient consultation is provided in towns by psychiatrists or psycho-neurologists; these provide high-quality help in a psycho-neurological dispensary polyclinic or a psychiatric hospital.

Non-Governmental Organizations NGOs are involved with mental health in the country. They are mainly involved in advocacy, promotion and prevention.

Information Gathering System There is mental health reporting system in the country.
The country has no data collection system or epidemiological study on mental health.

Programmes for Special Population There are no special services.

Therapeutic Drugs The following therapeutic drugs are generally available at the primary health care level of the country: carbamazepine, ethosuximide, phenobarbital, phenytoin sodium, sodium valproate, amitriptyline, chlorpromazine, diazepam, fluphenazine, haloperidol, lithium, biperiden, carbidopa, levodopa.

Other Information

Additional Sources of Information

Wasserman, D., Varnik, A. (1998) Reliability of statistics on violent death and suicide in the former USSR, 1970-1990. Acta Psychiatrica Scandinavica, Supplement 394, 34-41.

Wasserman, D., Varnik, A., Dankowicz, M. (1998) Regional differences in the distribution of suicide in the former Soviet Union during perestroika, 1984-1990. Acta Psychiatrica Scandinavica, Supplement 394, 5-12.

Romania

GENERAL INFORMATION

Romania is a country with an approximate area of 238 thousand sq. km. (UNO, 2001). Its population is 22.28 million, and the sex ratio (men per hundred women) is 95 (UNO, 2004). The proportion of population under the age of 15 years is 16% (UNO, 2004), and the proportion of population above the age of 60 years is 19% (WHO, 2004). The literacy rate is 99% for men and 97.3% for women (UNESCO/MoH, 2004).

The country is a lower middle income group country (based on World Bank 2004 criteria). The proportion of health budget to GDP is 6.5%. The per capita total expenditure on health is 460 international $, and the per capita government expenditure on health is 365 international $ (WHO, 2004).

The main language(s) used in the country is (are) Romanian. The largest ethnic group(s) is (are) Romanian (nine-tenths), and the other ethnic group(s) are (is) Hungarian and Roma. The largest religious group(s) is (are) Orthodox Christian (seven-tenths), and the other religious group(s) are (is) Protestant, Roman Catholic and Unite Catholic.

The life expectancy at birth is 68 years for males and 75 years for females (WHO, 2004). The healthy life expectancy at birth is 61 years for males and 65 years for females (WHO, 2004).

EPIDEMIOLOGY

Grecu et al (1990) found that the mortality index (1.97%) for patients with alcohol dependence (n=5580) was significantly higher than the index (0.36%) for other psychiatric patients (n=46 591). Berlescu et al (1995) reviewed hospital data on mental disorder occurring or aggravating during pregnancy or the postpartum period (n=642). Mental disorders in this period were associated with lower education level, labile biological and psychological structure, abortions and high post-natal complications. Ionescu and Popescu (1989) assessed a group of depressed students (n=111) and found that 70% had a concurrent personality disorder. Unstable, obsessive, hysteric, dysthymic and mixed personality disorders were more prevalent. Personality disorders were associated with earlier onset, severity, recurrence and non-reactivity of depression. Makinen (2000) found that patterns in suicide and their causes varied between countries of Eastern Europe and former republics that formed the USSR. A model consisting of general stress, democratization, alcohol consumption and social disorganization (with a period-dependent effect) predicted fairly accurately the changes in the suicide rates in 16 out of the 28 Eastern Bloc countries in 1984-1989 and 1989-1994, but it failed to do so for Romania. Voracek et al (2002) compared data for suicide by hanging in a county for 1990-98 and 1980-89 and found that there was no decrease in seasonality of suicide, nor was there a shift in location for suicide peak and trough months. Pluye et al (2001) assessed 508 children selected randomly from homes for children based on a clinical evaluation protocol. Using ICD-10 criteria, 54% of the children had a diagnosis of mental or behavioural disorder. Scripcaru et al (1991) found behavioural problems in 33% and post-school integration problems in 70% of the 1029 children cared for in orphanages. Kaler and Freeman (1994) assessed a representative group of Romanian orphans between the ages of 23 and 50 months. Deficits in cognitive and social functioning were present across all domains and were often severe. The deficits were unrelated to length of time in the orphanage, age at entrance, Apgar scores or birthweight. Indredavik et al (1991) studied 154 children in an institution for mentally retarded and found evidence of deprivation, anxiety and behavioural maladjustment suggesting physical, psychological, pedagogic and social neglect. Iftene et al (2000) reviewed records of 1467 adolescents (14-16 year olds) seen in 1995-2000 and 1985-90 and found a three-fold increase in number of offences. The increase in prevalence of delinquent acts was associated with locality (urban), gender (girls), age (reduction in age of onset) and unemployment in families. A change in offence profile was also noticed, with a greater degree of sexual offences, driving without license and forging money. Lupu et al (2002) interviewed 500 school-teenagers from 3 different districts with a structured questionnaire that included the 20 questions of the American Anonymous Gambling Association. They found that 6.8% of the teenagers were pathological gamblers, with a male to female ratio of 4.6:1. The majority (82.4%) preferred group gambling. Gambling was responsible for school absenteeism in 64.7% and modest results at school in 52.9% of subjects.

MENTAL HEALTH RESOURCES

Mental Health Policy A mental health policy is absent.

Substance Abuse Policy A substance abuse policy is present. The policy was initially formulated in 1998. There is a legal ban on smoking in public places.

National Mental Health Programme A national mental health programme is present. The programme was formulated in 1999. The programme was developed mainly due to the efforts of the Romanian League for Mental Health and Romanian Psychiatric Association, but it is not yet promulgated. It is based on the analysis of the mental health assessment (morbidity and mortality figures) in Romania. It incorporates ideas on prevention and rehabilitation, health care system, community psychiatry, administration and legislation and coordination with other health care sectors. Within the national mental health programmes established and financed by the Ministry of Health and Family (according to Law no. 100/1998 concerning public health assistance) there is a 'National Programme of Mental Health and Prophylaxis and Psycho-Social Pathology'..Details about its implementation are not available. A national programme for the treatment of schizophrenia and depression is in place.

National Therapeutic Drug Policy/Essential List of Drugs A national therapeutic drug policy/essential list of drugs is present. It was formulated in 1994.
The new draft national drug policy was launched in 2000.

Mental Health Legislation Experts from WHO have made recommendations in the process of elaboration of the law. Currently, a commission is working to establish the implementation norms for this law. The law includes provisions for the use of the least restrictive alternative, confidentiality, informed consent and establishes detailed rules for involuntary hospitalization, with concern for protection of the civil rights of the patient. It prohibits discrimination in general and at workplace and in health insurance and disability benefits, in particular.
The latest legislation was enacted in 2002.

Mental Health Financing There are budget allocations for mental health.
The country spends 3% of the total health budget on mental health.
The primary sources of mental health financing in descending order are social insurance and out of pocket expenditure by the patient or family.
In 1998, the Health Insurance Scheme was introduced. It is based on a social health insurance fund, where the employers and the employees contribute 14% of gross salary incomes (7% each of them). The state provides funds for some activities, e.g. prevention. Through these systems, free health care services are guaranteed for all employees and their families, pensioners, self-employed, unemployed, children up to the age of 14 and pregnant women. Both state and private pharmacies are reimbursed for issuing approved free or subsidized drugs. For employees and their families, 50% of the price is reimbursed and for pensioners and unemployed 65%.
The country has disability benefits for persons with mental disorders. Persons with mental illness can take early retirement just like any other illness. Recently, the Labour and Social Protection Department has started providing some financial support to families/ caregivers of the chronically ill with handicap (including those with dementia) who are treated at home.

Mental Health Facilities Mental health is a part of primary health care system. Actual treatment of severe mental disorders is not available at the primary level.
Regular training of primary care professionals is not carried out in the field of mental health. A programme for training of general practitioners in depression and schizophrenia was elaborated by the Ministry of Health in 2001, but it has been implemented only partially.
There are no community care facilities for patients with mental disorders. Community-based care including sheltered homes is mainly provided by the NGOs, foundations and religious organizations. Some day care centres are available and a proportion (around 10%) of designated mental health laboratories provide ambulatory services. Geographical disparities in community services are marked (some counties do not have any outpatient facilities) and coordination between services is limited. In 2003 a programme to provide domiciliary care to elderly with mental disorders and dementia was started.

Psychiatric Beds and Professionals

Total psychiatric beds per 10 000 population	7.6
Psychiatric beds in mental hospitals per 10 000 population	5.5
Psychiatric beds in general hospitals per 10 000 population	2
Psychiatric beds in other settings per 10 000 population	0.2
Number of psychiatrists per 100 000 population	4.1
Number of neurosurgeons per 100 000 population	1
Number of psychiatric nurses per 100 000 population	8.9
Number of neurologists per 100 000 population	3
Number of psychologists per 100 000 population	4.5
Number of social workers per 100 000 population	

The territorial distribution of services is uneven. About 7% of the beds are located in day hospitals, 3.5% in secure units and about 1% are allocated for treatment of drug abuse. Some beds are also earmarked for geriatric and child and adolescent services. There are no private psychiatry hospitals. There are around 260 child and adolescent psychiatrists in the country, which forms more than one-fourth of the psychiatry workforce. Geriatric Psychiatry was recognized as a sub-speciality by the Ministry in 2001. Some psychiatrists work in private ambulatory clinics with authorization from the Ministry of Health. The Human Resources Department of the Ministry has begun the complex task of classification and categorization of medical staff employed in the mental health services. The Department in cooperation with the medical education authorities is trying to develop a training programme for psychiatrists. The profession of psychiatric nurse was officially recognized by the Ministry of Health in 2003. There are few trained social workers and occupational therapists. The practice of psychotherapy is not regulated.

Non-Governmental Organizations NGOs are involved with mental health in the country. They are mainly involved in advocacy, promotion, prevention, treatment and rehabilitation. The Romanian League for Mental Health was the first organization involved in mental health promotion. It has developed a long term programme for changing perceptions about mental health and developed models of practice. Since 2000, large media campaigns on topics like domestic violence, child abuse, stigma and discrimination, depression and anxiety problems, child and adolescent mental health problems and alcohol abuse are being implemented by NGOs, with European Union assistance. A school for psychiatric nurses was initiated in 1993 by NGOs from Romania and Belgium. More than 250 nurses have already graduated from this school. In 2002, the first user organization was established, but the user/carer movement is not strong at present.

Information Gathering System There is mental health reporting system in the country. The health reporting system is based on ICD-10. The country has no data collection system or epidemiological study on mental health.

Programmes for Special Population The country has specific programmes for mental health for minorities, refugees, disaster affected population, indigenous population, elderly and children. Mental health services are provided for the populations mentioned above, but they are insufficient.
At least 1-2 physicians specialized in child neuropsychiatry are posted in each region. The labour and social protection department and the education department also provide special schools and homes for mentally challenged and delinquent children and adolescents. However, many of these services are understaffed or staffed by under-qualified personnel and are handicapped by lack of complementary services. NGOs are also active in this sector and provide social assistance for street children and abandoned, neglected and abused children.

Therapeutic Drugs The following therapeutic drugs are generally available at the primary health care level of the country: carbamazepine, ethosuximide, phenobarbital, phenytoin sodium, amitriptyline, chlorpromazine, diazepam, fluphenazine, haloperidol, lithium, carbidopa, levodopa.
Though a number of newer psychotropics have been included, they are not easily available at primary level.

Other Information A mental health audit for Romania was organized by the WHO Regional Office for Europe together with the Romanian Ministry of Health, WHO Liaison Office for Romania and the Romanian League for Mental Health.

Additional Sources of Information

Assessment of the mental health situation in Romania.

Berlescu, M. E., Pricop, F., Butureanu, S., et al (1995) The psycho-relational aspects of the psychopathological dynamics and profile in postpartum mental disorders in the county of Iasi in 1988-1993. Revista Medico-Chirurgicala a Societatii de Medici Si Naturalisti Din Iasi, 99, 63-69.

Grecu, G., Grecu-Gabos, M., Grecu-Gabos, I. (1990) Observations on deaths in alcoholism. Revista de Medicina-Interna, Neurologie, Psihiatrie, Neurochirurgie, Dermato-Venerologie – Neurologie, Psihiatrie, Neurochirurgie, 35, 41-50.

Iftene, F., Siserman, C., Siserman, A., et al. (2000) The juvenile delinquency in the transition period in the district of Cluj. Romanian Journal of Legal Medicine, 8, 367-373.

Indredavik, M. S., Skranes, J., Skranes, J., et al (1991) Assistance work in Romania. A multidisciplinary study of institutionalized children. Tidsskrift for Den Norske Laegeforening, 111, 2109-2113.

Ionescu, R., Popescu, C. (1989) Personality disorders in students with depressive pathology. Neurologie et Psychiatrie, 27, 45-55.

Kaler, S. R., Freeman, B. J. (1994) Analysis of environmental deprivation: cognitive and social development in Romanian orphans. Journal of Child Psychology & Psychiatry & Allied Disciplines, 35, 769-781.

Lupu, V., Onaca, E., Lupu, D. (2002) The prevalence of pathological gambling in Romanian teenagers. Minerva Medica, 93, 413-418.

Makinen, I. H. (2000) Suicide mortality in the Eastern European transition. Sociologisk Forskning, 37, 180-209.

Ministerul Sanatatii. Program de Sanatate.

Mircea, T. (1999) Child and adolescent psychiatry in Romania. In: H. Remschmidt, H. van Engeland (Eds). Child and Adolescent Psychiatry in Europe. Historical Development, Current Situation and Future Perspectives. Darmstadt, Steinkopff. pp261-270.

Pluye, P., Lehingue, Y., Aussilloux, C., et al. (2001) Child out of home care in Romania: mental and behavioural disorders. Sante, 11, 5-12.

Scripcaru, G., Pirozynski, T., Astarastoae, V., et al (1991) Sociopathy: genesis and development. Revista Medico-Chirurgicala a Societatii de Medici Si Naturalisti Din Iasi, 95, 49-51.

Tataru, N. (2004) Psychiatry and geriatric psychiatry in Romania. International Psychiatry (in press).

Voracek, M., Vintila, M., Fisher, M.L., et al (2002) Evidence for lack of change in seasonality of suicide from Timis County, Romania. Perceptual & Motor Skills, 94, 1071-1078.

Russian Federation

GENERAL INFORMATION

Russian Federation is a country with an approximate area of 17075 thousand sq. km. (UNO, 2001). Its population is 142.397 million, and the sex ratio (men per hundred women) is 88 (UNO, 2004). The proportion of population under the age of 15 years is 15% (UNO, 2004), and the proportion of population above the age of 60 years is 18% (WHO, 2004). The literacy rate is 99.7% for men and 99.5% for women (UNESCO/MoH, 2004).

The country is a lower middle income group country (based on World Bank 2004 criteria). The proportion of health budget to GDP is 5.4%. The per capita total expenditure on health is 454 international $, and the per capita government expenditure on health is 310 international $ (WHO, 2004).

The main language(s) used in the country is (are) Russian. The largest ethnic group(s) is (are) Russian. The largest religious group(s) is (are) Russian Orthodox (three-fourths), and the other religious group(s) are (is) Muslim.

The life expectancy at birth is 58.3 years for males and 71.8 years for females (WHO, 2004). The healthy life expectancy at birth is 53 years for males and 64 years for females (WHO, 2004).

EPIDEMIOLOGY

Bogdan (1998) found the prevalence of borderline minor psychiatric disorders in primary care samples to vary between 1.7% and 21%. Gavrilova and Kalyn (2002) identified psychiatric disorders (ICD-10 diagnoses) in 36.6% (6.1% psychotic disorders) of a sample of elderly subjects (n=1109). Bobak et al (1999) interviewed 1599 adults and found that 10% of men and 2% of women drank alcohol several times a week. Alcohol consumption was associated with smoking, unmarried status, unemployment and poor health among men. In women, higher education, widowed status, not smoking and poor health was associated with less alcohol consumption. Malyutina et al (2001) assessed about 3000 subjects in 1985/86 and 1994/95 and found that the proportion of men who drank at least once a week increased from 27% to 38% and among women from 0.6% to 6.5%. Lisenko and Richards (1994) found that alcohol dependence/alcoholic psychosis rates in Siberia and the Far East increased from 20/10 000 in 1965 to 250/10 000 in 1985. Gafarov and Gagulin (2000) found a reduction in smoking in a representative sample of urban adult males (about 700) who were assessed at two points in time in the 1990s. In a sample of 7093 students, Rozenfel'd and Kharisova (1990) found the following prevalence rates for use of various substances: alcohol (49.4%), tobacco (24.2%) and illicit drugs (9.8%). In a sample of 385 adolescents, Kemppainen et al (2002) reported that 29% of males and 7% of females smoked daily. Dershem (1996) administered the Centre for Epidemiological Studies – Depression scale (CES-D) to 263 rural subjects. Prevalence of depression was associated with age (elderly), gender (women), health (poor) and marital status (divorced/separated). Herrman et al (2002) reported the findings of the multi-country Longitudinal Investigation of Depression Outcomes (LIDO) study in which primary care subjects (n=18 489) were assessed using the Center for Epidemiologic Studies Depression Scale (cut-off 15/16). Nearly 37% (range 24-55% at different sites) met the criterion for caseness. As a part of the same study, Simon et al (2002) interviewed 968 depressed patients using the Composite International Diagnostic Interview and CES-D at baseline and 9 months. In this period only one third of patients had complete remission. Those with favourable outcome reported less work disability. Maksimova et al (1997) assessed 4000 people and found that the incidence of sleep disorders was about 30% in different regions of Russia. The rate varied from 5% in the 20-24 years age group to 40% in the elderly (above 60 years). Bogoyavlenskiy (2002) and Varnik et al (1998) reported that in the 1980s and 1990s the rate of suicide in Russia was among the highest in the world. Suicide rates were higher among men and had two peaks (at 50 and 70 years). In women, suicide rates increased after 70 years of age. Varnik and Wasserman (1992) reported that the overall rates of suicide in the former USSR increased from 17.1 per 10 0000 inhabitants in 1965 to 29.6 in 1984. Rates were higher in the rural areas. The rate of suicide in the year 2002 was 38.6 per 100 000 population (Goscomstat of Russian Federation, 2004). Voitsekhovich and Red'ko (1996) found that the rate of suicide was associated with gender (male), age (over 60 years), marital status (divorced and widowed), isolation, occupation (temporary), illnesses (mental and alcohol use disorders) and disability. Analyses of trends in suicide rate have shown marked regional variation across the republics of the former USSR and the regions within the Russian Federation and an increase in the number of suicides in Russia over every decade of the 20th century with a sharp dip (almost by a third for men and a fifth for women) during the perestroika period in the late 1980s (Varnik & Wasserman 1992; Varnik et al, 1998; Bogoyavlenskiy, 2002). Varnik and Wasserman (1992) noted that the rate of suicide was low in regions with traditional lifestyles and strong family relationships (the Caucasus and Central Asia) and high in regions facing major sociopolitical changes (Baltic States and Russia). Burdeinyi et al (1991) evaluated 1179 rural children (7-14 years) and found mental deficiency in 5.7% of boys and 3.9% of girls in the highlands and 3.6% of boys and 2.1% of girls in lowlands. Neurotic disorders were common in all the subgroups (1.6% to 4.7%), and boys had a higher rate of overall psychiatric morbidity. Knyazev et al (2002) found that behavioural problems and school adjustment were associated in a study on 446 Russian adolescents (12-16 years).

MENTAL HEALTH RESOURCES

Mental Health Policy A mental health policy is present. The policy was initially formulated in 1992.
The components of the policy are promotion, prevention, treatment and rehabilitation. The mental health policy is developed by the Ministry of Health in the form of statements/orders to be carried out by the governmental and non-governmental bodies.

Substance Abuse Policy A substance abuse policy is present. The policy was initially formulated in 1995. The substance abuse policy is developed by the Ministry of Health in the form of statements/orders to be carried out by the governmental and non-governmental bodies.

National Mental Health Programme A national mental health programme is present. The programme was formulated in 1995. The programme exists on sectoral level (in charge of the Ministry of Health). A national mental health programme for 1995-1997 was adopted by the Government and methodical recommendations on structural reorganization in psychiatric care were developed but the funds allotted to it were limited. At present a mid-term programme for 2005-2008 to introduce the above recommendations into practice is under preparation. Regional mental health programmes have been developed in several regions.

National Therapeutic Drug Policy/Essential List of Drugs A national therapeutic drug policy/essential list of drugs is present. It was formulated in 1993.
The order of the Ministry of Health is considerably renewed.

Mental Health Legislation The Law of Russian Federation on Psychiatric Assistance and Rights of Patients provides details about the rights of psychiatrists and patients regarding examination, ethics, types of services, patients' rights, social protection of the mentally ill, admission and discharge procedures and monitoring facilities. In 1999, many new additions and changes were made to the existing law and presented to the Government for further consideration and adoption in the Parliament. Forensic psychiatry is regulated by the following laws – Criminal Code, Criminal-legal Code, Civil-legal Code and two documents, 'The instruction for the forensic psychiatric assessment in the USSR' and 'The regulation concerning the outpatient forensic psychiatric expert commission. New laws have been proposed. The concept of limited responsibility has been introduced by the Criminal Code of 1997. From 2004, the Law of Psychiatric Care is the part of the Principles of Legislation of Health Protection of Citizens (of 22.07.1993 No. 5487-1 in version of 22.08.2004 No. 22).
The latest legislation was enacted in 1992.

Mental Health Financing There are no budget allocations for mental health.
Details about expenditure on mental health are not available.
The primary source of mental health financing is tax based.
State psychiatric service on the whole is funded by the state, but is not covered by the obligatory state insurance. Regional (Municipal) financial support is an additional resource for psychiatric institutions. The programme of State Guaranties is the basis of free medication for disabled mentally ill, those admitted in hospitals, and for people suffering from schizophrenia and epilepsy. But the list of free medicines for outpatients is limited to inexpensive medicines.
The country has disability benefits for persons with mental disorders. Monetary assistance is allocated from the Ministry of Social Assistance's budget.

Mental Health Facilities Mental health is a part of primary health care system. Actual treatment of severe mental disorders is not available at the primary level. The practice of recognition and treatment of depression in primary care is developing in several regions.
Regular training of primary care professionals is carried out in the field of mental health. In the last two years, about 720 personnel were provided training.
There are community care facilities for patients with mental disorders. A social rehabilitation system including workshops, rehabilitation units in industrial firms and residential homes (for about 125 000 persons) exists. Day care facilities are available for almost 15 000 persons. Home care is also provided in some cases. The University of Calgary and the Moscow Research Institute of Psychiatry have collaborated to develop two projects "Community Mental Health Rehabilitation" and "Russia Mental Health System Reform". The first project trained trainers for community care, developed curricula for community mental health care, led to some policy changes and initiated the process of creating a parent support organization. The second project helped in the development of support for consumer organizations, rehabilitation centres and vocational training centres and training of human resources. Russian Orthodox church also provides some services particularly in the drug abuse field. Some churches have opened in large psychiatric hospitals in St. Petersburg.

Psychiatric Beds and Professionals

Total psychiatric beds per 10 000 population	11.5
Psychiatric beds in mental hospitals per 10 000 population	10.1
Psychiatric beds in general hospitals per 10 000 population	0.5
Psychiatric beds in other settings per 10 000 population	1
Number of psychiatrists per 100 000 population	13.3
Number of neurosurgeons per 100 000 population	1.7
Number of psychiatric nurses per 100 000 population	50
Number of neurologists per 100 000 population	1.58
Number of psychologists per 100 000 population	1.9
Number of social workers per 100 000 population	1.2

The system of Russian Ministry of Health consists of 278 mental hospitals, 164 psycho-neurological outpatient clinics (dispensaries) that include day-hospitals as separate wards in their structure (each dispensary provides sectorized coverage to a population of approximately 25 000 people); 2010 psychoneurological consulting rooms in rural areas; 1117 psychotherapeutic rooms, mostly in primary care facilities. There are also beds in 442 hostels, nursing homes and 'internats' under the authority of the Ministry of Social Protection. There is a 10-fold variation in the availability of beds in different regions (minimum – Altai, maximum – Kostroma). About 6% of beds have been allocated to child and adolescent mental health services. Three types of forensic units are available under the Ministry of Health, which differ according to the security level. Besides these, psychiatric hospitals managed by the Ministry of Justice also exist within the correctional system for treatment of inmates suffering from minor or temporary mental disorders. More than half of psychiatrists work in outpatient services. The territorial unevenness in professional manpower is almost 10-fold between Ingush republic and Moscow. The Code of Professional Ethics of the Russian Society of Psychiatrists, which is influenced by international conventions was adopted in 1994. Most mental health care psychologists work at specialized health facilities at companies or professional unions. Every 5 years a psychologist must undergo CME courses for 144 to 288 hours. Psychologists do not have prescription privileges. Salaries are very low, e.g. a physician gets the equivalent of $50 to $200 per month.

Non-Governmental Organizations NGOs are involved with mental health in the country. They are mainly involved in advocacy, promotion, prevention and rehabilitation. About 10 NGOs are dealing with mental health in the country. Social support is also provided by religious organizations (e.g. Russian Orthodox Church). The volume of care rendered by the organizations of care consumers themselves, acting mainly at regional levels, has increased (in approximately 20 regions).

Information Gathering System There is mental health reporting system in the country.
The country has data collection system or epidemiological study on mental health. The Ministry of Health has the Unit of Statistics in the Department of Development of Medical Care. The function of this Unit is to collect information, about morbidity in the country, including mental illness.

Programmes for Special Population The country has specific programmes for mental health for refugees, disaster affected population and elderly. Programmes on refugees and disaster victims are carried out by the Ministry of Emergency Situations (EMERCOM). Elderly population are looked after by the Ministry of Social Protection.
In large dispensaries there are specialized units of geriatric psychiatry, epilepsy, sexopathology and psychotherapeutic units. Each psychiatrist for children and adolescents administers psychiatric care over the catchment area with 15 000 children. As a rule, child psychoneurological units are situated in the local child primary-care system. Narcological dispensaries and hospitals (or, less often, narcological departments in psychiatric institutions), render care for alcohol and drug abusers. Psychiatric (as well as narcological) hospitals have close connections with the dispensaries. Various programmes for the examination, support and treatment of trauma affected persons have been implemented. Care for children with mental disorders is divided into three departments: Public Health (outpatient, inpatient and day care), Education (services for mentally challenged and delinquent children) and Social Protection (about 30 000 children with severe disability including mental retardation have been provided residential facilities, vocational training is also available). Psychologists are being increasingly used in school based care. Offenders suffering from mental illness are either subjected to compulsory outpatient care in dispensaries or inpatient care in either the dispensaries or specialized hospitals with high security.

Therapeutic Drugs The following therapeutic drugs are generally available at the primary health care level of the country: carbamazepine, ethosuximide, phenobarbital, phenytoin sodium, sodium valproate, amitriptyline, chlorpromazine, diazepam, fluphenazine, haloperidol, lithium, biperiden, carbidopa, levodopa.
The Ministry of Health and Social Assistance approved the list of mentally ill who would receive free medication in 1993, the funds for which were to be allocated by local institutions.

Other Information

Additional Sources of Information

Balachova, T. N., Levy, S., Isurina, G. L., et al (2001) Medical Psychology in Russia. Journal of Clinical Psychology in Medical Settings, 8, 61-68.

Blum, R. W., Blum, L., Phillips, S., et al (1996) Adolescent health in Russia: a view from Moscow and St. Petersburg. Journal of Adolescent Health, 19, 308-314.

Bobak, M., McKee, M., Rose, R., et al (1999) Alcohol consumption in a national sample of the Russian population. Addiction, 94, 857-866.

Bogdan, M. N. (1998) The epidemiological aspect of the problem of diagnosing borderline mental disorders. Zhurnal Nevrologii i Psikhiatrii Imeni S.S. Korsakova, 98, 35-38.

Bogoyavlenskiy, D. D. (2002) Russian suicides and Russian reforms. Sotsiologicheskie Issledovaniya, 28, 76-80.

Burdeinyi, A. F., Krasnopol'skaia, I. I., Burdelnyi, V. A., et al (1991) Mental health of children living in rural high- and low-altitude areas of the Ivano-Frankovsk district (clinico-epidemiological study). Zhurnal Nevropatologii i Psikhiatrii Imeni S-S-Korsakova, 91, 85-87.

Community Rehabilitation and Disability Studies (2002). http://www.crds.org/regional/russia

Dershem, L. D., Patsiorkovski, V. V., O'Brien, D. (1996) The use of the CES-D for measuring symptoms of depression in three rural Russian villages. Social Indicators Research, 39, 89-108.

Gafarov, V. V., Gagulin, I. V. (2000) Population study of ischemic heart disease socio-psychological risk factors in male population of Novosibirsk. Terapevticheskii Arkhiv, 72, 40-43.

Gavrilova, S. I., Kalyn, I.B. (2002) Social and environmental factors and mental health in the elderly. Vestnik Rossiiskoi Akademii Meditsinskikh Nauk, 9, 15-20.

Goscomstat of Russian Federation, State Committee of Statistics of Russian Federation (2004).

Herrman, H., Patrick, D. L., Diehr, P., et al (2002) Longitudinal investigation of depression outcomes in primary care in six countries: the LIDO study. Functional status, health service use and treatment of people with depressive symptoms. Psychological Medicine, 32, 889-902.

Kemppainen, U., Tossavainen, K., Vartiainen, E., et al (2002) Smoking patterns among ninth-grade adolescents in the Pitkaranta district (Russia) and in eastern Finland. Public Health Nursing, 19, 30-39.

Kinsey, D. (1994) The new Russian law on psychiatric care. Perspectives in Psychiatric Care, 30, 15-19.

Knyazev, G. G., Slobodskaya, H. R., Safronova, M. V., et al (2002) School adjustment and health in Russian adolescents. Psychology Health & Medicine, 7, 143-155.

Krasnov, V. N. (1998) The provision of mental health care in the Russian Federation. In: Manage or Perish? The challenges of managed mental health care in Europe. J. Guimon, N Sartorius (Eds). NY: Kluwer. pp. 173-180.

Lisenko, V. P., Richards, B. (1994) Substance abuse problems in the Magadan Region of the Russian Far East. Alaska Medicine, 36, 168-172.

Makarov, I. V., Rubina, L. P. (2002) Mental disorders in hospitalized children. Problemy Sotsialnoi Gigieny i Istoriia Meditsiny, 5, 16-18.

Maksimova, T. M., Romanov, A. I., Kakorina, E. P., et al (1997) Social-hygienic evaluation of the prevalence of sleep disorders. Problemy Sotsialnoi Gigieny i Istoriia Meditsiny, 6, 14-17.

Malyutina, S., Bobak, M., Kurilovitch, S., et al (2001) Alcohol consumption and binge drinking in Novosibirsk, Russia, 1985-95. Addiction, 987-995.

Polubinskaya, S. V., Bonnie, R. J. (1996) The Code of Professional Ethics of the Russian Society of Psychiatrists. International Journal of Law and Psychiatry, 19, 143-172.

Poloshij, B., Saposhnikova, I. (2001) Psychiatric reform in Russia. Acta Psychiatrica Scandinavica, 104 (suppl. 410), 56-62.

Polubinskaya, S.V. (2000) Reform in Psychiatry in Post-Soviet Countries. Acta Psychiatrica Scandanavia, Supplementum. 101 (Supplementum 399), 106-108.

Rozenfel'd, L. G., Kharisova, I. M. (1990) Complex analysis of a sociological study of harmful habits among college students. Sovetskoe Zdravookhranenie, 11, 35-38.

Ruchkin, V. V. (2000). The forensic psychiatric system of Russia. International Journal of Law and Psychiatry, 23, 555-565.

Severny, A. A., Shevchenko, Y. S., Kazakovtsev, B. A., et al (1999) Child and adolescent psychiatry in Russia. In: H. Remschmidt, H. van Engeland, H. (Eds). Child and Adolescent Psychiatry in Europe. Historical Development, Current Situation and Future Perspectives. Darmstadt, Steinkopff. pp271-284.

Simon, G. E., Chisholm, D., Treglia, M., et al (2002) Course of depression, health services costs, and work productivity in an international primary care study. General Hospital Psychiatry, 24, 328-335.

Varnik, A., Wasserman, D. (1992) Suicides in the former Soviet republics. Acta Psychiatrica Scandinavica, 86, 76-78.

Varnik, A., Wasserman, D., Dankowicz, M., et al (1998) Age-specific suicide rates in the Slavic and Baltic regions of the former USSR during perestroika, in comparison with 22 European countries. Acta Psychiatrica Scandinavica, Supplement 394, 20-25.

Voitsekhovich, B. A., Red'ko, A. N. (1996) Suicide from the standpoint of social medicine. Problemy Sotsialnoi Gigieny i Istoriia Meditsiny, 216-219.

Wasserman, D., Varnik, A., Dankowicz, M. (1998) Regional differences in the distribution of suicide in the former Soviet Union during perestroika, 1984-1990. Acta Psychiatrica Scandinavica, Supplement 394, 5-12.

Rwanda

GENERAL INFORMATION

Rwanda is a country with an approximate area of 26 thousand sq. km. (UNO, 2001). Its population is 8.481 million, and the sex ratio (men per hundred women) is 91 (UNO, 2004). The proportion of population under the age of 15 years is 45% (UNO, 2004), and the proportion of population above the age of 60 years is 4% (WHO, 2004). The literacy rate is 75.3% for men and 63.4% for women (UNESCO/MoH, 2004).

The country is a low income group country (based on World Bank 2004 criteria). The proportion of health budget to GDP is 5.5%. The per capita total expenditure on health is 44 international $, and the per capita government expenditure on health is 24 international $ (WHO, 2004).

The main language(s) used in the country is (are) Kinyarwanda, French, English and Swahili. The largest religious group(s) is (are) Roman Catholic, and the other religious group(s) are (is) Protestant and Muslim.

The life expectancy at birth is 41.9 years for males and 46.8 years for females (WHO, 2004). The healthy life expectancy at birth is 36 years for males and 40 years for females (WHO, 2004).

EPIDEMIOLOGY

There is a paucity of epidemiological data on mental illnesses in Rwanda in internationally accessible literature. Bolton et al (2002) estimated the prevalence of major depressive disorder among Rwandans 5 years after a civil war. They interviewed a random sample of 368 adults living in a rural community with the Hopkins Symptom Checklist and a locally developed functional impairment instrument. Using DSM-IV criteria they found that 15.5% met Criteria A, C, and E for current major depression. Depressive symptoms were strongly associated with functional impairment in most major roles for men and women. The authors conclude that a significant part of this population has seriously disabling depression. Keogh et al (1994) interviewed a group of 55 HIV infected women in 1988 and again in 1991 and found some differences in needs for services and noticed an increased acceptance by families of the status of the patient.

MENTAL HEALTH RESOURCES

Mental Health Policy A mental health policy is present. The policy was initially formulated in 1995.
The components of the policy are advocacy, promotion, prevention and treatment.

Substance Abuse Policy A substance abuse policy is present. The policy was initially formulated in 1995.

National Mental Health Programme A national mental health programme is present. The programme was formulated in 1995.

National Therapeutic Drug Policy/Essential List of Drugs A national therapeutic drug policy/essential list of drugs is present. It was formulated in 2000.

Mental Health Legislation The draft of the mental health legislation is being prepared with WHO's support.
Details about the year of enactment of the mental health legislation are not available.

Mental Health Financing There are budget allocations for mental health.
The country spends 1% of the total health budget on mental health.
The primary sources of mental health financing in descending order are private insurances, social insurance, out of pocket expenditure by the patient or family and tax based.
The country does not have disability benefits for persons with mental disorders.

Mental Health Facilities Mental health is a part of primary health care system. Actual treatment of severe mental disorders is available at the primary level. At the primary care level, the patients are diagnosed, referred and followed up.
Regular training of primary care professionals is carried out in the field of mental health. In the last two years, about 60 personnel were provided training.
There are community care facilities for patients with mental disorders. Motivating staff to work in the community and reinforcing pro-community behaviour continues to be somewhat difficult.

Psychiatric Beds and Professionals

Total psychiatric beds per 10 000 population	0.2
Psychiatric beds in mental hospitals per 10 000 population	0.2
Psychiatric beds in general hospitals per 10 000 population	0
Psychiatric beds in other settings per 10 000 population	0
Number of psychiatrists per 100 000 population	0.03
Number of neurosurgeons per 100 000 population	0.02
Number of psychiatric nurses per 100 000 population	0.8
Number of neurologists per 100 000 population	0
Number of psychologists per 100 000 population	0.3
Number of social workers per 100 000 population	0

There are 200 other mental health personnel.

Non-Governmental Organizations NGOs are involved with mental health in the country. They are mainly involved in advocacy, promotion, prevention and rehabilitation.

Information Gathering System There is no mental health reporting system in the country.
The country has data collection system or epidemiological study on mental health. The district hospitals send quarterly reports to the central level.

Programmes for Special Population There are no special services available.

Therapeutic Drugs The following therapeutic drugs are generally available at the primary health care level of the country: carbamazepine, phenobarbital, sodium valproate, amitriptyline, chlorpromazine, diazepam, haloperidol, biperiden.

Other Information Rwanda's mental health delivery system is a tiered set-up. At the bottom are the community workers and health centres, followed by the district hospitals with capabilities to manage mental disorders. The third tier is formed by different speciality hospitals like the Ndera which is the main neuropsychiatric set-up.

N–R

Additional Sources of Information

Bolton, P., Neugebauer, R., Ndogoni, L. (2002) Prevalence of depression in rural Rwanda based on symptom and functional criteria. Journal of Nervous & Mental Disease, 190, 631-637.

Gatarayiha, F., Baro, F., Wagenfeld, M.O. et al (1991) The development of mental health services in Sub-Saharan Africa: the case of Rwanda. Journal of Sociology & Social Welfare, 18, 25-40.

Keogh, P., Allen, S., Almedal, C., et al (1994) The social impact of HIV infection on women in Kigali, Rwanda: a prospective study. Social Science & Medicine, 38, 1047-1053.

Mental Health Policy. (Government document).

Saint Kitts and Nevis*

GENERAL INFORMATION

Saint Kitts and Nevis is a country with an approximate area of 0.36 thousand sq. km. (UNO, 2001). Its population is 0.046 million, and the sex ratio (men per hundred women) is 99 (UNO, 2004). The proportion of population under the age of 15 years is 31% (UNO, 2004), and the proportion of population above the age of 60 years is 10% (WHO, 2004). The literacy rate is 97% for men and 98% for women (UNESCO/MoH, 2004).

The country is a higher middle income group country (based on World Bank 2004 criteria). The proportion of health budget to GDP is 4.8%. The per capita total expenditure on health is 576 international $, and the per capita government expenditure on health is 382 international $ (WHO, 2004).

The main language(s) used in the country is (are) English.

The life expectancy at birth is 68.7 years for males and 72.2 years for females (WHO, 2004). The healthy life expectancy at birth is 60 years for males and 63 years for females (WHO, 2004).

EPIDEMIOLOGY

There is a paucity of epidemiological data on mental illnesses in Saint Kitts and Nevis in internationally accessible literature.

MENTAL HEALTH RESOURCES

Mental Health Policy Details about the mental health policy are not available.

Substance Abuse Policy Details about the substance abuse policy are not available.

National Mental Health Programme Details about the national mental health programme are not available.

National Therapeutic Drug Policy/Essential List of Drugs Details about the national therapeutic drug policy/essential list of drugs are not available.

Mental Health Legislation Details about the mental health legislation are not available.

Mental Health Financing Details about disability benefits for mental health are not available.
Details about expenditure on mental health are not available.
Details about sources of financing are not available.
Details about disability benefits for mental health are not available.

Mental Health Facilities Details about mental health facilities at the primary care level are not available.
Details about training facilities are not available.
Details about community care facilities in mental health are not available.

Psychiatric Beds and Professionals

Total psychiatric beds per 10 000 population
Psychiatric beds in mental hospitals per 10 000 population
Psychiatric beds in general hospitals per 10 000 population
Psychiatric beds in other settings per 10 000 population
Number of psychiatrists per 100 000 population
Number of neurosurgeons per 100 000 population
Number of psychiatric nurses per 100 000 population
Number of neurologists per 100 000 population
Number of psychologists per 100 000 population
Number of social workers per 100 000 population

In the past, patients were kept in geriatric homes. Nowadays, the mentally ill patients receive treatment through a seven bedded psychiatric unit and a network of health centres scattered all over the islands.

Non-Governmental Organizations Details about NGO facilities in mental health are not available.

Information Gathering System Details about mental health reporting systems are not available.
Details about data collection system or epidemiological study on mental health are not available.

Programmes for Special Population Details about specific mental health programmes are not available.

Therapeutic Drugs The following therapeutic drugs are generally available at the primary health care level of the country: unknown.

Other Information * The verification of this country profile is still being awaited from the Ministry of Health of Saint Kitts and Nevis.

Additional Sources of Information

S

Saint Lucia

GENERAL INFORMATION

Saint Lucia is a country with an approximate area of 0.62 thousand sq. km. (UNO, 2001). Its population is 0.15 million, and the sex ratio (men per hundred women) is 97 (UNO, 2004). The proportion of population under the age of 15 years is 30% (UNO, 2004), and the proportion of population above the age of 60 years is 8% (WHO, 2004). The literacy rate is 65% for men and 69% for women (UNESCO/MoH, 2004).

The country is a higher middle income group country (based on World Bank 2004 criteria). The proportion of health budget to GDP is 4.5%. The per capita total expenditure on health is 272 international $, and the per capita government expenditure on health is 176 international $ (WHO, 2004).

The main language(s) used in the country is (are) English and Patois. The largest ethnic group(s) is (are) African. The largest religious group(s) is (are) Roman Catholic.

The life expectancy at birth is 69.8 years for males and 74.4 years for females (WHO, 2004). The healthy life expectancy at birth is 61 years for males and 64 years for females (WHO, 2004).

EPIDEMIOLOGY

There is a paucity of epidemiological data on mental illnesses in Saint Lucia in internationally accessible literature. Perks and Jameson (1999) assessed 60 students using the teacher-rated Revised Behaviour Problem Checklist (RBPC) and the self-rated Reynolds Child Depression Scale (RCDS) or the Reynolds Adolescent Depression Scale (RADS). Students whose parents were experiencing violent marital discord had significantly greater depression and behavioural problems. Exposed children exhibited more behavioural problems but less depressive symptomatology than adolescents.

MENTAL HEALTH RESOURCES

Mental Health Policy A mental health policy is absent.
A mental health policy is presently being developed by the Ministry of Health.

Substance Abuse Policy A substance abuse policy is absent.

National Mental Health Programme A national mental health programme is absent.

National Therapeutic Drug Policy/Essential List of Drugs A national therapeutic drug policy/essential list of drugs is present. It was formulated in 1986.

Mental Health Legislation The Mental Hospital Act is the latest legislation on mental health.
The latest legislation was enacted in 1957.

Mental Health Financing There are budget allocations for mental health.
The country spends 4% of the total health budget on mental health.
The primary source of mental health financing is tax based.
The country does not have disability benefits for persons with mental disorders. Benefits are given on a case by case basis.

Mental Health Facilities Mental health is a part of primary health care system. Actual treatment of severe mental disorders is not available at the primary level. Cases are referred to the mental health clinics.
Regular training of primary care professionals is not carried out in the field of mental health.
There are no community care facilities for patients with mental disorders. Community mental heath services are provided through four health centres. The Government of St Lucia has recently signed a tripartite agreement with the Pan American Health Organization and the UK based AMKAM Foundation to strengthen community mental health services in on the western part of the island.

Psychiatric Beds and Professionals

Total psychiatric beds per 10 000 population	10.7
Psychiatric beds in mental hospitals per 10 000 population	10.7
Psychiatric beds in general hospitals per 10 000 population	0
Psychiatric beds in other settings per 10 000 population	0
Number of psychiatrists per 100 000 population	1.9
Number of neurosurgeons per 100 000 population	
Number of psychiatric nurses per 100 000 population	2.6
Number of neurologists per 100 000 population	
Number of psychologists per 100 000 population	0
Number of social workers per 100 000 population	0.7

Mental health services are provided at the Golden Hope Hospital (Mental Health Facility) in the north of the island and at St Jude Hospital (General Hospital) in the south of the island. The services at the Golden Hope Hospital comprise clinical services inclusive of referral and intervention, assessment, domiciliary treatment and outpatient services. The adjunctive services include psychotherapy and occupational therapy. A drug rehabilitation centre provides specialized services. There are two consultant psychiatrists at the mental health facility who are responsible for the clinical services. There is one psychiatric nurse, nine registered nurses, seven nursing assistants and two occupational therapists at the facility. A consultant psychiatrist provides psychiatric services in the south of the island.

Non-Governmental Organizations NGOs are involved with mental health in the country. They are mainly involved in promotion and prevention.

Information Gathering System There is no mental health reporting system in the country.
The country has no data collection system or epidemiological study on mental health.

Programmes for Special Population The country has specific programmes for mental health for elderly and children.

Therapeutic Drugs The following therapeutic drugs are generally available at the primary health care level of the country: carbamazepine, phenobarbital, phenytoin sodium, sodium valproate, amitriptyline, chlorpromazine, diazepam, fluphenazine, haloperidol, lithium, carbidopa, levodopa.

Other Information

Additional Sources of Information

Jameson, M., Perks, S. M. (1999) The effects of witnessing domestic violence on behavioural problems and depressive symptomatology. A community sample of pupils from Saint Lucia. West Indian Medical Journal, 48, 208-11.

Perks, S. M., Jameson, M. (1999) The effects of witnessing domestic violence on behavioural problems and depressive symptomatology. A community sample of pupils from St Lucia. West Indian Medical Journal, 48, 208-211.

S

Saint Vincent and the Grenadines

GENERAL INFORMATION

Saint Vincent and the Grenadines is a country with an approximate area of 0.39 thousand sq. km. (UNO, 2001). Its population is 0.121 million, and the sex ratio (men per hundred women) is 101 (UNO, 2004). The proportion of population under the age of 15 years is 30% (UNO, 2004), and the proportion of population above the age of 60 years is 9% (WHO, 2004). The literacy rate is 96% for men and 96% for women (UNESCO/MoH, 2004).

The country is a higher middle income group country (based on World Bank 2004 criteria). The proportion of health budget to GDP is 6.1%. The per capita total expenditure on health is 358 international $, and the per capita government expenditure on health is 227 international $ (WHO, 2004).

The main language(s) used in the country is (are) English and French. The largest ethnic group(s) is (are) African, and the other ethnic group(s) are (is) European, East Indian and Carib Indian. The largest religious group(s) is (are) Anglican, and the other religious group(s) are (is) Methodist and Roman Catholic.

The life expectancy at birth is 67.8 years for males and 71.9 years for females (WHO, 2004). The healthy life expectancy at birth is 60 years for males and 62 years for females (WHO, 2004).

EPIDEMIOLOGY

There is a paucity of epidemiological data on mental illnesses in Saint Vincent and the Grenadines in internationally accessible literature.

MENTAL HEALTH RESOURCES

Mental Health Policy A mental health policy is present. The policy was initially formulated in 1998.
The components of the policy are advocacy, prevention, treatment and rehabilitation.

Substance Abuse Policy A substance abuse policy is present. The policy was initially formulated in 2000.

National Mental Health Programme A national mental health programme is present. The programme was formulated in 2000.
The mental health programme is reviewed and updated every year.

National Therapeutic Drug Policy/Essential List of Drugs A national therapeutic drug policy/essential list of drugs is present.
Details about the year of formulation are not available.

Mental Health Legislation There is an Act (No. 56), which is related to mental health.
The latest legislation was enacted in 1989.

Mental Health Financing There are budget allocations for mental health.
The country spends 4.6% of the total health budget on mental health.
The primary source of mental health financing is tax based.
The country has disability benefits for persons with mental disorders. Patients suffering from severe mental illnesses receive public disability benefits.

Mental Health Facilities Mental health is a part of primary health care system. Actual treatment of severe mental disorders is available at the primary level. District medical officers are trained to handle mental health issues and are experienced in administering psychotropic medication.
Regular training of primary care professionals is carried out in the field of mental health. In the last two years, about 25 personnel were provided training.
There are community care facilities for patients with mental disorders. Community mental health services are available in all districts. Psychiatric nurses are involved in these activities.

Psychiatric Beds and Professionals

Total psychiatric beds per 10 000 population	10.6
Psychiatric beds in mental hospitals per 10 000 population	9.7
Psychiatric beds in general hospitals per 10 000 population	0.9
Psychiatric beds in other settings per 10 000 population	0
Number of psychiatrists per 100 000 population	0.9
Number of neurosurgeons per 100 000 population	0
Number of psychiatric nurses per 100 000 population	14.2
Number of neurologists per 100 000 population	0
Number of psychologists per 100 000 population	1.8
Number of social workers per 100 000 population	2.7

Non-Governmental Organizations NGOs are involved with mental health in the country. They are mainly involved in promotion, prevention and rehabilitation.

Information Gathering System There is mental health reporting system in the country.
The country has no data collection system or epidemiological study on mental health.

Programmes for Special Population The country has specific programmes for mental health for elderly.

Therapeutic Drugs The following therapeutic drugs are generally available at the primary health care level of the country: carbamazepine, ethosuximide, phenobarbital, phenytoin sodium, sodium valproate, amitriptyline, chlorpromazine, diazepam, fluphenazine, haloperidol, lithium, carbidopa, levodopa.
Currently, only 2 children are on treatment with ethosuximide, so the drug is dispensed from the central pharmacy.

Other Information

Additional Sources of Information

Samoa

GENERAL INFORMATION

Samoa is a country with an approximate area of 3 thousand sq. km. (UNO, 2001). Its population is 0.18 million, and the sex ratio (men per hundred women) is 109 (UNO, 2004). The proportion of population under the age of 15 years is 40% (UNO, 2004), and the proportion of population above the age of 60 years is 6% (WHO, 2004). The literacy rate is 98.9% for men and 98.4% for women (UNESCO/MoH, 2004).

The country is a lower middle income group country (based on World Bank 2004 criteria). The proportion of health budget to GDP is 5.8%. The per capita total expenditure on health is 199 international $, and the per capita government expenditure on health is 164 international $ (WHO, 2004).

The main language(s) used in the country is (are) Samoan and English. The largest ethnic group(s) is (are) Samoan. The largest religious group(s) is (are) Christian.

The life expectancy at birth is 66.8 years for males and 69.7 years for females (WHO, 2004). The healthy life expectancy at birth is 59 years for males and 60 years for females (WHO, 2004).

EPIDEMIOLOGY

There is a paucity of epidemiological data on mental illnesses in Samoa in internationally accessible literature. Booth (1999) reviewed data from thirteen Pacific Island nations and showed that the Pacific countries had very high reported suicide rates. Among youth, females committed more suicide than males in Western Samoa. Paraquat ingestion was the commonest mode of self-poisoning, especially among females, in Western Samoa. Societal stresses were the commonest causal factors. Cribb (1999) ascertained variations in Western Samoan women's responses to domestic violence in three different contexts, in rural and urban Western Samoa and in New Zealand. On interviewing family, religious and community leaders and 90 women, the researchers found that social relations, changes in women's economic independence and differences in levels of formal support for battered women were probable causes for differences in women's responses to abuse in the three areas.

MENTAL HEALTH RESOURCES

Mental Health Policy A mental health policy is absent.

Substance Abuse Policy A substance abuse policy is absent. There is a felt need for developing a substance abuse policy in view of the problems being faced by the country with respect to rising alcohol and other substance used disorders.

National Mental Health Programme A national mental health programme is absent.

The need for a programme is felt acutely. It is hoped that in future, programmes would be developed incorporating treatment, prevention and promotion. It is proposed to establish a multi-sectoral, multi-disciplinary national committee on mental health as a sub-committee of the national non-communicable diseases committee. This body would have specific functions and would include suicide and alcohol and drug use related problems. The committee would include experts from the Government, non-governmental organizations, international organizations, donors, etc.

National Therapeutic Drug Policy/Essential List of Drugs A national therapeutic drug policy/essential list of drugs is present. It was formulated in 1994.

There is a drug policy approved in 2001 and awaiting an implementation plan.

Mental Health Legislation There is a mental health law. The law is based on New Zealand's mental health laws of the 1960s and needs to be updated. Mental impairment is not clearly identified in disability legislation. Substance Abuse laws and regulations are enforced mainly in relation to marijuana. The licensing of the sale of paraquat to farmers was introduced by the Ministry of Agriculture, Forestry, Fisheries and Meteorology.

The latest legislation was enacted in 1961.

Mental Health Financing There are no budget allocations for mental health.

Details about expenditure on mental health are not available.

The primary source of mental health financing is tax based.

The country does not have disability benefits for persons with mental disorders. There are no disability benefits for mental illness or disabilities.

Mental Health Facilities Mental health is a part of primary health care system. Actual treatment of severe mental disorders is available at the primary level.

Regular training of primary care professionals is not carried out in the field of mental health. However, family care givers are receiving training. Community nurses working in the field have received focused short term (3 weeks) training sessions in 1998/99. The Mental Health Unit staff provide outreach support to district health centres and the village sub-centres, working with the district nurses and doctors.

There are community care facilities for patients with mental disorders. Community mental health care is family focussed and is completely provided by nurses. The services were started during the late 80's and 90's, but they face some problems like lack of specialist psychiatrist back-up for the community staff, limited availability of medicines, uncertain policy regarding distribution of medicines by nurses, limited diagnosis, referral and follow-up for people with mental disorders, poor transportation facilities in the rural areas and absence of any alcohol and drug use related services.

Psychiatric Beds and Professionals

Total psychiatric beds per 10 000 population	0.2
Psychiatric beds in mental hospitals per 10 000 population	0
Psychiatric beds in general hospitals per 10 000 population	0
Psychiatric beds in other settings per 10 000 population	0.2
Number of psychiatrists per 100 000 population	0
Number of neurosurgeons per 100 000 population	0
Number of psychiatric nurses per 100 000 population	0.5
Number of neurologists per 100 000 population	0
Number of psychologists per 100 000 population	0
Number of social workers per 100 000 population	0

Patients can be admitted in general medical wards, under joint supervision of staff from the mental unit and the hospital ward staff. Psychiatric nursing is a component of the graduate course on nursing in Samoa. Nurses have prescription privileges.

Non-Governmental Organizations NGOs are not involved with mental health in the country. NGOs are involved in counselling and suicide awareness groups. The Traditional Healers' Organization (THO) in association with NGOs and the church provide some mental health services. The Faataua le Ola (Suicide Prevention/Awareness Group and International Lifeline) a multisectoral organization was founded in 2001 with Government support. It has a few trained counsellors. It conducts lifeline counselling, face-to-face crisis counselling, counsellor training and public education.

Information Gathering System There is mental health reporting system in the country. There was an Annual Report by the Department of Health in 1997 and 1998.
The country has data collection system or epidemiological study on mental health. A report is prepared every month and sent to the health planning and information section.
A database on suicide has been maintained since 1970 through the individual effort of Galumalemana S. Percival. The Government, with the collaboration of Inclusion International, is completing a disability census.

Programmes for Special Population The country has specific programmes for mental health for indigenous population, elderly and children. There are programmes to look after dementias in elderly and mental retardation and developmental problems in children and also victims of abuse and suicide.
It is proposed that school mental health programmes should be developed. There are programmes for awareness of epilepsy. Related Government departments, Village Council of Chiefs, NGOs and Churches address issues of substance abuse. A youth suicide prevention campaign was launched by the National University of Samoa in 2001 with support of donor agencies.

Therapeutic Drugs The following therapeutic drugs are generally available at the primary health care level of the country: carbamazepine, ethosuximide, phenobarbital, phenytoin sodium, sodium valproate, amitriptyline, chlorpromazine, diazepam, fluphenazine, haloperidol, lithium, carbidopa, levodopa.
The supply of drugs is not uniform.

Other Information Samoa is the first country in the Western Pacific Region that has shown interest in starting a mental health promotion programme. This programme would be linked to other prevention programmes for suicide and programmes aimed at reducing stigma and discrimination against mental illness.

Additional Sources of Information

Booth, H. (1999) Pacific Island suicide in comparative perspective. Journal of Biosocial Science, 31, 433-448.

Cribb, J. (1999) Being bashed: Western Samoan women's responses to domestic violence in Western Samoa and New Zealand. Gender, Place & Culture, 6, 49-65.

S

San Marino

GENERAL INFORMATION

San Marino is a country with an approximate area of 0.06 thousand sq. km. (UNO, 2001). Its population is 0.027 million, and the sex ratio (men per hundred women) is 96 (UNO, 2004). The proportion of population under the age of 15 years is 15% (UNO, 2004), and the proportion of population above the age of 60 years is 24% (WHO, 2004). The literacy rate is 97% for men and 95% for women (UNESCO/MoH, 2004).

The country is a high income group country (based on World Bank 2004 criteria). The proportion of health budget to GDP is 6.8%. The per capita total expenditure on health is 1711 international $, and the per capita government expenditure on health is 1334 international $ (WHO, 2004).

The main language(s) used in the country is (are) Italian. The largest ethnic group(s) is (are) Sammarinese and Italian. The largest religious group(s) is (are) Roman Catholic.

The life expectancy at birth is 77.2 years for males and 84 years for females (WHO, 2004). The healthy life expectancy at birth is 71 years for males and 76 years for females (WHO, 2004).

EPIDEMIOLOGY

There is substantial epidemiological data on mental illnesses in San Marino in internationally accessible literature. No attempt was made to include this information here.

MENTAL HEALTH RESOURCES

Mental Health Policy A mental health policy is absent.
The Republic of San Marino refers to the EU guidelines.

Substance Abuse Policy A substance abuse policy is absent. The Republic of San Marino refers to the EU guidelines.

National Mental Health Programme A national mental health programme is absent.

National Therapeutic Drug Policy/Essential List of Drugs A national therapeutic drug policy/essential list of drugs is absent.
The Republic of San Marino refers to the EU guidelines.

Mental Health Legislation The current mental health legislation is being updated. A mixed commission, made up of judges and psychiatrists, is working to adapt the present legislation on mental health to new needs of both the citizens and the services. In particular, the aim is to reconciliate the demands of individual freedom and liberty of choice with the need for intervention in the care of mental disorder. A further matter of great relevance here is to respect patients' privacy.
Details about the year of enactment of the mental health legislation are not available.

Mental Health Financing There are no budget allocations for mental health.
Details about expenditure on mental health are not available.
The primary source of mental health financing is tax based.
The country has disability benefits for persons with mental disorders. There is a possibility to obtain both economic benefits and a job with the public administration.

Mental Health Facilities Mental health is a part of primary health care system. Actual treatment of severe mental disorders is available at the primary level.
Regular training of primary care professionals is not carried out in the field of mental health.
There are community care facilities for patients with mental disorders. The mental health service is the only agency dealing with mental health. It is a multidisciplinary service and is based on the teamwork of psychiatrists, psychologists, social workers and nurses. Health and social care services are offered both at centres and in the patients' homes, schools and places of work.

Psychiatric Beds and Professionals

Total psychiatric beds per 10 000 population	3.8
Psychiatric beds in mental hospitals per 10 000 population	0
Psychiatric beds in general hospitals per 10 000 population	3.8
Psychiatric beds in other settings per 10 000 population	0
Number of psychiatrists per 100 000 population	15
Number of neurosurgeons per 100 000 population	0
Number of psychiatric nurses per 100 000 population	0
Number of neurologists per 100 000 population	19
Number of psychologists per 100 000 population	96
Number of social workers per 100 000 population	54

In 1969, the Neuro-Psychiatric Service (SNP) was created and in 1977 became part of the social services. The SNP or neuropsychiatric service is made up of psychiatrists, psychologists, neurologists, social workers, nurses, technicians of electrophysiology and a secretary. In 1980, a section dealing with alcohol-related problems and drug abuse was created within the SNP. Since there is no psychiatric department in the hospital, psychiatric admissions go to the department of general medicine or, if necessary, to an Italian psychiatric clinic.

Non-Governmental Organizations NGOs are not involved with mental health in the country.

Information Gathering System There is mental health reporting system in the country.
The country has data collection system or epidemiological study on mental health. The system is conducted by the neuropsychiatric services.

Programmes for Special Population The country has specific programmes for mental health for elderly and children.

Therapeutic Drugs The following therapeutic drugs are generally available at the primary health care level of the country: carbamazepine, ethosuximide, phenobarbital, phenytoin sodium, sodium valproate, amitriptyline, chlorpromazine, diazepam, fluphenazine, haloperidol, lithium, biperiden, carbidopa, levodopa.
All the drugs are provided free of cost by the Government at the primary care level.

Other Information The three matters of both concern and progress in San Marino are considered to be: destigmatization and social prejudice towards mental illness, improving the relationship between the mental health service and other structures, better collaboration between the mental health service, schools and the political and judicial spheres.

Additional Sources of Information

S

Sao Tome and Principe

GENERAL INFORMATION

Sao Tome and Principe is a country with an approximate area of 1 thousand sq. km. (UNO, 2001). Its population is 0.164 million, and the sex ratio (men per hundred women) is 98 (UNO, 2004). The proportion of population under the age of 15 years is 41% (UNO, 2004), and the proportion of population above the age of 60 years is 6% (WHO, 2004). The literacy rate is 85% for men and 62% for women (UNESCO/MoH, 2004).

The country is a low income group country (based on World Bank 2004 criteria). The proportion of health budget to GDP is 2.3%. The per capita total expenditure on health is 22 international $, and the per capita government expenditure on health is 15 international $ (WHO, 2004).

The main language(s) used in the country is (are) Portuguese. The largest ethnic group(s) is (are) Foro and Angolare, and the other ethnic group(s) are (is) Minuye and Capeverdins. The largest religious group(s) is (are) Roman Catholic.

The life expectancy at birth is 61.7 years for males and 63.6 years for females (WHO, 2004). The healthy life expectancy at birth is 54 years for males and 55 years for females (WHO, 2004).

EPIDEMIOLOGY

There is a paucity of epidemiological data on mental illnesses in Sao Tome and Principe in internationally accessible literature.

MENTAL HEALTH RESOURCES

Mental Health Policy A mental health policy is absent.

Substance Abuse Policy A substance abuse policy is absent.

National Mental Health Programme A national mental health programme is present. The programme was formulated in 1993.

National Therapeutic Drug Policy/Essential List of Drugs A national therapeutic drug policy/essential list of drugs is present. It was formulated in 2000.

Mental Health Legislation The latest legislation was enacted in 1963.

Mental Health Financing There are budget allocations for mental health.
Details about expenditure on mental health are not available.
The primary source of mental health financing is tax based.
The country has disability benefits for persons with mental disorders.

Mental Health Facilities Mental health is a part of primary health care system. Actual treatment of severe mental disorders is available at the primary level.
Regular training of primary care professionals is not carried out in the field of mental health.
There are no community care facilities for patients with mental disorders.

Psychiatric Beds and Professionals

Total psychiatric beds per 10 000 population	2.2
Psychiatric beds in mental hospitals per 10 000 population	0
Psychiatric beds in general hospitals per 10 000 population	2.2
Psychiatric beds in other settings per 10 000 population	0
Number of psychiatrists per 100 000 population	0
Number of neurosurgeons per 100 000 population	1
Number of psychiatric nurses per 100 000 population	0.3
Number of neurologists per 100 000 population	0
Number of psychologists per 100 000 population	3
Number of social workers per 100 000 population	0.001

Non-Governmental Organizations NGOs are involved with mental health in the country. They are mainly involved in promotion and prevention.

Information Gathering System There is no mental health reporting system in the country.
The country has data collection system or epidemiological study on mental health.

Programmes for Special Population There are no special services.

Therapeutic Drugs The following therapeutic drugs are generally available at the primary health care level of the country: phenobarbital, phenytoin sodium, amitriptyline, chlorpromazine, diazepam, haloperidol.

Other Information

Additional Sources of Information

S

Saudi Arabia

GENERAL INFORMATION

Saudi Arabia is a country with an approximate area of 2150 thousand sq. km. (UNO, 2001). Its population is 24.919 million, and the sex ratio (men per hundred women) is 116 (UNO, 2004). The proportion of population under the age of 15 years is 39% (UNO, 2004), and the proportion of population above the age of 60 years is 4% (WHO, 2004). The literacy rate is 84.1% for men and 69.5% for women (UNESCO/MoH, 2004).

The country is a higher middle income group country (based on World Bank 2004 criteria). The proportion of health budget to GDP is 4.6%. The per capita total expenditure on health is 591 international $, and the per capita government expenditure on health is 441 international $ (WHO, 2004).

The main language(s) used in the country is (are) Arabic and English. The largest ethnic group(s) is (are) Arab, and the other ethnic group(s) are (is) Afro-Asian. The largest religious group(s) is (are) Muslim.

The life expectancy at birth is 68.4 years for males and 73.9 years for females (WHO, 2004). The healthy life expectancy at birth is 60 years for males and 63 years for females (WHO, 2004).

EPIDEMIOLOGY

Al-Khatami and Ogbeide (2002) evaluated 609 adults, selected randomly from a family and community clinic at an Armed Forces hospital, using the Rahim Anxiety-Depression Scale. The prevalence of minor mental morbidity was 18.2% (women: 22.2%, men: 13.7%). Rates were higher among the young (15-29 years: 23.2%), divorcees and widows (more than 40%) and among those suffering from bronchial asthma (28.3%). El Rufaie et al (1999) estimated the prevalence of somatized mental disorder (SMD) and psychologized mental disorder (PMD) in a sample of primary health care patients using the 12-item General Health Questionnaire and the Clinical Interview Schedule. SMD and PMD constituted 48% and 42% of those identified with a psychiatric disorder, respectively. The estimated prevalence rate of SMD was 12% and it was associated with less education and less severe disorders. The most common ICD-10 psychiatric diagnoses among both the groups were mixed anxiety and depressive disorder, generalized anxiety disorder and mood and adjustment disorders. Recurrent depressive disorder and dysthymia were significantly more prevalent in the PMD group. El-Rufaie et al (1988) used the Arabic version of the Hospital Anxiety and Depression Scale (HAD) in primary care patients and found the prevalence rate of depression and anxiety to be 26% (17% had depression and 16% had anxiety). The rate of depression was higher among females and that of anxiety among males. Al-Shammari and Al-Subaie (1999) assessed 7970 elderly (above 60 years) subjects who were selected from primary health care in five administrative regions by a stratified two-stage sampling procedure using the Geriatric Depression Scale (GDS) and clinical evaluation. Depressive symptoms were reported by 39%, with 8.4% having severe depression. Depression was associated with gender (female), education (low), unemployment, marital status (divorced or widowed), locality (rural), housing arrangements (poor), isolation, financial constraints, life events (loss), participation in recreational activities (limited), medical illness (especially faecal or urinary incontinence), medication, perception of poor health and dependence on others for daily activities. Elfawal (1999) reviewed hospital data on suicides and estimated its prevalence to be 1.1/100 000 population. It was associated with gender (male:female ratio was 4.5:1), age (30 to 39 years: 44.3%), ethnicity (all immigrants: 77%, Indians: 43%). The most common means of suicide were hanging (63%). Malik et al (1996) found that more than four fifths of drug overdose cases (n=57) were self-inflicted (parasuicide). Parasuicide was associated with age (more than 95% were below 40 years), ethnicity (Saudi: 89%) and gender (females: 78%). Psychiatric illnesses were diagnosed in 74.4% of cases, with depression (39.5%) and personality disorders (34.9%) being common. Abolfotouh (1997) assessed 305 schoolboys aged 8-12 years using the Rutter Children's Behaviour Questionnaire. The prevalence of behaviour disorders was 13.4% and it was associated with family size, crowding index, parents' education, birth order, parental death, social class and poor academic performance of index child. These factors jointly contributed to 12.8% of the variance in total behaviour score. However, mother's illiteracy was the only significant predictor of maladjusted children. Al-Subaie et al (1996) validated the Arabic version of the Eating Attitude Test (EAT-26) and assessed a representative stratified random sample of grade 7-12 urban female students (n=129). Twenty-five were identified by EAT-26 as having abnormal eating attitudes. One case was identified as having anorexia nervosa and no cases of bulimia were found. Milaat et al (2001) assessed children (below 15 years) selected through a multistage sampling of households (n=875) using the ten questions survey. The point prevalence of any disability was 3.7%. Three-fifths of cases had a single disability, one-fifth had two conditions and one-fifth had three or more conditions. Speech, motor and mental disabilities were the commonest disabilities identified.

MENTAL HEALTH RESOURCES

Mental Health Policy A mental health policy is present. The policy was initially formulated in 1989.
The components of the policy are advocacy, promotion, prevention, treatment and rehabilitation.

Substance Abuse Policy A substance abuse policy is present. The policy was initially formulated in 2000.

National Mental Health Programme A national mental health programme is present. The programme was formulated in 1989. The national mental health programme aims at integrating mental health into primary and community care, developing a model keeping in view the social, cultural and religious values of the country in perspective, using mental health principles in promoting social health, decreasing untoward impact of social and economic development on society like drug abuse, smoking, delinquency and crime.

National Therapeutic Drug Policy/Essential List of Drugs A national therapeutic drug policy/essential list of drugs is present. It was formulated in 1988.

Mental Health Legislation A mental health act is awaiting approval. The General Directorate for Mental Health has developed a manual of procedures and regulations for mental health institutions in the country until the mental health act is approved.
Details about the year of enactment of the mental health legislation are not available.

Mental Health Financing There are budget allocations for mental health.
Details about expenditure on mental health are not available.
The primary source of mental health financing is tax based.
Development of psychiatric services is incorporated in the budget of general health services.
The country has disability benefits for persons with mental disorders.

Mental Health Facilities Mental health is a part of primary health care system. Actual treatment of severe mental disorders is available at the primary level. All anti-depressants and neuroleptics and some anti-epileptics are exempt from control and so all primary care physicians can prescribe most of the drugs.
Regular training of primary care professionals is carried out in the field of mental health. The General Directorate for Mental Health has a well designed training programme for the mental health component of primary health care. There are training manuals and workshops for psychiatrists on methods how to train primary care personnel. All medical staff of primary care services are required to attend training programmes on the recognition and management of common mental disorders. The immediate and post-training evaluations of the trainees show favourable changes in their attitude and knowledge and enhanced motivation to practice psychiatry at primary health care centres. A system of ongoing training is needed because the majority of primary care doctors are expatriates (predominantly from neighbouring Arab states).
There are community care facilities for patients with mental disorders. Rehabilitative services were planned following a Royal decree in 1988 but it mainly concentrated among private organizations and self help groups like the Patients' Friends Committee, etc.

Psychiatric Beds and Professionals

Total psychiatric beds per 10 000 population	1.18
Psychiatric beds in mental hospitals per 10 000 population	0.8
Psychiatric beds in general hospitals per 10 000 population	0.04
Psychiatric beds in other settings per 10 000 population	0.34
Number of psychiatrists per 100 000 population	1.1
Number of neurosurgeons per 100 000 population	0.5
Number of psychiatric nurses per 100 000 population	6.4
Number of neurologists per 100 000 population	0.07
Number of psychologists per 100 000 population	0.97
Number of social workers per 100 000 population	2.4

There are 22 other mental health staff belonging to different categories. There are three Amal hospitals which take care of patients with problems with drug abuse. They collectively have 840 beds. Some beds have been earmarked for mentally retarded individuals and mentally ill offenders. About three fourths of the psychiatrists and a majority of nurses are expatriates. Traditional healers and religious healers play an important part in mental health care.

Non-Governmental Organizations NGOs are involved with mental health in the country. They are mainly involved in advocacy, promotion, prevention, treatment and rehabilitation.

Information Gathering System There is mental health reporting system in the country.
The country has data collection system or epidemiological study on mental health. There are no epidemiological studies, but data are available for all services.

Programmes for Special Population The country has specific programmes for mental health for children. Child psychiatric services are mainly provided as out-patient care and emergency cases are admitted in paediatric hospitals or general hospitals. Six school units are operational in Riyadh.

Therapeutic Drugs The following therapeutic drugs are generally available at the primary health care level of the country: carbamazepine, ethosuximide, phenobarbital, phenytoin sodium, sodium valproate, amitriptyline, chlorpromazine, diazepam, fluphenazine, haloperidol, lithium, biperiden, carbidopa, levodopa.

Other Information Till 1983, mental health care was mainly provided by the Taif mental hospital, but since then smaller hospitals and outpatient clinics have been set up. The next phase would involve integration of mental health into primary care.

Additional Sources of Information

Abolfotouh, M. A. (1997) Behaviour disorders among urban schoolboys in south-western Saudi Arabia. Eastern Mediterranean Health Journal, 3, 274-283.

Al-Faris, E., Al-Subaie, A., Khoja, T., et al (1997) Training primary health care physicians in Saudi Arabia to recognize psychiatric illness. Acta Psychiatrica Scandinavica, 96, 439-444.

Al-Khathami, A. D., Ogbeide, D. O. (2002) Prevalence of mental illness among Saudi adult primary-care patients in Central Saudi Arabia. Saudi Medical Journal, 23, 721-724.

Al-Shammari, S. A, Al-Subaie, A. (1999) Prevalence and correlates of depression among Saudi elderly. International Journal of Geriatric Psychiatry, 14, 739-747.

Al-Subaie, A., Al-Shammari, S., Bamgboye, E., et al (1996) Validity of the Arabic version of the Eating Attitude Test. International Journal of Eating Disorders, 20, 321-324.

Elfawal, M. A. (1999) Cultural influence on the incidence and choice of method of suicide in Saudi Arabia. American Journal of Forensic Medicine & Pathology, 20, 163-168.

El-Rufaie, O. E., Albar, A. A., Al-Dabal, B. K. (1988) Identifying anxiety and depressive disorders among primary care patients: a pilot study. Acta Psychiatrica Scandinavica, 77, 280-282.

El-Rufaie, O. E. F., Al Sabosy, M. M. A., Bener, A., et al (1990) Somatized mental disorder among primary care Arab patients: I. Prevalence and clinical and sociodemographic characteristics. Journal of Psychosomatic Research, 46, 549-555.

Malik, G. M., Bilal, A., Mekki, T. E., et al (1996) Drug overdose in the Asir region of Saudi Arabia. Annals of Saudi Medicine, 16, 33-36.

Milaat, W. A., Ghabrah, T. M., Al-Bar, H. M. S., et al (2001) Population-based survey of childhood disability in Eastern Jeddah using the ten questions tool. Disability & Rehabilitation, 23, 199-203.

Qureshi, N. A., Al-Ghamady, S., Al-Haddad, N. S., et al. (2001) Integration of mental health care into primary care. Saudi Medical Journal, 22, 899-906.

The National Scientific Committee of Mental Health in Primary Health Care (1996) National Manual for Primary Mental Health Care.

Senegal

GENERAL INFORMATION

Senegal is a country with an approximate area of 197 thousand sq. km. (UNO, 2001). Its population is 10.339 million, and the sex ratio (men per hundred women) is 99 (UNO, 2004). The proportion of population under the age of 15 years is 43% (UNO, 2004), and the proportion of population above the age of 60 years is 4% (WHO, 2004). The literacy rate is 49% for men and 29.7% for women (UNESCO/MoH, 2004).

The country is a low income group country (based on World Bank 2004 criteria). The proportion of health budget to GDP is 4.8%. The per capita total expenditure on health is 63 international $, and the per capita government expenditure on health is 37 international $ (WHO, 2004).

The main language(s) used in the country is (are) French, Wolof and Serer. The largest ethnic group(s) is (are) Wolof, and the other ethnic group(s) are (is) Fulani, Serer, Toucouleur, Diola and Manding. The largest religious group(s) is (are) Muslim (approximately 95%).

The life expectancy at birth is 54.3 years for males and 57.3 years for females (WHO, 2004). The healthy life expectancy at birth is 47 years for males and 49 years for females (WHO, 2004).

EPIDEMIOLOGY

In a study done in the primary care setting, Diop et al (1982) used a 10-item screening questionnaire to assess 545 children (5-15 years) and the 24-item Self-Reporting Questionnaire (SRQ) to assess 933 adults. Almost 17% of children had emotional/behavioural or neuro-psychiatric disorders and 16% of adults had psychiatric illnesses. Beiser et al (1976) developed an emic questionnaire to tap symptoms of psychiatric distress. In a sample of more than 400 subjects, they found that the idiom of expressing distress was not limited to the somatic, and they were able to discriminate between mentally ill and well people in the local frame of reference. Seck et al (1994) reported on findings from a UNESCO study on epidemiology of drug abuse in young people. Drug use was common among the youth and was associated with certain religious practices, curiosity, ignorance of harmful effects and lack of education. Gueye et al (1998) identified erectile dysfunction in 16% of diabetic outpatients (n=431). Complications of diabetes (especially neurological) and duration of diabetes were associated with the risk of erectile dysfunction. Thiam et al (1998) assessed 1025 psychiatric out-patients. Schizophrenia and hysteria were the commonest diagnoses made. The occurrence of hysteria was associated with disturbances in interpersonal relationships (49.6%) and difficulties of daily life. Big Charcot attacks were seen in 10% of the patients. Hysterical personality type was common in these patients (85.1%). Reitter et al (1996) reviewed the hospital records of 450 persons with suicide attempts. Such attempts were common among young (particularly in young women) and the commonest cause was family problems (all problems: 42%, marital problems: 15%).

MENTAL HEALTH RESOURCES

S

Mental Health Policy A mental health policy is present. The policy was initially formulated in 1980.
The components of the policy are advocacy, promotion, prevention, treatment and rehabilitation.

Substance Abuse Policy A substance abuse policy is present. The policy was initially formulated in 1997. The Law number 97 – 18 of 1st December 1997 serves as the policy for substance abuse.

National Mental Health Programme A national mental health programme is absent.
The draft of the National Mental Health Plan is ready and it will be put up for approval in January 2005.

National Therapeutic Drug Policy/Essential List of Drugs A national therapeutic drug policy/essential list of drugs is present. Details about the year of formulation are not available.

Mental Health Legislation The most recent laws in mental health are law 75-80 of 9th July 1975, Decree 75-1092 of 23 October 1975 and Decree 75-1023 of 23 October 1975. The Law number 97 – 18 of 1st December 1997 also has mental health implications.
The latest legislation was enacted in 1975.

Mental Health Financing There are budget allocations for mental health.
The country spends 9% of the total health budget on mental health.
The primary sources of mental health financing in descending order are private insurances, social insurance, out of pocket expenditure by the patient or family and tax based.
The country does not have disability benefits for persons with mental disorders.

Mental Health Facilities Mental health is a part of primary health care system. Actual treatment of severe mental disorders is available at the primary level. The programme for primary mental health care was developed in 1975 with the assistance of WHO. Regular training of primary care professionals is carried out in the field of mental health. In the last two years, about 350 personnel were provided training. Out of the 200 personnel trained over the last two years, 100 were nurses and the remaining physicians. There are community care facilities for patients with mental disorders. Community care is provided by private clinics and traditional healers.

Psychiatric Beds and Professionals

Total psychiatric beds per 10 000 population	0.3
Psychiatric beds in mental hospitals per 10 000 population	0.15
Psychiatric beds in general hospitals per 10 000 population	0.1
Psychiatric beds in other settings per 10 000 population	0.05
Number of psychiatrists per 100 000 population	0.16
Number of neurosurgeons per 100 000 population	0.06
Number of psychiatric nurses per 100 000 population	0.06
Number of neurologists per 100 000 population	0.1
Number of psychologists per 100 000 population	0.04
Number of social workers per 100 000 population	0.035

Non-Governmental Organizations NGOs are involved with mental health in the country. They are mainly involved in advocacy, promotion, prevention, treatment and rehabilitation.

Information Gathering System There is mental health reporting system in the country.
The country has data collection system or epidemiological study on mental health.

Programmes for Special Population The country has specific programmes for mental health for children.

Therapeutic Drugs The following therapeutic drugs are generally available at the primary health care level of the country: carbamazepine, phenobarbital, sodium valproate, amitriptyline, chlorpromazine, diazepam, haloperidol, lithium.

Other Information

Additional Sources of Information

Beiser, M., Benfari, R. C., Collomb, H., et al (1976) Measuring psychoneurotic behavior in cross-cultural surveys. Journal of Nervous & Mental Disease, 163, 10-23.

Diop, B., Collignon, R., Gueye, M., et al (1982) Diagnosis and symptoms of mental disorder in a rural area of Senegal. African Journal of Medicine & Medical Sciences, 11, 95-103.

Gueye, S. M., Diop, S. N., Ba, M., et al (1998) Erectile dysfunction in diabetics. Epidemiological profile in Senegal. Progrès en Urologie, 8, 377-381.

Reitter, M., Vilane, A., Sylla, A. (1996) Suicidal attempts without borders? Médecine Tropicale, 56, 430-432.

Seck, B., Choquet, M., Sarr, L., et al (1994) Attitude and behavior of the youth of Senegal toward drugs. Dakar Medical, 39, 17-22.

Thiam, M. H., Gueye, M. (1998) Clinical aspects of hysteria at the psychiatric clinic of the Fann University Hospital Center. Apropos of a prospective study of 121 cases. Dakar Medical, 43, 41-44.

Serbia and Montenegro

GENERAL INFORMATION

Serbia and Montenegro is a country with an approximate area of 102 thousand sq. km. (UNO, 2001). Its population is 10.519 million*, and the sex ratio (men per hundred women) is 99 (UNO, 2004). The proportion of population under the age of 15 years is 19% (UNO, 2004), and the proportion of population above the age of 60 years is 18% (WHO, 2004).

The country is a higher middle income group country (based on World Bank 2004 criteria). The proportion of health budget to GDP is 8.2%. The per capita total expenditure on health is 616 international $, and the per capita government expenditure on health is 488 international $ (WHO, 2004).

The main language(s) used in the country is (are) Serbian. The largest ethnic group(s) is (are) Serb. The largest religious group(s) is (are) Orthodox Christian.

The life expectancy at birth is 69.7 years for males and 74.9 years for females (WHO, 2004). The healthy life expectancy at birth is 63 years for males and 65 years for females (WHO, 2004).

EPIDEMIOLOGY

Eric et al (1988) did an assessment of mental health among fresh medical students (n=523) in one area and found that 16.1% had psychiatric disorders and that two years later the rate had increased to 17.5%. The incidence rate was 5.3% per year with neuroses being the most frequent diagnoses (3.5%). Based on a register of treated alcohol dependent patients, Saponja et al (1996) suggested that there was a decrease in incidence, prevalence and risk of morbidity in the population of the examined territory during 1991-1993. Plavljanic and Mijic (1997) found that the alcohol abuse was 3.7 times more frequent in participants of combat actions compared to those who did not have such assignment in an investigated base on retrospective analysis of medical documentation. Durmisevic et al (1999) studied 208 primary school pupils and 232 secondary school pupils to assess drug use pattern. Prevalence of smoking, use of alcohol and use of narcotics was found to be 0.9%, 5.8%, and 0.9% among primary school children, 28%, 28.8% and 10.6% among secondary school students and 42.9%, 41.1% and 13.5% in the last two years of secondary school. Milic (2000a) assessed a group of primary and secondary school students (one-fifth of students from concerned classes in 17 schools were selected) and found that one in 30 students used psychoactive substances, with males using them more frequently. Among males, almost 52.9% of those who used alcohol and tobacco also used other drugs. Roncevic et al (1989) reviewed data related to poisoning and intoxication in children aged 0-15 years from 11 hospitals (n=795). Almost 6.5% of children had ethanol intoxication. Ethanol intoxication was associated with gender (male) and age. Starcevic and Bogojevic (1997) examined 90 consecutive day clinic patients with panic disorder and agoraphobia (PDA) who were administered the SCID-III-R (modified for DSM-IV). The overall comorbidity rate for simple phobia (SP) was 65.6%. The most frequent subtypes of SP were situational phobia and dental phobia, followed by natural environment phobia, death related phobia and blood-injection-injury phobia. Mandic et al (1994) assessed the prevalence of psychogenic headache in 150 displaced persons. Nearly 70% suffered from headaches (female to male ratio 2.5:1). Among males the common causes were depression (43%) and conversion (8.3%), and among females depression (66%), anxiety (10.7%) and conversion (4.3%). Headache was correlated with the severity of trauma and employment status (before and after displacement). Milcinski and Mrevlje (1990) found very high suicide rates in northern parts of erstwhile Yugoslavia e.g. Vojvodina and very low rates in southern parts, e.g. Kosovo (2.4 per 100 000). Petrovich et al (2001) studied suicide rates (between 1987-99) in a Serbian region using death certificates. The average annual suicide rate (per 100 000) in the region during the period 1987/1989 (economic/political stability) was 14.8 among males and 6.8 among females, and in 1999 (economic/political crisis) it was 13.8 among males and 3.7 among females. This was despite a rise in the rates of suicide and homicide during the war (1991-1994) (Biro & Selakovic-Bursic, 1996). During this period the rate of suicides committed by fire arms increased (from 8.1% to 14.5%), while there was a decrease in cases of poisoning. Milic (2000b) reviewed data obtained from the Ministry of Internal Affairs of Serbia and medical records from the psychiatry center for the years 1991-1995. Three-fifths of those attempting suicide were unemployed. There was a significant difference in the age of suicide attempters (average: 41.23 years) and suicide completers (average: 59.50 years). The suicide rate in the age groups above 45 years was approximately 27.2 per 100 000 population. Unemployment was related to suicide among the 15-24 and 55-64 age groups. The rate of suicide in 2002 was 19.3 per 100 000 population (9 National Committee for Mental Health of Serbia and National Committee for Mental Health of Montenegro, 2003)

MENTAL HEALTH RESOURCES

Mental Health Policy A mental health policy is absent.

The new policy of health care system reforms is described in the following document: Ministry of Health of Republic of Serbia: Better Health for All in Third Millennium – Health Policy, Vision of System of Health Care in Serbia; Strategy and Action Plan of Reform of System of Health Care in Republic of Serbia – draft version, Belgrade, 10/2003. Mental Health Policy and Action Plan has been drafted by the National Committee for Mental Health of Serbia in October 2004.

Substance Abuse Policy A substance abuse policy is present. The policy was initially formulated in 1991. Montenegro has a plan and programme for prevention of substance abuse (multidisciplinary) which was implemented in 2001.

National Mental Health Programme A national mental health programme is absent.

National Therapeutic Drug Policy/Essential List of Drugs A national therapeutic drug policy/essential list of drugs is present. Details about the year of formulation are not available.

Mental Health Legislation Mental health legislation includes provisions on protection of the rights of people with mental disorders. These are distributed between stipulations of the Health Care Law (articles 1, 7 and 10), Out-of-court Proceedings Law, Marriage and Family Relations Law and Execution of Criminal Sanctions Law. A new law on mental health and protection of rights of mentally disabled persons has been drafted by the National Committee for Mental Health in October 2004.
The latest legislation was enacted in 1931.

Mental Health Financing There are budget allocations for mental health.
Details about expenditure on mental health are not available.
The primary source of mental health financing is social insurance.
Mental health care is financed from the obligatory insurance, like general health.
Details about disability benefits for mental health are not available.

Mental Health Facilities Mental health is a part of primary health care system. Actual treatment of severe mental disorders is available at the primary level. Mental health care is quite well integrated with the primary health care system, at least in larger cities that have mental health sections and developmental counseling units within municipal health centers (which represent the primary organizational form of the primary health care system). However, some parts of Serbia do not have such mental health care units within municipal health centres (mainly because of the lack of adequate personnel). The mental health sector is also quite well integrated with the somatic health care sector, through the municipal health care centers, general hospitals or medical centers that have psychiatric outpatient services or psychiatric departments.
Regular training of primary care professionals is carried out in the field of mental health. Continuous education of primary care physicians started in 2000, by the Institute of Mental Health (supported by the Committee for Human Rights, Norwegian Medical Association). So far, four courses have been organized, the last two in cooperation with the colleagues from Sarajevo. Programmes were conducted by the use of the same teaching modules and were followed by an evaluation.
There are community care facilities for patients with mental disorders. Some elements of community mental health services have existed in various forms for years: psychiatric departments within general hospitals, day hospitals, outpatient services within stationary psychiatric institutions, mental health sections within municipal health centers, social work centers with their facilities for psychotherapeutic work with some categories of beneficiaries (the young suffering from behavioural disorders; the young delinquents, etc.), cooperation with pre-school and school institutions and various non-governmental and humanitarian organizations, in the field of prevention and some forms of psychosocial counselling. Mental health care is also integrated with welfare services through the cooperation of centres for mental health care and psychiatric departments with regional centres for social work which exist in each municipality of Serbia. There is also a good cooperation with other welfare institutions, such as retirement homes and orphanages, and there are some joint projects in the fields of prevention and therapy.

Psychiatric Beds and Professionals

Total psychiatric beds per 10 000 population	9.6
Psychiatric beds in mental hospitals per 10 000 population	4.5
Psychiatric beds in general hospitals per 10 000 population	
Psychiatric beds in other settings per 10 000 population	
Number of psychiatrists per 100 000 population	12.8
Number of neurosurgeons per 100 000 population	
Number of psychiatric nurses per 100 000 population	19
Number of neurologists per 100 000 population	6
Number of psychologists per 100 000 population	1.2
Number of social workers per 100 000 population	0.5

Until 1993, doctors were educated about neuropsychiatry, but since then the specialities of psychiatry and neurology have divided and there are further courses for child psychiatry and neurology. Psychiatric day hospitals have capacity of 495 patients. Forensic services in Serbia have capacity of 700 beds. Prison hospitals are managed by the Ministry of Justice. About 5% of psychiatrists are engaged in the practice of child and adolescent psychiatry.

Non-Governmental Organizations NGOs are involved with mental health in the country. They are mainly involved in rehabilitation. Non-governmental and paraprofessional groups have had an increasing role within the mental health system, most of all through various psychosocial programmes, but also through cooperation and common projects with the mental health, social and educational sectors. Child Advocacy International established a comprehensive child and adolescent mental health service (CAMHS) in Kosovo in the postwar situation, when psychiatric services in the region were in a state of disarray. Clinics were located in primary

S

health care facilities and home visits were made as necessary. It also provided a training base for future child and adolescent mental health specialists.

Information Gathering System There is mental health reporting system in the country. Non-affective and affective psychoses as well as epilepsy are reported.
The country has data collection system or epidemiological study on mental health.

Programmes for Special Population The country has specific programmes for mental health for refugees, elderly and children. During the years of crisis, many programmes for mental health care of refugees and internally displaced people were developed, as well as programmes for rehabilitation of torture victims. These programmes were conducted by the governmental organizations and NGOs and supported by many organizations (UNHCR, UNICEF). The Stress Clinic, the Psychotrauma Center and the Center for Abused Children were established within the Institute of Mental Health. The Trauma Center of International Aid Network (IAN) has been established in 1997 and the Center for Rehabilitation of Torture Victims within this centre in 2000. International cooperation has been achieved through various multicentric research on posttraumatic stress disorder (STOP, CONNECT, supported by the EU).

Therapeutic Drugs The following therapeutic drugs are generally available at the primary health care level of the country: carbamazepine, phenobarbital, amitriptyline, chlorpromazine, diazepam, fluphenazine, haloperidol, lithium, biperiden, carbidopa, levodopa.
Social insurance fully covers the cost of most of the above therapeutic drugs.

Other Information * Its population excluding Kosovo is 7.498 million (National Politics Census, 2002). The population of Montenegro is 0.672 Million (National Politics Census, 2003).

Additional Sources of Information

Agani, F. (2001) Mental health challenges in postwar Kosova. JAMA, 285, 1217.

Black, M. (1993) Letter from Serbia and Montenegro: collapsing health care in Serbia and Montenegro. British Medical Journal, 307, 1135-1137.

Biro, M., Selakovic-Bursic, S. (1996) Suicide, aggression and war. Archives of Suicide Research, 2, 75-79.

Durmisevic, S., Huseinagic, S., Imamovic, D., et al (1999) The prevalence of smoking, alcohol consumption and drug abuse in school children and adolescents. Medicinski Arhiv, 53, 105-107.

Eric, L., Radovanovic, Z., Jevremovic, I. (1988) Mental disorders among Yugoslav medical students. British Journal of Psychiatry, 152, 127-129.

Ispanovic-Radojkovic, V., Tadic, N. (1999) Child and adolescent psychiatry in Serbia. In: H. Remschmidt, H. van Engeland (Eds). Child and Adolescent Psychiatry in Europe. Historical Development, Current Situation and Future Perspectives. Darmstadt, Steinkopff. pp285-297.

Jones, L., Rrustemi, A., Shahini, M., et al. (2003) Mental health services for war-affected children. Report from a survey in Kosovo. British Journal of Psychiatry, 183, 540-546.

Mandic, N., Ebling, Z., Delalle-Zebic, M., et al (1994) Headache in displaced persons from east Slavonia. Lijecnicki Vjesnik, 116, 291-294.

Milcinski, L., Mrevlje, G. (1990) Epidemiology of suicide in Yugoslavia--methodological questions. Medicinski Pregled, 43, 453-456.

Milic, C. T. (2000a) Characteristics of the use and abuse of psychoactive substances. Vojnosanitetski Pregled, 57, 49-53.

Milic, C. T. (2000b) General characteristics of suicide in the region of Kragujevac. Vojnosanitetski Pregled, 57, 677-681.

Ministry of Health of Republic Serbia (2003) Better Health for All in the Third Millennium – Health Policy, Vision of System of Health Care in Serbia; Strategy and Action Plan of Reform of System of Health Care in Republic of Serbia – Draft version, Belgrad.

Petrovich, B., Tiodorovich, B., Kocich, B., et al (2001) Influence of socio-economic crisis on epidemiological characteristic of suicide in the region of Nis (southeastern part of Serbia, Yugoslavia). European Journal of Epidemiology, 17, 183-187.

Plavljanic, R., Mijic, R. (1997) Alcohol abuse in soldiers of the Herzegovina Corps of the Republic of Serbia Army during the 1992-1994 war. Vojnosanitetski Pregled, 54, 469-472.

Roberts, H. (2003) Serbia and Montenegro's state services behind rest of Europe. Lancet, 361, 316-317.

Roncevic, N., Konstantinidis, G., Stevanovic, V. (1989) Acute alcoholic intoxication in children in Vojvodina. Arhiv Za Higijenu Rada i Toksikologiju, 40, 47-55.

Saponja, N., Vuckovic, N., Misic-Pavkov, G., et al (1996) Sociodemographic and epidemiologic characteristics of hospitalized alcoholics in Vojvodina. Medicinski Pregled, 49, 119-124.

Starcevic, V., Bogojevic, G. (1997) Comorbidity of panic disorder with agoraphobia and specific phobia: relationship with the subtypes of specific phobia. Comprehensive Psychiatry, 38, 315-320.

National Committee for Mental Health of Serbia and National Committee for Mental Health of Montenegro. Study on Mental Health Policy and Legislation, Belgrade and Podgorica, November 2003.

Zivkovic-Sulovic, M. (2003) Analysis of organisation and work of services for mental health in Republic of Serbia in 2002. Institute for Health Protection,'Dr Milan Jovanovic Batut', Belgrade.

Seychelles

GENERAL INFORMATION

Seychelles is a country with an approximate area of 0.45 thousand sq. km. (UNO, 2001). The country is an archipelago consisting of more than 100 islands. Its population is 0.081 million, and the sex ratio (men per hundred women) is 97 (UNO, 2004). The proportion of population under the age of 15 years is 28% (UNO, 2004), and the proportion of population above the age of 60 years is 9% (WHO, 2004). The literacy rate is 91.4% for men and 92.3% for women (UNESCO/MoH, 2004).

The country is a higher middle income group country (based on World Bank 2004 criteria). The proportion of health budget to GDP is 6%. The per capita total expenditure on health is 770 international $, and the per capita government expenditure on health is 525 international $ (WHO, 2004).

The main language(s) used in the country is (are) English, French and Seselwa. The largest ethnic group(s) is (are) Seychellois. The largest religious group(s) is (are) Roman Catholic (five-sixths).

The life expectancy at birth is 67 years for males and 77.2 years for females (WHO, 2004). The healthy life expectancy at birth is 57 years for males and 65 years for females (WHO, 2004).

EPIDEMIOLOGY

There is a paucity of epidemiological data on mental illnesses in Seychelles in internationally accessible literature. Myers and Davidson (1998) conducted a large controlled longitudinal study on the neurotoxicity of methylmercury in a population consuming seafood. No adverse associations were found in the Seychelles, where exposure is mainly from fish consumption. The study did not support the hypothesis that consumption of such fish during pregnancy places the fetus at increased neuro-developmental risk.

MENTAL HEALTH RESOURCES

Mental Health Policy A mental health policy is present. The policy was initially formulated in 1992.
The components of the policy are advocacy, promotion, prevention, treatment and rehabilitation. The policy was revised in 1995.

Substance Abuse Policy A substance abuse policy is absent. A National Alcohol Policy was formulated in 2003.

National Mental Health Programme A national mental health programme is present. The programme was formulated in 1989.
The national mental health programme for the period 2000-2004 has been drafted for approval.

National Therapeutic Drug Policy/Essential List of Drugs A national therapeutic drug policy/essential list of drugs is present. It was formulated in 2001.
The essential drug list is being drafted. The essential drugs are compiled in the National Drug Formulary (NDF). The present NDF (Third Edition, 2000) is being reviewed and updated.

Mental Health Legislation The existing law on mental health, the Mental Treatment Act, has been reviewed and submitted for enactment in 2001.
The latest legislation was enacted in 1906.

Mental Health Financing There are budget allocations for mental health.
The country spends 2.8% of the total health budget on mental health.
The primary sources of mental health financing in descending order are tax based and private insurances.
The health services are free of charge to every citizen.
The country has disability benefits for persons with mental disorders. There are provisions for invalidity benefit by the social security funding.

Mental Health Facilities Mental health is a part of primary health care system. Actual treatment of severe mental disorders is not available at the primary level. Follow-up maintenance treatment is available with the support of the community psychiatry nurse along with other specialists and primary health workers. Since the return of the Seychellois psychiatrist in October 2003, the patients in the community are also being reviewed every 3 months by the psychiatrist.
Regular training of primary care professionals is carried out in the field of mental health. Training is provided to health workers as an ongoing continuous programme. Primary care doctors also attend seminars on mental health twice a year.
There are community care facilities for patients with mental disorders. Community care is provided by the community psychiatry nurse with help from the primary health care workers and other specialists.

Psychiatric Beds and Professionals

Total psychiatric beds per 10 000 population	7.7
Psychiatric beds in mental hospitals per 10 000 population	6
Psychiatric beds in general hospitals per 10 000 population	1.7
Psychiatric beds in other settings per 10 000 population	0
Number of psychiatrists per 100 000 population	2
Number of neurosurgeons per 100 000 population	0
Number of psychiatric nurses per 100 000 population	8
Number of neurologists per 100 000 population	1
Number of psychologists per 100 000 population	1
Number of social workers per 100 000 population	48

There are only 3 occupational therapists working in psychiatry though there is an established network of them. The social workers are employed by different ministries. One social worker is working in mental health. There is no medical school or university, so most of the doctors are expatriates. Since February 2004, an 18-month diploma course in mental health nursing was started. Twelve nurses are enrolled in the programme.

Non-Governmental Organizations NGOs are involved with mental health in the country. They are mainly involved in advocacy, promotion and rehabilitation.

Information Gathering System There is mental health reporting system in the country.
The country has data collection system or epidemiological study on mental health. Mental disorders are included in epidemiological morbidity data.

Programmes for Special Population The country has specific programmes for mental health for elderly and children. Support for the special population is available only when asked for and is not an outreach programme. There are also programmes for the mentally retarded.

Therapeutic Drugs The following therapeutic drugs are generally available at the primary health care level of the country: carbamazepine, ethosuximide, phenobarbital, phenytoin sodium, sodium valproate, amitriptyline, chlorpromazine, diazepam, haloperidol, lithium, carbidopa, levodopa.
Some drugs which are not there in the primary health care can be dispensed if prescribed by consultants.

Other Information

S

Additional Sources of Information

Islam, R. (1999). Mental health services in the Seychelles. Psychiatric Bulletin, 23, 565-567.

Myers, G. J., Davidson, P. W. (1998) Prenatal methylmercury exposure and children: neurologic, developmental, and behavioral research. Environmental Health Perspectives, 106, 841-847.

Sierra Leone

GENERAL INFORMATION

Sierra Leone is a country with an approximate area of 72 thousand sq. km. (UNO, 2001). Its population is 5.169 million, and the sex ratio (men per hundred women) is 97 (UNO, 2004). The proportion of population under the age of 15 years is 44% (UNO, 2004), and the proportion of population above the age of 60 years is 5% (WHO, 2004). The literacy rate is 45% for men and 18% for women (UNESCO/MoH, 2004).

The country is a low income group country (based on World Bank 2004 criteria). The proportion of health budget to GDP is 4.3%. The per capita total expenditure on health is 26 international $, and the per capita government expenditure on health is 16 international $ (WHO, 2004).

The main language(s) used in the country is (are) English. The largest ethnic group(s) is (are) African. The largest religious group(s) is (are) Muslim, and the other religious group(s) are (is) indigenous groups and Christian.

The life expectancy at birth is 32.4 years for males and 35.7 years for females (WHO, 2004). The healthy life expectancy at birth is 27 years for males and 30 years for females (WHO, 2004).

EPIDEMIOLOGY

There is a paucity of epidemiological data on mental illnesses in Sierra Leone in internationally accessible literature. Lacoux et al (2002) reported on the experience of 40 upper limb amputees (11 bilateral) with regard to stump pain, phantom sensation and phantom pain. All the patients lost their limbs as a result of violent injuries and were assessed 10-48 months after the injury. All amputees reported stump pain in the month prior to the interview and ten of the 11 bilateral amputees had bilateral pain. Phantom sensation was common (92.5%), but phantom pain was only present in 32.5% of amputees. Problems in translation and explanation may have influenced the low incidence of phantom pain and high incidence of stump pain. In the bilateral amputees, phantom sensation, phantom pain and telescoping all showed bilateral concordance, whereas stump pain and neuromas did not show concordance. There is one study on the problems of refugees from Sierra Leone living in camps in Gambia, which has been included in studies from Gambia.

MENTAL HEALTH RESOURCES

Mental Health Policy A mental health policy is absent.

A Mental Health Coordination Group has been formed with the participation of various stakeholders, e.g. inter-governmental organizations, NGOs and the Government. This group is chaired by the Ministry of Health and seconded by WHO. It is charged with the responsibility of developing a Mental Health and Substance Abuse Policy, a modern mental health legislation and national mental health programme including a plan of action for short and long term initiatives. It is also responsible for developing models for decentralized community-based services and human resource development for all levels of care.

Substance Abuse Policy A substance abuse policy is absent.

National Mental Health Programme A national mental health programme is absent.

National Therapeutic Drug Policy/Essential List of Drugs A national therapeutic drug policy/essential list of drugs is absent. Both, the national therapeutic drug policy and the essential drug list are in the process of being developed.

Mental Health Legislation The Sierra Leone Mental Health Act is present.

Details about the year of enactment of the mental health legislation are not available.

Mental Health Financing There are no budget allocations for mental health.

Details about expenditure on mental health are not available.

The primary source of mental health financing is tax based.

The country does not have disability benefits for persons with mental disorders.

Mental Health Facilities Mental health is a part of primary health care system. Actual treatment of severe mental disorders is available at the primary level.

Regular training of primary care professionals is not carried out in the field of mental health.

There are no community care facilities for patients with mental disorders. Some traditional healers and general practitioners provide mental health care in the community setting.

Psychiatric Beds and Professionals

Total psychiatric beds per 10 000 population	0.47
Psychiatric beds in mental hospitals per 10 000 population	0.32
Psychiatric beds in general hospitals per 10 000 population	0.11
Psychiatric beds in other settings per 10 000 population	0.03
Number of psychiatrists per 100 000 population	0.02
Number of neurosurgeons per 100 000 population	0
Number of psychiatric nurses per 100 000 population	0.04
Number of neurologists per 100 000 population	0.02
Number of psychologists per 100 000 population	0
Number of social workers per 100 000 population	0.06

There are 200 psychiatric assistants.

Non-Governmental Organizations NGOs are involved with mental health in the country. They are mainly involved in treatment and rehabilitation.

Information Gathering System There is no mental health reporting system in the country.
Details about data collection system or epidemiological study on mental health are not available. The first Systematic Needs Assessment on Mental Health and Substance Abuse Survey in post-conflict Sierra Leone was undertaken in October 2002 with the support of WHO under the direction of the MOH. In the random sample, 2% of subjects had psychosis, 4% had severe depression, 4% had prominent substance abuse, 1% had mentally retardation and 1% had epilepsy. Almost 85% of the population never took alcohol (97% of secondary school students) and even fewer had experimented with/abused drugs.

Programmes for Special Population The country has specific programmes for mental health for refugees.

Therapeutic Drugs The following therapeutic drugs are generally available at the primary health care level of the country: phenobarbital, chlorpromazine, diazepam, haloperidol, biperiden.

Other Information

Additional Sources of Information

Lacoux, P. A., Crombie, I. K., Macrae, W. A. (2002) Pain in traumatic upper limb amputees in Sierra Leone. Pain, 99, 309-312.

S

Singapore

GENERAL INFORMATION

Singapore is a country with an approximate area of 0.62 thousand sq. km. (UNO, 2001). Its population is 4.315 million, and the sex ratio (men per hundred women) is 101 (UNO, 2004). The proportion of population under the age of 15 years is 20% (UNO, 2004), and the proportion of population above the age of 60 years is 11% (WHO, 2004). The literacy rate is 96.6% for men and 88.6% for women (UNESCO/MoH, 2004).

The country is a high income group country (based on World Bank 2004 criteria). The proportion of health budget to GDP is 3.9%. The per capita total expenditure on health is 993 international $, and the per capita government expenditure on health is 333 international $ (WHO, 2004).

The main language(s) used in the country is (are) Malay, Chinese (Mandarin), Tamil and English. The largest ethnic group(s) is (are) Chinese, and the other ethnic group(s) are (is) Malays and Indian. The largest religious group(s) is (are) Buddhist, and the other religious group(s) are (is) Christian, Muslim and Taoist.

The life expectancy at birth is 77.4 years for males and 81.7 years for females (WHO, 2004). The healthy life expectancy at birth is 69 years for males and 71 years for females (WHO, 2004).

EPIDEMIOLOGY

There is substantial epidemiological data on mental illnesses in Singapore in internationally accessible literature. No attempt was made to include this information here.

MENTAL HEALTH RESOURCES

Mental Health Policy A mental health policy is present. The policy was initially formulated in 1952.

The components of the policy are advocacy and treatment. This has been further supplemented with the National Disease Control Plan for Major Mental Disorders which was formulated in January 2001. This policy framework identifies key mental diseases for Singapore, prioritizes the areas for action and formulates national level strategic initiatives for improving mental health. It also sets in place medium to long term targets for control of major mental disorders such as depression, anxiety and schizophrenia.

Substance Abuse Policy A substance abuse policy is present. The policy was initially formulated in 1973.

National Mental Health Programme A national mental health programme is present. The programme was formulated in 1993. The national mental health programme present was significantly expanded in 2001 with the launch of the 'Mind Your Mind' (MYM) Programme. MYM, which is run by Institute of Mental Health and funded by the Health Promotion Board, aims to promote mental health among Singaporeans, create greater awareness about mental disorders in the general public, and destigmatize mental disorders. It also aims to improve the rate of early detection and treatment for depression, anxiety disorders and schizophrenia in Singapore. MYM started in 2001 with a focus on stress management, followed by destigmatization in 2002 and depression in 2003 and 2004.

National Therapeutic Drug Policy/Essential List of Drugs A national therapeutic drug policy/essential list of drugs is present. It was formulated in 1979.

The essential drug's list was reviewed in 2002.

Mental Health Legislation The Mental Disorders and Treatment Act was enacted in 1952 but the latest revision was in 1985.

The latest legislation was enacted in 1952.

Mental Health Financing There are budget allocations for mental health.

The country spends 6.1% of the total health budget on mental health.

The primary sources of mental health financing in descending order are tax based, out of pocket expenditure by the patient or family, social insurance and private insurances.

The National Savings Scheme helps individuals to put aside part of their incomes in their accounts to meet their personal and immediate family's hospitalization expenses, especially after retirement. For the poor there is an alternative fund set up by the Government (Medifund).

The country has disability benefits for persons with mental disorders.

Mental Health Facilities Mental health is a part of primary health care system. Actual treatment of severe mental disorders is available at the primary level. Mental health care is provided across the continuum of care, from primary to tertiary levels. Primary mental health care is provided by private general practitioners and at the polyclinics.

Regular training of primary care professionals is carried out in the field of mental health. In the last two years, about 400 personnel were provided training.

There are community care facilities for patients with mental disorders. Community-based mental health services are organized by the Institute of Mental Health and comprise Outpatient Services, Day Centres, a Community Psychiatric Nursing Service, an Assertive Community Treatment Programme, a Mobile Crisis Team and a Crisis Hotline Service.

Psychiatric Beds and Professionals

Total psychiatric beds per 10 000 population	6.1
Psychiatric beds in mental hospitals per 10 000 population	5.9
Psychiatric beds in general hospitals per 10 000 population	0.2
Psychiatric beds in other settings per 10 000 population	0
Number of psychiatrists per 100 000 population	2.3
Number of neurosurgeons per 100 000 population	0.5
Number of psychiatric nurses per 100 000 population	10.4
Number of neurologists per 100 000 population	1.1
Number of psychologists per 100 000 population	1
Number of social workers per 100 000 population	3

All personnel are only those working in the public health sector. Secondary and tertiary level specialist care is delivered mainly at the Institute of Mental Health. Most of the acute general hospitals also provide some specialist mental health care. Patients with severe, refractory psychoses requiring long-term inpatient stay are cared for at Woodbridge Hospital, which is part of the Institute of Mental Health.

Non-Governmental Organizations NGOs are involved with mental health in the country. They are mainly involved in advocacy, promotion, prevention and rehabilitation. Some day-care services are provided by NGOs. The Singapore Anglican Welfare Council (SAWC) has started an On-the-Job Training (OJT) programme and the Certificate in Office Skills (COS), both programmes approved by the Singapore Institute of Technical Education (ITE).

Information Gathering System There is mental health reporting system in the country.
The country has data collection system or epidemiological study on mental health.
Details can be obtained from the Quarterly Statistics Bulletin of the Ministry of Health.

Programmes for Special Population The country has specific programmes for mental health for elderly and children.
There is a Child Guidance Clinic (CGC) run by the Institute of Mental Health. It is located in the community and provides psychiatric services to children and adolescents mainly in an outpatient setting. CGC has strong links with both mainstream schools and schools for the mentally challenged. CGC has set up a 'Children One-Stop Educational Service' (COPES), which is a comprehensive, non-categorical educational centre for children with learning disabilities. CGC also operates a 20-bed inpatient unit for children and adolescents with severe, acute psychiatric illnesses. Older persons, aged 65 years and above, with a variety of psychiatric and emotional problems have access to a dedicated care at the Department of Geriatric Psychiatry of the Institute of Mental Health. A multidisciplinary team at the department provides for the psychosocial as well as physical care needs of these persons. The Institute of Mental Health runs an Early Psychosis Intervention Programme (EPIP). EPIP improves the outcome of patients with early psychosis by emphasizing early detection and intervention as well as establishing strong links with available community resources to provide carers with optimal support. The Community Addictions Management Programme (CAMP) is a programme run by the Institute of Mental Health to provide an integrated, comprehensive range of medical services (that span from prevention to rehabilitation) in the community for persons with addictions. CAMP also educates the public on addiction-related issues, provides treatment that is specific and relevant to the needs of special groups, develops resources in the community to support the recovery process and provides training to professionals in the field. Patients requiring an intensive in-patient detoxification programme are admitted to a dedicated 24-bed ward in the hospital.

Therapeutic Drugs The following therapeutic drugs are generally available at the primary health care level of the country: carbamazepine, ethosuximide, phenobarbital, phenytoin sodium, sodium valproate, amitriptyline, chlorpromazine, diazepam, fluphenazine, haloperidol, lithium, carbidopa, levodopa.
Other drugs like fluoxetine and fluvoxamine are available.

Other Information

Additional Sources of Information

Chew, K., Eu, P.,Lee, E. (1994) The community psychiatric nurse in Singapore. Singapore Medical Journal, 35, 93-95.

Fung, D. S. S., Aw, S. C. (1999) A clinical study of 100 new admissions to an adolescent psychiatric inpatient unit in Singapore. Singapore Medical journal, 40, http://www.sma.org.sg/smj/4002/articles/4002a8.html

Ministry of Health (2000) A Guide to Medisave.

Ministry of Health (1999) A Guide to Medifund.

Thio, S. (2001) Rehabilitation for people with psychiatric disabilities: from care-role to payroll. Psychiatric Rehabilitation Journal, 25, 74-76.

S

Slovakia

GENERAL INFORMATION

Slovakia is a country with an approximate area of 49 thousand sq. km. (UNO, 2001). Its population is 5.407 million, and the sex ratio (men per hundred women) is 94 (UNO, 2004). The proportion of population under the age of 15 years is 17% (UNO, 2004), and the proportion of population above the age of 60 years is 16% (WHO, 2004). The literacy rate is 99.7% for men and 99.7% for women (UNESCO/MoH, 2004).

The country is a higher middle income group country (based on World Bank 2004 criteria). The proportion of health budget to GDP is 5.7%. The per capita total expenditure on health is 681 international $, and the per capita government expenditure on health is 608 international $ (WHO, 2004).

The main language(s) used in the country is (are) Slovak. The largest ethnic group(s) is (are) Slovak, and the other ethnic group(s) are (is) Hungarian, Czech, Romani, Ukrainian, and German. The largest religious group(s) is (are) Roman Catholic (more than half), and the other religious group(s) are (is) Protestant.

The life expectancy at birth is 69.8 years for males and 78.3 years for females (WHO, 2004). The healthy life expectancy at birth is 63 years for males and 69 years for females (WHO, 2004).

EPIDEMIOLOGY

Heretik et al (2003) applied the Mini International Neuropsychiatric Interview (MINI) and the shortened form of Beck Depression Inventory (BDI) to an adult population selected through quota sampling from across Slovakia (n=1212). They found that the 6-month prevalence of major depression was 12.8%, and that of minor depression was 5.1%. Regional differences in the prevalence of depression was noted. Depression was associated with ethnicity (Hungarian), availability of mental health services, residence (urban), gender (female), occupation (unemployed, students, disabled), marital status (widowed), social support (living alone) and life events (family and health related). Baska et al (2000) assessed more than 2400 students in five universities for smoking and eating habits. The results showed that 19.6% of males and 12.3% of females were regular smokers (min 1 cig/day) and 16.1% of males and 15.1% of females were occasional smokers. Smoking was associated with urban locality and alcohol consumption in males. One sixth of males were overweight (BMI>=25) and 8.5 % of females were grossly underweight (BMI<=17.5). Geckova et al (2002) assessed 1370 boys and 1246 girls (mean age 15 years) and found that adolescents from lower socio-economic strata were likely to exhibit health risk behaviour, except that a higher frequency of alcohol consumption was noted among girls whose parents were more educated. Okruhlica et al (2001) administered a questionnaire to 215 patients with heroin dependence (three-quarters of whom were males) and a control group of 231 adolescent students (one-quarter of whom were males). Gender specific analyses did not support the hypothesis that sports would help in the prevention of drug use. Okruhlica (1997) reviewed hospital records and noted that there has been a sharp rise in drug use since 1990. New patients consisted mainly of unemployed young (15-24 years) males (>70%). Intravenous use increased from 34% in 1993 to 72% in 1995. Okruhlica et al (2002) followed up more than 350 patients of opioid dependence after 3 years of treatment. Nearly 30% of patients had been abstinent for at least 6 months, 6% had been abstinent less than 6 months, 10% were on substitution treatment and 25% were regular heroin users. Patients were more likely to remain abstinent if they were going to work or school at the time of intake. Horazd'ovsky (1993) investigated trends in suicide rate in Czechoslovakia in 1975-1990 using national statistical databases. Suicide rates had decreased in both Czech and Slovak Republics. The rate was 13.4 per 100 000 in 2003, with the male to female ratio being 6.2:1 (Statistical Office of the Slovak Republic, 2004). Makinen (2000) discussed changing suicide patterns in Eastern Europe and former republics that formed the USSR. They found that the trends in suicide and their causes varied between countries. A model consisting of general stress, democratization, alcohol consumption and social disorganization (with a period-dependent effect) predicted fairly accurately the changes in the suicide rates in 16 out of the 28 Eastern Bloc countries in 1984-1989 and 1989-1994, but it failed to do so for Slovakia. Boehnke and Bergs-Winkels (2002) surveyed 42 independent samples of seventh graders from East and West Germany, Poland, Russia, Bulgaria, Slovakia, Hungary, Czechia and Greece in the years 1992-1995. Data on deviant school behaviour, delinquent drift, nurturant parenting and subjective feelings of justice in public were obtained from 7282 13- to 14-year-olds. Analyses showed that delinquent drift was a valid predictor of deviant school behaviour only on the individual level. The extent to which adolescents engage in pro-delinquent peer activities depends more on the cultural context in which adolescents live than on their personal experience in the family and in public. However, nurturant parenting co-varied negatively with deviant school behaviour irrespective of level of analysis.

MENTAL HEALTH RESOURCES

Mental Health Policy A mental health policy is absent.

There is no official mental health policy, but a Programme for Psychiatric Care exists which was formulated in 1997. It is based on the work of a large group of psychiatrists in the beginning of the 1990s: The Reform of Psychiatric Care. There are recommended numbers for all kinds of services. It was accepted by the Government but it lacked a time frame. The reform was based on the regional (or catchment area) principle, with units of 100 000 to 150 000 inhabitants, in which all the required services should function. The emphasis was placed on the balance of inpatient and outpatient care, including restructuring the profile of beds (closing beds in mental hospitals and opening new wards in general hospitals). The development of new outpatient services and forms of

S

care such as day centres, rehabilitation facilities, sheltered workshops and sheltered housing were also included. Non-regional facilities were to be used for special forms of treatment (addiction, children, forensic units, etc.).

Substance Abuse Policy A substance abuse policy is present. The policy was initially formulated in 1995.

National Mental Health Programme A national mental health programme is absent.
The national mental health programme was approved by the Government on October 6th 2004 as a basic document. It has to be elaborated in details as the intersectoral programme until October 31, 2005.

National Therapeutic Drug Policy/Essential List of Drugs A national therapeutic drug policy/essential list of drugs is present.
Details about the year of formulation are not available.
The essential drugs list is still to be approved.

Mental Health Legislation Completely new health care legislation (6 health care laws) was approved by the parliament on October 21, 2004. This forms the basis for the reform of health care. There is no single mental health law. It is included in laws concerning health, social care and others. The general health care laws have a special section which deals with psychiatry, mainly with involuntary admissions. The courts have to decide on individual cases.
The latest legislation was enacted in 2004.

Mental Health Financing There are budget allocations for mental health.
The country spends 5% of the total health budget on mental health.
The primary sources of mental health financing in descending order are social insurance and out of pocket expenditure by the patient or family.
Efforts to transform the health care system began with the change in the political system. The Governmental budget system was replaced by an insurance system requiring compulsory payments by both employees and employers. The Government paid insurance only for those without jobs. Primary care was virtually completely privatized, as general practitioners entered into contracts with insurance companies. Direct cash payments by patients remained rare, as salaries for most of the population were very low. Employers and Government failed to pay insurance companies, who in turn failed to pay providers (e.g. private doctors, hospitals and pharmacies). As a result, hospitals were unable to pay for drugs, power, or food; a hospital's debts sometimes reached as high as its annual budget.
The country has disability benefits for persons with mental disorders.

Mental Health Facilities Mental health is a part of primary health care system. Actual treatment of severe mental disorders is available at the primary level.
Regular training of primary care professionals is not carried out in the field of mental health.
There are community care facilities for patients with mental disorders. Most patients admitted to the ward are referred by outpatient psychiatrists. If the patient does not need inpatient treatment, he/she can be admitted to the day centre (18 in number), but most patients in the day centre come through the inpatient department.

Psychiatric Beds and Professionals

Total psychiatric beds per 10 000 population	9
Psychiatric beds in mental hospitals per 10 000 population	6
Psychiatric beds in general hospitals per 10 000 population	3
Psychiatric beds in other settings per 10 000 population	0
Number of psychiatrists per 100 000 population	10
Number of neurosurgeons per 100 000 population	1
Number of psychiatric nurses per 100 000 population	32
Number of neurologists per 100 000 population	9
Number of psychologists per 100 000 population	3
Number of social workers per 100 000 population	1

There are 60 other mental health personnel. Over the last decade, a 10% increase in the number of beds in general hospitals and a 10% reduction in the number of beds in psychiatry hospitals has occurred. However, a true transformation of the entire system has not been achieved. The restructuring of hospitals, including the closure of unnecessary ones, failed to occur. It had been accepted that standard psychiatric care should be according to region, made generally accessible and diversified so it can care for the whole spectrum of patients with mental disorders within all age-categories. Special centres for drug dependence treatment have been opened. Some self-help groups have also started. About 320 beds have been allocated to child and adolescent psychiatry. Most psychiatrists and clinical psychologists work on a private basis.

Non-Governmental Organizations NGOs are involved with mental health in the country. They are mainly involved in advocacy and treatment.

Information Gathering System There is mental health reporting system in the country. The annual health report is not published but a statistical report of general health with psychiatry in it is published.
The country has data collection system or epidemiological study on mental health. A statistical list compiling number and types of services, treatment, demographical data on suicide and drug users are prepared.

Programmes for Special Population No special care programmes exist but children have outpatient child psychiatry clinics and services for the elderly are available in outpatient and inpatient care facilities in a limited way.
Child and adolescent psychiatric services are available in cities, but facilities are particularly limited in east Slovakia. Some of these centres offer day care services. Complementary services outside the health system include counselling centres in each district (under Ministry of Education), special schools and residential facilities (about 4500 places) for mentally challenged children and short-term stay centres for children with conduct problems and abused or neglected children prior to foster placement.

Therapeutic Drugs The following therapeutic drugs are generally available at the primary health care level of the country: carbamazepine, ethosuximide, phenobarbital, phenytoin sodium, sodium valproate, amitriptyline, chlorpromazine, diazepam, haloperidol, lithium, biperiden, levodopa.
The drugs are divided into 3 categories, and the first category is fully reimbursed by the insurance.

Other Information

Additional Sources of Information

Baska, T., Straka, S., Mad'ar, R. (2000) Smoking habits in university students in Slovakia. Central European Journal of Public Health, 8, 245-248.

Boehnke, K., Bergs-Winkels, D. (2002) Juvenile delinquency under conditions of rapid social change. Sociological Forum, 17, 57-79.

Geckova, A., van Dijk, J.P., Groothoff, J.W., et al (2002) Socio-economic differences in health risk behaviour and attitudes towards health risk behaviour among Slovak adolescents. Sozial- und Präventivmedizin, 47, 233-239.

Heretik, A. S. sr., Heretik, A. Jr., Novotný, V. et al (2003) EPID. Epidemiológia depresie na Slovensku (EPID – Epidemiology of Depression in Slovakia). Nové Zámky: Psychoprof.

Horazd'ovsky, V. (1993) The suicide rate in Czechoslovakia 1975-1990. Ceskoslovenska Psychiatrie, 89, 233-238.

Makinen, I. H. (2000) Suicide mortality in the eastern European transition. Sociologisk Forskning, 37, 180-209.

Okruhlica, L. (1997) Epidemic of heroin use in Slovakia. European Addiction Research, 3, 83-86.

Okruhlica, L., Kaco, J., Klempova, D. (2001) Sports activities in the prevention of heroin dependency. European Addiction Research, 7, 83-86.

Okruhlica, L., Mihalkova, A., Klempova, D., et al (2002) Three-year follow-up study of heroin users in Bratislava. European Addiction Research, 8, 103-106.

Pecenak, J. (1999) Child and adolescent psychiatry in Slovakia. In: H. Remschmidt, H. van Engeland (Eds). Child and Adolescent Psychiatry in Europe. Historical Development, Current Situation and Future Perspectives. Darmstadt, Steinkopff. pp299-312.

Statistical Office of the Slovak Republic, 2004

Slovenia

GENERAL INFORMATION

Slovenia is a country with an approximate area of 20 thousand sq. km. (UNO, 2001). Its population is 1.982 million, and the sex ratio (men per hundred women) is 95 (UNO, 2004). The proportion of population under the age of 15 years is 14% (UNO, 2004), and the proportion of population above the age of 60 years is 20% (WHO, 2004). The literacy rate is 99.7% for men and 99.6% for women (UNESCO/MoH, 2004).

The country is a high income group country (based on World Bank 2004 criteria). The proportion of health budget to GDP is 8.4%. The per capita total expenditure on health is 1545 international $, and the per capita government expenditure on health is 1157 international $ (WHO, 2004).

The main language(s) used in the country is (are) Slovenian. The largest ethnic group(s) is (are) Slovene. The largest religious group(s) is (are) Roman Catholic.

The life expectancy at birth is 72.8 years for males and 80.5 years for females (WHO, 2004). The healthy life expectancy at birth is 67 years for males and 72 years for females (WHO, 2004).

EPIDEMIOLOGY

There is substantial epidemiological data on mental illnesses in Slovenia in internationally accessible literature. No attempt was made to include this information here.

MENTAL HEALTH RESOURCES

Mental Health Policy A mental health policy is absent.

Substance Abuse Policy A substance abuse policy is absent. The Drug Office at the Slovenian Government is presently working on the National Programme for Prevention of Drug Misuse and a new strategy plan is under development.

National Mental Health Programme A national mental health programme is absent.

Though a national programme of mental health has not yet been adopted, it is the responsibility of the Council for Health, a Government advisory body which includes experts from the fields of both health and social security. However, national programmes have been suggested for preventing suicide and dependence on alcohol and drugs.

National Therapeutic Drug Policy/Essential List of Drugs A national therapeutic drug policy/essential list of drugs is present. It was formulated in 1999.

A Medicinal Product and Medical Device Act was adopted in 1999.

Mental Health Legislation The Mental Health Act is in under Government evaluation. The Involuntary Commitment Law, Section 7 of 1986 and the Act on Legal Proceedings of 1999 deal with mental health. The different legislation on substance abuse are: Prevention of the Use of Illicit Drugs and Dealing with Consumers of Illicit Drugs Act (1999), Production and Trade in Illicit Drugs Act (1999), and the Law on Precursors for Illicit Drugs Act (1999). The Ministry of Health, together with competent experts from the field, the Ministry of Labour, Family and Social affairs and the Ministry of Justice are drafting a new mental health legislation which will include: voluntary and involuntary admission to treatment, emergency admission, prolonged detention, early discharge, patient rights, advocacy and care planning.

The latest legislation was enacted in 1999.

Mental Health Financing There are no budget allocations for mental health.

Details about expenditure on mental health are not available.

The primary sources of mental health financing in descending order are tax based, social insurance, private insurances and out of pocket expenditure by the patient or family.

Part of the problems in the development of community mental health programmes in the country is related to the fact that insurance agencies finance hospital beds rather than programmes. Rehabilitation services are funded partly by health care and partly by the social care system.

The country has disability benefits for persons with mental disorders. The essential socioeconomic provisions for people with mental disorders, include disability allowance, social support, free medications and no restrictions in the number of outpatient psychiatry consultation. Retirement benefits are present for chronically mentally ill patients.

Mental Health Facilities Mental health is a part of primary health care system. Actual treatment of severe mental disorders is available at the primary level. Psychiatrists can be employed at a primary health care level.

Regular training of primary care professionals is carried out in the field of mental health. In the last two years, about 50 personnel were provided training. Though courses, mostly on depression, have been provided, most such practitioners do not have adequate mental health training.

There are community care facilities for patients with mental disorders. There are some attempts by psychiatric institutions and NGOs, but no system for community mental health approach has been developed as yet. In Ljubljana (the capital), a rehabilitation service has been created within the framework of the psychiatric service, which is intended to provide better coordination with outside collaborators and introduce rehabilitation principles in treatment. The psychiatric rehabilitation service should enable suitable referral of patients and coordination among the so far poorly linked non-governmental and social services as well as GP services. The University Psychiatric Hospital in Ljubljana also gives professional and material support to non-governmental organizations that provide outpatient community care for its patients. It serves as a national tertiary referral centre. User organizations and associations of interested experts have been founded. The largest are ŠENT, ALTRA; OZARA; PARADOKS which, together with the psychiatric profession, are involved in preventive, mainly anti-stigma programmes. Among the psychosocial services offered are housing facilities with support (about 1800 places), day centres, vocational rehabilitation development, sheltered employments and education facilities for patients and carers.

Psychiatric Beds and Professionals

Total psychiatric beds per 10 000 population	8.46
Psychiatric beds in mental hospitals per 10 000 population	7.2
Psychiatric beds in general hospitals per 10 000 population	1.26
Psychiatric beds in other settings per 10 000 population	0
Number of psychiatrists per 100 000 population	5.35
Number of neurosurgeons per 100 000 population	0
Number of psychiatric nurses per 100 000 population	5.8
Number of neurologists per 100 000 population	0.8
Number of psychologists per 100 000 population	1.65
Number of social workers per 100 000 population	0.45

There are altogether six regional psychiatric hospitals including the university psychiatric hospital and the Psychiatric Clinic. All have wards for general psychiatry, psycho-geriatrics and the treatment of alcohol dependency. The Psychiatric Clinic also has wards for adolescent psychiatry, drug dependency and psychotherapy. There is also the Child Psychiatry Ward in the Paediatric Clinic. About 30 beds have been allocated for child and adolescent psychiatry. Deinstitutionalization has not taken place significantly in Slovenia. Also, there are no psychiatric hospitals in the southern region. There are 24 child and adolescent psychiatrists in the country. In addition, 35 clinical psychologists, 25 educational psychologists, 42 social workers and a number of other professionals are involved in provision of child and adolescent mental health services. Some psychiatrists have started working as private practitioners following the implementation of the national insurance scheme.

Non-Governmental Organizations NGOs are involved with mental health in the country. They are mainly involved in advocacy, promotion, prevention, treatment and rehabilitation. From 1997-98, there was an attempt to strengthen the civil initiatives in the country, initially with the help of the Netherlands MATRA funds. And education programmes for patients, carers and professionals were created. These helped to increase awareness regarding mental disorders, treatment facilities, psychosocial rehabilitation facilities, which in turn helped in reducing stigma. The network of organizations and services outside psychiatry which could support preventive activities – mainly early recognition and treatment of mental disorders – is weak. A national organization of relatives of people with severe mental illness called Forum of carers was established in 1999 and many self-help groups are functioning.

Information Gathering System There is mental health reporting system in the country. Details can be obtained from the Health Statistics Yearbook of Slovenia 1999, Institute of Public Health.
The country has data collection system or epidemiological study on mental health.

Programmes for Special Population The country has specific programmes for mental health for minorities, refugees, disaster affected population, elderly and children.
Preventive education programmes for recognizing suicidal tendencies take place constantly. Therapeutic work is done with the suicide survivors, individually and in groups, and some preventive work has been done with GPs and teachers to recognize and react with depressed and suicidal individuals. The Institute for Health Protection organizes numerous preventive programmes against smoking, other addictions and infection with AIDS. Health programmes are also organized at schools and kindergarten. A part of mental health services for children and adolescents is provided within the framework of education and social care programme. Most schools in Slovenia have one or more school counsellors, who often collaborate with social workers at regional centres for social care. Centres for social care supervise and run dwellings for adolescents with dysfunctional families. Child guidance clinics are also available and are usually staffed by psychologists.

Therapeutic Drugs The following therapeutic drugs are generally available at the primary health care level of the country: carbamazepine, ethosuximide, phenobarbital, amitriptyline, diazepam, fluphenazine, haloperidol, lithium, biperiden, levodopa.
The anti-epileptics prescribed most often are carbamazepine, valproic acid and gabapentin. The anti-parkinsonians, used most often are biperiden, levodopa and decarboxylase inhibitor and entacapone. The most popular anxiolytics/hypnotics in terms of prescription support are bromazepam, alprazolam and zolpidem; and the most popular anti-depressants are citalopram, sertraline and fluoxetine.

Other Information

Additional Sources of Information

Brecelj, M., Marusic, A. (2000) Psychiatry in Slovenia: a high suicide rate and cirrhosis rates country. Psychiatric Bulletin, 24, 385-387.

Marusic, A., Turein, A. (2004) Mental health reforms in Slovenia awaited. Mental Health Reforms, 18-20.

Dernovsek, M. Z., Marusic, A., Tavcar, R. (2003) How to avoid community psychiatry. International Journal of Psychiatry, 49, 5-7.

Svab, V., Tomori, M. (2002). Mental health in Slovenia. International Journal of Social Psychiatry, 48, 177-188.

Tomori, M. (1999) Child and adolescent psychiatry in Slovenia. In: H.Remschmidt, H. van Engeland (Eds). Child and Adolescent Psychiatry in Europe. Historical Development, Current Situation and Future Perspectives. Darmstadt, Steinkopff. pp313-328.

Zakon O Zdravilih. Medicinal Products Act. (Government document).

Solomon Islands

GENERAL INFORMATION

Solomon Islands is a country with an approximate area of 29 thousand sq. km. (UNO, 2001). The country is an archipelago of about 1000 mountainous islands and low-lying coral atolls. Its population is 0.491 million, and the sex ratio (men per hundred women) is 106 (UNO, 2004). The proportion of population under the age of 15 years is 42% (UNO, 2004), and the proportion of population above the age of 60 years is 4% (WHO, 2004). The literacy rate is 85% for men and 68% for women (UNESCO/MoH, 2004).
The country is a low income group country (based on World Bank 2004 criteria). The proportion of health budget to GDP is 5%. The per capita total expenditure on health is 133 international $, and the per capita government expenditure on health is 124 international $ (WHO, 2004).
The main language(s) used in the country is (are) English and Solomon Pijin. The largest ethnic group(s) is (are) Melanesian. The largest religious group(s) is (are) Christian.
The life expectancy at birth is 63.6 years for males and 67.4 years for females (WHO, 2004). The healthy life expectancy at birth is 55 years for males and 57 years for females (WHO, 2004).

EPIDEMIOLOGY

There is a paucity of epidemiological data on mental illnesses in Solomon Islands in internationally accessible literature. Dohan et al (1984) reviewed multiple data sources and found only two cases of schizophrenia in Pacific Islands including Solomon Islands during the historical epoch when the islanders were unfamiliar with gluten containing cereals (e.g. wheat), when the expected number based on population estimates was 130. Later, when the eating habits of this region approached patterns common in Europe, the prevalence of schizophrenia also reached European levels. From this, the researchers inferred a role for grain glutens in the onset of schizophrenia.

MENTAL HEALTH RESOURCES

Mental Health Policy A mental health policy is absent.
An initial draft of mental health policy is ready. Further progress could not be made because of absence of consultants to guide and advise on the development of the policy. The policy on mental health is expected to be finalized by January 2006.

Substance Abuse Policy A substance abuse policy is absent. There is no substance abuse programme, although it is a part of the national mental health programme.

National Mental Health Programme A national mental health programme is present. The programme was formulated in 1999. It is a six year plan. Part of it was incorporated in the Ministry of Health's National Health Policies and Development Plans 1999-2003. The draft plan for the next 10-years is ready for approval of the Ministry.

National Therapeutic Drug Policy/Essential List of Drugs A national therapeutic drug policy/essential list of drugs is present. Details about the year of formulation are not available.
The national drug policy was drafted in 1999 but has still not been ratified. However, it is being applied in functions related to the essential drug programme, dangerous drugs and psychotherapy, administration and reporting, poison registration and pharmaceutical personnel development and training.

Mental Health Legislation There is a Mental Treatment Act. This act consolidates the law relating to persons of unsound mind and makes further and better provision for the care of persons suffering from mental disorders and for custody of persons and the management and control of mental hospitals. There is now an attempt to include community and primary care facilities incorporated into the act. The Act was amended in 1995 by two consultants and attempts are being made to get it passed by the parliament. It is a part of the mental health programme.
The latest legislation was enacted in 1970.

Mental Health Financing There are budget allocations for mental health.
The country spends 1.4% of the total health budget on mental health.
The primary source of mental health financing is tax based.
The country does not have disability benefits for persons with mental disorders. There is no public disability benefit. The insurance system does not insure against mental illness.

Mental Health Facilities Mental health is a part of primary health care system. Actual treatment of severe mental disorders is not available at the primary level. There is a basic continuum of service from acute care at the outpatient clinics to outreach services, but the links are erratic.
Regular training of primary care professionals is carried out in the field of mental health. In the last two years, about 62 personnel were provided training. Some psychiatric health coordinators have been trained and the plan is to train all registered nurses and nursing aides throughout the country over a five year period. A one-month training programme funded by WHO trained 12 nurse coordinators (4 underwent a full psychiatric nursing training later) who are now functioning in 7 out of 9 provinces. Similarly, about 50 nurse aids were trained in courses funded by the Health Institute Strengthening Project from the Australian Government. In addi-

tion to their regular duties, the nurse coordinators carry out psychiatric tours of remote areas, where they educate the public and give mental health talks to nurses and doctors besides providing clinical care and referral. Nurse coordinators do not have prescribing privileges.
There are no community care facilities for patients with mental disorders. Nurses give injections to patients in rural areas. There are plans to start a day care centre.

Psychiatric Beds and Professionals

Total psychiatric beds per 10 000 population	0.26
Psychiatric beds in mental hospitals per 10 000 population	0.26
Psychiatric beds in general hospitals per 10 000 population	0
Psychiatric beds in other settings per 10 000 population	0
Number of psychiatrists per 100 000 population	0
Number of neurosurgeons per 100 000 population	0
Number of psychiatric nurses per 100 000 population	0.9
Number of neurologists per 100 000 population	0
Number of psychologists per 100 000 population	0
Number of social workers per 100 000 population	0

There is a lack of specialists because of difficulties in getting through the advertisement and recruitment process. The appointment of an overseas psychiatrist is expected this year. The psychiatric ward at the National Psychiatric Unit was closed in 2002 following a shortage of medicines and daily necessities. Patients with suicide attempts/overdose are admitted in medical wards. The nurses are in psychiatric nursing training in Papua New Guinea, and a doctor has been sent for overseas training as a psychiatrist.

Non-Governmental Organizations NGOs are not involved with mental health in the country. Churches offer counselling, and the Richmond Fellowship has expressed a willingness to help in mental health services.

Information Gathering System There is no mental health reporting system in the country. Currently, mental health is not included in the Monthly Clinic Report System (Health Information System) but it would be reported in future and is a programme under the mental health programme. There is an annual mental health report by the Mental Health Division Heads which use standard reporting systems.
The country has no data collection system or epidemiological study on mental health. A prevalence survey was tried unsuccessfully and would be retried again.

Programmes for Special Population There are no special services available.

Therapeutic Drugs The following therapeutic drugs are generally available at the primary health care level of the country: carbamazepine, phenobarbital, phenytoin sodium, chlorpromazine, diazepam, fluphenazine, lithium.
Only chlorpromazine is stocked to area health centres and to some rural health centres. Other drugs such as fluphenazine, haloperidol and benzhexol are supplied to the patients who have been discharged from the hospital. Supplies are ordered against patients names to ensure patients have enough supply stocked in the rural clinics. Other drugs like trifluoperazine, benzhexol and fluoxetine are also available for use in primary care.

Other Information Training programmes are being conducted for community leaders, relatives and carers, police and those in the legal profession. The World Mental Health Day is celebrated to generate awareness on mental health issues.

Additional Sources of Information

Dohan, F. C., Harper, E. H., Clark, M. H., et al (1984) Is schizophrenia rare if grain is rare? Biological Psychiatry, 19, 385-399.

Somalia

GENERAL INFORMATION

Somalia is a country with an approximate area of 638 thousand sq. km. (UNO, 2001). Its population is 10.312 million, and the sex ratio (men per hundred women) is 99 (UNO, 2004). The proportion of population under the age of 15 years is 48% (UNO, 2004), and the proportion of population above the age of 60 years is 4% (WHO, 2004). The literacy rate is 25.1% for men and 13.4% for women (UNESCO/MoH, 2004).

The country is a low income group country (based on World Bank 2004 criteria). The proportion of health budget to GDP is 2.6%. The per capita total expenditure on health is 15 international $, and the per capita government expenditure on health is 7 international $ (WHO, 2004).

The main language(s) used in the country is (are) Somali, Arabic, English and Italian. The largest ethnic group(s) is (are) Somali (five-sixths), and the other ethnic group(s) are (is) Bantu. The largest religious group(s) is (are) Muslim.

The life expectancy at birth is 43 years for males and 45.7 years for females (WHO, 2004). The healthy life expectancy at birth is 36 years for males and 38 years for females (WHO, 2004).

EPIDEMIOLOGY

There is a paucity of epidemiological data on mental illnesses in Somalia in internationally accessible literature. Elmi (1983) conducted an epidemiological research on khat chewing in a random sample of about 7500 people. He suggested that the prevalence of the khat chewing has continuously increased in all social groups and that the excessive use of khat may create considerable problems of social, health and economic nature.

MENTAL HEALTH RESOURCES

Mental Health Policy A mental health policy is absent.
There is no unified health policy.

Substance Abuse Policy A substance abuse policy is absent.

National Mental Health Programme A national mental health programme is absent.

National Therapeutic Drug Policy/Essential List of Drugs A national therapeutic drug policy/essential list of drugs is absent.

Mental Health Legislation Details about the mental health legislation are not available.

Mental Health Financing There are no budget allocations for mental health.
Details about expenditure on mental health are not available.
The primary source of mental health financing is grants.
The financing of mental health services is almost entirely dependent on grants from WHO and NGOs.
The country does not have disability benefits for persons with mental disorders.

Mental Health Facilities Mental health is not a part of primary health care system. Actual treatment of severe mental disorders is not available at the primary level. Recently, a Mental Health Coordinator was appointed for North West Somalia to initiate integration of mental health care in primary health care and training of primary health care personnel.

Regular training of primary care professionals is not carried out in the field of mental health. The voluntary workers of GAVO have been trained about the principles of psychiatric interview, introduced to DSM-IV, given training about psychopharmacology, psychosocial rehabilitation and hospital management. The training had lasted for 2 years and is not on a regular basis.

There are no community care facilities for patients with mental disorders. Limited community care through NGOs and WHO are available in very limited areas of one region in northwest Somalia. A psychosocial centre was established in Berbera in 1990.

Psychiatric Beds and Professionals

Total psychiatric beds per 10 000 population	0.398
Psychiatric beds in mental hospitals per 10 000 population	
Psychiatric beds in general hospitals per 10 000 population	
Psychiatric beds in other settings per 10 000 population	
Number of psychiatrists per 100 000 population	0.06
Number of neurosurgeons per 100 000 population	
Number of psychiatric nurses per 100 000 population	0.03
Number of neurologists per 100 000 population	
Number of psychologists per 100 000 population	0
Number of social workers per 100 000 population	0.19

There are only three centres for psychiatry, the mental hospital in Berbera and the general psychiatric wards in Hargesia and Mogadishu. Until the arrival of the NGO from Italy, the condition of the mental hospital was appalling. Patients were kept in chains, and supply of food was largely dependent on charity. UNDP is supporting the psychiatric ward in Hargesia in terms of structural facilities and supplies. There is no private psychiatric inpatient facility though there are a few private clinics in Mogadishu and Hargesia. There is no specialized drug abuse treatment centre and there is no mental health training facility in the country. Only limited data about one area of Somalia, Somaliland is available. Psychiatrists have private clinics.

Non-Governmental Organizations NGOs are involved with mental health in the country. They are mainly involved in advocacy, promotion, prevention, treatment and rehabilitation. The whole mental health set-up of Somalia is based on the efforts of NGOs – GRT-UNA of Italy and General Assistance and Volunteer Association (GAVO), a local Somali NGO. They help in the provision of services to mental patients and street children and provide training for primary health care personnel.

Information Gathering System There is no mental health reporting system in the country.
The country has no data collection system or epidemiological study on mental health.

Programmes for Special Population No programmes for special population exist.
UNDP and NGOs are supporting the Government's plans for reintegration of militia including those that are mentally ill into the mainstream through projects involving occupation.

Therapeutic Drugs The following therapeutic drugs are generally available at the primary health care level of the country: unknown.

Other Information

Additional Sources of Information

Elmi, A. S. (1983) The chewing of khat in Somalia. Journal of Ethnopharmacology, 8, 163-176.

Mental Health in Somaliland. (Government document).

Omar, M. A. (1986) Developments in mental health services in Somalia. NIMHANS Journal, 4, 131-132.

S

South Africa

GENERAL INFORMATION

South Africa is a country with an approximate area of 1221 thousand sq. km. (UNO, 2001). Its population is 45.214 million, and the sex ratio (men per hundred women) is 95 (UNO, 2004). The proportion of population under the age of 15 years is 33% (UNO, 2004), and the proportion of population above the age of 60 years is 6% (WHO, 2004). The literacy rate is 86.7% for men and 85.3% for women (UNESCO/MoH, 2004).

The country is a lower middle income group country (based on World Bank 2004 criteria). The proportion of health budget to GDP is 8.6%. The per capita total expenditure on health is 652 international $, and the per capita government expenditure on health is 270 international $ (WHO, 2004).

The main language(s) used in the country is (are) eleven, with English being important for commerce. The largest ethnic group(s) is (are) African, and the other ethnic group(s) are (is) European and Asian. The largest religious group(s) is (are) Christian, and the other religious group(s) are (is) Hindu and Muslim.

The life expectancy at birth is 48.8 years for males and 52.6 years for females (WHO, 2004). The healthy life expectancy at birth is 43 years for males and 45 years for females (WHO, 2004).

EPIDEMIOLOGY

Rumble et al (1996) conducted a two-stage survey in a rural community (n=481) using the Self-Reporting Questionnaire (SRQ) and the Present State Examination (PSE). The weighted prevalence of psychiatric morbidity was 27.1%. Depression and anxiety disorder were common. Bhagwanjee et al (1998) assessed 354 rural adults with SRQ-20 and standardized instruments following a two-stage procedure. The weighted prevalence for DSM-IV generalized anxiety and depressive disorders was 23.9% (generalized anxiety: 3.7%, major depression: 4.8%, dysthymia: 7.3% and major depression and dysthymia: 8.2%). Michalowsky et al (1989) evaluated 1239 respondents from 3 mining areas. According to GHQ, the number of cases varied from 14.1% to 23.8%, and between 23.2% and 31.2% of respondents drank alcohol at least once a day. Women had more psychosocial illnesses in comparison to men. Ben-Arie et al (1983) examined 139 non-institutionalized coloured elderly (above 65 years) persons using the PSE and the Mini Mental State Examination (MMSE). Dementia (8.6%, severe: 3.6%), other psychiatric disorders (24%, depression: 16.5%) and alcohol dependence (15% of men) were common. Parry et al (2002) reported the findings of the South African Community Epidemiology Network on Drug Use (SACENDU) project. Between 1997-99, alcohol was the most commonly used drug (51.1% – 77% in various regions) and use of alcohol was associated with trauma and comorbid psychiatric disorders. School surveys showed a harmful drinking pattern in 36% to 53.3% of male students. Use of cannabis and methaqualone was also common. There was a significant increase in cocaine and heroin use during the period. Flisher et al (2002) assessed 2930 students of grades 8 and 11. Lifetime prevalence rates of substance use were: 42.1% for tobacco, 43.8% for alcohol, 12.3% for cannabis and 3.6% for methaqualone, ecstasy or crack. London (2000) reported problem drinking and dangerous drinking according to CAGE and a shortened version of the Michigan Alcoholism Screening Test (MAST) in about two-thirds and 9.3%, respectively, of a sample of farm workers. In a rural general practice (n=858), 15.6% of the subjects had major depression (Strauss et al, 1995). Cooper et al (1999) found depression (as per DSM-IV) in 34.7% of 147 women who had delivered two months previously. Maternal depression was associated with poor support from partners and insensitive engagement with the infants. Allwood et al (2001) reported an incidence rate of 2-3 per 1000 births for puerperal psychosis (n=381) and that it was associated with primiparity and family or past history of psychiatric or medical illnesses. Flisher and Parry (1994) analysed the suicide mortality data from the national registry (1984-1986). Suicides accounted for 1.3% of deaths, with higher rates among the Whites, but suicide were very common among young Asian women. The most common method of committing suicide in Whites was firearms and in others hanging. Sukhai et al (2002) reviewed the National Injury Mortality Surveillance System register and police and hospital records (1996-2000) and found that suicides accounted for 5.6% of deaths. The majority of suicides were reported for black women in their thirties. In a sample of 7340 school children, Flisher et al (1993) found that during the previous 12 months, 19% of students had suicidal thoughts and 7.8% had attempted suicide. Mhlongo and Peltzer (1999) found parasuicidal behaviour in 10% of young patients (15-24 years) attending a regional hospital. Robertson and Juritz (1998) found that 17.6% to 21% of 10-13 year-old children according to parents' reports, and 9.5% to 10.5% of children according to teachers' reports met the criteria for behaviour disorders. Behaviour disorders were associated with gender (boys), age (older), IQ (below 100) and learning disability. Robertson et al (1999) administered the Xhosa Diagnostic Interview Schedule for Children Version 2.3 to children and adolescents aged 6-16 years (n=500) in an informal settlement area. Psychiatric disorder with impairment was found in 15.2% of the children and adolescents. Peltzer (1999) assessed 148 secondary school children using the Children's Posttraumatic Stress Disorder Inventory and the Reporting Questionnaire for Children and found that two-thirds of the children had experienced a traumatic situation and 8.4% met a diagnosis of PTSD. In a sample of 7516 Black primary school children, Cartwright et al (1981) found that 22.4% had a learning problem and 8.7% had a physical or mental handicap. Couper (2002) found a prevalence rate of 6% for various disabilities in a two-stage survey (n=2036) of children (<10 years). Perceptual or learning disabilities were common. Christianson et al (2002) assessed 6692 rural children (2-9 years old) following a two stage procedure and found a rate of 3.6% for intellectual disability (severe – 0.6% and mild – 2.9%). The male:female ratio was 3:2.

MENTAL HEALTH RESOURCES

Mental Health Policy A mental health policy is present. The policy was initially formulated in 1997.
The components of the policy are advocacy, promotion, prevention, treatment and rehabilitation. The White Paper for the Transformation of the Health System in South Africa (1997) sets out the policy direction for the development and transformation of mental heath services.

Substance Abuse Policy A substance abuse policy is absent. The substance abuse policy is in the process of being finalized.

National Mental Health Programme A national mental health programme is present. The programme was formulated in 1997. The mental health programme is different for each province. The present move is towards establishing community-based services, with the integration of mental health services into primary health care. Concerted efforts are also being made to assist with preventive and promotive aspects of mental health.

National Therapeutic Drug Policy/Essential List of Drugs A national therapeutic drug policy/essential list of drugs is present. It was formulated in 1998.

Mental Health Legislation The existing legislation, the Mental Health Act, is old. The Mental Health Care Act, was passed by Parliament in 2002. It will be promulgated in 2004. The main aims of the Act are to promote human rights of people with disabilities; improve mental health services through a primary health care approach and an emphasis on community care; protect the health and safety of the public in circumstances where a person with mental disabilities may be a danger to him/herself or others; set out the framework and statutory roles with respect to voluntary users, assisted users, involuntary users, state patients and mentally ill prisoners. Current legislation will allow the possibility of non-medical practitioners having the right to prescribe (CRTP) medication in South Africa.
The latest legislation was enacted in 2002.

Mental Health Financing There are budget allocations for mental health.
Details about expenditure on mental health are not available.
The primary sources of mental health financing in descending order are tax based, private insurances, out of pocket expenditure by the patient or family and social insurance.
Quite recently, a study was commissioned to calculate the expenditure on mental health. The study provided highly disputed figures as it failed to calculate the cost of the integrated mental health care. A patient advocacy NGO, the Depression and Anxiety Support Group, found evidence of discrimination against mental illnesses in South African medical aids and state-funded health systems. Specifically, some aids refused to cover hospitalization for suicide attempts and substance use disorders.
The country has disability benefits for persons with mental disorders.

Mental Health Facilities Mental health is a part of primary health care system. Actual treatment of severe mental disorders is available at the primary level. Care is provided in some cases by a psychiatric nurse and in others by a primary health care worker. The current psychiatric practice is varied and a new patient can be initially seen by either a psychiatrist or a community nurse or a primary nurse depending on the place. The patient is then either treated at that place or is immediately referred to a secondary facility. The aim is to make the system more efficient so that there is a comprehensive mental care facility at the community level. However the integration of mental health into primary health care services is sub-optimal.
Regular training of primary care professionals is carried out in the field of mental health. In the last two years, about 450 personnel were provided training. Primary health care practitioners, e.g. nurses undergo integrated training that provides for knowledge and skills needed to handle psychosocial issues. This is supplemented by further training in additional or contemporary mental health issues like crisis intervention/trauma counselling, phacotherapy, management of substance abuse etc. Evaluation of components of these programmes have shown that the interventions have been successful.
There are community care facilities for patients with mental disorders. Other than giving medical care, community care is very limited.

Psychiatric Beds and Professionals

Total psychiatric beds per 10 000 population	4.5
Psychiatric beds in mental hospitals per 10 000 population	4
Psychiatric beds in general hospitals per 10 000 population	0.38
Psychiatric beds in other settings per 10 000 population	0.12
Number of psychiatrists per 100 000 population	1.2
Number of neurosurgeons per 100 000 population	0.3
Number of psychiatric nurses per 100 000 population	7.5
Number of neurologists per 100 000 population	0.3
Number of psychologists per 100 000 population	4
Number of social workers per 100 000 population	20

The staff-patient ratios cited above may be an over-estimation due to the high rate of emigration of health personnel and the employment of mental health professionals in other sectors. There are 109 occupational therapists, 89 medical officers and 28 community health workers besides a number of trainee mental health professionals working in the mental health services. About a quarter of the beds are acute beds and three quarters medium-long stay beds. There are large differences between bed strengths in each province, with Mpumalanga, North-West Province and Northen Cape having few beds and Gauteng and Northern Province having many beds for mental health care. In some province downsizing has occurred, but it was not accompanied by the development of residential and ambulatory care in the community. The only province to report residential care facilities in the community was Gauteng, which reported a total of 305 places. Most mental health professionals are concentrated in the Cape Town and Guateng (Johannesburg-Pretoria) region. The North-West Province has no psychiatrist, and Northern Cape and Mpumalanga have only one each. These regions have a low concentration of other mental health professionals also. About 56% of psychiatrists in South Africa work in private set-ups. They provide services to about 20% of the population, the majority of whom are funded by medical insurance. Only 4.7% of psychiatrists are practicing in the rural setting. Most psychiatrists are biologically oriented and the few who practice psychotherapy use cognitive-behavioural models in most situations. However, Jungian School of analytical psychotherapy is practised by some in Cape Town. Limited private practice is permitted to psychiatrists in the Government set-up. A substantial proportion of psychiatrists recruited to English-speaking countries are from South Africa. Not many black doctors have been attracted to psychiatry; as a result only 10.8% of South African psychiatrists are able to communicate fluently in one or more African languages.

Non-Governmental Organizations NGOs are involved with mental health in the country. They are mainly involved in advocacy, promotion, prevention, treatment and rehabilitation. At least 14 support groups are functioning in South Africa. However, 10 areas have no support groups. They rendered assistance in advocacy, providing for basic needs of their members, life skills teaching, crisis intervention and counselling. Rural support groups provide advocacy, treatment and rehabilitation.

Information Gathering System There is no mental health reporting system in the country. The national indicators do not include information on the prevalence of mental disorders. At the district level, data on clinical consultations is collected.
The country has data collection system or epidemiological study on mental health. Data are collected from hospital and community services. A national epidemiological study is under way. The South African Demographic Health Survey conducted in 1998 and the First South African Youth Risk Behaviour Survey (2002) contributed important findings on mental health of populations.

Programmes for Special Population The country has specific programmes for mental health for children. Some of the programmes are run by NGOs and the Government has also started working in some areas. There are some programmes for victims of violence.
Child and adolescent, geriatric and neuropsychiatric services are available, but dedicated staff and facilities are available at only a few centres. Some community psychiatric nurses have been given special training in child and adolescent mental health issues. As a part of the National Crime Prevention strategy, the mental health directorate has taken responsibility for training general health workers in 'victim empowerment', setting up 'violence referral centres' in disadvantaged areas, setting up violence prevention programmes in schools and developing mother-infant bonding programmes for violence prevention in poor communities. As a part of the national initiative to prevent the spread of HIV among school children, teachers in every school are being trained to teach HIV/AIDS-related and substance abuse-related life skills at primary and secondary school levels. The need for pre-test and post-test counselling on HIV/AIDS will lead to the deployment of counsellors in every clinic in a five-year period. A Mental Health Information Centre has been started to provide psychoeducation.

Therapeutic Drugs The following therapeutic drugs are generally available at the primary health care level of the country: carbamazepine, ethosuximide, phenobarbital, sodium valproate, amitriptyline, chlorpromazine, diazepam, fluphenazine, haloperidol, lithium, biperiden, carbidopa, levodopa.
The acquisition costs of new psychotropics is considerably greater than those of their predecessors.

Other Information In 1978, the APA compiled a report criticizing the racial bias in psychiatric practice. Similar reports were filed by the Royal College of Psychiatrists in 1983. Isolation from international forums followed from 1987. Though currently racial bias is not present in treatment issues, a recent study (Lee et al, 1999) found that the better centres tended to be utilized more by the white community. This was due to the availability of better services in the white population dominated areas, and the conclusion was to extend some of these services to the poorer sections of the community without compromising the existing structure present in the more affluent white community. In response to the gross violation of human rights in the past, the post-apartheid Government established a Truth and Reconciliation (TRC) in a move to promote national unity and reconciliation. Mental health professionals provided advice regarding the manner in which testimony should be taken, and provided psychological support when necessary to those who testified. TRC members were trained in issues relevant to psychological support, and some of the TRC commissioners were mental health professionals.

Additional Sources of Information

Allwood, C. W., Berk, M., Bodemer, W. (2000) An investigation into puerperal psychoses in black women admitted to Baragwaneth Hospital. South African Medical Journal, 90, 518-520.

Ben-Arie, O., Swartz, L., Teggin, A. F., et al (1983) The coloured elderly in Cape Town-a psychosocial, psychiatric and medical community survey. Part II. Prevalence of psychiatric disorders. South African Medical Journal, 64, 1056-1061.

Bhagwanjee, A., Parekh, A., Paruk, Z., et al (1998) Prevalence of minor psychiatric disorders in an adult African rural community in South Africa. Psychological Medicine, 28, 1137-1147.

Cartwright, J. D., Jukes, C., Wilson, A., et al (1981) A survey of learning problems in black primary school children. South African Medical Journal, 59, 488-490.

Christianson, A. L., Zwane, M. E., Manga, P., et al (2002) Children with intellectual disability in rural South Africa: prevalence and associated disability. Journal of Intellectual Disability Research, 46, 179-186.

Couper, J. (2002) Prevalence of childhood disability in rural KwaZulu-Natal. South African Medical Journal, 92, 549-552.

Cooper, P. J., Tomlinson, M., Swartz, L., et al (1999) Post-partum depression and the mother-infant relationship in a South African peri-urban settlement. British Journal of Psychiatry, 175, 554-558.

Emsley, R. (2001) Focus on psychiatry in South Africa. British Journal of Psychiatry, 178, 382-386.

Flisher, A. J., Parry, C. D. (1994) Suicide in South Africa. An analysis of nationally registered mortality data for 1984-1986. Acta Psychiatrica Scandinavica, 90, 348-353.

Flisher, A. J., Parry, C. D. H., Muller, M., et al (2002) Stages of substance use among adolescents in Cape Town, South Africa. Journal of Substance Use, 7, 162-167.

Flisher, A. J., Riccitelli, G., Jhetam, N., et al (1997) A survey of professional activities of psychiatrists in South Africa. Psychiatric Services, 48,707-709.

Flisher, A. J., Ziervogel, C. F., Chalton, D. O., et al (1993) Risk-taking behaviour of Cape Peninsula high-school students. Part II. Suicidal behaviour. South African Medical Journal, 83, 474-476

Lee, T., Freeman, M., Vivian, W. (1999). Evaluation of mental health services in the Free State. Part I. Quality of outpatient care. South African Medical Journal, 89, 302-305.

Lee, T., Freeman, M., Vivian, W. (1999). Evaluation of Mental Health Services in the Free State. Part II. Training, Attitudes and Practices of Generalist and Psychiatric Nurses. 15. South African Medical Journal, 89, 306-310.

Lindegger, G. (1999). Psychologists' right to prescribe – should prescribing privileges be granted to South African psychologists? South African Medical Journal, 89, 69-75.

London, L. (2000) Alcohol consumption amongst South African farm workers: a challenge for post-apartheid health sector transformation. Drug & Alcohol Dependence, 59, 199-206.

Lund, C., Flisher, A. J. (2002) Staff-bed and staff-patient ratios in South African public sector mental health services. South African Medical Journal, 92, 157-161.

Lund, C., Flisher, A. J.(2002) Staff-population ratios in South African public sector mental health services. South African Medical Journal, 92, 161-164.

Lund, C., Flisher, A. J., Porteus, K., et al. (2002) Bed-population ratios in South African public sector mental health services. Social Psychiatry & Psychiatric Epidemiology, 37, 346-349.

Mhlongo, T., Peltzer, K. (1999) Parasuicide among youth in a general hospital in South Africa. Curationis, 22, 72-76.

Michalowsky, A. M., Wicht, C. L., Moller, A. T. (1989) The psychosocial effects of living in an isolated community. A community health study. South African Medical Journal, 75, 532-534.

Parry, C. D., Bhana, A., Pluddemann, A., et al (2002) The South African Community Epidemiology Network on Drug Use (SACENDU): description, findings (1997-99) and policy implications. Addiction, 97, 969-976.

Peltzer, K. (1999) Posttraumatic stress symptoms in a population of rural children in South Africa. Psychological Reports, 85, 646-650.

Pillay, A. L., Lockhat, M. R. (1997). Developing community mental health services for children in South Africa. Social Science and Medicine, 45, 1493-1501.

Robertson, B. A., Ensink, K., Parry, C. D., et al (1999) Performance of the Diagnostic Interview Schedule for Children Version 2.3 (DISC-2.3) in an informal settlement area in South Africa. Journal of the American Academy of Child & Adolescent Psychiatry, 38, 1156-1164.

Robertson, B. A., Juritz, J. M. (1988) Behavioural screening of 10- and 13-year-old pupils in selected schools in the Cape Peninsula. South African Medical Journal, 73, 24-25.

Rumble, S., Swartz, L., Parry, C., et al (1996) Prevalence of psychiatric morbidity in the adult population of a rural South African village. Psychological Medicine, 26, 997-1007.

Strauss, P. R., Gagiano, C. A., van Rensburg, P. H., et al (1995) Identification of depression in a rural general practice. South African Medical Journal, 85, 755-759.

Sukhai, A., Harris, C., Moorad, R. G., et al (2002) Suicide by self-immolation in Durban, South Africa: a five-year retrospective review. American Journal of Forensic Medicine & Pathology, 23, 295-298.

Thom R. (2000) Mental health services. A review of Southern African literature 1967-1999. Monograph 69. Centre for Health Policy. University of the Witwatersrand. Johannesburg.

Spain

GENERAL INFORMATION

Spain is a country with an approximate area of 506 thousand sq. km. (UNO, 2001). Its population is 41.128 million, and the sex ratio (men per hundred women) is 96 (UNO, 2004). The proportion of population under the age of 15 years is 14% (UNO, 2004), and the proportion of population above the age of 60 years is 22% (WHO, 2004). The literacy rate is 98.5% for men and 96.8% for women (UNESCO/MoH, 2004).

The country is a high income group country (based on World Bank 2004 criteria). The proportion of health budget to GDP is 7.5%. The per capita total expenditure on health is 1607 international $, and the per capita government expenditure on health is 1148 international $ (WHO, 2004).

The main language(s) used in the country is (are) Spanish. The largest religious group(s) is (are) Roman Catholic.

The life expectancy at birth is 76.1 years for males and 83 years for females (WHO, 2004). The healthy life expectancy at birth is 70 years for males and 75 years for females (WHO, 2004).

EPIDEMIOLOGY

There is substantial epidemiological data on mental illnesses in Spain in internationally accessible literature. No attempt was made to include this information here.

MENTAL HEALTH RESOURCES

Mental Health Policy A mental health policy is present. The policy was initially formulated in 1985.

The components of the policy are advocacy, promotion, prevention, treatment and rehabilitation. Although in a strict sense, there exists no official policy on mental health issues at a national level, a mental health plan does exist in each of the 17 Autonomous Communities, framed in the health plan of each Community. However, it can be considered that the last reference at a national level to mental health are the recommendations of the Commission for the Psychiatric Reform (1985), and the General Health Law (1986). Each Autonomous Community has published a plan on mental health, the first ones dates from the late 1980s and the last ones from the 2003s.They include all the components listed above. Social insertion is also a part of the mental health policy. Details about the components of the policy can be obtained from the different Plans on Mental Health documents.

Substance Abuse Policy A substance abuse policy is present. The policy was initially formulated in 1985. Details can be obtained from the document-'Estrategia Nacional Sobre Drogas, 2000-2008.

National Mental Health Programme A national mental health programme is absent.

There is no national mental health programme but there are mental health plans formulated by each Autonomous Community. Although being very similar in their theoretical formulation they are not as similar in their practical application, there are marked differences with regards to funding of resources for psychiatric care among them. There are also no psychiatric care programmes at a national level making that the responses of each one of the Autonomous Community with regards to concrete problems on mental health differs.

National Therapeutic Drug Policy/Essential List of Drugs A national therapeutic drug policy/essential list of drugs is present. It was formulated in 1994.

Mental Health Legislation The General Health Law has a chapter on mental health. The Commission for the Psychiatric Reform includes in its conclusion the need to substitute the old model of care giving, centred on psychiatric hospitals by an integral care of mental pathologies, outpatient and community based, recommending the replacement of psychiatric hospitals by hospitalization units for severe cases in general hospitals, the creation of outpatient mental health units, of intermediate and rehabilitation mechanisms. The Civil and Penal code have incorporated modifications to protect the rights of psychiatric patients and improve conditions for penal sentences for offenders with mental illness. As a part of these reforms prison hospitals were closed and special units under the National health Care were started. The latest civil legislation was enacted in 2000.

The latest legislation was enacted in 1986.

Mental Health Financing There are no budget allocations for mental health.

Details about expenditure on mental health are not available.

The primary sources of mental health financing in descending order are tax based, out of pocket expenditure by the patient or family and private insurances.

Some Autonomous Communities have a budget line for mental health. In the financing model currently in force, the Autonomous Communities receive from the State a final budget for health care calculated according to capitative criteria, with small correction criteria. Hospitals are financed through a global budget, calculated according to the volume and complexity of the foreseen activities, although some experiences of financing per capita have started to be introduced, a model reserved until now only for primary health. The overall health budget is provided through the central administration, the local bodies and private spending. In all it amounts to 7.8% of the GNP. In the frame of the private health care sector, the care of severe psychiatric pathologies is covered by all insurance companies, although they do establish maximum limits to the length of psychiatric hospialization. Psychotropic drugs

(including newer ones) are subsidized by the social security system. A relatively small proportion of the population has additional health insurance, allowing them more freedom of choice for their health care. The care of severe psychiatric illness is covered by all private insurance companies, although they lay down maximum limits to the length of psychiatric hospitalization.
The country has disability benefits for persons with mental disorders. Psychiatric illnesses are considered as a transitory working disability and also a definitive one. In both cases its recognition gives right to an economic compensation, for the first case only if previously working and in the second case with different amounts, depending on whether the patient did contribute before or not to the social security system.

Mental Health Facilities Mental health is a part of primary health care system. Actual treatment of severe mental disorders is available at the primary level.
Regular training of primary care professionals is not carried out in the field of mental health. Specialists in Family and Community Medicine receive short training (two months) in mental health facilities. Several NGOs, international organizations, such as WPA and WHO Collaborating Centres promote the training of primary care physicians in mental health.
There are community care facilities for patients with mental disorders. The community care is provided by mental health centres, which were initially developed as support units for the primary care and are integrated in the network of psychiatric facilities (there is an exception of Cataluña where the mental health centres are included in primary care level).

Psychiatric Beds and Professionals

Total psychiatric beds per 10 000 population	4.4
Psychiatric beds in mental hospitals per 10 000 population	3.7
Psychiatric beds in general hospitals per 10 000 population	0.6
Psychiatric beds in other settings per 10 000 population	0.1
Number of psychiatrists per 100 000 population	3.6
Number of neurosurgeons per 100 000 population	0.9
Number of psychiatric nurses per 100 000 population	4.2
Number of neurologists per 100 000 population	2.5
Number of psychologists per 100 000 population	1.9
Number of social workers per 100 000 population	

There are 3913 other mental health professionals belonging to different categories. Until the adoption of the Commission for Psychiatric Reform the psychiatric care was mainly in the hands of local authorities (Diputaciones Provinciales or Local Councils) and religious orders, owners of the old psychiatric hospitals and university hospitals with psychiatric departments. In the last years of the 1970s, the first psychiatric units in general hospitals were opened although sometimes with minimal facilities sometimes limited to liaison consultation with other specialities. Since the 1980s, there has been an increase in development of new organizational structure for mental health, integration of psychiatry in general health care system (e.g. psychiatry departments have been established in all public hospitals with more than 200 beds), creation of an extensive community network and better public awareness about mental health along with adoption of legislation to improvement of patients rights. However, there needs a lot to be done in the sphere of intermediate community care (Garcia et al, 1999). Details can be obtained from the document 'Sistema de Informacion en Salud Mental Indicadores' (1996). Most psychologists work in the private sphere.

Non-Governmental Organizations NGOs are involved with mental health in the country. They are mainly involved in advocacy, promotion, treatment and rehabilitation.

Information Gathering System There is mental health reporting system in the country. Details can be obtained from the CMBD National Report 1999 and INSALUD CMBD Report 2002.
The country has no data collection system or epidemiological study on mental health. Some records are available from certain Autonomous Communities and other regions.

Programmes for Special Population The country has specific programmes for mental health for children. Besides facilities for children there are facilities for drug addiction and for eating disorders.

Therapeutic Drugs The following therapeutic drugs are generally available at the primary health care level of the country: carbamazepine, phenobarbital, phenytoin sodium, sodium valproate, amitriptyline, chlorpromazine, diazepam, fluphenazine, haloperidol, lithium, biperiden, carbidopa, levodopa.
Psychopharmacological drugs, including the new anti-psychotics, neuroleptics and anti-depressants, are financed by the social security system and are given for free to pensioners and many of them at subsidized rates for active population, who in the worst of cases have to contribute 40% of the cost.

Other Information Custodial care continued till 1977, but due to increasing costs, poor conditions of the mental hospitals and professional awareness about community care, Autonomous Communities were created and health care was transferred into the hands of decentralized units. With the publication of the report of the 'Commission of Psychiatric Reform' in 1985, a large number of beds were established in general hospitals and community care units were set up in the Autonomous Communities. Sheltered accommodation, rehabilitation centres and centres for social integration also started functioning. The limitations are: uneven course of reform with lot of variability between communities, inadequate integration with general health system, especially where knowledge about psychological management is concerned, lack of support for families and carers of patients, a strong tendency to maintain mental hospitals in some form and lack of a national mental health information system and a national assessment system. Two years ago a Mental Health National Report was published, including the data of different Autonomous Communities (24). The EPSILON Group found that Santander has very few acute hospital residential care and day care services for patients suffering from schizophrenia. There were no self-help groups and non professional services. However, community services were present.

Additional Sources of Information

Becker T., Hullsmann, S., Knudsen, H. C. et al & the EPSILON Group (2002) Provision of services for people with schizophrenia in five European regions. Journal of Social Psychiatry and Psychiatric Epidemiology, 37, 465-474.

Conjunto Mínimo Básico de Datos. Hospitales del INSALUD 2001. Instituto Nacional de la Salud. Subdirección General de Coordinación Administrativa. Madrid. 2002.

Comelles, J. M., Hernaez, A. M. (1994) The dilemmas of chronicity: The transition of care policies from the authoritarian state to the wefare state in Spain. International Journal of Social Psychiatry, 40, 283-295.

Decreto 389/1994 de 15 de diciembre de Regulación de la Salud mental de Galicia. Conselleria de Sanidad. Xunta de Galicia.

Del Barrio, V., Carpintero, H. (2003) Clinical psychology in Spain. Journal of Clinical Psychology, 59, 687-699.

Garcia, J., Vazquez-Barquero, J. (1999) Deinstitutionalization and psychiatric reform in Spain. Actas Espanolas de Psiquiatrica en Espana, 27, 281-291.

Informe de la Comisión Ministerial para la Reforma de la Salud Mental en España. Ministerio de Sanidad (1995).

II Plan de Salud de Castilla y León 1998-2007. Junta de Castilla y León. Valladolid 1998.

Informe de Situación de Salud Mental. Ministerio de Sanidad y Consumo 2003. http://www.msc.es/Diseno/informacionProfesional/profesional_observatorioSNS.htm

Ministerio del Interior (2000) Estrategia Nacional Sobre Drogas 2000 – 2008. (Spain National Substance Abuse Policy).

Ministerio de Sanidad y Consumo (1998) Sistema de Informacion en Salud Mental Indicadores Añoo 1996 – Tablas 1991 – 1996.

Mnoz, C. G., Mateu, F. N., Departmento de Slaud Mental del S. M. S. (1999) Plan de Salud Mental de la Region de Murcia. (National Mental Health Program).

Plan Autonómico de Salud Mental (1998) Conselleria de Sanitat I Consum. Gobierno de las Islas Baleares.

Plan de Asistencia Psiquiátrica y Salud Mental 2003-2008. Comunidad de Madrid. Consejería de Sanidad.

Plan de Salud de Canarias. Boletín Oficial de Canarias (BOC), 357. Decreto 3/1997 de 21 de enero. BOC de 31 de marzo de 1997.

Plan de Salud Mental de Cantabria. Análisis de situación y perspectivas de futuro 1998-2001. Gobierno de Cantabria. Consejería de Sanidad, Consumo y Servicios Sociales. Santander, 2002.

Plan de Salud Mental de Castilla- La Mancha 2000-2004. Junta de Comunidades de Castilla –La Mancha.

Plan de Salut de Catalunya 1999-2001. Generalitat de Catalunya. Departament de Sanitat y Seguretat Social.

Plan de Salud mental de la Comunidad Autónoma de Extremadura. Junta de Extremadura. Dirección General de Salud Pública y Consumo. Mérida, 1996.

Plan de Salud Mental de La Rioja. Gobierno de La Rioja. Consejería de Salud, Consumo y Bienestar Social, 1999.

Plan de Salud Mental del País Vasco. Consejería de Sanidad del País Vasco, 1990.

Plan estratégico para el desarrollo de los servicios de salud mental 2001-2003. Principado de Asturias. Consejería de Sanidad, 2000.

Plan Director de Salud mental y asistencia psiquiátrica de la Comunidad Valenciana. Generalitat Valenciana. Conselleria de Sanitat. Conselleria de Bienestar social. Generalitat Valenciana, 2001.

Plan Estratégico 2002-2010 de Atención a la salud mental en la Comunidad autónoma de Aragón. Departamento de Salud, Consumo y Servicios Sociales. Gobierno de Aragón, 2002.

Sistema Nacional de Salud. Año 1999. Explotación de las bases del CMBD. Estadísticas de referencia estatal de los sistemas de agrupación de registros de pacientes GDRs. Ministerio de Sanidad y Consumo, 2002.

Vazquez-Barquero, J. L., Garcia, J., Torres-Gonzalez, F. (2001) Spanish psychiatric reform: what can be learned from two decades of experience? Acta Psychiatrica Scandinavica. 104 (suppl 410), 89-95.

Sri Lanka

GENERAL INFORMATION

Sri Lanka is a country with an approximate area of 66 thousand sq. km. (UNO, 2001). Its population is 19.218 million, and the sex ratio (men per hundred women) is 107 (UNO, 2004). The proportion of population under the age of 15 years is 24% (UNO, 2004), and the proportion of population above the age of 60 years is 10% (WHO, 2004). The literacy rate is 94.7% for men and 89.6% for women (UNESCO/MoH, 2004).

The country is a lower middle income group country (based on World Bank 2004 criteria). The proportion of health budget to GDP is 3.6%. The per capita total expenditure on health is 122 international $, and the per capita government expenditure on health is 60 international $ (WHO, 2004).

The main language(s) used in the country is (are) Sinhala. The largest ethnic group(s) is (are) Sinhalese, and the other ethnic group(s) are (is) Tamil. The largest religious group(s) is (are) Buddhist (seven-tenths), and the other religious group(s) are (is) Hindu, Christian and Muslim.

The life expectancy at birth is 67.2 years for males and 74.3 years for females (WHO, 2004). The healthy life expectancy at birth is 59 years for males and 64 years for females (WHO, 2004).

EPIDEMIOLOGY

Wijesinghe et al (1978) conducted a community survey of a semi-urban population (n=7653) with a two-stage screening method. The 6-month period prevalence for all psychiatric disorders was 4.6%, with psychoses accounting for 0.7% (males 0.6%, females 0.8%) and neuroses for 2.5% (males 1.0%, females 4.1%). They also found a rate of 0.5% for possession and trance states (Wijesinghe et al, 1976). De Silva and Gunatilake (2002) found that 8.7% of subjects in a sample of 380 subjects over the age of 65 years from a semi-urban community had cognitive impairment (scored less than 18 points) when assessed with the Sinhalese version of the Mini Mental State Examination (MMSE). Somasundaram and Sivayokan (1994) interviewed one member each from 101 randomly selected families from a primary health area with the Stress Impact Questionnaire. The vast majority of the respondents had suffered numerous traumas. Common diagnoses reported were PTSD (27%), anxiety disorder (26%), major depression (25%) and alcohol and drug misuse (15%). Functional disability was reported in 18%. Somasundaram (1996) assessed a refugee population within two months of being exposed to aerial bombing (n=15). Nearly 74% had experienced an immediate but transient stress reaction. Subsequently, PTSD, anxiety, depressive and somatic symptoms were common and 44% met the DSM-III diagnostic criteria for PTSD. Reppesgaard (1997) conducted a study among a Tamil population affected by trauma. Surprisingly, the results showed that subjects in non-war zones had a significantly higher frequency of serious PTSD, depression and somatoform disorder as per DSM-III-R than subjects in war zones. The number of moderately affected was significantly higher in war zones. The young and the middle-aged groups had higher scores on serious manifestations than the older group. La Vecchia et al (1994) analysed suicide mortality for 57 countries on the basis of the World Health Organization mortality database. Sri Lanka has the second highest male suicide rate (49.6/100 000 population) and the highest female suicide rate (19.0/100 000 population). Sri Lanka also had an unfavourable trend over time, unlike most other developing countries. Ganesvaran et al (1984) found that the suicide rate was 53.5 per 100 000 population in a town in the northern region. The rate of suicide was increasing among the 15-34 age group. The commonest method was self-poisoning by agrochemicals and insecticides of organophosphorus type. Similar findings were reported by Berger (1998) who compared the rate of suicide in Sri Lanka and USA. Somasundaram and Rajadurai (1995) reported a decline in suicide rate during the civil war 1980-89, notably among males and youth. An inverse relationship between suicide and homicide rates was shown. The use of agrochemicals for suicidal purposes declined during war, while alary seeds (?) became more popular. Eddleston et al (1998) reported that ingestion of yellow oleander seeds has recently become a popular method of deliberate self-harm in northern Sri Lanka. Four hundred and fifteen cases were admitted to a general hospital in Sri Lanka's north central province during 11 months. Nearly half of the ingesters were less than 21 years old. The mortality rate was more than 6%.

MENTAL HEALTH RESOURCES

Mental Health Policy A mental health policy is absent.

Steps have been taken to gather evidence for policy formulation, and a committee has been appointed to formulate draft policy and legislation.

Substance Abuse Policy A substance abuse policy is absent. A substance abuse policy has been developed but is still to be ratified by the parliament.

National Mental Health Programme A national mental health programme is present. The programme was formulated in 1966. The current mental health programme is based on the WHO recommendations given in the World Health Report 2001 and the National Strategic Mental Health Plan formulated in 2001 with the assistance of WHO. It emphasizes equity and accessibility of services. The long-term goals are described under 5 broad categories of patient care and follow-up, rehabilitation, prevention and promotion, management and research. The public health approach of delivering mental health care integrated into general health services, primary health care services and community care is envisaged. The main strategies are to improve material resources, human resources in the periphery and to downsize specialized mental health hospitals. Linkages to promote intra- and inter-sectoral

S

collaboration for improved care of people with mental health needs is envisaged. A referral system and continuity-of-care system is to be developed with a good information system for effective monitoring and evaluation.

National Therapeutic Drug Policy/Essential List of Drugs A national therapeutic drug policy/essential list of drugs is present. It was formulated in 1985.
The new mental health policy will consider the issue of inclusion of newer anti-psychotics in the essential drug list.

Mental Health Legislation The current legislation dates back to the Mental Disease Ordinance of 1873 (amended in 1956). Efforts to formulate a new Mental Health Act have started since the year 2000. The act will emphasize community mental health services and rights of people with mental disorders.
The latest legislation was enacted in 1956.

Mental Health Financing There are budget allocations for mental health.
The country spends 1.6% of the total health budget on mental health.
The primary sources of mental health financing in descending order are tax based, out of pocket expenditure by the patient or family and private insurances.
There are budget allocations for mental health, but mostly for the mental hospital. Individual general hospitals meet their own mental health care expenses. Drugs are provided free of charge to those receiving services from the Government sector.
The country does not have disability benefits for persons with mental disorders. Mental illness is considered a disability, but is not entitled for benefits.

Mental Health Facilities Mental health is a part of primary health care system. Actual treatment of severe mental disorders is not available at the primary level. Primary care workers in some regions carry out mental health work including dispensing of medication.
Regular training of primary care professionals is carried out in the field of mental health. In the last two years, about 1500 personnel were provided training.
There are no community care facilities for patients with mental disorders. Up to the year 2000, psychiatry services were available only at tertiary care level. Appointment of Medical Officers Mental Health to 30 base hospitals made mental health services available at secondary care level. Outreach, liaison, community mental health and school mental health services have been launched. With the assistance of the Nations for Mental Health Programme of WHO, attempts have been made to resettle long-stay patients from mental hospitals in the community. Recently, the Ministry of Health has initiated a programme to develop intermediate-stay units at a regional level. Ten such units provide rehabilitation services to patients with disability, discharged from the psychiatry units at tertiary care level. Day care services and community care services are also provided from these centres. Health camps are conducted by the Ministry of Health medical teams in the community to provide holistic treatments including medication, counselling etc. A few NGOs (e.g. Sahanaya) also provide residential facilities and conduct rehabilitation programmes in the community. A special effort is being given towards developing primary and community care incorporating policies and programmes that would facilitate the alleviation of the problem of high suicide rates. Though community facilities are not uniformly distributed, different kind of services are often available in different areas.

Psychiatric Beds and Professionals

Total psychiatric beds per 10 000 population	1.8
Psychiatric beds in mental hospitals per 10 000 population	1.4
Psychiatric beds in general hospitals per 10 000 population	0.3
Psychiatric beds in other settings per 10 000 population	0
Number of psychiatrists per 100 000 population	0.2
Number of neurosurgeons per 100 000 population	0.03
Number of psychiatric nurses per 100 000 population	1.8
Number of neurologists per 100 000 population	0.06
Number of psychologists per 100 000 population	0.02
Number of social workers per 100 000 population	0.07

Most of the non-medical mental health professionals do not have formal training in mental health. The mental health facilities are mainly located in the urban areas. Both the Government and the private sector are involved in providing services. Almost three-fourth of the beds are in Colombo. There is only one private hospital providing inpatient services. Most of the psychiatrists work in the public sector, but almost all of them have private clinics also. Most mental health professionals are stationed in urban areas. Sahanaya (NGO) with the support of the Ministry of Health has initiated a 3-year training programme for general physicians (post-graduate training in psychiatry takes 5 years). This has led to the placement of 40 medical officers in mental health at secondary care hospitals. Later, a one-year training programme was also initiated.

S

Non-Governmental Organizations NGOs are involved with mental health in the country. They are mainly involved in advocacy, promotion, prevention, treatment and rehabilitation. Many non-governmental organizations provide mental health care in certain areas. Sahanaya provides day care services to those in need and training to mental health professionals. BasicNeeds, which is a UK based NGO, implements a community mental health project in the southern part of Sri Lanka. Horticulture Therapy Project initiated and supported by BasicNeeds is helping many of the long term inpatients at specialized mental hospitals to recover from their illness and to find self-employment. Local NGOs like Navajeevana and Gides help BasicNeeds to provide care to the mentally ill. Voluntary Services Overseas, another UK based organization provides psychiatry nurses, occupational therapists and management volunteers for mental health programmes. NGOs are also involved in community-based interventions in the areas of suicide prevention, disasters, mental retardation, alcohol related problems and mental disorders in elderly population. NGOs work in close collaboration with the Ministry of Health.

Information Gathering System There is mental health reporting system in the country. Only hospital data is reported.
The country has no data collection system or epidemiological study on mental health.

Programmes for Special Population The country has specific programmes for mental health for children. Occasional focussed projects are held for the special population but for limited periods of time.
The country has specific programmes for mental health for trauma victims. However, they are not adequate. The maternal and child health programme and school health programme have components of child and adolescent mental health. Two child psychiatrists provide specialized services in the capital. Homes for children with severe learning and behavioural disorders are available. There has also been a steady growth of counselling centres in the private and NGO sectors. Counselling on war-related issues is done by NGOs in the northern and eastern regions.

Therapeutic Drugs The following therapeutic drugs are generally available at the primary health care level of the country: carbamazepine, ethosuximide, phenobarbital, phenytoin sodium, sodium valproate, amitriptyline, chlorpromazine, diazepam, carbidopa, levodopa.

Other Information A WHO (SEARO) Expert Committee Meeting in 2000 helped in defining some of the critical issues related to the development of mental health care in Sri Lanka. WHO is involved in a project to encourage a process of deinstitutionalization of psychiatric patients and promotion of reintegration in the community.

Additional Sources of Information

Berger, L. R. (1988) Suicides and pesticides in Sri Lanka. American Journal of Public Health, 78, 826-828.

Department of Mental Health Care (2000) Critical Issues – WHO Expert Committee Meeting Report.

de Silva, D. (2002) Psychiatric service delivery in an Asian country: the experience of Sri Lanka. International Review of Psychiatry, 14, 66-70.

de Silva, H. A., Gunatilake, S. B. (2002) Mini Mental State Examination in Sinhalese: a sensitive test to screen for dementia in Sri Lanka. International Journal of Geriatric Psychiatry, 17, 134-139.

de Silva, H. J., Kasturiaratchi, N., Seneviratner, S. L., et al. (2000) Suicide in Sri Lanka: points to ponder. Ceylon Medical Journal, 45, 17-24.

Eddleston, M., Rezvi Sheriff, M. H., Hawton, K. (1998) Deliberate self harm in Sri Lanka: an overlooked tragedy in the developing world. British Medical Journal, 317, 133-135.

Fernandopulle, S., Thalagala, N., Barraclough, S. (2002) Mental health in Sri Lanka: challenges for primary health care. Australian Journal of Primary Health – Interchange, 8, 31-38.

Ganesvaran, T., Subramaniam, S., Mahadevan, K. (1984) Suicide in a northern town of Sri Lanka. Acta Psychiatrica Scandinavica, 69, 420-425.

La Vecchia, C., Lucchini, F., Levi, F. (1994) Worldwide trends in suicide mortality, 1955-1989. Acta Psychiatrica Scandinavica, 90, 53-64.

Mendis N. (2004) Mental health services in Sri Lanka. International Psychiatry, 3, 10-12.

Reppesgaard, H. O. (1997) Studies on psychosocial problems among displaced people in Sri Lanka. European Journal of Psychiatry, 11, 223-234.

Somasundaram, D. J. (1996) Post-traumatic responses to aerial bombing. Social Science & Medicine, 42, 1465-1471.

Somasundaram, D. J., Rajadurai, S. (1995) War and suicide in northern Sri Lanka. Acta Psychiatrica Scandinavica, 91, 1-4.

Somasundaram, D. J., Sivayokan, S. (1994) War trauma in a civilian population. British Journal of Psychiatry, 165, 524-527.

WHO (2002) Working with countries: mental health policy and service development projects. WHO. Geneva. WHO/MSD/MPS/02.1.

Wijesinghe, C. P., Dissanayake, S. A., Dassanayake, P. V. (1978) Survey of psychiatric morbidity in a semi-urban population in Sri Lanka. Acta Psychiatrica Scandinavica, 58, 413-441.

Wijesinghe, C. P., Dissanayake, S. A., Mendis, N. (1976) Possession trance in a semi-urban community in Sri Lanka. Australian & New Zealand Journal of Psychiatry, 10, 135-139.

Sudan

GENERAL INFORMATION

Sudan is a country with an approximate area of 2506 thousand sq. km. (UNO, 2001). Its population is 34.333 million, and the sex ratio (men per hundred women) is 101 (UNO, 2004). The proportion of population under the age of 15 years is 39% (UNO, 2004), and the proportion of population above the age of 60 years is 6% (WHO, 2004). The literacy rate is 70.8% for men and 49.1% for women (UNESCO/MoH, 2004).

The country is a low income group country (based on World Bank 2004 criteria). The proportion of health budget to GDP is 3.5%. The per capita total expenditure on health is 39 international $, and the per capita government expenditure on health is 7 international $ (WHO, 2004).

The main language(s) used in the country is (are) Arabic and English. The largest ethnic group(s) is (are) Arab and African. The largest religious group(s) is (are) Muslim, and the other religious group(s) are (is) indigenous groups and Christian.

The life expectancy at birth is 54.9 years for males and 59.3 years for females (WHO, 2004). The healthy life expectancy at birth is 47 years for males and 50 years for females (WHO, 2004).

EPIDEMIOLOGY

Rahim and Cederblad (1989) evaluated a sample of 204 subjects aged 22-35 years using the Self-Rating Questionnaire, the Eysenck Personality Inventory and a Sudanese rating scale of anxiety and depression, a psychiatric interview and a medical examination. Results showed that 16.6% of the subjects had at least one disorder as per DSM-III. The most common were depression (8.4%) and generalized anxiety (3.4%). Alcohol abuse was rare (0.4%). There was no sex difference in the prevalence of mental disorders. Cederblad and Rahim (1989) re-interviewed 104 randomly chosen subjects in 1983 (from the original pool of 197 children examined in 1964-1965). The overall psychiatric impairment was 14% (males 18%; females 8%). In an earlier study they evaluated the psychological effect of urbanization on children aged 3-15 years living in a sub-urban community that transformed from a rural to urban economy between 1965 and 1980. Interviews done in 1965 and 1980 showed an increase in behaviour problems in boys aged 7-15, while there was an improvement in physical health and nutrition. Behaviour problems were associated with factors related to parents (blue-collar workers, maternal anxiety/depression, harsh corporal punishment) and children (dropping out of school, poor somatic health) (Rahim & Cederblad, 1986). Cederblad (1988) assessed behaviour disorders in children of different ages in Sweden, Sudan and Nigeria. The similarities of frequencies of behaviourally disturbed children were more striking than the differences. Rural children generally had less behaviour problems than urban ones. However, in another multi-country study, carried out in a primary care setting (n=925), that employed a two-stage screening process, Giel et al (1981) found the prevalence of mental disorders among children to range from 12% to 29%. Rahim and Cederblad (1986) and Cederblad et al (1986) evaluated the prevalence of enuresis in 8462 children aged 3-15 living in the suburban area. 88% wetted their beds at least several times per week. The prevalence of enuresis was higher in boys than in girls. Only 5% of the children above 7 years of age had secondary enuresis. An intensive study of 245 children selected through stratified sampling did not reveal any association between enuresis and somatic, developmental, behavioural, socio-economic or child rearing (including bladder-training) factors.

MENTAL HEALTH RESOURCES

Mental Health Policy A mental health policy is present. The policy was initially formulated in 1998.
The components of the policy are advocacy, promotion, prevention, treatment and rehabilitation.

Substance Abuse Policy A substance abuse policy is present. The policy was initially formulated in 1995.

National Mental Health Programme A national mental health programme is present. The programme was formulated in 1998. The national mental health programme aims to integrate with general health facilities along with promotion of comprehensive mental health care, train mental health personnel and establish a national organizational body for systematic coordination of related activities and the promotion of mental health.

National Therapeutic Drug Policy/Essential List of Drugs A national therapeutic drug policy/essential list of drugs is present. It was formulated in 1970.

Mental Health Legislation The most recent legislation is the state law 'Gezira Mental Health Law' of 1998. The mental health legislation forms a chapter of the Public Health Act of 1973, which was revised in 1985. The Mental Health Act has been drafted and has gone to the parliament for approval.
The latest legislation was enacted in 1998.

Mental Health Financing There are budget allocations for mental health.
Details about expenditure on mental health are not available.
The primary source of mental health financing is tax based.
The country has disability benefits for persons with mental disorders.

Mental Health Facilities Mental health is not a part of primary health care system. Actual treatment of severe mental disorders is not available at the primary level. Mental health has not been integrated with the primary care, and there is also a lack of personnel.

Regular training of primary care professionals is carried out in the field of mental health. In the last two years, about 40 personnel were provided training. Training facilities are present for primary care physicians, police and prison officers. The Gezira Mental Health Programme was aimed at modifying community concepts, attitudes and practices concerning mental health, ensuring community involvement and participation and extending mental health services by training primary health care staff. The evaluation of the programme showed that it helped in raising public awareness and community participation. Members of the health team and teachers who received training reported a better understanding of mental health problems and an improvement in their handling of the mental problems. Sudan has the experience of using traditional healers for provision of mental health services.
There are no community care facilities for patients with mental disorders. Community care is absent due to the lack of proper transportation, lack of social workers and poor health education.

Psychiatric Beds and Professionals

Total psychiatric beds per 10 000 population	0.2
Psychiatric beds in mental hospitals per 10 000 population	0.18
Psychiatric beds in general hospitals per 10 000 population	0.02
Psychiatric beds in other settings per 10 000 population	0
Number of psychiatrists per 100 000 population	0.09
Number of neurosurgeons per 100 000 population	0.007
Number of psychiatric nurses per 100 000 population	0.2
Number of neurologists per 100 000 population	0.014
Number of psychologists per 100 000 population	0.17
Number of social workers per 100 000 population	0.1

Many mental health professionals including most psychiatrists have left for other countries.

Non-Governmental Organizations NGOs are not involved with mental health in the country. Special attention has been given to migrants, elderly, refugees, displaced and homeless and children.

Information Gathering System There is no mental health reporting system in the country. Some mental health information particularly numbers related to admissions for major disorders are collected from a few hospitals in the general health data collection system, but the system has many limitations.
The country has no data collection system or epidemiological study on mental health. There are no funds or personnel to carry out epidemiological studies.

Programmes for Special Population These groups are supported by NGOs and UNICEF.
A school mental health programme is present.

Therapeutic Drugs The following therapeutic drugs are generally available at the primary health care level of the country: phenobarbital, phenytoin sodium.
Since mental health is not integrated in primary care level, most of the drugs are not available at primary care level. A list of essential neuropsychiatric drugs for all levels has been formulated.

Other Information

Additional Sources of Information

Cederblad, M. (1988) Behavioural disorders in children from different cultures. Acta Psychiatrica Scandinavica, Supplementum 344, 85-92.

Cederblad, M., Rahim, S. I. (1986) Epidemiology of nocturnal enuresis in a part of Khartoum, Sudan. II. The intensive study. Acta Paediatrica Scandinavica, 75, 1021-1027.

Cederblad, M., Rahim, S. I. (1989) A longitudinal study of mental health problems in a suburban population in Sudan. Acta Psychiatrica Scandinavica, 79, 537-543.

El Gaili, D. E., Magzoub, M., Schmidt, H. G. (2002) The impact of a community-oriented medical school on mental health services. Education for Health, 15, 149-157.

Giel, R., de Arango, M. V., Climent, C. E., et al (1981) Childhood mental disorders in primary health care: results of observations in four developing countries. A report from the WHO collaborative Study on Strategies for Extending Mental Health Care. Pediatrics, 68, 677-683.

Mohit, A. (2001) Mental health and psychiatry in the Middle East: historical development. Eastern Mediterranean Health Journal, 7, 336-347.

Rahim, S. I., Cederblad, M. (1986) Epidemiology of nocturnal enuresis in a part of Khartoum, Sudan. I. The extensive study. Acta Paediatrica Scandinavica, 75, 1017-1020.

Rahim, S. I., Cederblad, M. (1986) Effects of rapid urbanization on child behaviour and health in a part of Khartoum, Sudan--II. Psycho-social influences on behaviour. Social Science & Medicine, 22, 723-730.

Rahim, S. I., Cederblad, M. (1989) Epidemiology of mental disorders in young adults of a newly urbanized area in Khartoum, Sudan. British Journal of Psychiatry, 155, 44-47.

Suriname

GENERAL INFORMATION

Suriname is a country with an approximate area of 163 thousand sq. km. (UNO, 2001). Its population is 0.439 million, and the sex ratio (men per hundred women) is 98 (UNO, 2004). The proportion of population under the age of 15 years is 30% (UNO, 2004), and the proportion of population above the age of 60 years is 8% (WHO, 2004). The literacy rate is 90.2% for men and 82.3% for women (UNESCO/MoH, 2004).
The country is a lower middle income group country (based on World Bank 2004 criteria). The proportion of health budget to GDP is 9.4%. The per capita total expenditure on health is 398 international $, and the per capita government expenditure on health is 240 international $ (WHO, 2004).
The main language(s) used in the country is (are) Dutch and Surinamese. The largest ethnic group(s) is (are) East Indian and Creole, and the other ethnic group(s) are (is) Javanese and African. The largest religious group(s) is (are) Hindu, and the other religious group(s) are (is) Protestant, Roman Catholic and Muslim.
The life expectancy at birth is 64.4 years for males and 70.8 years for females (WHO, 2004). The healthy life expectancy at birth is 57 years for males and 61 years for females (WHO, 2004).

EPIDEMIOLOGY

There is a paucity of epidemiological data on mental illnesses in Suriname in internationally accessible literature. Hanoeman et al (2002) studied the incidence of schizophrenia among the Surinamese population in order to compare the results with those among Surinamese immigrants in the Netherlands who show a high incidence. The researchers examined the medical records of the sole psychiatric hospital in Suriname and found that the mean annual incidence rate of first admissions for schizophrenia or schizophreniform disorder (DSM-III-R criteria) in 1992 and 1993 was not low (1.6/10 000). These findings constitute a challenge to the hypothesis that selection explains the increased incidence in the migrants. The possibility of an increased incidence of the disorder in Surinam (which might also explain the increased incidence among migrants) could not be ruled out. Mahy (1993) reported on suicidal behaviour in different Caribbean countries where records suggest that the rate of suicide particularly by the use of agrochemicals has been steadily increasing in the East Indian community. Perriens et al (1989) studied records at the University Hospital that manages 83% of all cases of paraquat poisoning occurring throughout the country. For 1985 and 1986 the corrected incidence rates of paraquat poisoning were 211 and 68 cases/million population/year, among the highest reported worldwide. Paraquat poisoning was associated with gender (male) and ethnicity (Hindustani) and availability of the chemical (e.g. volume of monthly import of paraquat). Suicide attempts accounted for 76% of the cases. The overall case fatality rate was 71% and it was associated with gender (male) and age. In 2001, 72 deaths by suicide were noted (Punwasi, 2003). Of the deceased subjects, four-fifths were Hindustani, three-fourths were male and two-thirds were under 45 years of age. Regional variation was marked with projected figures for the population per district ranging from 5.55 to 55.06 per 100 000 population. The analysis in 2000 showed a similar pattern.

MENTAL HEALTH RESOURCES

Mental Health Policy A mental health policy is present. The policy was initially formulated in 2000.
The components of the policy are treatment and rehabilitation.

Substance Abuse Policy A substance abuse policy is present. The policy was initially formulated in 1996.

National Mental Health Programme A national mental health programme is present. The programme was formulated in 2000.

National Therapeutic Drug Policy/Essential List of Drugs A national therapeutic drug policy/essential list of drugs is present. It was formulated in 1984.

Mental Health Legislation There is a Mental Health Act.
The latest legislation was enacted in 1912.

Mental Health Financing There are budget allocations for mental health.
The country spends 4.2% of the total health budget on mental health.
The primary sources of mental health financing in descending order are tax based, social insurance, out of pocket expenditure by the patient or family and private insurances.
The country has disability benefits for persons with mental disorders. Benefits are present but limited.

Mental Health Facilities Mental health is not a part of primary health care system. Actual treatment of severe mental disorders is not available at the primary level.
Regular training of primary care professionals is not carried out in the field of mental health.
There are no community care facilities for patients with mental disorders.

Psychiatric Beds and Professionals

Total psychiatric beds per 10 000 population	5.2
Psychiatric beds in mental hospitals per 10 000 population	5.2
Psychiatric beds in general hospitals per 10 000 population	0
Psychiatric beds in other settings per 10 000 population	0
Number of psychiatrists per 100 000 population	1.25
Number of neurosurgeons per 100 000 population	0.2
Number of psychiatric nurses per 100 000 population	15
Number of neurologists per 100 000 population	0.83
Number of psychologists per 100 000 population	0.2
Number of social workers per 100 000 population	0.62

Non-Governmental Organizations NGOs are involved with mental health in the country. They are mainly involved in advocacy and promotion.

Information Gathering System There is no mental health reporting system in the country.
The country has no data collection system or epidemiological study on mental health.

Programmes for Special Population There are no facilities for special population groups.

Therapeutic Drugs The following therapeutic drugs are generally available at the primary health care level of the country: carbamazepine, phenobarbital, phenytoin sodium, sodium valproate, chlorpromazine, diazepam, fluphenazine, haloperidol, lithium, biperiden, levodopa.

Other Information

Additional Sources of Information

Hanoeman, M., Selten, J.-P., Kahn, R. S. (2002) Incidence of schizophrenia in Surinam. Schizophrenia Research, 54, 219-221.

Mahy, G. (1993) Suicide behaviour in the Caribbean. International Review of Psychiatry, 5, 261-269.

Perriens, J., Van der Stuyft, P., Chee, H., et al (1989) The epidemiology of paraquat intoxications in Surinam. Tropical & Geographical Medicine, 41, 266-269.

Punwasi, W. (2003) Causes of Death in Suriname 2001. BOG (MOH).

S

Swaziland

GENERAL INFORMATION

Swaziland is a country with an approximate area of 17 thousand sq. km. (UNO, 2001). Its population is 1.083 million, and the sex ratio (men per hundred women) is 92 (UNO, 2004). The proportion of population under the age of 15 years is 43% (UNO, 2004), and the proportion of population above the age of 60 years is 5% (WHO, 2004). The literacy rate is 82% for men and 80% for women (UNESCO/MoH, 2004).

The country is a lower middle income group country (based on World Bank 2004 criteria). The proportion of health budget to GDP is 3.3%. The per capita total expenditure on health is 167 international $, and the per capita government expenditure on health is 115 international $ (WHO, 2004).

The main language(s) used in the country is (are) English and Swazi. The largest ethnic group(s) is (are) African. The largest religious group(s) is (are) Christian (more than half), and the other religious group(s) are (is) indigenous groups.

The life expectancy at birth is 36.9 years for males and 40.4 years for females (WHO, 2004). The healthy life expectancy at birth is 33 years for males and 35 years for females (WHO, 2004).

EPIDEMIOLOGY

Guinness (1992) conducted a survey of 2040 senior secondary school students in different types of school (rural, urban and elite) with open-ended questions and SRQ-24. Symptom prevalence was generally higher among the rural and semi-urban schools in comparison to the schools in the city. The SRQ-24 items screening for psychosis were associated with a range of spontaneous symptoms representing anxiety. Neurotic symptoms were expressed in the form of 'spiritual' problems and it was concluded that under stress these could cause transient reactive psychosis. In a study on school-going adolescents and young adults from a combined sample from clinics and the community, Guinness (1992) found that the common presentations of psychopathology were somatized anxiety (brain fag), depressive neurosis characterized by hypochondriasis, cognitive complaints, dissociative states, culturally determined paranoid ideation and brief reactive psychosis. There was a temporal relationship between transient psychosis and the school calendar. Anxiety or depression often predated the florid psychotic reaction which served as a form of help-seeking behaviour or defence in intolerable stress. In a hospital based study, Guiness (1992) compared patients with brief reactive psychosis with patients of schizophreniform disorder, schizophrenia and manic-depressive psychosis. Brief reactive psychosis was found to be a composite syndrome with 50% showing a preceding history of depression. Of those with prodromal anxiety, most were precipitated by a major life event and a few showed a recurrent pattern. Schizophrenia occurred months or years later in 10-20%. The schizophreniform group comprised of symptoms intermediate between the transient and major psychoses. The pattern of precipitants and the over-representation of education and paid employment in the acute syndromes, compared with the major psychoses, in a society which was largely first-generation educated, suggested a link with rapid social change. Stephens et al (1999) compared eating behaviours of university students from Australia and Swaziland using EAT 26. The results did not support the hypothesis that more Australian students than Swazi students would display eating disorder symptoms.

MENTAL HEALTH RESOURCES

Mental Health Policy A mental health policy is absent.
A draft policy is available.

Substance Abuse Policy A substance abuse policy is absent.

National Mental Health Programme A national mental health programme is present. Details about the year of formulation of the programme are not available.
The current focus of the mental health programme is on the development of standardized guidelines for diagnosis and management of common mental health disorders.

National Therapeutic Drug Policy/Essential List of Drugs A national therapeutic drug policy/essential list of drugs is present. It was formulated in 2002.

Mental Health Legislation There is a Mental Health Act.
The latest legislation was enacted in 1978.

Mental Health Financing There are budget allocations for mental health.
The country spends 0.3% of the total health budget on mental health.
The primary sources of mental health financing in descending order are out of pocket expenditure by the patient or family, private insurances, social insurance and tax based.
Mental health services are free.
The country does not have disability benefits for persons with mental disorders.

Mental Health Facilities Mental health is a part of primary health care system. Actual treatment of severe mental disorders is not available at the primary level. The great majority of severe mental disorders are transferred to the National Psychiatric Centre. Regular training of primary care professionals is not carried out in the field of mental health.
There are community care facilities for patients with mental disorders. Lack of transport and shortage of staff have adversely affected the functionality of community outreach services for patients with mental disorders.

Psychiatric Beds and Professionals

Total psychiatric beds per 10 000 population	2
Psychiatric beds in mental hospitals per 10 000 population	2
Psychiatric beds in general hospitals per 10 000 population	0
Psychiatric beds in other settings per 10 000 population	0
Number of psychiatrists per 100 000 population	0.1
Number of neurosurgeons per 100 000 population	0
Number of psychiatric nurses per 100 000 population	10
Number of neurologists per 100 000 population	0
Number of psychologists per 100 000 population	0.1
Number of social workers per 100 000 population	0.1

Mental health services are mainly managed by nurses. There is only one hospital, the National Psychiatric Centre, fully dedicated to mental health. In addition, two general hospitals have functional psychiatric units and capacity to admit severe mental health patients. Beds have been earmarked for women patients.

Non-Governmental Organizations NGOs are involved with mental health in the country. They are mainly involved in promotion, prevention and rehabilitation.

Information Gathering System There is no mental health reporting system in the country. Mental health reporting is not well established but is presently being addressed.
The country has no data collection system or epidemiological study on mental health.

Programmes for Special Population A special programme addresses the needs of epileptic patients.
Counselling services and offered, but they are hampered by the shortage of trained staff. Mental health talks are delivered at health facilities, schools and tinkhundla centres.

Therapeutic Drugs The following therapeutic drugs are generally available at the primary health care level of the country: carbamazepine, phenobarbital, phenytoin sodium, amitriptyline, chlorpromazine, diazepam, fluphenazine, haloperidol, lithium, biperiden.
These drugs are not routinely available at the primary health care level.

Other Information

Additional Sources of Information

Guinness, E. A. (1992a) Brief reactive psychosis and the major functional psychoses: descriptive case studies in Africa. British Journal of Psychiatry, Supplementum 16, 24-41.

Guinness, E. A. (1992b) Profile and prevalence of the brain fag syndrome: psychiatric morbidity in school populations in Africa. British Journal of Psychiatry, Supplementum 16, 42-52.

Guinness, E. A. (1992c) Relationship between the neuroses and brief reactive psychosis: descriptive case studies in Africa. British Journal of Psychiatry, Supplementum 16, 12-23.

Stephens, N. M., Schumaker, J. F., Sibiya, T. E. (1999) Eating disorders and dieting behavior among Australian and Swazi university students. Journal of Social Psychology, 139, 153-158.

Ministry of Health and Welfare. Swaziland. National psychiatric centre. Http://www.gov.sz/home.asp?pid=212.

Sweden

GENERAL INFORMATION

Sweden is a country with an approximate area of 450 thousand sq. km. (UNO, 2001). Its population is 8.886 million, and the sex ratio (men per hundred women) is 98 (UNO, 2004). The proportion of population under the age of 15 years is 17% (UNO, 2004), and the proportion of population above the age of 60 years is 23% (WHO, 2004). The literacy rate is 99% for men and 99% for women (UNESCO/MoH, 2004).

The country is a high income group country (based on World Bank 2004 criteria). The proportion of health budget to GDP is 8.7%. The per capita total expenditure on health is 2270 international $, and the per capita government expenditure on health is 1935 international $ (WHO, 2004).

The main language(s) used in the country is (are) Swedish. The largest ethnic group(s) is (are) European. The largest religious group(s) is (are) Evangelical Lutheran.

The life expectancy at birth is 78 years for males and 82.6 years for females (WHO, 2004). The healthy life expectancy at birth is 72 years for males and 75 years for females (WHO, 2004).

EPIDEMIOLOGY

There is substantial epidemiological data on mental illnesses in Sweden in internationally accessible literature. No attempt was made to include this information here.

MENTAL HEALTH RESOURCES

Mental Health Policy A mental health policy is absent.

Substance Abuse Policy A substance abuse policy is absent.

National Mental Health Programme A national mental health programme is absent.

Mental health care reforms directed towards individuals suffering from severe and long-standing mental illness was initiated in 1995. Sweden has a comprehensive national suicide prevention programme.

National Therapeutic Drug Policy/Essential List of Drugs A national therapeutic drug policy/essential list of drugs is absent.

Mental Health Legislation The fundamental legislation for psychiatric health and sickness are the Health and Illness Act (HSL), the Compulsory Psychiatric Care Act (LPT) and the Forensic Psychiatric Care Act (LRV). Guidance is also provided by the 1991 UN Resolution, supported by Sweden, concerning the principles for the protection of the mentally ill. The latest legislations are the Law on Compulsory Care and the Law on Forensic Psychiatry Care. The Swedish National Board on Forensic Medicine is responsible for the assessment of offenders with mental illness. Treatment is carried out in special wards within the civil psychiatric hospitals in each county or in special forensic psychiatric hospitals. The latest legislation was enacted in 2000.

Mental Health Financing There are budget allocations for mental health.

The country spends 11% of the total health budget on mental health.

The primary sources of mental health financing in descending order are tax based, social insurance, out of pocket expenditure by the patient or family and private insurances.

The Municipal Financial Responsibility Act makes it incumbent upon the municipalities to pay for the care of patients who have to remain in hospitals because of lack of community services. As a part of the Mental Health Reform (1995), the counties themselves receive a state subsidy in order to ease the transition from life in an institution to living in the community. In addition, there were specified subsidies for provision of case managers, severely mentally ill drug abusers, family programmes and for supporting user associations. Community services now account for about 15% of the budget of psychiatric care organizations.

The country has disability benefits for persons with mental disorders. The objective of the Swedish Disability Act and Assistance Compensation Act is to provide comprehensive and equal benefits to patients with physical or mental illness. Under these laws the individual is allowed counselling, personal assistance, housing with special services, contact people and companions. The municipalities are obligated to conduct outreach care facilities including rehabilitation for the elderly and disabled. The Municipal Financial Responsibility Act makes it compulsory for the municipalities to pay for the treatment of patients, who after 3 consecutive months of inpatient care are deemed treated but still require hospital care as they are not able to lead independent lives within a community care system. Disability benefits are reaching between 10-30% of those who need them, but the proportion is likely to rise as case management becomes more frequent.

Mental Health Facilities Mental health is a part of primary health care system. Actual treatment of severe mental disorders is available at the primary level.

Regular training of primary care professionals is not carried out in the field of mental health. There are some local and regional training programmes.

There are community care facilities for patients with mental disorders. Community care is primarily carried out by social services. As a result of the 1995 reforms, approximately 4000 patients and 400 rehabilitation programmes were transferred from psychiatric care organizations to municipal social services. Furthermore, nearly 900 projects related to employment and rehabilitation were financed with state subsidies and about 300 educational projects directed towards the staff of the social services were launched. There are, however, regional variations in services. Day care facilities are currently available for about 50% of those in need. Mobile teams are operational in more than 50% of the catchment areas.

Psychiatric Beds and Professionals

Total psychiatric beds per 10 000 population	6
Psychiatric beds in mental hospitals per 10 000 population	
Psychiatric beds in general hospitals per 10 000 population	6
Psychiatric beds in other settings per 10 000 population	
Number of psychiatrists per 100 000 population	20
Number of neurosurgeons per 100 000 population	1
Number of psychiatric nurses per 100 000 population	32
Number of neurologists per 100 000 population	4
Number of psychologists per 100 000 population	76
Number of social workers per 100 000 population	

In Sweden, there has been sectorization, where the psychiatric service unit of a particular catchment area was responsible for comprehensive psychiatric care of the whole population belonging to that area. However, a referral is not required for contacting specialized services. There has been a reduction of inpatient beds (by almost 85% over a 25 year period starting in 1962) and an increase in community based treatment. Most of the stand-alone mental hospitals have closed. Regional differences in resources for care, methods of care and use of care have been noted. There are, specially in the northern part of Sweden, long distances between the municipalities, and as it is sparsely populated it is hard to fund the adequate resources needed. Individual care plans are drafted in consultation with patients and their relatives. Other than psychiatrists, the number of other mental health professionals, seem to be adequate. Most are employed by the municipalities. Sub-specialization in forensic and geriatric psychiatry is possible.

Non-Governmental Organizations NGOs are involved with mental health in the country. They are mainly involved in advocacy, promotion, prevention and rehabilitation. NGOs play an important part in suicide prevention programmes. Increased user influence through well-informed and participating patients and relatives is an important development. Under the mental health reform movement of 1995, financial support was provided for user and carer organizations and these were able to launch about 170 projects.

Information Gathering System There is mental health reporting system in the country. Reports of county council for inpatient care is available.
The country has data collection system or epidemiological study on mental health.
As required by the mental health reform, approximately 85% of the municipalities have conducted surveys to identify people with mental disabilities living in their communities and the needs these persons have for social assistance.

Programmes for Special Population The country has specific programmes for mental health for elderly and children. There is a Swedish National Programme to develop suicide prevention with the objectives: to decrease the number of successful and unsuccessful suicide attempts; early detection and management of high risk cases; public education on management of suicide both by laymen and professional staff. There is also a National Council for Suicide Prevention.
Specialized sub-systems exist for child, adolescent and forensic (there are six regional forensic hospitals) patients. Mobile teams are providing outreach, health care, food and other services for the homeless.

Therapeutic Drugs The following therapeutic drugs are generally available at the primary health care level of the country: carbamazepine, ethosuximide, phenobarbital, phenytoin sodium, sodium valproate, amitriptyline, chlorpromazine, diazepam, fluphenazine, haloperidol, lithium, biperiden, carbidopa, levodopa.
Carbidopa is available in combination with levodopa (200 mg).

Other Information In 1967, the responsibility of care was shifted from the state to the counties. The 1970s saw the creation and reorganization of community centres in catchment areas and promulgation of the National Board on Health and Welfare's policies concerning deinstitutionalization, development of out-patient care, intersectoral collaboration and involvement of families in services development. In 1992, a parliamentary commission reported that much more needed to be done and the Mental Health Care Reform of 1995 provided the required mandate to municipal social services for providing mental health care.

Additional Sources of Information

Belfrage, H., Fransson, G. (2000) Swedish forensic psychiatry. International Journal of Law and Psychiatry, 23, 509-514.

Centre for Epidemiology (1996) The Swedish Hospital Discharge Register 1987-1996 – Quality and Contents.

Stefansson, C-G., Hansson, L. (2001) Mental health care reform in Sweden, 1995. Acta Psychiatrica Scandinavica, 104 (suppl. 410), 82-88.

Silfverhielm, H., Kamis-Gould, E.(2000) The Swedish mental health system. International Journal of Law and Psychiatry, 23, 293-307.

The National Council for Suicide Prevention (1996) Support in Suicidal Crises – The Swedish National Programme to Develop Suicide Prevention.

Westrin, C. G. (1991) Strategies implemented but goals not attained: some comments on an evaluation of the Swedish mental health services. Scandinavian Journal of Social Medicine, 19, 53-56.

Switzerland

GENERAL INFORMATION

Switzerland is a country with an approximate area of 41 thousand sq. km. (UNO, 2001). Its population is 7.163 million, and the sex ratio (men per hundred women) is 98 (UNO, 2004). The proportion of population under the age of 15 years is 16% (UNO, 2004), and the proportion of population above the age of 60 years is 22% (WHO, 2004). The literacy rate is 99% for men and 99% for women (UNESCO/MoH, 2004).

The country is a high income group country (based on World Bank 2004 criteria). The proportion of health budget to GDP is 11%. The per capita total expenditure on health is 3322 international $, and the per capita government expenditure on health is 1897 international $ (WHO, 2004).

The main language(s) used in the country is (are) German (with several dialects), French, Italian and Romansh. The largest religious group(s) is (are) Roman Catholic and Protestant.

The life expectancy at birth is 77.7 years for males and 83.3 years for females (WHO, 2004). The healthy life expectancy at birth is 71 years for males and 75 years for females (WHO, 2004).

EPIDEMIOLOGY

There is substantial epidemiological data on mental illnesses in Switzerland in internationally accessible literature. No attempt was made to include this information here.

MENTAL HEALTH RESOURCES

Mental Health Policy A mental health policy is absent.

Substance Abuse Policy A substance abuse policy is present. The policy was initially formulated in 1990.

National Mental Health Programme A national mental health programme is absent.

National Therapeutic Drug Policy/Essential List of Drugs A national therapeutic drug policy/essential list of drugs is absent.

Mental Health Legislation The law regarding 'deprivation of liberty for assistance purpose' (Art: 397 ZGB) is a federal law concerning mental health. Its implementation is accomplished in accordance to Cantonal laws.

The latest legislation was enacted in 1981.

Mental Health Financing There are no budget allocations for mental health.

Details about expenditure on mental health are not available.

The primary sources of mental health financing in descending order are social insurance, tax based and out of pocket expenditure by the patient or family.

Mental health insurance does not cover the services of non-medical psychotherapists, unless they are employed and supervised by licensed physicians or psychiatrists.

The country has disability benefits for persons with mental disorders.

Mental Health Facilities Mental health is a part of primary health care system. Actual treatment of severe mental disorders is available at the primary level.

Regular training of primary care professionals is not carried out in the field of mental health.

There are community care facilities for patients with mental disorders. Communities are free to organize care for the mentally ill.

In 1977, the canton Bern took the decision to decentralize the existing system and community oriented institutions and psychiatric departments in some general hospitals were started. Since then it has been observed that an increasing number of patients are managed on an outpatient care basis and there has been a free flow of patients between private and public sectors for further management as and when required (Saameli et al, 1990).

Psychiatric Beds and Professionals

Total psychiatric beds per 10 000 population	13.2
Psychiatric beds in mental hospitals per 10 000 population	13.2
Psychiatric beds in general hospitals per 10 000 population	0
Psychiatric beds in other settings per 10 000 population	0
Number of psychiatrists per 100 000 population	23
Number of neurosurgeons per 100 000 population	0.8
Number of psychiatric nurses per 100 000 population	46
Number of neurologists per 100 000 population	3.4
Number of psychologists per 100 000 population	40.8
Number of social workers per 100 000 population	106

2616 non-medical psychotherapists are available; most of them (85%) have a psychology background. Among nurses, about half are in full-time employment and the other half in part-time employment. Among social workers, one-third are in full-time employ-

S

ment and two-thirds in part-time employment. Instead of housing long-term patients, psychiatric centres now cater to patients requiring short-term admissions for different mental disorders. Two-thirds of Swiss psychiatrists are involved in private practice. Those in private practice are more psychoanalytically oriented whereas those in universities are more biologically oriented (Guimon et al, 2000). There has been a lack of junior research scientists in psychiatry (Buddeberg et al, 1994). Since 1980, non-medical psychotherapists have been permitted to practice independently. Currently, they provide almost half of psychotherapy services provided.

Non-Governmental Organizations NGOs are involved with mental health in the country. They are mainly involved in advocacy, promotion, prevention, treatment and rehabilitation.

Information Gathering System There is no mental health reporting system in the country.
The country has no data collection system or epidemiological study on mental health. Data collection occurs at the cantonal level for insurance systems or as a part of health surveys, but these are not reported annually.

Programmes for Special Population The country has specific programmes for mental health for minorities, refugees, elderly and children.
There is a lack of facilities for admission of adolescents and towards this end the first adolescent psychiatry department was opened in Basel in 1993 as an open ward where milieutherapy, psychotherapy and pharmacotherapy work hand-in-hand.

Therapeutic Drugs The following therapeutic drugs are generally available at the primary health care level of the country: carbamazepine, ethosuximide, phenobarbital, phenytoin sodium, sodium valproate, amitriptyline, chlorpromazine, diazepam, fluphenazine, haloperidol, lithium, biperiden, carbidopa, levodopa.
Almost all kind of drugs are available at the primary health care level and practically all are available in clinics (Government and private). Prices are usually higher than in the neighbouring countries, but 90% of the costs are covered by the health insurance. The usual practice is to prescribe low therapeutic doses, there are however some exceptions.

Other Information

Additional Sources of Information

Beeler, I., Lorenz, S., Szucs, T. D. (2003) Provision and remuneration of psychotherapeutic services in Switzerland. Sozial- und Praventivmedizin, 48, 88-96.

Ernst, C., Angst, J. (1996) The Burgholzli Clinic. American Journal of Psychiatry, 153, 816.

Guimon, J. (2000) New forms of psychiatric education: the Geneva experience. European Journal of Psychiatry, 14, 52-60.

Guimon, J., Fischer, W., Zbinden, E., et al (1998) Therapeutic practice profiles, work settings and activities of Swiss psychiatrists. Schweizer Archiv für Neurologie und Psychiatrie, 149, 29-39.

Guimon, J, Goerg, D., Fischer, W. et al (1997) Theoretical trends among Swiss psychiatrists. Annales Medico-Psychologiques, 155, 184-201.

Guimon, J., Goerg, D., Fischer, W. et al (2000) Private psychiatry in Switzerland. International Journal of Psychiatry in Clinical Practice, 4, 227-232.

Meng, H., Burgin, D. (1998) Department of adolescent psychiatry: building up and first experiences. Psychiatrische Praxis, 25, 61-66.

Saameli, W., Kopp, W. (1990) Decentralized psychiatry – an evaluation of the first 5 years of a general hospital-based psychiatric service. Psychiatrische Praxis, 17, 191-199.

Syrian Arab Republic

GENERAL INFORMATION

Syrian Arab Republic is a country with an approximate area of 185 thousand sq. km. (UNO, 2001). Its population is 18.223 million, and the sex ratio (men per hundred women) is 102 (UNO, 2004). The proportion of population under the age of 15 years is 37% (UNO, 2004), and the proportion of population above the age of 60 years is 5% (WHO, 2004). The literacy rate is 91% for men and 74.2% for women (UNESCO/MoH, 2004).

The country is a lower middle income group country (based on World Bank 2004 criteria). The proportion of health budget to GDP is 5.4%. The per capita total expenditure on health is 427 international $, and the per capita government expenditure on health is 188 international $ (WHO, 2004).

The main language(s) used in the country is (are) Arabic, French and English. The largest ethnic group(s) is (are) Arab. The largest religious group(s) is (are) Muslim (nine-tenths).

The life expectancy at birth is 68.8 years for males and 73.6 years for females (WHO, 2004). The healthy life expectancy at birth is 60 years for males and 63 years for females (WHO, 2004).

EPIDEMIOLOGY

There is a paucity of epidemiological data on mental illnesses in Syrian Arab Republic in internationally accessible literature. Maziak et al (2002) recruited a sample of 412 women from 8 randomly selected primary care centres in one area. A special questionnaire was prepared for the study purpose consisting of SRQ-20 non-psychotic items and questions about background information considered relevant to the mental health of women in the studied population. Direct individual interviews were also conducted. The prevalence of psychiatric distress was 55.6%. The following factors were found to predict women's mental health on logistic regression: physical abuse, education (illiteracy), polygamy, residence, age and age of marriage. Among those predictors, women's illiteracy, polygamy and physical abuse were the strongest determinants of mental distress leading to the worse outcomes.

MENTAL HEALTH RESOURCES

Mental Health Policy A mental health policy is present. The policy was initially formulated in 2001.

Substance Abuse Policy A substance abuse policy is present. The policy was initially formulated in 1993.

National Mental Health Programme A national mental health programme is present. The programme was formulated in 2001.

National Therapeutic Drug Policy/Essential List of Drugs A national therapeutic drug policy/essential list of drugs is present. It was formulated in 1990.

Mental Health Legislation The legislation concerns organizing the admission and discharge of patients in Government psychiatric hospitals.

The latest legislation was enacted in 1965.

Mental Health Financing There are budget allocations for mental health.

Details about expenditure on mental health are not available.

Details about sources of financing are not available.

The country has disability benefits for persons with mental disorders.

Mental Health Facilities Mental health is a part of primary health care system. Actual treatment of severe mental disorders is available at the primary level.

Regular training of primary care professionals is carried out in the field of mental health. About 110 nurses and general physicians have been trained in the last ten years.

There are no community care facilities for patients with mental disorders.

Psychiatric Beds and Professionals

Total psychiatric beds per 10 000 population	0.8
Psychiatric beds in mental hospitals per 10 000 population	0.78
Psychiatric beds in general hospitals per 10 000 population	0.02
Psychiatric beds in other settings per 10 000 population	0
Number of psychiatrists per 100 000 population	0.5
Number of neurosurgeons per 100 000 population	0.6
Number of psychiatric nurses per 100 000 population	0.5
Number of neurologists per 100 000 population	0.9
Number of psychologists per 100 000 population	0
Number of social workers per 100 000 population	0

Beds have been earmarked for female patients. Forensic beds are available.

S

Non-Governmental Organizations NGOs are not involved with mental health in the country.

Information Gathering System There is no mental health reporting system in the country. Only statistical admission data of psychiatric hospitals are reported.
The country has no data collection system or epidemiological study on mental health.

Programmes for Special Population The country has specific programmes for mental health for refugees and elderly.
Services for mentally challenged and delinquents are available.

Therapeutic Drugs The following therapeutic drugs are generally available at the primary health care level of the country: carbamazepine, phenobarbital, phenytoin sodium, sodium valproate, amitriptyline, chlorpromazine, diazepam, fluphenazine, haloperidol, carbidopa, levodopa.

Other Information

Additional Sources of Information

Maziak, W., Asfar, T., Mzayek, F., et al (2002) Socio-demographic correlates of psychiatric morbidity among low-income women in Aleppo, Syria. Social Science & Medicine, 54, 1419-1427.

S

Tajikistan

GENERAL INFORMATION

Tajikistan is a country with an approximate area of 143 thousand sq. km. (UNO, 2001). Its population is 6.297 million, and the sex ratio (men per hundred women) is 99 (UNO, 2004). The proportion of population under the age of 15 years is 35% (UNO, 2004), and the proportion of population above the age of 60 years is 7% (WHO, 2004). The literacy rate is 99.7% for men and 99.3% for women (UNESCO/MoH, 2004).

The country is a low income group country (based on World Bank 2004 criteria). The proportion of health budget to GDP is 3.3%. The per capita total expenditure on health is 43 international $, and the per capita government expenditure on health is 12 international $ (WHO, 2004).

The main language(s) used in the country is (are) Tajik. The largest ethnic group(s) is (are) Tajik, and the other ethnic group(s) are (is) Uzbek. The largest religious group(s) is (are) Sunni Muslim (five-sixths).

The life expectancy at birth is 61 years for males and 66.5 years for females (WHO, 2004). The healthy life expectancy at birth is 53 years for males and 56 years for females (WHO, 2004).

EPIDEMIOLOGY

There is a paucity of epidemiological data on mental illnesses in Tajikistan in internationally accessible literature. Bochkov et al (1971) conducted a clinico-genealogical investigation of the population of some small villages and found olygophrenia (0.4%), epilepsy (0.5%) and schizophrenia (0.7%) in the population. These indices did not differ significantly from those for other regions of the erstwhile USSR. There was an absence of genetic forms of olygophrenia. Services data (MoH, 2004) suggest lower figures for these conditions (0.3%, 0.4% and 0.6%, respectively) as expected because some patients may not come in contact with treatment services. Wasserman et al (1998) reported on the changing pattern of suicide across different countries that were a part of erstwhile USSR between 1984-90 prior to its break-up. Suicide rates varied greatly between different regions. It was 11.8 per 100 000 in Central Asia (Kazakhstan, Kirgizia, Turkmenistan, Uzbekistan and Tajikistan). Correspondence between the Ministry of Internal Affairs and Ministry of Health suggest that the suicide rate in Tajikistan has recently increased up to 19.9 per 100 000, perhaps due to the civil war and the resultant devastation, increase in unemployment, domestic violence, etc.

MENTAL HEALTH RESOURCES

Mental Health Policy A mental health policy is absent.

Substance Abuse Policy A substance abuse policy is absent. The 'National Program on Substance Abuse Prevention and Rehabilitation of Drug-dependants by 2010' was submitted for consideration to the legislative body in 2004.

National Mental Health Programme A national mental health programme is absent.
The national mental health programme has been drafted.

National Therapeutic Drug Policy/Essential List of Drugs A national therapeutic drug policy/essential list of drugs is present. It was formulated in 1999.
Therapy is based on outdated Russian books. Old and outdated modes of treatment are still used. Often there are no drugs to treat the patients (Veeken, 1997).

Mental Health Legislation The new law on mental health was discussed and recommended for approval by the Geneva Initiative on Psychiatry. A draft law in Russian is available.
Details about the year of enactment of the mental health legislation are not available.

Mental Health Financing Details about disability benefits for mental health are not available.
Details about expenditure on mental health are not available.
Details about sources of financing are not available.
The health care system is funded by the state in principle but depended largely on foreign aid. In 2004, the budget for mental health reached 2 416 278 USD, but it may be insufficient for covering even essential needs. Foreign financing stopped in 2003 due to completion of MSF-Holland activity in Tajikistan.
The country has disability benefits for persons with mental disorders. Disability benefits consist of pension funds and keeping right to the living property for institutionalized disabled.

Mental Health Facilities Mental health is a part of primary health care system. Actual treatment of severe mental disorders is not available at the primary level. About 50 primary health care facilities have access for mental health services.
Regular training of primary care professionals is not carried out in the field of mental health. A few NGOs are dealing with training in mental health. Their activity has to be coordinated with mental health state institutions.
There are no community care facilities for patients with mental disorders.

Psychiatric Beds and Professionals

Total psychiatric beds per 10 000 population	2.47
Psychiatric beds in mental hospitals per 10 000 population	2.47
Psychiatric beds in general hospitals per 10 000 population	
Psychiatric beds in other settings per 10 000 population	
Number of psychiatrists per 100 000 population	1.8
Number of neurosurgeons per 100 000 population	0.9
Number of psychiatric nurses per 100 000 population	3.6
Number of neurologists per 100 000 population	3.7
Number of psychologists per 100 000 population	0.1
Number of social workers per 100 000 population	

There are a few psychiatric institutes and they lack drugs, food, bedding, clothes, equipment and transport. Lack of heating is a problem during winter months. There is a lack of specialist staff. The salaries are extremely low. A psychiatrist is paid the equivalent of $3 a month.

Non-Governmental Organizations Details about NGO facilities in mental health are not available.

Information Gathering System Details about mental health reporting systems are not available.
Details about data collection system or epidemiological study on mental health are not available.

Programmes for Special Population There are children homes but the conditions are unsatisfactory.

Therapeutic Drugs The following therapeutic drugs are generally available at the primary health care level of the country: carbamazepine, phenobarbital, amitriptyline, chlorpromazine, diazepam, fluphenazine, haloperidol, levodopa.

Other Information There is almost no contact with international psychiatry. However, in August 1997, after an initial assessment of the mental health infrastructure by the Médecins Sans Frontières of Holland a three year project called 'Support for Inpatients of Mental Health Institutions and Dispensaries in the Republic of Tajikistan' has been undertaken with the aim of reducing the mortality rate in the two large psychiatric hospitals (Leninsky and Lakkon) and at the Child and Adolescent Centre. Since then, the programme has been extended to 14 psychoneurological dispensaries. The MSF has also rehabilitated two mental health institutions, one in the capital and the other in the north of the country. Besides improving the infrastructure it has provided training to personnel and has developed a community-based programme for treating individuals suffering from trauma.

Additional Sources of Information

Baibabayev, A., Cunningham, D., de Jong, K. (2000) Update on the state of mental health in Tajikistan. Mental Health Reforms, 5, 14-16.

Bochkov, N. P., Anfalova, T. V., Dement'eva, E. S., et al (1971) Medical genetic study of the population of the western Pamir. I. Sex ratio, hereditary neuropsychiatric diseases, and general anthropogenetic traits. Soviet Genetics, 7, 669-674.

Médecins Sans Frontières (2002) http://www.doctorswithoutborders.org

Veeken, H. (1997) Tajikistan: no pay, no care. British Medical Journal, 315, 1460-1461.

Wasserman, D., Varnik, A., Dankowicz, M. (1998) Regional differences in the distribution of suicide in the former Soviet Union during perestroika, 1984-1990. Acta Psychiatrica Scandinavica, Supplement 394, 5-12.

Thailand

GENERAL INFORMATION

Thailand is a country with an approximate area of 513 thousand sq. km. (UNO, 2001). Its population is 63.465 million, and the sex ratio (men per hundred women) is 96 (UNO, 2004). The proportion of population under the age of 15 years is 25% (UNO, 2004), and the proportion of population above the age of 60 years is 9% (WHO, 2004). The literacy rate is 94.9% for men and 90.5% for women (UNESCO/MoH, 2004).

The country is a lower middle income group country (based on World Bank 2004 criteria). The proportion of health budget to GDP is 3.7%. The per capita total expenditure on health is 254 international $, and the per capita government expenditure on health is 145 international $ (WHO, 2004).

The main language(s) used in the country is (are) Thai, Chinese and English. The largest ethnic group(s) is (are) Thai, and the other ethnic group(s) are (is) Chinese. The largest religious group(s) is (are) Buddhist (almost 95%).

The life expectancy at birth is 66 years for males and 72.7 years for females (WHO, 2004). The healthy life expectancy at birth is 58 years for males and 62 years for females (WHO, 2004).

EPIDEMIOLOGY

Bonyawongvirot et al (2004) conducted a two-stage survey (n=11 700) using the Alcohol Use Disorder Identification Test (AUDIT) and Mini International Neuropsychiatric Interview (MINI). The following disorders were common: alcohol use disorder (28.5%), major depression disorder (3.2%), generalized anxiety disorder (1.85%), psychotic disorders (1.76%), dsythymia disorders (1.18%), agoraphobia (0.89%), panic disorder (0.75%) and bipolar disorder (mnia: 0.65%). Thavichachart et al (2001) assessed 3000 adults selected through a multi-stage random sampling procedure using modified Composite International Diagnostic Interview (CIDI/DSM-IV). The life time prevalence of mental disorders was: schizophrenia (1.3%), manic episode (9.3%), major depressive episode (9.9%), dysthymia (1%), anxiety disorders (10.2%), mental retardation (1.8%), epilepsy (1.3%), suicidal idea (7.1%), drug and substances use disorders (11.2%) and alcohol use disorders (18.4%). Jitapunkal et al (2001) conducted a country wide survey of more than 4000 elders (over 60 years) using CMT (cut-off score < 15) and impairment as criteria to diagnose dementia. They found the overall prevalence of dementia to be 3.3% (1% in 60-64 years to 31.3% in the over 90 years age group). Senanarong et al (2001a) found that the prevalence of dementia (diagnosed according to Thai Mental State Examination score below 25th percentile and an impairment criterion) in a countrywide survey involving 3177 elderly people over 60 years to be in the 9.9%. In another study, Senanarong et al (2001b) found cognitive impairment in 52.7% of subjects in a community sample of 550 elderly subjects (age > 55 years) examined with the Thai Mental State Examination (cut off < 25). Cognitive impairment was associated with age, blood pressure, serum cholesterol, liver function parameters, haemoglobin, neutrophil counts and weight. Srisurapanont and Intaprasert (1999) mailed the Seasonal Pattern Assessment Questionnaire (SPAQ) to 520 randomly selected subjects and found the prevalence of summer SAD, sub-syndromal summer SAD and winter SAD to be 6.2%, 8.3% and 1%, respectively. Kongkanand (2000) assessed 1250 individuals in an urban area using pre-tested questionnaires and found that the rate of erectile dysfunction was associated with age, hypertension, diabetics or heart disease, smoking, alcohol and caffeine consumption. Eungprabhanth (1975) examined autopsy reports of 581 suicidal cases and found that the male:female ratio was 6:4 and the highest incidence was in the 20-39 years age group. Girls predominate among adolescents (0-19 years). Farmers showed the highest suicide rate, and poisoning (with parathion) was the commonest method of suicide. Wacharasindhu and Panyyayong (2002) assessed 1698 children (8-11 years old) in a two stage survey using Thai Youth Checklist (TYC) – Parent and Teacher form and the Child and Adolescent Psychiatric Assessment (CAPA). The overall prevalence rate of child psychiatric disorders was 37.6% with anxiety (10.8%), specific phobia (9.7%), depression (7.1%), conduct disorder (5.5%), ADHD (5.1%) and separation anxiety disorder (5%) being the common diagnoses. Cederblad et al (2001) evaluated 483 Thai children and youths, aged 7-18 years, using the Child Behavior Checklist (CBCL) and the Teacher's Report Form (TRF). Older children living in urban areas had higher problem scores than other groups. Boys showed more 'externalizing' and delinquent behaviour on both the CBCL and the TRF. Benjasuwantep et al (2002) assessed 353 school students (grades 1 to 6) using Connor's Rating Scale and behavioural observation in classroom. A DSM-IV diagnosis of ADHD was made in 6.5%. Mollica et al (1997) assessed 182 refugee adolescents aged 12-13 years based on a multistage probability sample of 1000 households using the Child Behavior Checklist (CBCL) and the Youth Self-Report (YSR). Nearly 54% had total problem scores in the clinical range by parent report on the CBCL and 26.4% by adolescent report on the YSR. The dose-effect relationship between cumulative trauma and symptoms was strong for total problems on CBCL and subscales for Anxious/Depressed and Attention Problems on both the YSR and CBCL. Mollica et al (1998) found that cumulative trauma continued to affect psychiatric symptom levels a decade after the original trauma events, especially for symptom categories of depression, PTSD and dissociative and culturally dependent symptoms. Savin et al (1996) found that PTSD endured in a sample of Khmer youths who had survived conflict as children. Sub-clinical forms of PTSD were found in those who reported their worst trauma during life in the camp, while the full PTSD syndrome was found in those who reported trauma related to the conflict. Extremely high rates of depressive disorder was also reported, which was interpreted as related to the impending repatriation back to Cambodia. In a sample of 486 primary students who did not have mental deficiency, Roongpraiwan et al (2002) found the prevalence of dyslexia and probable dyslexia to be 6.3% and 12.6%, respectively, with males affected 3.4 times more often than females. Nearly 90% of the affected students showed soft neurological signs and 8.7% had comorbid ADHD.

MENTAL HEALTH RESOURCES

Mental Health Policy A mental health policy is present. The policy was initially formulated in 1995.

The components of the policy are advocacy, promotion, prevention, treatment and rehabilitation. Administration and technical development is also a component of the policy. The mental health policy plans to promote mental health and prevent mental health problems, to expand and develop the service system of treatment and rehabilitation, to develop mental health knowledge and technology, to develop the management system for reformation of all aspects of mental health, to develop people's co-operation in order to achieve the goal of taking care of one's mental health by applying local wisdom to family assistance, community programmes, etc. and to develop modern psychosocial and other technical knowledge in order to apply them fruitfully to Thailand's mental health situation.

Substance Abuse Policy A substance abuse policy is present. The policy was initially formulated in 1998. On substance abuse there was an initial law from 1988 which dealt with Drugs Prevention and Suppression Policy. This was implemented under the strategy of state-civil alliance against drugs, which unites the power of civil and state agencies to continually and seriously fight against drug abuse under more systematic and cooperative administration. The more recent policy on Reformation of Addicts Treatment and Rehabilitation System guides all rural and urban centres to undertake programmes to look into the management issues of addicts. National institutes are urged to develop advanced technologies to tackle the treatment and rehabilitation of such addicts in cooperation with international agencies. It also specifies that the provincial health doctor would act as the chief of treatment and rehabilitation centres at provincial levels.

National Mental Health Programme A national mental health programme is present. The programme was formulated in 1997.

National Therapeutic Drug Policy/Essential List of Drugs A national therapeutic drug policy/essential list of drugs is present. Details about the year of formulation are not available.
The National Drug Committee policy encourages general practitioners to use only drugs available from the National List of Essential Drugs. The Department of Mental Health has recently developed the practice guideline on the care of patients with mood disorders.

Mental Health Legislation There is no mental health legislation.
Details about the year of enactment of the mental health legislation are not available.

Mental Health Financing There are budget allocations for mental health.
The country spends 2.5% of the total health budget on mental health.
The primary sources of mental health financing in descending order are tax based, out of pocket expenditure by the patient or family and social insurance.
Universal health care insurance is not available, but there are several types of limited coverage available. For Government officials, health coverage is extensive. Employees of private companies are usually covered by the company's health benefits. Such benefits are also available, to a more limited extent, to blue-collar workers or labourers whose companies are registered by the labour department. For citizens with low income, a special health insurance plan provided free of charge by the Government covers hospitalization for acute psychotic episodes for up to 15 days in Government hospitals. Drug use disorders in general are not covered by health benefit plans. Psychological assessment and therapy are not reimbursable.
The country has disability benefits for persons with mental disorders.

Mental Health Facilities Mental health is a part of primary health care system. Actual treatment of severe mental disorders is not available at the primary level.
Regular training of primary care professionals is carried out in the field of mental health. In the last two years, about 300 personnel were provided training. Training of trainers has been organized for mental health professionals. About 300 general practitioners were trained in the last two years on mental health. Mental health home visit project trains staff in caring for patients at home. A range of training manuals have been prepared.
There are no community care facilities for patients with mental disorders. It is planned to develop home health care centres and other community programmes. A total of 182 telephone counselling services, 470 counselling centres and 327 stress-relief clinics provide community services. A pilot project for vocational rehabilitation of mentally challenged and mentally ill persons is under way. A few halfway houses are available.

Psychiatric Beds and Professionals

Total psychiatric beds per 10 000 population	1.4
Psychiatric beds in mental hospitals per 10 000 population	1.4
Psychiatric beds in general hospitals per 10 000 population	
Psychiatric beds in other settings per 10 000 population	
Number of psychiatrists per 100 000 population	0.6
Number of neurosurgeons per 100 000 population	0.4
Number of psychiatric nurses per 100 000 population	2.7
Number of neurologists per 100 000 population	0.2
Number of psychologists per 100 000 population	0.2
Number of social workers per 100 000 population	0.6

There are 17 occupational therapists. More than half of the beds are in Bangkok and the central region. Three-fifths of psychiatrists are located in Bangkok, even though three-fourths are in Government service. More than two-fifths of social workers are also placed in the central region. Psychologists and psychiatric nurses are distributed more evenly. Psychologists are active in the designing and implementation of training programmes and development of educational material.

Non-Governmental Organizations NGOs are involved with mental health in the country. They are mainly involved in advocacy, promotion and prevention. The NGO sector is quite active in opening mental health centres, funding campaigns, telephone counselling, child right and protection issues, etc.

Information Gathering System There is mental health reporting system in the country.
The country has data collection system or epidemiological study on mental health.
A database on mental health issues related to elderly is being built.

Programmes for Special Population The country has specific programmes for mental health for elderly and children.
The Government supports programmes for prevention of family mental health problems, for mental health education in institutions, for elderly, for physically challenged and underprivileged children.

Therapeutic Drugs The following therapeutic drugs are generally available at the primary health care level of the country: carbamazepine, ethosuximide, phenobarbital, phenytoin sodium, sodium valproate, amitriptyline, chlorpromazine, diazepam, fluphenazine, haloperidol, lithium.

Other Information Quite a few projects are being implemented. The notable ones being the promotion of Buddhist monks' role in mental health, psychosocial care for the depressed, mental health prevention and support for the risk groups to suicide, mental health projects for the physically handicapped and underprivileged children, projects for prisoners and prison officers, model development of community participation in preventing substance abuse, programmes for the elderly and family, model programmes to look into the psychiatric mental health care in general hospitals, etc. The Department of Mental Health in the Ministry of Public Health has undertaken a quality inspection of agencies under its charge and has developed quality guidelines. Six of its hospitals have attained ISO 9002 quality certification. Many projects involving international collaboration are also under way. Studies on cost-effectiveness of services are being carried out.

Additional Sources of Information

Benjasuwantep, B., Ruangdaraganon, N., Visudhiphan, P. (2002) Prevalence and clinical characteristics of attention deficit hyperactivity disorder among primary school students in Bangkok. Journal of the Medical Association of Thailand, 85, 1232-1240.

Bunyawongwirot, P., Siriwanarungsun, P., Kongsuk, T., et al. (2004) Prevalence of mental disorders in Thailand: a national survey. Proceeding of the 17th National Epidemiology Seminar, Bangkok, Thailand, May 20th 2004.

Cederblad, M., Pruksachatkunakorn, P., Boripunkul, T., et al (2001) Behaviour problems and competence in Thai children and youths: Teachers', parents' and subjects' perspectives. Transcultural Psychiatry, 38, 64-79.

Department of Mental Health (2003) Mental Health in Thailand 2002-2003. Bangkok: Department of Mental Health, Ministry of Public Health.

Eungprabhanth, V. (1975) Suicide in Thailand. Forensic Science, 5, 43-51.

Jitapunkul, S., Kunanusont, C., Phoolcharoen, W., et al (2001) Prevalence estimation of dementia among Thai elderly: a national survey. Journal of the Medical Association of Thailand, 84, 461-467.

Kongkanand, A. (2000) Prevalence of erectile dysfunction in Thailand. Thai Erectile Dysfunction Epidemiological Study Group. International Journal of Andrology, 23, 77-80.

Ministry of Health. General Report on State of Mental Health and Associated Services in Thailand.

Ministry of Public Health, Narcotics Control Board. Strategies and Guidelines on Drugs Prevention and Treatment.

Mollica, R. F., Poole, C., Son, L., et al (1997) Effects of war trauma on Cambodian refugee adolescents' functional health and mental health status. Journal of the American Academy of Child & Adolescent Psychiatry, 36, 1098-1106.

Mollica, R. F., McInnes, K., Poole, C., et al (1998) Dose-effect relationships of trauma to symptoms of depression and post- traumatic stress disorder among Cambodian survivors of mass violence. British Journal of Psychiatry, 173, 482-488.

National List of Psychotherapeutic Drugs (Government document).

Roongpraiwan, R., Ruangdaraganon, N., Visudhiphan, P., et al (2002) Prevalence and clinical characteristics of dyslexia in primary school students. Journal of the Medical Association of Thailand, 85, 1097-1103.

Savin, D., Sack, W. H., Clarke, G. N., et al (1996) The Khmer adolescent project: III. A study of trauma from Thailand's Site II refugee camp. Journal of the American Academy of Child & Adolescent Psychiatry, 35, 384-391.

Senanarong, V., Jamjumrus, P., Harnphadungkit, K., et al (2001b) Risk factors for dementia and impaired cognitive status in Thai elderly. Journal of the Medical Association of Thailand, 84, 468-474.

Senanarong, V., Poungvarin, N., Sukhatunga, K., et al (2001a) Cognitive status in the community dwelling Thai elderly. Journal of the Medical Association of Thailand, 84, 408-416.

Siriwanarangsan, P., Liknapichitkul, D., Khandelwal, S. K. (2004) Thailand mental health country profile. International Review of Psychiatry, 16, 150-158.

Srisurapanont, M., Intaprasert, S. (1999) Seasonal variations in mood and behaviour: epidemiological findings in the north tropics. Journal of Affective Disorders, 54, 97-99.

Sukying, C. (2000) Pharmacotherapy of depression in Thailand: country report 1999. Singapore Medical Journal, 41, 53-54.

Tapanya, S. (2001) Psychology in medical settings in Thailand. Journal of Clinical Psychology in Medical Settings, 8, 69-72.

Thavichachart, N., Intoh, P., Thavichachart, T., et al (2001) Epidemiological survey of mental disorders and knowledge attitude practice upon mental health among people in Bangkok Metropolis. Journal of the Medical Association of Thailand, 84, 118-126.

Wacharasindhu, A., Panyyayong, B. (2002) Psychiatric disorders in Thai school-aged children: I Prevalence. Journal of the Medical Association of Thailand, 85, 125-136.

T–Z

The former Yugoslav Republic of Macedonia

GENERAL INFORMATION

The former Yugoslav Republic of Macedonia is a country with an approximate area of 26 thousand sq. km. (UNO, 2001). Its population is 2.066 million, and the sex ratio (men per hundred women) is 100 (UNO, 2004). The proportion of population under the age of 15 years is 21% (UNO, 2004), and the proportion of population above the age of 60 years is 15% (WHO, 2004). The literacy rate is 97% for men and 91% for women (UNESCO/MoH, 2004).

The country is a lower middle income group country (based on World Bank 2004 criteria). The proportion of health budget to GDP is 6.8%. The per capita total expenditure on health is 331 international $, and the per capita Government expenditure on health is 281 international $ (WHO, 2004).

The main language(s) used in the country is (are) Macedonian and Albanian. The largest ethnic group(s) is (are) Macedonian, and the other ethnic group(s) are (is) Albanian, Turkish, Roma, Vlachs and Serb. The largest religious group(s) is (are) Macedonian Orthodox Christian (three-fourths), and the other religious group(s) are (is) Muslim and Roman Catholic.

The life expectancy at birth is 69 years for males and 75.1 years for females (WHO, 2004). The healthy life expectancy at birth is 62 years for males and 65 years for females (WHO, 2004).

EPIDEMIOLOGY

There is a paucity of epidemiological data on mental illnesses in The Former Yugoslav Republic of Macedonia in internationally accessible literature. Milcinski and Mrevlje (1990) compared the rate of suicide across different regions. The study showed that there was a wide variation in rates of suicide, with the northern region having very high rates (among the highest in Europe) and the southern and eastern regions including Macedonia having very low rates (among the lowest in Europe).

MENTAL HEALTH RESOURCES

Mental Health Policy A mental health policy is absent.

A mental health policy has been reviewed and it is in the process of being adopted by the Government. The document is constituted of three parts, namely National Policy, Strategy with Action Plan and Legislation on Mental Health.

Substance Abuse Policy A substance abuse policy is present. The policy was initially formulated in 1999. A substance abuse action plan is available, launched for the period 1999-2002, by the Inter-ministerial National Commission for Prevention of Illegal Drug Trafficking and Abuse.

National Mental Health Programme A national mental health programme is absent.

A National Master Mental Health Plan is already prepared by the National Task Force Team (assigned by the Minister of Health) in collaboration with WHO. It is expected to be adopted shortly by the Government.

National Therapeutic Drug Policy/Essential List of Drugs A national therapeutic drug policy/essential list of drugs is present. Details about the year of formulation are not available.

There is a list of essential drugs covered by the Health Insurance Fund as part of the health insurance scheme. Currently, this list is under revision to reflect prevailing needs.

Mental Health Legislation Currently, some of the legislative regulation is incorporated in the Law on Health Protection, and some under criminal law, but little relates to human rights of people with mental disorders and compulsory hospitalization. The mental health legislation is in a draft form. Compulsory hospitalization is under review with the aim to reflect international trends.

Details about the year of enactment of the mental health legislation are not available.

Mental Health Financing There are budget allocations for mental health.

Details about expenditure on mental health are not available.

The primary source of mental health financing is social insurance.

There are budget allocations for mental health services as part of the Law for Health Protection and Law for Health Insurance (Government budget and Health Insurance Fund).

The country has disability benefits for persons with mental disorders. Mental health patients according to the newly developed law are treated in the same way regarding employment as persons with somatic disabilities. There are examples from practice in cities of Gevgelia and Skopje where there are companies that facilitate the employment possibilities of mentally ill persons, an issue that previously was available only for persons with somatic disabilities.

Mental Health Facilities Mental health is a part of primary health care system. Actual treatment of severe mental disorders is not available at the primary level. Severe disorders are mainly treated at secondary and tertiary level.

Regular training of primary care professionals is carried out in the field of mental health. Regular training of primary care professionals is carried out in the field of mental health. A training programme for primary health care persons has been organized by the World Bank in 2000 and by the WHO since 2001.

There are community care facilities for patients with mental disorders. The country had a traditional hospital-based mental health services. New policy developments recognize the need for reform in this sector especially towards decentralization and community-based services. Current developments of the community based mental health programme and services are due to the joint endeavour of the Ministry of Health and WHO, with support from the international community. A National Board for promotion and implementation of community-based services on mental health has been created.

Psychiatric Beds and Professionals

Total psychiatric beds per 10 000 population	8.2
Psychiatric beds in mental hospitals per 10 000 population	6.2
Psychiatric beds in general hospitals per 10 000 population	2
Psychiatric beds in other settings per 10 000 population	0
Number of psychiatrists per 100 000 population	7.5
Number of neurosurgeons per 100 000 population	1
Number of psychiatric nurses per 100 000 population	24
Number of neurologists per 100 000 population	5
Number of psychologists per 100 000 population	2
Number of social workers per 100 000 population	1.5

There are 320 administrators. The country has traditional hospital-based mental health services, which are not efficient and largely depend on a centralized organization; they have not been able to meet these extensive needs. The services are unsatisfactory from the medical, psychological, human, outcome, efficiency or economic points of view. Over the last 20 years a 20% reduction in the number of beds in psychiatric hospitals has been achieved. Forty mental health professionals have been trained in a one-year post-graduate course entitled, 'Psychosocial and traumatic stress – understanding, prevention, treatment'.

Non-Governmental Organizations NGOs are involved with mental health in the country. They are mainly involved in advocacy, promotion and rehabilitation. The NGOs are also working in the field of legislation formulation and fight against stigma.

Information Gathering System There is mental health reporting system in the country. Information is collected as part of Annual National Statistics by the Republican Institute for Health Protection.
The country has no data collection system or epidemiological study on mental health.

Programmes for Special Population The country has specific programmes for mental health for children.
The host families, local health and social services, the local communities and society in general are all involved in tackling the refugee and internally displaced persons problem. Some effort has been put into prevention of substance abuse, child abuse and domestic violence, mostly by NGOs, as well as in schools with the cooperation of NGOs and the Ministry of Education.

Therapeutic Drugs The following therapeutic drugs are generally available at the primary health care level of the country: carbamazepine, ethosuximide, phenobarbital, phenytoin sodium, sodium valproate, amitriptyline, chlorpromazine, diazepam, fluphenazine, haloperidol, lithium, biperiden, carbidopa, levodopa.
A list of drugs are covered by the health insurance, which is constantly changing the so-called positive list (with drugs covered by the national fund). Drugs like risperidone and sertraline are available in the positive list.

Other Information The four challenges facing the country are: elaboration of a national programme for mental health; adoption of mental health legislation; preparation of a national register of mental disorders, a database and epidemiological research.

Additional Sources of Information

Milcinski, L., Mrevlje, G. (1990) Epidemiology of suicide in Yugoslavia--methodological questions. Medicinski Pregled, 43, 453-456.
Ministry of Health.
Republic Institute for Statistic.
Republic Institute for Health Protection.
WHO, Country Office Skopje – Mental Health Programme.

Timor-Leste

GENERAL INFORMATION

Timor-Leste is a country with an approximate area of 15 thousand sq. km. (UNO, 2001). Its population is 0.82 million, and the sex ratio (men per hundred women) is 108 (UNO, 2004). The proportion of population under the age of 15 years is 34% (UNO, 2004), and the proportion of population above the age of 60 years is 5% (WHO, 2004).
The country is a low income group country (based on World Bank 2004 criteria). The proportion of health budget to GDP is 9.8%. The main language(s) used in the country is (are) Tetum and Portuguese.
The life expectancy at birth is 54.8 years for males and 60.5 years for females (WHO, 2004). The healthy life expectancy at birth is 48 years for males and 52 years for females (WHO, 2004).

EPIDEMIOLOGY

There is a paucity of epidemiological data on mental illnesses in Timor-Leste in internationally accessible literature. Modvig et al (2000) carried out a national psychosocial needs assessment. An estimated 750 000 individuals from over 1000 households in 13 districts were interviewed. One respondent was selected from each household. Almost all (97%) respondents said they had experienced at least one traumatic event like direct exposure to combat situation, lack of shelter and ill health with no access to medical care. Death of parents, spouse and children and the stress of having to take over responsibility of the family was a common occurrence. Torture appears to have been widespread. Two-fifths of the respondents said that they had been tortured, but a larger number (57%) said they had experienced at least one of the six forms of torture included in the study instrument. One-third were diagnosed to have PTSD, based on a cut-off score of 2.5 or greater in the Harvard Trauma Questionnaire Symptoms Checklist.

MENTAL HEALTH RESOURCES

Mental Health Policy A mental health policy is absent.
The health policy suggests that mental health care would be provided by the public sector. The services would be centralized to facilitate uniform development across the country. The services would be free and sustainable. A mental health policy has been drafted in 2003. It has components of advocacy, promotion, prevention and treatment.

Substance Abuse Policy A substance abuse policy is absent.

National Mental Health Programme A national mental health programme is absent.
The Ministry of Health has approved the National Project of Mental Health to increase the capacity of the Ministry to provide mental health care. The proposed components of the project are: policy development and service delivery; training and workforce development; community involvement and mental health promotion; effective project management.

National Therapeutic Drug Policy/Essential List of Drugs A national therapeutic drug policy/essential list of drugs is present. It was formulated in 2004.
Psychotropic drug procurement and distribution systems were set up.

Mental Health Legislation There is no mental health legislation. The courts usually follow Indonesian laws.
Details about the year of enactment of the mental health legislation are not available.

Mental Health Financing Details about disability benefits for mental health are not available.
Details about expenditure on mental health are not available.
Details about sources of financing are not available.
The Government has reached an agreement with the AusAID to fund a nation-wide mental health programme over the next 3 years.
The country does not have disability benefits for persons with mental disorders.

Mental Health Facilities Details about mental health facilities at the primary care level are not available.
Details about training facilities are not available. Psychosocial Recovery and Development in East Timor (PRADET) has trained local workers, mainly nurses, who established outreach clinics in and around Dili. Mobile outreach clinics extended the work to the most disrupted communities in the west of the country. Till now, 15 specialized mental health workers, 130 general health workers and 60 sub-divisional managers have been trained. Fifty more workers are being trained in 2004/5.
Details about community care facilities in mental health are not available.

Psychiatric Beds and Professionals

Total psychiatric beds per 10 000 population
Psychiatric beds in mental hospitals per 10 000 population
Psychiatric beds in general hospitals per 10 000 population
Psychiatric beds in other settings per 10 000 population
Number of psychiatrists per 100 000 population
Number of neurosurgeons per 100 000 population
Number of psychiatric nurses per 100 000 population
Number of neurologists per 100 000 population
Number of psychologists per 100 000 population
Number of social workers per 100 000 population

There are no dedicated hospital beds for people with mental illness. Some of the key trainees were lost to mental health services as they were moved to other posts in the health system.

Non-Governmental Organizations NGOs are involved with mental health in the country. They are mainly involved in advocacy, promotion, prevention, treatment and rehabilitation. Close links were established between the emerging Ministry of Health, key NGOs and other service providers.

Information Gathering System There is mental health reporting system in the country. Mental health service has its own data recording system. Data is given to MOH every month.
The country has data collection system or epidemiological study on mental health.

Programmes for Special Population The country has specific programmes for mental health for disaster affected population. The entire population can be considered post-conflict and therefore at a potential for increased mental distress.
Meetings, pamphlets and radio broadcasts were made to normalize stress, destigmatize mental illness, and encourage community support for families affected by mental illness. A consultation service to assist prison staff to manage incarcerated persons with identified mental health disorders was developed.

Therapeutic Drugs The following therapeutic drugs are generally available at the primary health care level of the country: carbamazepine, sodium valproate, amitriptyline, chlorpromazine, diazepam, fluphenazine, haloperidol.
Lithium was available but was discontinued because of non-availability of testing. Cogentin is used for side-effects of neuroleptics. Cost of psychotropic drugs and blood testing is prohibitive.

Other Information Since May 2000, AusAID has conducted the Program for Psychosocial Recovery and Development (PRADET), especially in the field of emergency psychiatry. There are a number of outreach centres attached with this programme. They provide services at health centers, homes and prisons.

Additional Sources of Information

Anonymous (2002) East Timor National Mental Health Project Design document. Executive summary.
Anonymous (2002) Ministers approve Timor becoming World Bank Member. www.un.org.
Modvig, J., Pagaduan-Lopez, J., Rodenburg, J., et al (2000) Torture and trauma in post-conflict East Timor. Lancet, 18, 356.
Povey, G., Mercer, M. A. (2002) East Timor in transition: health and health care. International Journal of Health Services, 32, 607-623.
Zwi, A. B., Silove, D. (2002) Hearing the voices: mental health services in East Timor. Lancet, 360, 45-46.

Togo

GENERAL INFORMATION

Togo is a country with an approximate area of 57 thousand sq. km. (UNO, 2001). Its population is 5.017 million, and the sex ratio (men per hundred women) is 98 (UNO, 2004). The proportion of population under the age of 15 years is 43% (UNO, 2004), and the proportion of population above the age of 60 years is 5% (WHO, 2004). The literacy rate is 74.3% for men and 45.4% for women (UNESCO/MoH, 2004).

The country is a low income group country (based on World Bank 2004 criteria). The proportion of health budget to GDP is 2.8%. The per capita total expenditure on health is 45 international $, and the per capita government expenditure on health is 22 international $ (WHO, 2004).

The main language(s) used in the country is (are) French, Ewé, Mina, Kabyé and Cotocoli. The largest religious group(s) is (are) indigenous groups (half), and the other religious group(s) are (is) Christian and Muslim.

The life expectancy at birth is 50 years for males and 53.3 years for females (WHO, 2004). The healthy life expectancy at birth is 44 years for males and 46 years for females (WHO, 2004).

EPIDEMIOLOGY

There is a paucity of epidemiological data on mental illnesses in Togo in internationally accessible literature. Balogou et al (2001) used a WHO research protocol to study the prevalence of neurological disorders in two rural areas. The first survey was conducted in July-August 1989 on 19 241 inhabitants in one area. The second area was surveyed in January-February 1995 and involved 4182 subjects. The prevalence of epilepsy was 1.2% and 1.3% and that of psychomotor retardation was 0.3% and 0.8% in the two areas. The prevalence of neurological cretinism was 1.0%, while that of myxoedematous cretinism was 3.1% in the region that has a high prevalence of goiter (43% in females and 26.1% in males). Patients suffering from epilepsy commonly reported the occurrence of anxiety and depression, which led to significant interference with their quality of life (Nubukpo et al, 2004). Certain hereditary diseases (Huntington disease) that lead to dementia were reported to be relatively common in families living inshore (Grunitzky, 1995).

MENTAL HEALTH RESOURCES

Mental Health Policy A mental health policy is present. The policy was initially formulated in 1994.
The components of the policy are advocacy, promotion, prevention, treatment and rehabilitation.

Substance Abuse Policy A substance abuse policy is present. The policy was initially formulated in 1994.

National Mental Health Programme A national mental health programme is present. The programme was formulated in 1994.

National Therapeutic Drug Policy/Essential List of Drugs A national therapeutic drug policy/essential list of drugs is present. Details about the year of formulation are not available.

Mental Health Legislation There is a legislation on mental health. The mental health legislation as a whole will now be included in the new Health Code of Togo.
The latest legislation was enacted in 1999.

Mental Health Financing There are budget allocations for mental health.
The country spends 0.2% of the total health budget on mental health.
The primary sources of mental health financing in descending order are out of pocket expenditure by the patient or family and private insurances.
The country does not have disability benefits for persons with mental disorders.

Mental Health Facilities Mental health is a part of primary health care system. Actual treatment of severe mental disorders is available at the primary level. Primary care is available only at the district level where the staff has been trained.
Regular training of primary care professionals is carried out in the field of mental health. In the last two years, about 70 personnel were provided training. Doctors and health workers have been trained in the last 2 years.
There are no community care facilities for patients with mental disorders.

Psychiatric Beds and Professionals

Total psychiatric beds per 10 000 population	0.4
Psychiatric beds in mental hospitals per 10 000 population	0.3
Psychiatric beds in general hospitals per 10 000 population	0.1
Psychiatric beds in other settings per 10 000 population	0
Number of psychiatrists per 100 000 population	0.04
Number of neurosurgeons per 100 000 population	0.02
Number of psychiatric nurses per 100 000 population	0
Number of neurologists per 100 000 population	0.1
Number of psychologists per 100 000 population	0.2
Number of social workers per 100 000 population	0

Non-Governmental Organizations NGOs are involved with mental health in the country. They are mainly involved in advocacy, promotion, prevention and rehabilitation.

Information Gathering System There is mental health reporting system in the country.
The country has no data collection system or epidemiological study on mental health.

Programmes for Special Population The country has specific programmes for mental health for children. No specific programme exists.
Some services for children and adolescents exist.

Therapeutic Drugs The following therapeutic drugs are generally available at the primary health care level of the country: carbamazepine, ethosuximide, phenobarbital, phenytoin sodium, sodium valproate, amitriptyline, chlorpromazine, diazepam, fluphenazine, haloperidol, carbidopa, levodopa.
These drugs are available only in the capital.

Other Information

Additional Sources of Information

Balogou, A. A., Doh, A., Grunitzky, K. E. (2001) Neurological disorders and endemic goiter: comparative analysis of 2 provinces in Togo. Bulletin de la Société de Pathologie Exotique, 94, 406-410.

Dassa, K., Djassoa, G., Seck, B., et al. (2000) Perspectives for child and adolescent psychiatry in sub-Saharan Africa: a report from Togo. Neuropsychiatrie de l Enfance et de l Adolescence, 48, 284-288.

Grunitzky, E., et al (1995) Huntington disease in a large family in southern Togo. Annals Medicine Interne (Paris), 146, 581-583.

Nubukpo, P. et al. (2004) Psychosocial issues in people with epilepsy in Togo and Benin (West Africa). Part I. Anxiety and depression measured using Goldberg's scale. Part II. Quality of life measured using the QOLIE-31 scale. Epilepsy & Behavior, 5, 722-734.

Tonga

GENERAL INFORMATION

Tonga is a country with an approximate area of 0.75 thousand sq. km. (UNO, 2001). It consists of almost 150 islands, of which about a fifth are inhabited. Its population is 0.104 million, and the sex ratio (men per hundred women) is 103 (UNO, 2004). The proportion of population under the age of 15 years is 36% (UNO, 2004), and the proportion of population above the age of 60 years is 8% (WHO, 2004). The literacy rate is 98.8% for men and 98.9% for women (UNESCO/MoH, 2004).
The country is a lower middle income group country (based on World Bank 2004 criteria). The proportion of health budget to GDP is 5.5%. The per capita total expenditure on health is 223 international $, and the per capita government expenditure on health is 138 international $ (WHO, 2004).
The main language(s) used in the country is (are) Tongan and English. The largest ethnic group(s) is (are) Polynesian. The largest religious group(s) is (are) Christian.
The life expectancy at birth is 70 years for males and 71.4 years for females (WHO, 2004). The healthy life expectancy at birth is 62 years for males and 62 years for females (WHO, 2004).

EPIDEMIOLOGY

There is a paucity of epidemiological data on mental illnesses in Tonga in internationally accessible literature. Murphy and Taumoepeau (1980) have reported that psychoses are genuinely infrequent in this relatively stable agricultural society.

MENTAL HEALTH RESOURCES

Mental Health Policy A mental health policy is absent.

Substance Abuse Policy A substance abuse policy is absent.

National Mental Health Programme A national mental health programme is absent.

National Therapeutic Drug Policy/Essential List of Drugs A national therapeutic drug policy/essential list of drugs is present. It was formulated in 2000.
The National Drug Policy has three principal objectives: to ensure the consistent availability within the country of medicinal drugs which are of acceptable quality, safety and efficacy; to provide equity of access to medicinal drugs; and to ensure that medicinal drugs are used rationally by prescribers, other health professionals and consumers.

Mental Health Legislation There is a Mental Health Act. It details the powers of the Minister and the mental health welfare officer. It also provides guidelines for compulsory admission, detention and release of mentally ill patients.
The latest legislation was enacted in 1992.

Mental Health Financing There are budget allocations for mental health.
The country spends 0.5% of the total health budget on mental health.
The primary source of mental health financing is tax based.
The country does not have disability benefits for persons with mental disorders. There is no state disability benefit.

Mental Health Facilities Mental health is a part of primary health care system. Actual treatment of severe mental disorders is available at the primary level.
Regular training of primary care professionals is carried out in the field of mental health. In the last two years, about 14 personnel were provided training.
There are community care facilities for patients with mental disorders. Discharged patients are followed up through home visits if needed. Some social rehabilitation is provided by NGOs.

Psychiatric Beds and Professionals

Total psychiatric beds per 10 000 population	2.6
Psychiatric beds in mental hospitals per 10 000 population	0
Psychiatric beds in general hospitals per 10 000 population	2
Psychiatric beds in other settings per 10 000 population	0.6
Number of psychiatrists per 100 000 population	1
Number of neurosurgeons per 100 000 population	0
Number of psychiatric nurses per 100 000 population	1
Number of neurologists per 100 000 population	0
Number of psychologists per 100 000 population	0
Number of social workers per 100 000 population	6

There are ten psychiatric assistants and one mental health welfare officer.

Non-Governmental Organizations NGOs are involved with mental health in the country. They are mainly involved in advocacy, promotion, prevention, treatment and rehabilitation. Special education is coordinated by the Red Cross.

Information Gathering System There is mental health reporting system in the country.
The country has data collection system or epidemiological study on mental health.

Programmes for Special Population The country has specific programmes for mental health for indigenous population, elderly and children.

Therapeutic Drugs The following therapeutic drugs are generally available at the primary health care level of the country: carbamazepine, ethosuximide, phenobarbital, phenytoin sodium, sodium valproat, amitriptyline, chlorpromazine, diazepam, fluphenazine, haloperidol, lithium, carbidopa, levodopa.

Other Information Efforts have been made to study mental disorders in the country from the transcultural perspective.

Additional Sources of Information

An Act to deal with mental health in Tonga and mattes related there to. No 18 (1992) (Government document).

Japan International Cooperation Agency Planning and Evaluation Department (2002) Country profile on Disability. Kingdom of Tonga. http://www.worldbank.org/DISABILITY//Resources/Regions/East-Asia-Pacific/JICA_Tonga.pdf.

Jilek, W. (1988) Mental health, Ethnopsychiatry and traditional medicine in the Kingdom of Tonga. Curare, 11, 161-176.

Ministry of Health (2000) Kingdom of Tonga National Drug Policy.

Ministry of Health (1998) Standard Drug List Revisited.

Murphy, H. B., Taumoepeau, B. M. (1980) Traditionalism and mental health in the South Pacific: a re-examination of an old hypothesis. Psychological Medicine, 10, 471-482.

T–Z

Trinidad and Tobago

GENERAL INFORMATION

Trinidad and Tobago is a country with an approximate area of 5 thousand sq. km. (UNO, 2001). Its population is 1.307 million, and the sex ratio (men per hundred women) is 98 (UNO, 2004). The proportion of population under the age of 15 years is 22% (UNO, 2004), and the proportion of population above the age of 60 years is 10% (WHO, 2004). The literacy rate is 99% for men and 97.9% for women* (UNESCO/MoH, 2004).

The country is a higher middle income group country (based on World Bank 2004 criteria). The proportion of health budget to GDP is 2.5%. The per capita total expenditure on health is 388 international $, and the per capita government expenditure on health is 168 international $ (WHO, 2004).

The main language(s) used in the country is (are) English. The largest ethnic group(s) is (are) African, and the other ethnic group(s) are (is) East Indian. The largest religious group(s) is (are) Christian, and the other religious group(s) are (is) Hindu and Muslim.

The life expectancy at birth is 67.1 years for males and 72.8 years for females (WHO, 2004). The healthy life expectancy at birth is 60 years for males and 64 years for females (WHO, 2004).

EPIDEMIOLOGY

Neehall (1991) reviewed inpatient hospital data from a defined catchment area and suggested that the prevalence of mental disorders in the area was 0.5% with psychoses (38%), alcohol and drug use disorders (34%), affective disorders (15%) being the common diagnoses. Cembrowicz (1995) observed low rates of psychological disturbance as estimated by rates of recorded suicide, overdose and psychotropic drug use in Tobago. Singh et al (1991) conducted a questionnaire survey of 1603 secondary school students (14-18 years old). Prevalence of drug use was: alcohol (84%), tobacco (35%), marijuana (8%) and cocaine (2%). Those of Indian origin reported more frequent alcohol use, and those of African origin reported using marijuana more frequently. Alcohol use was associated with educational level, alcohol use by fathers and low religiosity. In a subsequent analysis, Singh and Mustapha (1994) found a significant association between substance abuse and the following factors: grades at school, religious involvement, pocket money, parental alcohol consumption, low self-esteem and low personal and parental educational expectations. Bhugra et al (1996) applied standardized diagnostic instruments to all new cases of psychosis presenting to various psychiatric services in two catchment areas. The incidence of broad schizophrenia and S+ schizophrenia was 2.2/1000 and 1.6/1000, respectively. These rates are similar to those from the WHO study in Honolulu and Aarhus and much lower than the rates for African-Caribbeans in London. The cases were followed up for one year and the poor outcome was observed in 19%. Hutchinson and Simeon (1997) noted a four-fold increase in male suicide rates, from 4.96/100 000 in 1978 to 20.8/100 000 in 1992 in an analysis based on national statistical data. Hutchison et al (1991) evaluated 270 patients who died at a general hospital over a 4.5 year period. Suicide was associated with gender (male), ethnicity (East Indian), age (half of the suicides occurred in the 11-34 years age group) and psychiatric morbidity (27.8%). Depression was the most common psychiatric illness diagnosed. Paraquat was used in 63.7% of the suicidal cases and other agrochemicals were used in another 20% of cases. Daisley and Simmons (1999) conducted a prospective autopsy study on deaths that occurred from poisoning (n=105). Suicide accounted for 94.29% of deaths, of which, 44.4% occurred in the 10-29 years age-group. The major poisons used were: paraquat (79%), organophosphate/carbamate insecticides (9%) and anti-psychotic drugs (5%). Ingestion of paraquat seems almost always fatal. Hutchison et al (1999) examined 48 cases of suicide in a defined region in a year; 81.3% were due to paraquat poisoning, yielding an incidence figure of 8.0 per 100 000. Among those who had ingested paraquat, half of the subjects were in the 25-34 years age group and nearly 90% were of East Indian origin. Neehall and Beharry (1994) suggested the rate of adolescent suicide for the catchment area of a general hospital to be 94/100 000 based on a sample of 102 adolescents seen over a 10 month period. Adolescent suicide was associated with gender (90% were girls), psychiatric morbidity (51%, mostly depression and adjustment disorders) and ethnicity (East Indians).

MENTAL HEALTH RESOURCES

Mental Health Policy A mental health policy is present. The policy was initially formulated in 2000.
The components of the policy are advocacy, promotion, prevention, treatment and rehabilitation. The formulation of the policy was supported by the WHO Regional Office for the Americas.

Substance Abuse Policy A substance abuse policy is absent. NGOs working in the field of substance abuse have developed guidelines related to activities in the field. A policy draft is nearing completion. There is a National Alcohol and Drug Abuse Prevention Programme.

National Mental Health Programme A national mental health programme is present. The programme was formulated in 2000. There is a new Mental Health Plan, and under this plan there is a National Mental Health Committee and Regional Mental Health Committees.

National Therapeutic Drug Policy/Essential List of Drugs A national therapeutic drug policy/essential list of drugs is present. It was formulated in 2000.
Research shows that in outpatients psychiatrists generally prefer tricyclic anti-depressants and phenothiazines and only moderately use anti-cholinergics.

Mental Health Legislation A draft Mental Health Act has been prepared and is being revised to replace the old Act of 1975. The Regional Health Authorities Act Number 5 of 1994 led to the establishment of health regions and provided support to a shift towards integration of specialist services with primary health care.
The latest legislation was enacted in 1975.

Mental Health Financing Details about disability benefits for mental health are not available.
Details about expenditure on mental health are not available.
The primary source of mental health financing is tax based.
The country has disability benefits for persons with mental disorders.

Mental Health Facilities Mental health is a part of primary health care system. Actual treatment of severe mental disorders is available at the primary level.
Regular training of primary care professionals is carried out in the field of mental health. Doctors are being trained and 23 mental health officers have received training in community care.
There are community care facilities for patients with mental disorders. Five sectors with multidisciplinary mental health teams were created. Regional hospitals were used for admissions. Outpatient clinics were set up in each sector, and there are at present 75 outpatient clinics. There is a proposal for a 40% reduction in mental hospital beds and an increase in general psychiatry beds, child psychiatry and drug abuse management beds in the general care setting, beds in extended care setting (10 for elderly and 20 for rehabilitation) and units for supported living, day care and occupational therapy.

Psychiatric Beds and Professionals

Total psychiatric beds per 10 000 population	10.29
Psychiatric beds in mental hospitals per 10 000 population	7.92
Psychiatric beds in general hospitals per 10 000 population	0.55
Psychiatric beds in other settings per 10 000 population	1.82
Number of psychiatrists per 100 000 population	1
Number of neurosurgeons per 100 000 population	0.31
Number of psychiatric nurses per 100 000 population	11.5
Number of neurologists per 100 000 population	0.5
Number of psychologists per 100 000 population	0.3
Number of social workers per 100 000 population	4

The others category is mainly comprised of nursing assistants. The island of Trinidad has one large mental hospital and a psychiatric unit at each of the two large general hospitals. The island of Tobago has a psychiatric unit but patients requiring long-term stay have to be referred to the mental hospital in Trinidad. Trinidad and Tobago have the highest number of trained mental health staff among the English speaking Caribbean countries, but distribution of staff is not adequate.

Non-Governmental Organizations NGOs are involved with mental health in the country. They are mainly involved in promotion and prevention.

Information Gathering System There is mental health reporting system in the country. Surveillance needs to be improved.
The country has data collection system or epidemiological study on mental health. Field studies are done for only data collection.

Programmes for Special Population The country has specific programmes for mental health for elderly. There is an Alzheimer's Disease Society.
The sub-specialities of forensic psychiatry, child psychiatry, geriatric psychiatry, alcohol and substance abuse need to be developed further.

Therapeutic Drugs The following therapeutic drugs are generally available at the primary health care level of the country: carbamazepine, ethosuximide, phenobarbital, phenytoin sodium, sodium valproate, amitriptyline, chlorpromazine, diazepam, fluphenazine, haloperidol, lithium, carbidopa, levodopa.
There is a wider range of psychotic drugs available at the present time, including three depot injections, fluphenozine dicanoate, pipothiozine-flucoclopenthixol.

Other Information A new mental health plan was approved in March 2000 and the implementation is to commence as part of a health sector reform with emphasis on promotion and primary care.
* According to the Ministry of Health (2004), the actual literacy rate is about 82%.

Additional Sources of Information

Bhugra, D., Hilwig, M., Hossein, B., et al (1996) First-contact incidence rates of schizophrenia in Trinidad and one-year follow-up. British Journal of Psychiatry, 169, 587-592.

Cembrowicz, S. (1995) Psychiatry on Tobago in 1989. Psychiatric Bulletin, 19, 421-426.

Daisley, H. Jr., Simmons, V. (1999) Forensic analysis of acute fatal poisonings in the southern districts of Trinidad. Veterinary & Human Toxicology, 41, 23-25.

Hutchinson, G., Daisley, H., Simmons, V., et al (1991) Suicide by poisoning. West India Medical Journal, 40, 69-73.

Hutchinson, G., Daisley, H., Simeon, D., et al (1999) High rates of paraquat-induced suicide in southern Trinidad. Suicide & Life-Threatening Behavior, 29, 186-191.

Hutchinson, G. A., Simeon, D. T. (1997) Suicide in Trinidad and Tobago: Associations with measures of social distress. International Journal of Social Psychiatry, 43, 269-275.

Moore, S., Jaime, L. K. M., Maharajh, H., et al (2002). The prescribing of psychotropic drugs in mental health services in Trinidad. Pan American Journal of Public Health, 12, 207-215.

Maharajh, H. D., Ali, A. (2004) The mental health policies of Trinidad and Tobago. International Psychiatry, 5, 13-16.

Neehall, J. (1991) An analysis of psychiatric inpatient admissions from a defined geographic catchment area over a one-year period. West Indian Medical Journal, 40, 16-21.

Neehall, J., Beharry, N. (1994) Demographic and clinical features of adolescent parasuicides. West Indian Medical Journal, 43, 123-126.

Singh, H., Maharaj, H.D., Shipp, M. (1991) Pattern of substance abuse among secondary school students in Trinidad and Tobago. Public Health, 105, 435-441.

Singh, H., Mustapha, N. (1994) Some factors associated with substance abuse among secondary school students in Trinidad and Tobago. Journal of Drug Education, 24, 83-93.

Tunisia

GENERAL INFORMATION

Tunisia is a country with an approximate area of 164 thousand sq. km. (UNO, 2001). Its population is 9.937 million, and the sex ratio (men per hundred women) is 101 (UNO, 2004). The proportion of population under the age of 15 years is 27% (UNO, 2004), and the proportion of population above the age of 60 years is 8% (WHO, 2004). The literacy rate is 83.1% for men and 63.1% for women (UNESCO/MoH, 2004).

The country is a lower middle income group country (based on World Bank 2004 criteria). The proportion of health budget to GDP is 6.4%. The per capita total expenditure on health is 463 international $, and the per capita government expenditure on health is 350 international $ (WHO, 2004).

The main language(s) used in the country is (are) Arabic and French. The largest ethnic group(s) is (are) Arab. The largest religious group(s) is (are) Muslim.

The life expectancy at birth is 69.5 years for males and 73.9 years for females (WHO, 2004). The healthy life expectancy at birth is 61 years for males and 64 years for females (WHO, 2004).

EPIDEMIOLOGY

A community epidemiological study carried out on a representative sample of 5000 adults in one region reported a life time prevalence of about 9% for major depression and 0.6% for schizophrenia (Hachmi et al, 1995). Fakhfakh et al (2000) assessed the use of tobacco (smoking) in Tunisia since 1970 using different sources. Cigarette smoking increased from 1981 to 1993 but decreased slightly after that. The prevalence of current tobacco smoking was 30.4% (52% for males and 6% for females). In young people, the prevalence was 29.2% (50% for males and 3.9% for females). Young people who attended school smoked less than those who did not (18.1% versus 38.4%). Most started smoking between 14 years and 18 years. Gassab et al (2002) conducted a retrospective study of depression in a clinical sample (n=155) of bipolar (n=86) and recurrent depressive disorder (n=59) patients, diagnosed according to the DSM-IV criteria. The following factors were correlated with bipolarity: separation/divorce, family history of psychiatric disorders (especially bipolar disorders), early onset, number of affective episodes, sudden onset of depressive episodes and psychotic features, catatonic features, hypersomnia and psychomotor inhibition. Somatic comorbidity (diabetes, hypertension, rheumatic diseases) and dysthymic disorders were predictors of non-bipolar depression. The bipolar family history criterion had the highest positive predictive validity, while the psychotic characteristics criterion had the lowest positive predictive validity. Moalla et al (2001) found that organic (somatic illnesses, epilepsy) and environmental (parental quarrels, poor family support) factors were associated with onset of mental disorders in a sample of more than 1400 child psychiatry out-patients. Ayadi et al (2002) found divorce to be associated with mental disorders in children (personality disorders, functional disturbance and depressive disturbance). Karoui and Karoui (1993) compared children with pica with children without pica in a day care centre and found that pica was associated with gender (male), family history of pica (positive in 57% of the cases), socioeconomic status (low) and locality (urban). The onset was between 12 and 18 months in most cases. Children of divorced parents had worse short- and medium-term outcomes in comparison to children of parents who were staying together, but the long-term outcome was similar.

MENTAL HEALTH RESOURCES

Mental Health Policy A mental health policy is present. The policy was initially formulated in 1986.

The components of the policy are advocacy, promotion, prevention, treatment and rehabilitation. There are committees and sub-committees looking into the training of personnel, preparation of manuals for physicians at the primary care level, visits of specialists to outpatient departments on a periodic basis, review of drug list, radio and television programmes and research. The main thrust of the policy are integration of mental health into primary care, training of non-psychiatric medical professionals in psychiatric care, creation of psychiatric services in general hospitals and sectorization of services.

Substance Abuse Policy A substance abuse policy is present. The policy was initially formulated in 1969. The substance abuse policy was revised in 1969 and 2000.

National Mental Health Programme A national mental health programme is present. The programme was formulated in 1990. The goals of the programme are to promote and protect mental health and to prevent, detect and treat mental disorders.

National Therapeutic Drug Policy/Essential List of Drugs A national therapeutic drug policy/essential list of drugs is present. It was formulated in 1979.

The national therapeutic drug policy/essential drugs list has been re-evaluated in 1993 and in 2000.

Mental Health Legislation Law No. 92-83 of 1992 on mental health and conditions of hospitalization of individuals with mental disorders was the first law in the field of mental health.

The latest legislation was enacted in 2003.

Mental Health Financing There are no budget allocations for mental health.

Details about expenditure on mental health are not available.

The primary sources of mental health financing in descending order are tax based, out of pocket expenditure by the patient or family, private insurances and social insurance.
The country has disability benefits for persons with mental disorders. Mental health patients are provided financial, treatment and transportation benefits.

Mental Health Facilities Mental health is a part of primary health care system. Actual treatment of severe mental disorders is available at the primary level. The general practitioners diagnose severe disorders and refer patients almost systematically to the second/third level care (a second level care is only available in a few regions) for treatment and monitoring.
Regular training of primary care professionals is carried out in the field of mental health. In the last two years, about 280 personnel were provided training. Though training has been provided to some primary care personnel, a system of follow-up has not been developed yet. A manual for training of physicians has been prepared.
There are community care facilities for patients with mental disorders. Some NGOs provide community based care for children under the aegis of the Social Affairs Ministry.

Psychiatric Beds and Professionals

Total psychiatric beds per 10 000 population	1.13
Psychiatric beds in mental hospitals per 10 000 population	0.85
Psychiatric beds in general hospitals per 10 000 population	0.27
Psychiatric beds in other settings per 10 000 population	0
Number of psychiatrists per 100 000 population	1.6
Number of neurosurgeons per 100 000 population	0.2
Number of psychiatric nurses per 100 000 population	0.2
Number of neurologists per 100 000 population	0.4
Number of psychologists per 100 000 population	0.6
Number of social workers per 100 000 population	

Two thirds of the specialists are based in the capital and along the coastline.

Non-Governmental Organizations NGOs are involved with mental health in the country. They are mainly involved in promotion, prevention and rehabilitation. Some NGOs are involved in the care and training of the mentally retarded children.

Information Gathering System There is no mental health reporting system in the country. Preparations are going on for some indicators in the annual health reporting system.
The country has data collection system or epidemiological study on mental health. A data collection document is in effect, though inadequate; one study on depression and schizophrenia is on-going.

Programmes for Special Population The country has specific programmes for mental health for indigenous population, elderly and children. There are services for delinquents, abandoned children, prostitutes and patients affected by HIV.
There are some facilities for children and adolescents in the form of day care hospitals, consultancy clinics and medico-school centres. There is also a school health programme. There are homes for the elderly and mentally challenged individuals.

Therapeutic Drugs The following therapeutic drugs are generally available at the primary health care level of the country: carbamazepine, sodium valproate, amitriptyline, chlorpromazine, diazepam, fluphenazine, haloperidol, lithium.
Drugs like cloimipramine form a part of the essential drug list.

Other Information

Additional Sources of Information

Ayadi, H., Moalla, Y., Ahmed, S. B., et al (2002) Parental divorce and psychopathologic unrests at the child and the teenager. Tunisian comparative study. Neuropsychiatrie de l'Enfance et de l'Adolescence, 50, 121-127.

Fakhfakh, R., Romdhane, H. B., Hsairi, M., et al (2000) Trends in tobacco consumption in Tunisia. Eastern Mediterranean Health Journal, 6, 678-686.

Gassab, L., Mechri, A., Gaha, L., et al (2002) Bipolarity correlated factors in major depression: about 155 Tunisian inpatients. Encephale, 28, 283-289.

Karoui, A., Karoui, H. (1993) Pica in Tunesian children. Results of a survey performed in a polyclinic of the tunisian social security national administration. Pediatrie, 48, 565-569.

Moalla, Y., Ayedi, H., Laaribi, H., et al (2001) What etiologic factors at the tunisian children? Timely an epidemiologic investigation. Neuropsychiatrie de l'Enfance et de l'Adolescence, 49, 343-351.

Hachmi et al. (1995) Epidémiologie des troubles dépressifs et de la schizophrénie dans le gouvernorat de l'ARIANA. Mémoire de psychiatrie. Library of the Faculty of medicine of Tunis: Srairi LYES.

Republique Tunisienne Ministere de la sante (1998). Programme National de Sante Mentale.

Turkey

GENERAL INFORMATION

Turkey is a country with an approximate area of 775 thousand sq. km. (UNO, 2001). Its population is 72.32 million, and the sex ratio (men per hundred women) is 101 (UNO, 2004). The proportion of population under the age of 15 years is 30% (UNO, 2004), and the proportion of population above the age of 60 years is 8% (WHO, 2004). The literacy rate is 94.4% for men and 78.5% for women (UNESCO/MoH, 2004).

The country is a lower middle income group country (based on World Bank 2004 criteria). The proportion of health budget to GDP is 5%. The per capita total expenditure on health is 294 international $, and the per capita government expenditure on health is 209 international $ (WHO, 2004).

The main language(s) used in the country is (are) Turkish. The largest ethnic group(s) is (are) Turkish, and the other ethnic group(s) are (is) Kurdish. The largest religious group(s) is (are) Muslim.

The life expectancy at birth is 67.9 years for males and 72.2 years for females (WHO, 2004). The healthy life expectancy at birth is 61 years for males and 63 years for females (WHO, 2004).

EPIDEMIOLOGY

Prevalence estimates varied widely (from more than 40% lifetime prevalence of any mental disorder in the Netherlands and the USA to 12% in Turkey) in a study done by the International Consortium in Psychiatric Epidemiology (ICPE) that used the Composite International Diagnostic Interview (CIDI). Findings suggested that mental disorders were often chronic, typically had early ages of onset, were associated with socioeconomic measures of disadvantage (low income and education, unemployment, unmarried status) and that the lifetime prevalence had increased in recent cohorts (Anonymous, 2000). In a sample of 13 665 high school girls (13-18 years), Vicdan et al (1996) found that 19.7% smoked cigarettes, 14.9% used alcohol and 0.63% used other drugs. Elbi et al (2002) surveyed 1749 subjects using the Seasonal Pattern Assessment Questionnaire. The prevalence of winter seasonal affective disorder (SAD) and summer SAD were reported to be 4.8% and 8.4%, respectively. Danaci et al (2002) assessed 257 randomly selected mothers who had delivered within the past 6 months using the Edinburgh Postnatal Depression Scale. Depression was identified in 14% and it was associated with living in a shanty, being an immigrant, number of children, baby's health problems, psychiatric history in parents and poor relationship with husband and in-laws. Basoglu et al (2002) administered the Screening Instrument for Traumatic Stress in Earthquake Survivors to 1000 subjects living in camps. The prevalence of PTSD and major depression were 43% and 31%, respectively. Traumatic stress symptoms were associated with female gender, more intense fear during the earthquake, having been trapped under the rubble, death of a family member, past psychiatric illness, having participated in rescue work and lower education level. In a representative urban sample (n=994) assessed with the Dissociative Experiences Scale (DES), the Dissociative Disorders Interview Schedule (DDIS) and a confirmatory clinical interview in a three-stage study, the prevalence of dissociative disorders was 0.4% (Akyuz et al, 1999). Akkus et al (2002) evaluated 1982 men selected by a stratified random method and found an age-adjusted prevalence of erectile dysfunction to be 69.2% (mild 33.2%, moderate 27.5%, severe 8.5%). In a multivariate model, moderate/severe ED was significantly associated with age, low socioeconomic status, low physical activity and medical illnesses. Based on national records, Sayil (1997) reported that the rates of suicide and suicide attempts were 3.3/100 000 and 145/100 000 population, respectively. Eskin (1999) assessed large samples of Swedish and Turkish school students (n>600) and found that between 2.7% to 9.4% of Swedish students and 4.6% to 10.9% of Turkish students had made previous suicide attempts. In the Turkish group, suicide attempts were associated with previous psychiatric contact, low perceived family support, suicide attempts and psychiatric disorder in the family. Past suicide attempts and low perceived family support were the most powerful and consistent predictors of current suicidal risk. Goksu et al (2002) found that 78.7% of poisoning cases admitted to a hospital were due to suicide attempts. Most of the suicide attempts were by females. Mattila et al (1987) found that among 1188 children (aged less than 17 years) admitted with a diagnosis of poisoning deliberate self-poisoning was reported in 12.8%. Suicide attempts were associated with gender (girls) and age group (among adolescents 79% of poisonings were self-induced). Cuhadaroglu et al (1999) assessed 434 school students with the Symptom Check List 90-Rand and found that psychiatric problems were associated with gender (female), age group (15-16 years) and socioeconomic status (low). In large samples of students (>800 subjects), Fichter et al (1988) found significantly higher GHQ-28 scores in Greeks and Turks in their homeland as compared to Greeks in Munich. In a similar study (>800 subjects), Bengi-Arslan et al (1997) found that immigrant Turkish children (4-18 years) had higher scores on at least five Child Behaviour Checklist (CBCL) scales in comparison to Dutch and Turkish children in their homeland. However, the differences in scores and the patterns of problem behaviours were small in the two Turkish samples. Studies that assessed nocturnal enuresis in large samples (>1700 subjects) of children (4-12 years) through parental questionnaires (Gumus et al, 1999; Oge et al, 2001) found that the prevalence rate was in the range of 11.6% to 13.7%. Enuresis was associated with gender (male), age (younger), deep sleep, poor toilet habits, urinary tract infections, large family size, low parental socioeconomic class and family history of enuresis.

MENTAL HEALTH RESOURCES

Mental Health Policy A mental health policy is present. The policy was initially formulated in 1983.
The components of the policy are advocacy, promotion, prevention, treatment and rehabilitation. The goal then was the integration of mental health into primary health care (i.e. a horizontal approach) with promotion and prevention activities in addition to the improvement of curative services. For inter-sectoral and inter-disciplinary coordination there were efforts to get the involvement of different ministries, universities and non-governmental organizations, with the support of the World Health Organization.

Substance Abuse Policy A substance abuse policy is present. The policy was initially formulated in 1983.

National Mental Health Programme A national mental health programme is present. The programme was formulated in 1987. A new programme is being developed by a project supported by the World Bank after the earthquake in 1999.

National Therapeutic Drug Policy/Essential List of Drugs A national therapeutic drug policy/essential list of drugs is present. Details about the year of formulation are not available.

Mental Health Legislation There is no existing legislation on mental health but a law on prevention of tobacco harm from 1996 does exist. The criminal law stipulates special conditions for the treatment of mentally ill offenders. Lack of an overall mental health law continues to be a concern for the mental health profession. The Psychiatric Association of Turkey has chosen to begin work on a draft law for the protection of the rights of psychiatric patients.
Details about the year of enactment of the mental health legislation are not available.

Mental Health Financing There are no budget allocations for mental health.
Details about expenditure on mental health are not available.
The primary sources of mental health financing in descending order are social insurance, private insurances, tax based and out of pocket expenditure by the patient or family.
The country has disability benefits for persons with mental disorders. After being approved by a mental health board as a chronic mental health patient, the patient can benefit from the social security services.

Mental Health Facilities Mental health is a part of primary health care system. Actual treatment of severe mental disorders is available at the primary level. Mental health in primary care is available in only some provinces.
Regular training of primary care professionals is carried out in the field of mental health. In the last two years, about 3000 personnel were provided training.
There are no community care facilities for patients with mental disorders.

Psychiatric Beds and Professionals

Total psychiatric beds per 10 000 population	1.3
Psychiatric beds in mental hospitals per 10 000 population	0.8
Psychiatric beds in general hospitals per 10 000 population	0.5
Psychiatric beds in other settings per 10 000 population	0
Number of psychiatrists per 100 000 population	1
Number of neurosurgeons per 100 000 population	1
Number of psychiatric nurses per 100 000 population	3
Number of neurologists per 100 000 population	1
Number of psychologists per 100 000 population	1
Number of social workers per 100 000 population	1

The number of child and adolescent psychiatrists per 100 000 is 0.3. Of the total beds available in the country about 2.5% are located in the private sector and 55 are under the charge of the Ministry of Social Security. Ethical rules for psychiatric practice were established in June 2002 by the Psychiatric Association of Turkey. Psychiatrists mainly work in the large cities and the western parts of the country. Almost two-thirds are located in Istanbul, Ankara and Izmir. Most psychologists work in private clinics. Within the government set-up, about two thirds of mental health staff are attached to general hospitals.

Non-Governmental Organizations NGOs are involved with mental health in the country. They are mainly involved in advocacy, promotion, prevention, treatment and rehabilitation. The Association for Child and Adolescent Mental Health is functioning as the main organization in the subjects related to children and adolescents. There are some newly founded associations that focus on the rights and welfare of psychiatric patients and their relatives, most of which are currently led by professionals who wish to promote 'consumer-led' services.

Information Gathering System There is mental health reporting system in the country.
The country has data collection system or epidemiological study on mental health.

Programmes for Special Population The country has specific programmes for mental health for disaster affected population and children. Services are limited.
Child and adolescent psychiatry has been a separate specialty since 1995. Committees on adolescence and ADHD within the Association for Child and Adolescent Mental Health are carrying on epidemiological research and interventional programmes. A child abuse and neglect team is functioning.

Therapeutic Drugs The following therapeutic drugs are generally available at the primary health care level of the country: carbamazepine, ethosuximide, phenobarbital, phenytoin sodium, sodium valproate, amitriptyline, chlorpromazine, diazepam, fluphenazine, haloperidol, lithium, biperiden, carbidopa, levodopa.
Drugs like thioridazine and imipramine are a part of the essential drug list.

Other Information The mental health department was established within the General Directorate of Primary Health Care of the Ministry in 1983 with the primary tasks of improving the mental health services, development and dissemination of preventive mental health services, integration of mental health with primary care, community education and protection of the community from harmful behaviours. The means of achieving these aims were through determination of standards, training programmes, data collection, research, creation of counselling and guiding units, creation of psychiatric clinics in state hospitals, assigning proper tasks to personnel, developing rehabilitation facilities, carrying out public education through the help of media, educating the public on harmful behaviour and taking care of those who succumb to those behaviours.

Additional Sources of Information

Akkus, E., Kadioglu, A., Esen, A., et al (2002) Prevalence and correlates of erectile dysfunction in Turkey: a population-based study. European Urology, 41, 298-304.

Akyuz, G., Dogan, O., Sar, V., et al (1999) Frequency of dissociative identity disorder in the general population in Turkey. Comprehensive Psychiatry, 40, 151-159.

Anonymous (2000) Cross-national comparisons of the prevalences and correlates of mental disorders. WHO International Consortium in Psychiatric Epidemiology. Bulletin of the World Health Organization, 78, 413-426.

Basoglu, M., Salcioglu, E., Livanou, M. (2002) Traumatic stress responses in earthquake survivors in Turkey. Journal of Traumatic Stress, 15, 269-276.

Bengi-Arslan, L., Verhulst, F. C., van der Ende J., et al (1997) Understanding childhood (problem) behaviors from a cultural perspective: comparison of problem behaviors and competencies in Turkish immigrant, Turkish and Dutch children. Social Psychiatry & Psychiatric Epidemiology, 32, 477-484.

Coskun, B. (2004) Psychiatry in Turkey. International Psychiatry, 3, 13-15.

Cuhadaroglu, F., Yazici, K. M. (1999) Psychiatric symptoms among Turkish adolescents. Turkish Journal of Pediatrics, 41, 307-313.

Danaci, A. E., Dinc, G., Deveci, A., et al (2002) Postnatal depression in Turkey: epidemiological and cultural aspects. Social Psychiatry & Psychiatric Epidemiology, 37, 125-129.

Elbi, H., Noyan, A., Korukoglu, S., et al (2002) Seasonal affective disorder in eight groups in Turkey: a cross-national perspective. Journal of Affective Disorders, 70, 77-84.

Eskin, M. (1999) Gender and cultural differences in the 12-month prevalence of suicidal thoughts and attempts in Swedish and Turkish adolescents. Journal of Gender, Culture, & Health, 4, 187-200.

Fichter, M. M., Elton, M., Diallina, M., et al (1988) Mental illness in Greek and Turkish adolescents. European Archives of Psychiatry & Neurological Sciences, 237, 125-134.

Goksu, S., Yildirim, C., Kocoglu, H., et al (2002) Characteristics of acute adult poisoning in Gaziantep, Turkey. Journal of Toxicology – Clinical Toxicology, 40, 833-837.

Gumus, B., Vurgun, N., Lekili, M., et al (1999) Prevalence of nocturnal enuresis and accompanying factors in children aged 7-11 years in Turkey. Acta Paediatrica, 88, 1369-1372.

Hincal, F., Hincal, A. A., Sarikayalar, F., et al. (1987) Self poisoning in children: a ten year survey. Journal of Toxicology – Clinical Toxicology, 25, 109-120.

Mental Health Department. Goals and Long Range Planning Document.

Oge, O., Kocak, I., Gemalmaz, H. (2001) Enuresis: point prevalence and associated factors among Turkish children. Turkish Journal of Pediatrics, 43, 38-43.

Ozkan, S., Yucel, B., Turgay, M. et al (1995) The development of psychiatric medicine at Istanbul Facility of Medicine and evaluation of 889 psychiatric referrals. General Hospital Psychiatry, 17, 216-223.

Oral, R., Can, D., Kaplan, S., et al (2001) Child abuse in Turkey. An experience in overcoming denial and a description of 50 cases. Child Abuse and Neglect, 25, 279-290.

Sayil, I. (1997) Review of suicide studies in Turkey. Crisis: Journal of Crisis Intervention & Suicide, 18, 124-127.

Vicdan, K., Kukner, S., Dabakoglu, T., et al (1996) Demographic and epidemiologic features of female adolescents in Turkey. Journal of Adolescent Health, 18, 54-58.

Turkmenistan

GENERAL INFORMATION

Turkmenistan is a country with an approximate area of 488 thousand sq. km. (UNO, 2001). Its population is 4.94 million, and the sex ratio (men per hundred women) is 98 (UNO, 2004). The proportion of population under the age of 15 years is 33% (UNO, 2004), and the proportion of population above the age of 60 years is 6% (WHO, 2004). The literacy rate is 99.3% for men and 98.3% for women (UNESCO/MoH, 2004).

The country is a lower middle income group country (based on World Bank 2004 criteria). The proportion of health budget to GDP is 4.1%. The per capita total expenditure on health is 245 international $, and the per capita government expenditure on health is 180 international $ (WHO, 2004).

The main language(s) used in the country is (are) Turkmen and Russian. The largest ethnic group(s) is (are) Turkmen, and the other ethnic group(s) are (is) Russian and Uzbek. The largest religious group(s) is (are) Muslim (nine-tenths).

The life expectancy at birth is 58.8 years for males and 66.9 years for females (WHO, 2004). The healthy life expectancy at birth is 52 years for males and 57 years for females (WHO, 2004).

EPIDEMIOLOGY

There is a paucity of epidemiological data on mental illnesses in Turkmenistan in internationally accessible literature. Suicide rates in the former USSR during 1984-1990 varied greatly between different regions. It was reported to be 11.8 in Central Asia (Kazakhstan, Kirgizia, Turkmenistan, Uzbekistan and Tajikistan) (Wasserman et al, 1998). Solov'eva et al (1997) compared emotional disturbances in patients suffering from gastrointestinal problems in cities in Russia and Turkmenistan. Psychological factors were common to all patients. Psychological factors were more prominent in children in Russia compared to children in Turkmenistan. Association of stress with peptic ulcers was stronger compared to other diseases. Similar association was noted for depression and chronic gastritis.

MENTAL HEALTH RESOURCES

Mental Health Policy A mental health policy is present. The policy was initially formulated in 1995.

The components of the policy are promotion, prevention, treatment and rehabilitation. The thrusts of the policy are on education, early detection and with timely assistance and treatment by family practitioners and specialists. In 1996, the president signed a decree 'Salt iodization and fortification of flour with iron', to prevent iodine deficiency diseases, that can lead to mental retardation of children and to improve mental capacity of adults. In 2001, the President adopted the 'National Plan on Fighting Illegal Trafficking of Narcotics and Medical Assistance to Substance users for 2001-2005'.

Substance Abuse Policy A substance abuse policy is present. The policy was initially formulated in 1996. In 2000, the Ministry of Health adopted the 'Improvement of Narcological Services' for prevention of substance abuse and treatment and rehabilitation of substance abusers.

National Mental Health Programme A national mental health programme is absent.

In 1997, the Ministry of Health adopted a programme 'Improvement of Psychiatric Assistance' on prevention of inappropriate imprisonment of the mentally ill and facilitation of their referral and transfer to specialized treatment centres. A national programme entitled 'Free Electricity, Gas, Water, and Salt Until 2020' was launched in 2003. The quantity of iodized salt provided free of charge is 4000 units per person per month.

National Therapeutic Drug Policy/Essential List of Drugs A national therapeutic drug policy/essential list of drugs is present. It was formulated in 1997.

The Ministry of Health has adopted a law on the sale of psychiatric drugs.

Mental Health Legislation There is a Law of Turkmenistan on Psychiatric Assistance. It is based on internal laws on human rights of persons with mental disorders. It stipulates that mentally ill people have the right to Government and social support in the form of free medical treatment, allowances for medication and pension funds. In 2004, the law 'On narcotics, psychotropic substances and illegal drug trafficking' was adopted.

The latest legislation was enacted in 1993.

Mental Health Financing There are no budget allocations for mental health.

Details about expenditure on mental health are not available.

Details about sources of financing are not available.

The country has disability benefits for persons with mental disorders. Disabled people receive a pension.

Mental Health Facilities Mental health is a part of primary health care system. Actual treatment of severe mental disorders is not available at the primary level. At primary level, family practitioners work with psychiatrists in providing emergency services to persons with mental disorders and in deciding whether hospitalization is needed. Specialized treatment is provided by psychiatrists in inpatient and outpatient setting.

Regular training of primary care professionals is carried out in the field of mental health. There are courses on psychiatry and narcology for family practitioners.

Details about community care facilities in mental health are not available.

Psychiatric Beds and Professionals

Total psychiatric beds per 10 000 population	3.5
Psychiatric beds in mental hospitals per 10 000 population	3.2
Psychiatric beds in general hospitals per 10 000 population	0.3
Psychiatric beds in other settings per 10 000 population	
Number of psychiatrists per 100 000 population	3
Number of neurosurgeons per 100 000 population	0.5
Number of psychiatric nurses per 100 000 population	
Number of neurologists per 100 000 population	4.2
Number of psychologists per 100 000 population	
Number of social workers per 100 000 population	

Continuing medical education of psychiatrists and narcologists is encouraged.

Non-Governmental Organizations NGOs are involved with mental health in the country. They are mainly involved in advocacy and prevention.

Information Gathering System There is mental health reporting system in the country.
The country has data collection system or epidemiological study on mental health.
Quarterly and annual reports are discussed in meetings of Ministerial Boards and medical industry. There are operational reports on psychiatry and narcology.

Programmes for Special Population There are no specific programmes.

Therapeutic Drugs The following therapeutic drugs are generally available at the primary health care level of the country: carbamazepine, phenobarbital, phenytoin sodium, amitriptyline, diazepam, haloperidol, levodopa.
Other drugs like cyclodol and aminazine are included in the essential list of psychotropics.

Other Information

Additional Sources of Information

Polubinskaya, S. V. (2000) Development of Legislation and Psychiatric Care in the New Independent States. Mental Health Reforms, 5, 12-13.

Solov'eva, A. D., Sheptulin, A. A., Annamamedova, R., et al (1997) Emotional-personality condition of patients with some gastroenterological diseases. Klinicheskaia.Meditsina, 75, 27-28.

Wasserman, D., Varnik, A., Dankowicz, M. (1998) Regional differences in the distribution of suicide in the former Soviet Union during perestroika, 1984-1990. Acta Psychiatrica Scandinavica, Supplement 394, 5-12.

T–Z

Tuvalu

GENERAL INFORMATION

Tuvalu is a country with an approximate area of 0.03 thousand sq. km. (UNO, 2001). The country consists of nine small islands. Its population is 0.01 million, and the sex ratio (men per hundred women) is 98 (UNO, 2004). The proportion of population under the age of 15 years is 41% (UNO, 2004), and the proportion of population above the age of 60 years is 7% (WHO, 2004). The literacy rate is 90% for men and 90% for women (UNESCO/MoH, 2004).

The country is a high income group country (based on World Bank 2004 criteria). The proportion of health budget to GDP is 5.4%. The per capita total expenditure on health is 673 international $, and the per capita government expenditure on health is 359 international $ (WHO, 2004).

The main language(s) used in the country is (are) Tuvaluan and English. The largest ethnic group(s) is (are) Polynesian. The largest religious group(s) is (are) Christian (Church of Tuvalu).

The life expectancy at birth is 60 years for males and 61.4 years for females (WHO, 2004). The healthy life expectancy at birth is 53 years for males and 53 years for females (WHO, 2004).

EPIDEMIOLOGY

There is a paucity of epidemiological data on mental illnesses in Tuvalu in internationally accessible literature.

MENTAL HEALTH RESOURCES

Mental Health Policy A mental health policy is present. The policy was initially formulated in 1978.

Substance Abuse Policy A substance abuse policy is absent.

National Mental Health Programme A national mental health programme is absent.

National Therapeutic Drug Policy/Essential List of Drugs A national therapeutic drug policy/essential list of drugs is absent. The essential drug list and the national therapeutic drug policy have been officially endorsed by the Government in 2004.

Mental Health Legislation There is a Mental Treatment Law.
The latest legislation was enacted in 1978.

Mental Health Financing There are no budget allocations for mental health.
Details about expenditure on mental health are not available.
Details about sources of financing are not available.
The mental health service is free of charge for every citizen.
The country does not have disability benefits for persons with mental disorders.

Mental Health Facilities Mental health is a part of primary health care system. Actual treatment of severe mental disorders is available at the primary level.
Regular training of primary care professionals is not carried out in the field of mental health.
There are no community care facilities for patients with mental disorders.

T–Z

Psychiatric Beds and Professionals

Total psychiatric beds per 10 000 population	2
Psychiatric beds in mental hospitals per 10 000 population	0
Psychiatric beds in general hospitals per 10 000 population	2
Psychiatric beds in other settings per 10 000 population	0
Number of psychiatrists per 100 000 population	0
Number of neurosurgeons per 100 000 population	0
Number of psychiatric nurses per 100 000 population	1000
Number of neurologists per 100 000 population	0
Number of psychologists per 100 000 population	0
Number of social workers per 100 000 population	1000

Psychiatric patients are managed by medical officers.

Non-Governmental Organizations NGOs are involved with mental health in the country. They are mainly involved in promotion, prevention and rehabilitation.

Information Gathering System There is no mental health reporting system in the country.
The country has no data collection system or epidemiological study on mental health.

Programmes for Special Population There are no special services available.

Therapeutic Drugs The following therapeutic drugs are generally available at the primary health care level of the country: carbamazepine, phenobarbital, phenytoin sodium, amitriptyline, chlorpromazine, diazepam, haloperidol.

Other Information

Additional Sources of Information

Government of Tuvalu (2000) Tuvalu Essential Drug List.

T–Z

Uganda

GENERAL INFORMATION

Uganda is a country with an approximate area of 241 thousand sq. km. (UNO, 2001). Its population is 26.699 million, and the sex ratio (men per hundred women) is 99 (UNO, 2004). The proportion of population under the age of 15 years is 50% (UNO, 2004), and the proportion of population above the age of 60 years is 4% (WHO, 2004). The literacy rate is 78.8% for men and 59.2% for women (UNESCO/MoH, 2004).

The country is a low income group country (based on World Bank 2004 criteria). The proportion of health budget to GDP is 5.9%. The per capita total expenditure on health is 57 international $, and the per capita government expenditure on health is 33 international $ (WHO, 2004).

The main language(s) used in the country is (are) English, Swahili, Luganda, Ateso and Luo. The largest ethnic group(s) is (are) Baganda, Basoga, Iteso, Langi and Acholi Banyankole/Bakiga, and the other ethnic group(s) are (is) Banyoro/Batoro, Yo'kwekyawa and Kwekubagiza. The largest religious group(s) is (are) Christian (two-thirds), and the other religious group(s) are (is) Muslim.

The life expectancy at birth is 47.9 years for males and 50.8 years for females (WHO, 2004). The healthy life expectancy at birth is 42 years for males and 44 years for females (WHO, 2004).

EPIDEMIOLOGY

Kasoro et al (2002) estimated the prevalence of psychiatric disorder in one district by interviewing members of randomly selected households and key informants and through focus group discussions. The estimated prevalence of mental disorders in adults was 30.7%. Orley and Wing (1979) conducted a survey in two small rural populations using standardized tools and methods of case identification and found that 20% suffered from a probable mental disorder and a further 5% from a definite disorder. Most suffered from depression, hypomania and anxiety. Cox (1979) examined 263 pregnant and 89 non-pregnant, non-puerperal women using a semi-structured psychiatric interview. A higher frequency of psychiatric morbidity was seen in pregnant women. Separated pregnant women were particularly at risk. Wilk and Bolton (2002) used ethnographic methods, free listing and key-informant interviews, among participants from two districts to examine the folk view of psychological consequences of the HIV epidemic in a severely affected community. Participants described two independent depression-like syndromes (Yo'kwekyawa and Okwekubaziga) resulting from the HIV epidemic. No syndromes similar to posttraumatic stress disorder were detected. Peltzer et al (1999) assessed the effects of trauma on the mental health of 323 refugees settled in Ugandan camps. One-third of adults and one-fifth of children had PTSD. Ex-soldiers had significant depression. While only a fifth of those seeking help from the formal health sector had psychiatric disorders, almost two-thirds of subjects visiting traditional healers had a psychiatric disorder (PTSD: 26% and depression: 39%). Drotar et al (1997) followed up 436 full-term infants (79 HIV-infected infants of HIV-infected mothers, 241 uninfected infants of HIV-infected mothers (seroreverters) and 116 uninfected infants of HIV-negative mothers) for 2 years. All evaluators were blinded to the HIV status of the child and family. Compared with controls, HIV-infected infants had more abnormalities in mental development at 6 and 18 months and an earlier onset of abnormalities. By 12 months, 26% of HIV-infected infants demonstrated cognitive abnormalities as compared with 6% in the other two groups. Information-processing abilities did not differ as a function of HIV infection. Home environments and infants' interactions with caretakers were similar across groups.

MENTAL HEALTH RESOURCES

Mental Health Policy A mental health policy is present. The policy was initially formulated in 2000.
The components of the policy are advocacy, promotion, prevention, treatment and rehabilitation.

Substance Abuse Policy A substance abuse policy is absent. There is no need for a separate substance abuse policy as mental health aspects of substance abuse are covered within the mental health policy

National Mental Health Programme A national mental health programme is present. The programme was formulated in 1996.
Mental health is one of the 12 key services to be provided as a part of the minimum health package at all levels of care.
Intersectoral collaboration is emphasized, though it is happening only at the national level at present.

National Therapeutic Drug Policy/Essential List of Drugs A national therapeutic drug policy/essential list of drugs is present. It was formulated in 1993.
The policy was reviewed in 1996 and 2001.

Mental Health Legislation The Mental Treatment Act is currently being reviewed. Enforcements of rights of patients is generally satisfactory in Government institutions. However, there is no specific body appointed to periodically review cases of involuntary admissions.
The latest legislation was enacted in 1964.

Mental Health Financing There are budget allocations for mental health.
The country spends 0.7% of the total health budget on mental health.
The primary sources of mental health financing in descending order are tax based, out of pocket expenditure by the patient or family, private insurances and social insurance.

Funding for health is mainly from economic aid and does not favour mental health. People with mental illness might spend on an average $57 per year on mental health care, a large amount given that the per capita income is $89. Most families and consumers report a worsening of their economic situation and productivity as a result of their contribution to patient care. NGOs are increasingly getting involved in funding of primary health care.
The country does not have disability benefits for persons with mental disorders. Disability benefits are low and even lower for mental health.

Mental Health Facilities Mental health is a part of primary health care system. Actual treatment of severe mental disorders is not available at the primary level. Treatment for severe mental disorders are available only at the 10 regional referral centres and the National Mental Referral Hospital. Mental health is an integral part of primary health care policy.
Regular training of primary care professionals is carried out in the field of mental health. Though training facilities for the primary care workers are not present, there is a training manual which can be obtained for purpose of training staff. There has been an effort to instil basic knowledge about mental disorders and its treatment among medical students so that they are able to identify the disorders and manage them in primary care level. Community-based programmes which combine the services of traditional medical practitioners with modern medical services in providing sustainable rural health care have been supported. Such clinics are staffed by a trained nurse and a pharmaceutical technician and visited by doctors. Traditional herbalists may refer patients to mental health care staff at these clinics. These clinics also provide community health education, which emphasizes hygiene and the appropriate use of local medicinal resources. Traditional health practitioners care for the emotional and spiritual as well as the physical well-being of their patients.
There are community care facilities for patients with mental disorders. All community health departments at all health units provide some form of community based care but it is still in its infancy. Secondary mental health services can be found at 10 regional referral hospitals where services are run by a resident psychiatrist who are supervised through visits by a psychiatrist on a quarterly basis. There is a provision of a psychiatrist at this level once adequate numbers are trained and are available.

Psychiatric Beds and Professionals

Total psychiatric beds per 10 000 population	0.44
Psychiatric beds in mental hospitals per 10 000 population	0.22
Psychiatric beds in general hospitals per 10 000 population	0.22
Psychiatric beds in other settings per 10 000 population	0.009
Number of psychiatrists per 100 000 population	1.6
Number of neurosurgeons per 100 000 population	0.009
Number of psychiatric nurses per 100 000 population	2
Number of neurologists per 100 000 population	0.1
Number of psychologists per 100 000 population	2
Number of social workers per 100 000 population	2

Out of the 55 other staff, 25 are psychiatric clinical officers. The bed strength in the Butabika National Mental Referral Hospital was reduced from 1000 to 450. With support of an ADB loan of USD 48 million, the Government has refurbished the Butabika National Mental Referral Hospital and constructed 6 Regional Mental Health Units with 35 beds each. There are 100 forensic beds, 50 beds for children and adolescents, 20 beds for psychologically traumatized patients and 10 beds for the treatment of drug abusers. Most health facilities try to segregate male and female patients. All qualified health workers are required to renew their registration – doctors every year and nurses every 3 years. All professionals are now prescribed minimum hours of exposure to continuing medical education for their reaccreditations, but the process is new and enforcement not particularly strict. There are few mental health professionals in the private sector, all of them are in the capital city. Trained specialists are found only in urban centres.

Non-Governmental Organizations NGOs are involved with mental health in the country. They are mainly involved in advocacy, promotion, prevention, treatment and rehabilitation. There is some increase in NGO participation in capacity building and primary mental health care provision. Consumer support groups for mental health are also emerging. They are involved particularly with psychosocial care to war-afflicted populations. NGOs are also carrying out research in mental health.

Information Gathering System There is mental health reporting system in the country. They are mentioned broadly as 'mental illness' without the break-up into different disorders.
The country has data collection system or epidemiological study on mental health. Monthly and quarterly reports are received from referral hospitals and NGOs. Some key psychiatric and monitoring items have been developed (including diagnoses) to collect data. Routine health management information forms list just 2 items under mental health, mental illness and epilepsy. Guidelines for monitoring mental health have been developed but have to be disseminated.

Programmes for Special Population The country has specific programmes for mental health for refugees, disaster affected population and children. There are psychosocial support programmes in war affected areas.
Limited services are available for children, elderly and those in prisons. There is an initiative to set up a substance abuse and trauma centre at the national hospital.

Therapeutic Drugs The following therapeutic drugs are generally available at the primary health care level of the country: carbamazepine, phenobarbital, phenytoin sodium, chlorpromazine, diazepam, haloperidol, lithium.
Some of the other drugs are available at referral centres only.

Other Information Academic psychiatry was started in the late 1960s when the Makerere University Department of Psychiatry was founded. Psychiatry suffered during the Amin regime, but over the years, there has been a lot of improvement. However, problems remain; there is a lack of resources and the legislation needs to be upgraded. HIV and PTSD place an added burden on Ugandan psychiatry.

Additional Sources of Information

Boardman, J., Ovuga, E. (1997) Rebuilding psychiatry in Uganda. Psychiatric Bulletin, 21, 649-655.

Cox, J. L. (1979) Psychiatric morbidity and pregnancy: a controlled study of 263 semi-rural Ugandan women. British Journal of Psychiatry, 134, 401-405.

Drotar, D., Olness, K., Wiznitzer, M., et al (1997) Neurodevelopmental outcomes of Ugandan infants with human immunodeficiency virus type 1 infection. Pediatrics, 100, E5.

Kasoro, S., Sebudde, S., Kabagambe-Rugamba, G., et al (2002) Mental illness in one district of Uganda. International Journal of Social Psychiatry, 48, 29-37.

Njenga, F. (2002) Focus on psychiatry in East Africa. British Journal of Psychiatry, 181, 354-359.

Orley, J., Wing, J. K. (1979) Psychiatric disorders in two African villages. Archives of General Psychiatry, 36, 513-520.

Ovuga, E. B. L., Buga, J., Oboke, H., et al (2002) Promoting psychiatry in the medical school. Psychiatric Bulletin, 26, 194-195.

Peltzer, K. (1999) Trauma and mental health problems of Sudanese refugees in Uganda. Central African Journal of Medicine, 45, 110-114.

Tumwesigye, O. (1996). Bumetha Rukararwe: integrating modern and traditional health care in southwest Uganda. Journal of Alternative and Contemprory Medicine, 2, 3-6.

Wilk, C. M., Bolton, P., et al (2002) Local perceptions of the mental health effects of the Uganda acquired immunodeficiency syndrome epidemic. Journal of Nervous & Mental Disease, 190, 394-397.

Ukraine

GENERAL INFORMATION

Ukraine is a country with an approximate area of 604 thousand sq. km. (UNO, 2001). Its population is 48.151 million, and the sex ratio (men per hundred women) is 87 (UNO, 2004). The proportion of population under the age of 15 years is 15% (UNO, 2004), and the proportion of population above the age of 60 years is 21% (WHO, 2004). The literacy rate is 99.8% for men and 99.5% for women (UNESCO/MoH, 2004).

The country is a lower middle income group country (based on World Bank 2004 criteria). The proportion of health budget to GDP is 4.3%. The per capita total expenditure on health is 176 international $, and the per capita government expenditure on health is 120 international $ (WHO, 2004).

The main language(s) used in the country is (are) Ukrainian. The largest ethnic group(s) is (are) Ukrainian, and the other ethnic group(s) are (is) Russian. The largest religious group(s) is (are) Orthodox Christian.

The life expectancy at birth is 61.7 years for males and 72.9 years for females (WHO, 2004). The healthy life expectancy at birth is 55 years for males and 64 years for females (WHO, 2004).

EPIDEMIOLOGY

Official statistics show that the prevalence of mental disorders reached 1 181 435 persons in 2003 or 2.47%. The incidence of mental disorders was 0.025% and 0.022% per year in urban and rural populations, respectively. The incidence of mental disorders among children was 0.049% and the prevalence 2.84%. About 0.53% were classified as having mental disability (Center of Medical Statistics of Ministry of Health, 2004). Buzanova (1981) did a comparative clinico-epidemiological study on a group of patients suffering from schizophrenia, living in urban and rural districts. The groups did not differ much with respect to age of onset and characteristics. In a clinical study done on a large number of patients (n=27 692), Dvirskii (1999) found that delirium tremens (DT) occurred in 8.1% of cases with alcohol dependence. Among patients with DT, 12.9% had more than one episode. Men were affected 5.3 times more than women. A number of studies have been done on different populations affected by the Chernobyl disaster. Most studies show that there is a significant increase in the prevalence of psychological problems and psychiatric disorders in the exposed population. Loganovsky and Loganovskaja (2000) examined the Chernobyl exclusion zone archives (1986-1997) and assessed 100 patients with acute radiation sickness and 100 exposed workers. They noted a significant increase in the incidence of schizophrenia in exclusion zone personnel in comparison to the general population (5.4 per 10 000 in the exclusion zone versus 1.1 per 10 000 in the rest of Ukraine) from the beginning of 1990. Those irradiated by moderate to high doses (more than 0.30 Sv or 30 rem) had significantly more left frontotemporal limbic and schizophreniform syndromes. Revonek (1991) showed that the rate of reactive psychosis was higher in inpatients affected by the disaster in comparison to the general group of inpatients. Napreenko and Loganovskii (1995) evaluated 476 subjects over a period of 8 years and found that mental disorders, especially psycho-organic (14.5%), neurotic (12.1%) and psychosomatic (58%) disorders were common. In a sample of 320 nonpsychotic patients, Panchenko et al (1996) found that five syndromes were common: astheno-neurotic (36.2%), astheno-depressive (28.8%), obsessive-phobic (17.8%), astheno-hypochondriac (10%) and hysteric-hypochondriac (7.2%). Revenok (1998) showed that personality and behavioural changes become predominant late in the course of organic brain affection. The rate of suicide has been reported to be in the range of 24.0-29.6 per 100 000 population over a 15 year period (1984 to 1998) and large regional variations have been noted (Mokhovikov & Donnets, 1996; Wassermann et al, 1998; Kryzhanovskaya & Pilyagina, 1999). In 2003, the rate of suicide was 26.1 per 100 000 (Center of Medical Statistics of Ministry of Health, 2004). Kryzhanovskaya and Pilyagina (1999) reported that the suicide rate had increased by 57% between 1988 and 1997. They also found that suicides were more prevalent in the industrially developed regions and that men committed suicide five times more often than women. Gadow et al (2000) conducted a study on ADHD in 10-12 year old urban children (n=600) in which parents, teachers and children were interviewed using standardized tools and DSM-IV criteria. They found the prevalence of ADHD to be 19.8% and that of inattentive, hyperactive-impulsive and combined subtypes to be 7.2%, 8.5% and 4.2%, respectively. Nyagu et al (1998) noted a significant increase in mental retardation, borderline and low range IQ, and emotional and behavioural disorders in children exposed to radiation prenatally (n=544) when compared to normal controls (n=759) in a study that involved examination of children and interviews with parents and teachers. However, these findings were not supported by Litcher et al's (2000) study, who examined the cognitive and neuropsychological functioning of children who had been less than 15 months of age or in utero at the time of the Chornobyl disaster (n=300).

MENTAL HEALTH RESOURCES

Mental Health Policy A mental health policy is present. The policy was initially formulated in 1988.
The components of the policy are prevention, treatment and rehabilitation.

Substance Abuse Policy A substance abuse policy is present. The policy was initially formulated in 1997.

National Mental Health Programme A national mental health programme is absent.
The project of national targets as a part of mental health programme has been prepared.

National Therapeutic Drug Policy/Essential List of Drugs A national therapeutic drug policy/essential list of drugs is present. It was formulated in 1998.

Mental Health Legislation There is a Law on Psychiatric Care. This was the first time in the history of the independent Ukrainian State that consideration was given by the supreme legislative body to a draft of a law by a non-governmental professional organization.
The latest legislation was enacted in 2000.

Mental Health Financing There are no budget allocations for mental health.
Details about expenditure on mental health are not available.
The primary sources of mental health financing in descending order are tax based and private insurances.
Though services are funded by the state, there are restrictions on the amount of free medication.
The country has disability benefits for persons with mental disorders.

Mental Health Facilities Mental health is a part of primary health care system. Actual treatment of severe mental disorders is not available at the primary level. There are some local experimental programmes at Kiev.
Regular training of primary care professionals is not carried out in the field of mental health.
There are no community care facilities for patients with mental disorders. There are experimental programmes only in some cities.
There are some polyclinics which take care of ambulant psychiatric patients, but no other psychiatric institution exists (Rupprecht et al, 2000).

Psychiatric Beds and Professionals

Total psychiatric beds per 10 000 population	9.6
Psychiatric beds in mental hospitals per 10 000 population	9.3
Psychiatric beds in general hospitals per 10 000 population	0.3
Psychiatric beds in other settings per 10 000 population	
Number of psychiatrists per 100 000 population	8.9
Number of neurosurgeons per 100 000 population	1.5
Number of psychiatric nurses per 100 000 population	34
Number of neurologists per 100 000 population	13
Number of psychologists per 100 000 population	0.06
Number of social workers per 100 000 population	0.4

Training of psychiatric nurses has been developed at Kiev. Training of social workers has been begun at the Kiev-Mogila Academy. There are 87 psychiatric hospitals in Ukraine. There is a trend to decrease the number of inpatient beds in hospitals. Almost one-sixth of psychiatric beds in Ukraine has been allocated for child and adolescent psychiatry.

Non-Governmental Organizations NGOs are involved with mental health in the country. They are mainly involved in advocacy, promotion, prevention, treatment and rehabilitation. The positive experience of interactions between state psychiatric services, non-governmental professional organizations and organizations of relatives and users has been an important factor. As a result of these projects, the approach of multidisciplinary teamwork and case management have been introduced into practice of some facilities at Kiev, Zhitomir and Donetsk.

Information Gathering System There is mental health reporting system in the country.
The country has data collection system or epidemiological study on mental health.

Programmes for Special Population The country has specific programmes for mental health for disaster affected population and children.
Each region has 1-3 child and 1-2 adolescent psychiatry departments. Special departments for drug dependent adolescents are also present. The Ministry of Social Security provides for boarding schools for mentally challenged children. A number of cities have also started municipal rehabilitation centres for disabled children.

Therapeutic Drugs The following therapeutic drugs are generally available at the primary health care level of the country: carbamazepine, ethosuximide, phenobarbital, phenytoin sodium, sodium valproate, amitriptyline, chlorpromazine, diazepam, fluphenazine, haloperidol, lithium, levodopa.
In place of biperiden other anti-parkinsonian drugs are used.

Other Information The provision of psychiatric care, with its planning and financing on the national level, are implemented by the Department on Disease Treatment and Prevention of the Ministry of Public Health of Ukraine. Currently, the most important problem for this working group is to develop a 'Conception of Mental Health Care in Ukraine'. Throughout the country, there are similar working groups, consisting of the leading specialists in the field of mental health within each region. In addition, there is a problem-solving commission within the structure of the Ministry of Public Health. Its main goal is to plan the directions of further scientific studies in the field of psychiatry.

Additional Sources of Information

Buzanova, V. E. (1981) Schizophrenia among urban and rural patients. Comparative clinico-demographic characteristics (according to the results of an epidemiologic study). Zhurnal Nevropatologii i Psikhiatrii Imeni S-S-Korsakova, 81, 729-734.

Center of Medical Statistics of Ministry of Health. (2004) Indicators of mental health disorders prevalence and work of psychiatric institutions in Ukraine in 2004. Kiev: Center of Medical Statistics of Ministry of Health, 2004.

Dvirskii, A. A. (1999) The role of genetic factors in the manifestation of delirium tremens. Zhurnal Nevrologii i Psikhiatrii Imeni S.S. Korsakova, 99, 48-50.

Gadow, K. D., Nolan, E. E., Litcher, L., et al (2000) Comparison of attention-deficit/hyperactivity disorder symptom subtypes in Ukrainian schoolchildren. Journal of the American Academy of Child & Adolescent Psychiatry, 39, 1520-1527.

Kryzhanovskaya, L., Pilyagina, G. (1999) Suicidal behavior in the Ukraine, 1988-1998. Crisis: Journal of Crisis Intervention & Suicide, 20, 184-190.

Levinsky, M., Aksentyev, S. (1999) Child and adolescent psychiatry in Ukraine. In: H. Remschmidt, H. van Engeland (Eds). Child and Adolescent Psychiatry in Europe. Historical Development, Current Situation and Future Perspectives. Darmstadt, Steinkopff. pp381-393.

Litcher, L., Bromet, E. J., Carlson, G., et al (2000) School and neuropsychological performance of evacuated children in Kyiv 11 years after the Chornobyl disaster. Journal of Child Psychology & Psychiatry & Allied Disciplines, 41, 291-299.

Loganovsky, K. N., Loganovskaja, T. K. (2000) Schizophrenia spectrum disorders in persons exposed to ionizing radiation as a result of the Chernobyl accident. Schizophrenia Bulletin, 26, 751-773.

Mokhovikov, A., Donets, O. (1996) Suicide in the Ukraine: epidemiology, knowledge, and attitudes of the population. Crisis: Journal of Crisis Intervention & Suicide, 17, 128-134.

Napreenko, A. K., Loganovskii, K.N. (1995) The systematics of mental disorders related to the sequelae of the accident at the Chernobyl Atomic Electric Power Station. Likarska Sprava, 5-6, 25-29.

Nyagu, A. I., Loganovsky, K. N., Loganovskaja, T. K. (1998) Psychophysiologic aftereffects of prenatal irradiation. International Journal of Psychophysiology, 30, 303-311.

Panchenko, O. A., Tabachnikov, S. I., Kut'ko, I. I. (1996) Mental disorders in the participants in the cleanup of the aftermath of the accident at the Chernobyl Atomic Electric Power Station. Zhurnal Nevropatologii i Psikhiatrii Imeni S-S-Korsakova, 96, 34-37.

Polubinskaya, S. V. (2000). Reform in psychiatry in post-Soviet countries. Acta Psychiatrica Scandanavia 101 (suppl. 399), 106-108.

Revenok, A. A. (1991) The structural-dynamic characteristics of the reactive psychoses in persons subjected to ionizing radiation exposure as a result of the accident at the Chernobyl Atomic Electric Power Station. Vrachebnoe.Delo, 83-86.

Revenok, A. A. (1998) Psychopathic-like disorders in persons with an organic brain lesion as a result of exposure to ionizing radiation. Likarska Sprava, 21-24.

Rupprecht, R., Hegerl, U. (2000) The state of psychiatry in the Ukraine – psychiatric hospitals in Kiev and Shitomir. Nervenartz, 71, 420-422.

Wasserman, D., Varnik, A., Dankowicz, M. (1998) Regional differences in the distribution of suicide in the former Soviet Union during perestroika, 1984-1990. Acta Psychiatrica Scandinavica, Supplement 394, 5-12.

T–Z

United Arab Emirates*

GENERAL INFORMATION

United Arab Emirates is a country with an approximate area of 84 thousand sq. km. (UNO, 2001). Its population is 3.051 million, and the sex ratio (men per hundred women) is 185 (UNO, 2004). The proportion of population under the age of 15 years is 25% (UNO, 2004), and the proportion of population above the age of 60 years is 2% (WHO, 2004). The literacy rate is 75.6% for men and 80.7% for women (UNESCO/MoH, 2004).

The country is a high income group country (based on World Bank 2004 criteria). The proportion of health budget to GDP is 3.5%. The per capita total expenditure on health is 921 international $, and the per capita government expenditure on health is 698 international $ (WHO, 2004).

The main language(s) used in the country is (are) Arabic. The largest ethnic group(s) is (are) South Asian, and the other ethnic group(s) are (is) Emiri and Iranian. The largest religious group(s) is (are) Muslim.

The life expectancy at birth is 71.3 years for males and 75.1 years for females (WHO, 2004). The healthy life expectancy at birth is 64 years for males and 64 years for females (WHO, 2004).

EPIDEMIOLOGY

There is substantial epidemiological data on mental illnesses in the United Arab Emirates in internationally accessible literature. No attempt was made to include this information here.

MENTAL HEALTH RESOURCES

Mental Health Policy A mental health policy is absent.

Substance Abuse Policy A substance abuse policy is present. Details about the year of formulation are not available.

National Mental Health Programme A national mental health programme is present. The programme was formulated in 1991. It aims at the universal provision of mental health and substance abuse services by their incorporation in primary health care. The strategies for realizing this aim are through training of personnel in mental health at all primary care levels, strengthening existing centres and opening new ones, streamlining referral services and providing essential drugs, linking community and other sectoral services to it and developing manpower.

National Therapeutic Drug Policy/Essential List of Drugs A national therapeutic drug policy/essential list of drugs is present. Details about the year of formulation are not available.

Mental Health Legislation There is a Federal Mental Health Act. It contains sections on definition of mental disorders, the role of authorities and police and on some details on detention and psychoses. The law needs to be reviewed. There is no specific mental health law on mentally abnormal offenders. The Sharia Islamic law addresses such issues. A national forensic psychiatric committee is being set up in collaboration with the ministries of health and justice. Attempted suicide is a crime.

The latest legislation was enacted in 1981.

Mental Health Financing Details about disability benefits for mental health are not available.

Details about expenditure on mental health are not available.

Details about sources of financing are not available.

Details about disability benefits for mental health are not available.

Mental Health Facilities Mental health is a part of primary health care system. Actual treatment of severe mental disorders is available at the primary level. There are extensive primary care services which cater to all kinds of mental disorders.

Regular training of primary care professionals is carried out in the field of mental health.

There are community care facilities for patients with mental disorders. Facilities for rehabilitation are available through CBR approach. Community care services are not well developed and this is compensated by the primary care services.

Psychiatric Beds and Professionals

Total psychiatric beds per 10 000 population	1.4
Psychiatric beds in mental hospitals per 10 000 population	
Psychiatric beds in general hospitals per 10 000 population	
Psychiatric beds in other settings per 10 000 population	
Number of psychiatrists per 100 000 population	2
Number of neurosurgeons per 100 000 population	
Number of psychiatric nurses per 100 000 population	11
Number of neurologists per 100 000 population	
Number of psychologists per 100 000 population	1
Number of social workers per 100 000 population	1.2

There are 7 occupational therapists. A psychiatric hospital opened in 1995 with facilities for general psychiatry, forensic psychiatry, addiction, emergency, child and adolescent psychiatry, consultation-liaison and community care. It has an attached day treatment centre. There are other psychiatric facilities in different cities. The private sector is well established. Most professionals work in the hospital in Abu Dhabi. In the other parts of the Emirate the number of personnel are limited and most have 1 or 2 psychiatrists only.

Non-Governmental Organizations Details about NGO facilities in mental health are not available.

Information Gathering System Details about mental health reporting systems are not available.
The country has data collection system or epidemiological study on mental health.
A central psychiatric register has been established by the Ministry of Health for collection of data and research statistics regarding mental health, and data from all over the Emirate would be pooled into this information system.

Programmes for Special Population The country has specific programmes for mental health for elderly and children. There are services for the mentally retarded and delinquents.
There are also school health centres in some areas which deal with early detection and intervention of psychological problems in school-children. Residential centres for delinquents are also present in some areas.

Therapeutic Drugs The following therapeutic drugs are generally available at the primary health care level of the country: unknown.

Other Information Psychiatric services are based on the public health system which is organized on an emirate by emirate basis. A federal ministry has a coordinating role. Abu Dhabi has the most extensive services followed by Dubai. A special committee was established to advise on planning and development of psychiatric services nation-wide.
* The verification of this country profile is still being awaited from the Ministry of Health of the United Arab Emirates.

Additional Sources of Information

Kraya, N. (2002) Thirty years on: psychiatric services in the United Arab Emirates. Australasian Psychiatry. 10, 168-171.

Kronfol, N.M. (1999) Perspectives on the health care system of the United Arab Emirates. Eastern Mediterranean Health Journal. 5, 149-167.

United Kingdom

GENERAL INFORMATION

The United Kingdom is a country with an approximate area of 243 thousand sq. km. (UNO, 2001). Its population is 59.428 million, and the sex ratio (men per hundred women) is 95 (UNO, 2004). The proportion of population under the age of 15 years is 18% (UNO, 2004), and the proportion of population above the age of 60 years is 21% (WHO, 2004). The literacy rate is 99% for men and 99% for women (UNESCO/MoH, 2004).

The country is a high income group country (based on World Bank 2004 criteria). The proportion of health budget to GDP is 5.8%. The per capita total expenditure on health is 1989 international $, and the per capita government expenditure on health is 1634 international $ (WHO, 2004).

The main language(s) used in the country is (are) English, Welsh, Scots Gaelic and South Asian languages. The largest ethnic group(s) is (are) English, and the other ethnic group(s) are (is) Scottish, Irish, Welsh and those from African Caribbean and South Asian backgrounds. The largest religious group(s) is (are) Anglican, and the other religious group(s) are (is) Roman Catholic and Muslim.

The life expectancy at birth is 75.8 years for males and 80.5 years for females (WHO, 2004). The healthy life expectancy at birth is 69 years for males and 72 years for females (WHO, 2004).

EPIDEMIOLOGY

There is substantial epidemiological data on mental illnesses in the United Kingdom in internationally accessible literature. No attempt was made to include this information here.

MENTAL HEALTH RESOURCES

Mental Health Policy A mental health policy is present. The policy was initially formulated in 1998.

The components of the policy are advocacy, promotion, prevention, treatment and rehabilitation. The policy focuses on primary care and access to services, effective services for people with severe mental illness, services for carers and action to reduce suicide. National Service Frameworks for older people and children have also recently been published.

Substance Abuse Policy A substance abuse policy is present. The policy was initially formulated in 2000.

National Mental Health Programme A national mental health programme is present. The programme was formulated in 1999. Details can be obtained from the documents 'National Service Framework for Mental Health, 1999' and 'NHS Plan, 2000' for England. The NHS Plan has three major priorities: (1) All people in a crisis will have access to crisis resolution/home treatment teams – by 2005; (2) All people with a first episode psychosis will have access to intensive treatment for the first three years from early intervention teams – by 2006; and (3) All people with intensive needs will have access to assertive outreach teams – by 2004. There is also a major new initiative attempting to reduce the social isolation experienced by people with mental health problems, 'Social Exclusion and Mental Health', produced by the Office of the Deputy Prime Minister (2004). 'The Framework for Mental Health Services in Scotland' was published in 1997' and 'Our National health: A plan for Action, a Plan for Change, in 2000'. 'The Way Forward for Northern Ireland' was published in 1995.

National Therapeutic Drug Policy/Essential List of Drugs A national therapeutic drug policy/essential list of drugs is present. It was formulated in 1979.

T–Z

Mental Health Legislation There is a Mental Health Act. There are proposals to reform it. Details can be obtained from the website: www.doh.gov.uk. The new proposal's focus is on managing risk and providing better health outcomes for patients in a way that strikes the right balance between public safety and the rights of individuals. One of the key changes proposed include extension of compulsory powers to the community – the 1983 Mental Health Act was exclusively concerned with detention in hospital, but services for people with mental disorder are increasingly being provided in the community. The new proposals would for the first time enable compulsory treatment to take place in the community. All patients would be formally assessed before compulsory treatment is imposed. One piece of legislation covers England and Wales, another Scotland (Mental health (Scotland) Act, 1984; The Mental Health (Public Safety and Appeals) (Scotland) Bill, 2001) and the third Northern Ireland (Mental Health Order, 1986). The Scottish legislation though historically different from the English legislation is similar in principle, however The Millan Committee (2001) has reviewed the Mental Health (Scotland) Act, 1984 and has suggested revisions.

The latest legislation was enacted in 1983.

Mental Health Financing There are budget allocations for mental health.

The country spends 10% of the total health budget on mental health.

The primary sources of mental health financing in descending order are tax based, private insurances, social insurance and out of pocket expenditure by the patient or family.

About 85% of the expenses for health and social care for mentally ill is borne by the NHS and the remainder by the local authorities. Scotland and Northern Ireland have heavier investment in health care in comparison to England and Wales. NHS services are provided free at the point of delivery. Though some local authority services are chargeable, they are provided free to people with

severe mental illnesses. Social care is partly provided by the Social Services Department of local authorities. Most residential care is provided by the independent (voluntary and private sector). Employment services are provided by a range of agencies.
The country has disability benefits for persons with mental disorders. Disability Discrimination Act 1995 introduced laws aimed at ending the discrimination that many disabled people face. It gave disabled people new rights in access to goods, facilities and services as well as in employment and buying or renting property. The Disability Living Allowance is an extra costs benefit for the physically and mentally disabled, which is tax free, non-contributory and not income related. DLA is based primarily on the disabled person's self-reporting of their condition. The person has to demonstrate that their disability is of a long standing nature. Welfare benefits are provided primarily by the Benefits Agency, which is linked to the Department for Social Security.

Mental Health Facilities Mental health is a part of primary health care system. Actual treatment of severe mental disorders is available at the primary level. The Government has set out clear national standards in the National Service Framework for Mental Health (1999), in which it sets out ways to get easy access to more effective primary care with support from specialized care wherever necessary. There are seven national standards covering mental health promotion, primary care access and services, effective services for people with mental illness, caring about carers and the action necessary to achieve the suicide target in 'Our Healthier Nation'. The standards 2 and 3 allows any person with mental disorder to be effectively treated at the primary care level and get access to complete services around the clock.
Regular training of primary care professionals is carried out in the field of mental health. Training facilities for mental health workers, general practitioners, social workers, community workers are to be strengthened in future through the NHS Plan. 'The HSC 1999/154 Continuing Professional development: Quality in the New NHS' stresses the importance of continuous training. Different bodies like the Primary Care Groups, Workforce Action Team are supposed to address the issue of training. The training for general practitioners is regulated through the NHS regulations of 1997. New guidance on the GP Registrar Scheme came into effect in April 2000 and set out enhanced arrangements for the management and delivery of general practice vocational training. Training for psychosocial intervention is also available, as are training facilities for community health nurses.
There are community care facilities for patients with mental disorders. Health care is provided largely by the National Health Service (NHS) and social care by local authorities in England and Wales. The Scottish care system is globally similar, but has a different legal system. In Northern Ireland, the health and social services are unified. There are at present more than 800 community care teams, but subject to wide geographic variation. There are over 300 work or employment rehabilitation schemes and over 50 000 residential places available. The regional distribution is uneven, with the proportion of provision that is hospital based as opposed to community based varying from one-fifth to half. Community care has traditionally not been integrated adequately, although the NHS Plan requires all areas to implement new teams and ensure consistent access for all. 400 new teams will be appointed.
Attempts have been made to establish systems of key workers and care planning-led health and social services. The Care Programme Approach (CPA) was introduced in 1991 as one of the cornerstones of the Government's mental health policy; it provides a framework for the care of people with mental illness. In collaboration with local social services departments, Mental Health Service units are required to initiate explicit, individually tailored care programmes. These are for all inpatients about to be discharged from mental illness hospitals and for all new patients accepted by the specialist psychiatric services. The essential elements of the CPA are: systematic assessment of health and social care needs; a care plan agreed between the relevant professional staff and the patient; the allocation of a key professional worker and regular review of the patient's progress. The key worker has the responsibility for coordinating care, keeping in touch with the patient, ensuring that the care plan is delivered and calling for reviews of the plan when required.

Psychiatric Beds and Professionals

Total psychiatric beds per 10 000 population	5.8
Psychiatric beds in mental hospitals per 10 000 population	
Psychiatric beds in general hospitals per 10 000 population	
Psychiatric beds in other settings per 10 000 population	
Number of psychiatrists per 100 000 population	11
Number of neurosurgeons per 100 000 population	1
Number of psychiatric nurses per 100 000 population	104
Number of neurologists per 100 000 population	1
Number of psychologists per 100 000 population	9
Number of social workers per 100 000 population	58

There are 15 040 occupational therapists, 594 psychotherapists, 856 psychiatric clinical assistants, 4 neurosurgeon clinical assistants, 39 neurologist clinical assistants. Not all of the above workers are attached to the mental health full time. Mental hospitals have mostly been phased out (about 110 mental hospitals were closed), so that the majority of acute beds are in general hospitals. The number of inpatient beds have declined by about 75% over the last 5 decades. Three high security hospitals (1500 beds), although these are reducing in size and a network of medium security units (1000 places), are present. A major problem facing the mental health services is in recruiting and retaining professionals.

Non-Governmental Organizations NGOs are involved with mental health in the country. They are mainly involved in advocacy, promotion, treatment and rehabilitation. User and carer movements have grown in a very significant way. Partnerships between user and carer agencies, voluntary organizations and professional groups often come together in influencing policy decisions.

Information Gathering System There is mental health reporting system in the country. ONS Annual Report provides mental health information.
The country has data collection system or epidemiological study on mental health.

Programmes for Special Population The country has specific programmes for mental health for minorities and elderly.
Separate services are available for children and adolescents, elderly and forensic patients. Programmes for homeless people who are mentally ill are available in the big cities. They provide assertive outreach, staffed hostels and ordinary move-on accommodation. Traditionally strong boundaries have existed between drug abuse and mental illness services. Some areas are now setting up specialist dual-diagnosis teams to tackle the problem of comorbidity.

Therapeutic Drugs The following therapeutic drugs are generally available at the primary health care level of the country: carbamazepine, ethosuximide, phenobarbital, phenytoin sodium, sodium valproate, amitriptyline, chlorpromazine, diazepam, fluphenazine, haloperidol, lithium, biperiden, carbidopa, levodopa.
All the drugs listed are available through the NHS. Some patients require to pay a standard prescription charge for each item prescribed by general practitioners.

Other Information During the 1960s and 1970s new medical and psychosocial methods of care evolved and this led to the Government to change its policies and call for the closure of asylums in a gradual fashion. Community care has increased during the same period, though some areas are better placed than others. There is a wide anti-stigma movement which embraces families, patients and the general public, in addition to experts.

Additional Sources of Information

Becker T., Hullsmann, S., Knudsen, H. C. et al & the EPSILON Group (2002) Provision of services for people with schizophrenia in five European regions. Journal of Social Psychiatry and Psychiatric Epidemiology, 37, 465-474.

British Medical Association (2000) British National Formulary. Royal Pharmaceutical Society of Great Britain.

Department of Health (1998) Modernising Mental Health Services.

Department of Health (1999) National Service Framework for Mental Health – Modern Standards and Service Models.

Department of Health (1999) Reform of the Mental Health Act 1983 – Proposals for Consultation.

Johnson, S., Zinkler, M., Priebe, S. (2001) Mental health service provision in England. Acta Psychiatrica Scandinavica, 104 (suppl. 410), 47-55.

Loudon, J., Coia, D. (2002) The Scottish scene. Psychiatric Bulletin, 26, 84-86.

McClelland, R., Webb, M., Mock, G. (2000) Mental health in Ireland. International Journal of Law and Psychiatry, 23, 309-328.

McCulloch, A., Muijen, M., Harper, H. (2000) New developments in mental health policy in the United Kingdom. International Journal of Law and Psychiatry, 23, 261-276.

National Health Service (2000) The NHS Plan – A Plan for Investment, A Plan for Reform.

Pierre, S. A. (2000) Psychiatry and Citizenship – The Liverpool Black Mental Health Service User's Perspective.

Smith, M. (2003) Devolution and 'public psychiatry in Scotland. Psychiatric Bulletin, 27, 41-43.

United Republic of Tanzania

GENERAL INFORMATION

The United Republic of Tanzania is a country with an approximate area of 945 thousand sq. km. (UNO, 2001). Its population is 37.671 million, and the sex ratio (men per hundred women) is 98 (UNO, 2004). The proportion of population under the age of 15 years is 45% (UNO, 2004), and the proportion of population above the age of 60 years is 4% (WHO, 2004). The literacy rate is 85.2% for men and 69.2% for women (UNESCO/MoH, 2004).

The country is a low income group country (based on World Bank 2004 criteria). The proportion of health budget to GDP is 4.4%. The per capita total expenditure on health is 26 international $, and the per capita government expenditure on health is 12 international $ (WHO, 2004).

The main language(s) used in the country is (are) Swahili and English. The largest ethnic group(s) is (are) African, and the other ethnic group(s) are (is) Arab. The largest religious group(s) is (are) Christian in the mainland and Muslim in Zanzibar, and the other religious group(s) are (is) Muslims and indigenous groups in the mainland.

The life expectancy at birth is 45.5 years for males and 47.5 years for females (WHO, 2004). The healthy life expectancy at birth is 40 years for males and 41 years for females (WHO, 2004).

EPIDEMIOLOGY

Bondestam et al (1990) conducted a population survey on 10 776 randomly selected subjects in Zanzibar and found epilepsy in 4.9/1000 and psychotic disorder in 3.2/1000 of the population. Matuja et al (1995) reported on the prevalence of psychiatric disorders among 205 consecutive patients referred to a psychiatric unit over a 2 year period. Classification was done according to ICD-10. The ratio of males to females was found to be 1.6:1. A large number of cases were referrals from other departments of the same hospital and the remaining were from dispensaries and other hospitals. A fifth of the patients had consulted traditional healers prior to referral which was often delayed. The commonest presentations were psychosis (36.6%, of which three fourth were schizophrenia), neurosis (19.5%), seizures (16.6%), substance abuse (8.8%) and organic mental disorders (5.3%). Headache, sexual disorders and conduct disorders were also seen. Comorbid physical illness was present in 17%. Ndosi and Mtawali (2002) studied puerperal psychosis among 86 hospital inpatients using standardized questionnaires and ICD-10 criteria. The study was conducted prospectively over 2 years, and clinical progress was monitored. The mean age of patients was 23.6 years; the majority was primiparous women. Anaemia and infection were the major comorbid physical illnesses. The prevalence of puerperal psychosis was 3.2/1000 births. Organic psychosis was found in four-fifths of the mothers and schizophrenia in 8.1%. Most mothers received social support from their extended families. Ndosi and Kisesa (1997) examined the clinical notes of deceased patients in the same psychiatric unit over a 5 year period and found that functional psychoses (52.7%), organic psychoses (37.6%), epilepsy (6.2%) and puerperal psychosis (2.1%) were the main diagnosis among those who died. Two-thirds of patients were males, and the main cause of mortality in about half the patients was infectious diseases.

MENTAL HEALTH RESOURCES

Mental Health Policy A mental health policy is present. The policy was initially formulated in 1990.
The components of the policy are advocacy, promotion, prevention, treatment and rehabilitation. The mental health policy is integrated into the national health policy of 1990.

Substance Abuse Policy A substance abuse policy is present. The policy was initially formulated in 1995. A substance abuse policy is a part of the drug control legislation.

National Mental Health Programme A national mental health programme is present. The programme was formulated in 1980. The programme was developed with the help of WHO and the Danish Development Agency.

National Therapeutic Drug Policy/Essential List of Drugs A national therapeutic drug policy/essential list of drugs is present. Details about the year of formulation are not available.

Mental Health Legislation A draft of an updated mental health legislation was initiated in 2000. The final draft has been placed before the parliament for approval in 2005.
The latest legislation was enacted in 1958.

Mental Health Financing There are budget allocations for mental health.
The country spends 7% of the total health budget on mental health.
The primary sources of mental health financing in descending order are tax based and grants.
A greater proportion of funding of mental health care is done by districts than was the case earlier. This makes the task of obtaining reliable figures on financing even more difficult.
The country has disability benefits for persons with mental disorders. Psychiatric patients are exempt from cost sharing charges for treatment.

Mental Health Facilities Mental health is a part of primary health care system. Actual treatment of severe mental disorders is available at the primary level. Most mental patients in Tanzania are initially seen in primary care facilities, dispensaries and health centres or traditional healing practices. Primary mental health care is provided by mental health nurses and general health workers. Some regions provide follow-up psychiatric care to patients as a part of primary health care.

Regular training of primary care professionals is carried out in the field of mental health.
There are community care facilities for patients with mental disorders. Regional mental health coordinators run community-based care for the mentally ill. There are 119 districts with district mental health coordinators. Psychiatric rehabilitation villages in 6 regions accommodate a total of between 80-100 patients at any given time. They provide 'agriculture psychiatric rehabilitation', sheltered living conditions for homeless psychiatric patients, continued treatment and training facilities in interpersonal relationships and a sheltered working place. The villages are managed by mental health nurse, nursing assistants, artisans and agriculturists who are responsible for the farms. A psychiatrist and medical social worker makes weekly visits. Each patient stays for an average period of 6 months with a range of 3 months to 2 years. Besides these, there is a network of traditional healers. The decentralized programme reaches about 20% of the population. External evaluation of the programme was carried out in 2 regions and it was found to be cost effective as it helped to decrease bed occupancy rates.

Psychiatric Beds and Professionals

Total psychiatric beds per 10 000 population	0.7
Psychiatric beds in mental hospitals per 10 000 population	0.36
Psychiatric beds in general hospitals per 10 000 population	0.04
Psychiatric beds in other settings per 10 000 population	0.3
Number of psychiatrists per 100 000 population	0.04
Number of neurosurgeons per 100 000 population	0.01
Number of psychiatric nurses per 100 000 population	2
Number of neurologists per 100 000 population	0.05
Number of psychologists per 100 000 population	0.005
Number of social workers per 100 000 population	0.2

In recent years, less than 50% of mental health nurses provide mental health care. There are 10 assistant medical officers in psychiatry. There are 3 centres at the tertiary care level. At this level, there is also a forensic psychiatric unit. In addition, there are 11 regions with psychiatric units with 30-50 general psychiatry beds, which provide care at the secondary level.

Non-Governmental Organizations NGOs are involved with mental health in the country. They are mainly involved in advocacy, promotion, prevention, treatment and rehabilitation.

Information Gathering System There is mental health reporting system in the country. All regions send yearly statistics of mental patients attended at regional hospitals. Audit of inpatient records for the years 2001-2003 showed that the following disorders were common: neuropsychiatric disorders (47.2%), functional psychosis (34.5%), anxiety disorders, intellectual disability and alcohol and drug abuse.
The country has data collection system or epidemiological study on mental health. The data collection system was developed for primary care facilities. In 2004, a pilot epidemiological study on mental health was conducted in Dar es Salaam.

Programmes for Special Population The country has specific programmes for mental health for refugees, disaster affected population and indigenous population. There are no specialized services for substance dependence or children.
Family life education programmes in schools have a component of prevention of substance abuse. Similar programmes are being extended into colleges and community institutions with the help of grants from UNDCP and the Government of Finland.

Therapeutic Drugs The following therapeutic drugs are generally available at the primary health care level of the country: phenobarbital, amitriptyline, chlorpromazine, diazepam.
Availability of psychotropics are variable. More psychotropics are available in large urban centres. There are very few drugs available in the primary care level.

Other Information An inventory that covers mental health services in Tanzania mainland has been completed. It covers all 20 regions' reports.

Additional Sources of Information

Bondestam, S., Garssen, J., Abdulwakil, A. I. (1990) Prevalence and treatment of mental disorders and epilepsy in Zanzibar. Acta Psychiatrica Scandinavica, 81, 327-331.

Kilonzo, G. P., Simmons, N. (1998) Development of mental health services in Tanzania: a reappraisal for the future. Social Science & Medicine, 47, 419-428.

Matuja, W. P., Ndosi, N. K., Collins, M. (1995) Nature of referrals to the psychiatric unit at Muhimbili Medical Centre, Dar es Salaam. East African Medical Journal, 72, 761-765.

Ndosi, N. K., Kisesa, A. F. (1997) Causes of death among mental patients at Muhimbili Medical Centre, Dar es Salaam. East African Medical Journal, 74, 82-84.

Ndosi, N. K., Mtawali, M. L. (2002) The nature of puerperal psychosis at Muhimbili National Hospital: its physical co-morbidity, associated main obstetric and social factors. African Journal of Reproductive Health, 6, 41-49.

Njenga, F.(2002) Focus on psychiatry in East Africa. British Journal of Psychiatry, 181, 354-359.

United States of America

GENERAL INFORMATION

The United States of America is a country with an approximate area of 9629 thousand sq. km. (UNO, 2001). Its population is 297.043 million, and the sex ratio (men per hundred women) is 97 (UNO, 2004). The proportion of population under the age of 15 years is 21% (UNO, 2004), and the proportion of population above the age of 60 years is 16% (WHO, 2004). The literacy rate is 97% for men and 97% for women (UNESCO/MoH, 2004).

The country is a high income group country (based on World Bank 2004 criteria). The proportion of health budget to GDP is 13.9%. The per capita total expenditure on health is 4887 international $, and the per capita government expenditure on health is 2168 international $ (WHO, 2004).

The main language(s) used in the country is (are) English and Spanish. The largest ethnic group(s) is (are) White (three-fourths of the population), and the other ethnic group(s) are (is) African-American and Hispanic-Latino (one-eighth, each). The largest religious group(s) is (are) Protestant (more than half of the population), and the other religious group(s) are (is) Roman Catholic (one fourth).

The life expectancy at birth is 74.6 years for males and 79.8 years for females (WHO, 2004). The healthy life expectancy at birth is 67 years for males and 71 years for females (WHO, 2004).

EPIDEMIOLOGY

There is substantial epidemiological data on mental illnesses in the United States of America in internationally accessible literature. No attempt was made to include this information here.

MENTAL HEALTH RESOURCES

Mental Health Policy A mental health policy is absent.

In 2002, the President of the United States of America convened the New Freedom Commission on Mental Health which issued a report in July 2003 entitled 'Achieving the Promise: Transforming Mental Health Care in America'. The vision put forth is "...a future when everyone with mental illness will recover..., mental illnesses are detected early..., and everyone with a mental illness at any stage of life has access to effective treatment and supports – essentials for living, working, learning, and participating fully in the community." The goals articulated by this report are that Americans understand that: mental health is essential to overall health, mental health care is consumer and family driven, disparities in mental health services are eliminated, early mental health screening, assessment and referral to services are common practice, excellent mental health care is delivered and research is accelerated and technology is used to access mental health care and information. In 2004, the US Center for Mental Health Services began working closely with the States to implement the six goals of this report.

Substance Abuse Policy A substance abuse policy is present. The policy was initially formulated in 1988.

National Mental Health Programme A national mental health programme is present. The programme was formulated in 1946. It was changed by the legislation in 1992 and is carried out by the Center for Mental Health Services (CMHS), Substance Abuse and Mental Health Services Administration (SAMHSA) and the National Institute of Mental Health (NIMH), National Institutes of Health (NIH).

National Therapeutic Drug Policy/Essential List of Drugs A national therapeutic drug policy/essential list of drugs is absent.

Mental Health Legislation The Public Health Service Act (2000) defines the functions of the NIMH and CMHS. The Health Insurance Portability and Accountability Act (1996) covered issues like confidentiality/privacy/security (with particular reference to electronic records and claims processing). The Mental Health Parity Act (1996) that required parity between mental health and health care benefits has 'sunsetted' meaning that new legislation will be required to continue these benefits. The Children's Health Act (2000) authorized the SAMHSA to carry out children and adolescent focused mental health programmes. The forensic psychiatric system in the US is a combination of civil and criminal laws, which vary between states in definition and practices, though remaining fundamentally similar. The civil commitment laws help in maintaining the dignity of offenders with mental illness. The criminal laws, on the other hand, help in ascertaining incompetency to stand trial because of mental illness and insanity defense. The latest legislation was enacted in 2000.

Mental Health Financing There are budget allocations for mental health.

The country spends 6% of the total health budget on mental health.

The primary sources of mental health financing in descending order are private insurances, tax based, out of pocket expenditure by the patient or family.

The United States of America does not have universal health insurance coverage (around one-sixth of the population is without any health insurance). In the 1980s, mental health care, on the federal level, began to be included in federal employees' insurance. Federal programmes, such as Medicaid and Social Security Disability Insurance were paid heavy attention to in the 1990s. The major focus was specifically on managed care, particularly to carve out plans where mental health benefits are separate from other medical benefits. However, public and private managed care plans are being developed independently. This multi-tiered system encourages dumping from one level to another (e.g. when private insurance benefits are exhausted, the consumer moves from the private to the public sector). Such dumping has the effect of keeping private sector insurance costs artificially low, while encouraging the development of a large public safety net of mental health services.

The country has disability benefits for persons with mental disorders. Disability entitles one to Federal Supplemental Security Income (SSI) for poor persons and Social Security Disability Insurance (SSDI) for workers and family members. Eligibility for the former results in eligibility for Medicaid; for the latter, eligibility for Medicare.

Mental Health Facilities Mental health is a part of primary health care system. Actual treatment of severe mental disorders is not available at the primary level. There are activities undertaken by the public speciality sector for children and adults.

Regular training of primary care professionals is not carried out in the field of mental health.

There are community care facilities for patients with mental disorders. Community care is organized by states, counties, localities, and private organizations, hence there are variations in the structure and quality of care. The 1950s saw the building of general hospital psychiatric units, outpatient clinics and halfway houses. The 1960s focussed on the philosophy of the least restrictive alternative. Comprehensive treatment became the primary focus of mental health services. Also, there was consolidation of services treatment for drug users, children and in impoverished areas. Case management and assertive community treatment are two relatively new forms of services. Evaluation of services began to be undertaken. Employment programs, travelling teams of professionals and pre-admission programs were developed. The message of the 1980s was that community services needed to be significantly improved for patients. The 1990s saw the U.S. focus shifting back to recidivism in the context of availability of community care. The other large foci of this decade concerned the homeless people who are mentally ill and the evolution of a recovery philosophy for consumer- and family-directed care. The latter focus has become even more pronounced in the first decade of the 21st century.

Psychiatric Beds and Professionals

Total psychiatric beds per 10 000 population	7.7
Psychiatric beds in mental hospitals per 10 000 population	3.1
Psychiatric beds in general hospitals per 10 000 population	1.3
Psychiatric beds in other settings per 10 000 population	3.3
Number of psychiatrists per 100 000 population	13.7
Number of neurosurgeons per 100 000 population	1.6
Number of psychiatric nurses per 100 000 population	6.5
Number of neurologists per 100 000 population	4.5
Number of psychologists per 100 000 population	31.1
Number of social workers per 100 000 population	35.3

There are other mental health professionals like mental health counsellors, psychosocial rehabilitation specialists, school psychologists, marriage and family therapists and pastoral counsellors. Currently, mental health care is provided in several types of settings: by mental health and substance abuse providers (5.9% of all adults are served); by primary care physicians (5.0% of all adults are served); and by social service providers or self-help groups (3.8% of all adults are served) (Manderscheid, et al, 1993). There are at present 4300 mental health organizations in the country. State and county and private mental hospitals and residential treatment centres for emotionally disturbed children form over one-fifth of the total. Mental health service organizations employ about 680 thousand people, with over three-fourth being patient care staff and nearly half qualifying as mental health professionals (Mental Health, United States, 2002).

Non-Governmental Organizations NGOs are involved with mental health in the country. They are mainly involved in advocacy, promotion and prevention.

Information Gathering System There is mental health reporting system in the country. The National Health Interview Survey conducted by the National Centre for Health Statistics collects information on mental disorders in adults and children.

The country has data collection system or epidemiological study on mental health. The data collection system is currently funded by NIMH. The CMHS is responsible for statistical information on mental health populations and services through the National Reporting System.

Programmes for Special Population The country has specific programmes for mental health for minorities, refugees, disaster affected population, indigenous population, elderly and children. CMHS is involved in coordinating relevant services for refugees and disaster-affected populations. Other groups are targeted as part of the SAMHSA Block Grant Programs in mental health and substance abuse. There are special programmes for HIV patients.

SAMHSA CMHS is charged with improving the quality of and access to mental health services, especially for underserved populations and people at greatest risk – adults with serious mental illnesses and children and adolescents with serious emotional disturbances. There are geographic disparities in mental health services delivery; it is particularly difficult to deliver these services in rural areas due in part to shortages of mental health providers. Specific funds were allotted to support demonstration programmes on community support for adults with serious mental illness (including those who were homeless) and to programmes of clinical training focusing on mental health for underserved populations, on HIV/AIDS, the Projects for Assistance in Transition from Homelessness (PATH) programme, the Protection and Advocacy Program, Employment Intervention Demonstration Program, and Comprehensive Community Mental Health Services for Children and Their Families Program. Currently, CMHS programmes are being transformed to address the recommendations of the President's New Freedom Commission on Mental Health.

Therapeutic Drugs The following therapeutic drugs are generally available at the primary health care level of the country: carbamazepine, ethosuximide, phenobarbital, phenytoin sodium, sodium valproate, amitriptyline, chlorpromazine, diazepam, fluphenazine, haloperidol, lithium, biperiden, carbidopa, levodopa.
Data on commonest strength and cost of medicines are based on responses to the 2001 Medical Expenditure Panel Survey (MEPS), a nationally representative sample of households that participated in the National Health Interview Survey, conducted by the National Center for Health Statistics, U.S. Department of Health and Human Services (DHHS). The MEPS is conducted by the Agency for Healthcare Research and Quality, DHHS. This is the mean price reported by consumers in the MEPS sample. The FDA approves all prescription drugs for usage by Americans including psycho-pharmacological agents. Some national data are available on prescription medications through the National Health Interview Survey. Recently, the Food and Drug Administration (FDA) has begun investigating the negative side effects of anti-depressants administered to children and adolescents and has asked manufacturers of all anti-depressant drugs to include in their labelling a boxed warning and expanded warning statements that alert health care providers to an increased risk of suicidality in children and adolescents being treated with these agents and additional information about the results of paediatric studies (http://www.fda.gov/cder/drug/antidepressants/default.htm).

Other Information In 1999, the Surgeon General of the United States issued 'Mental Health: A Report of the Surgeon General' (U.S. Department of Health and Human Services [HHS], 1999), which engaged the American public in a discussion about the importance of mental health and the status of research on services. In 2002, the President of the United States stated strong support for mental health insurance parity. He also signed an Executive Order creating the New Freedom Commission on Mental Health and charged it with issuing a report describing barriers to care within the mental health system, providing examples of successful community-based care models and suggesting ways to fix the problems. Both CMHS and the States are now beginning to implement the recommendations in this report. This effort has been facilitated through the planning requirements of the Community Mental Health Services Block Grant administered by SAMHSA CMHS. Similar planning has been initiated in the private sector around particular mental health benefit plans. Thus, current efforts could be said to reflect planning for particular population segments, without comprehensive planning for all persons in a geographical area. More comprehensive geographically based planning approaches can be expected in the future with the implementation of the recommendations in the President's Report.

Additional Sources of Information

Area Resource File from the Bureau of Health Professions, US Department of Health and Human Services

Arons, B., Searle, T., Sweetman, A., et al (2004) Chapter 1. SAMHSA's Center for Mental Health Services: A Decade of Achievement, 1992-2002. SAMHSA's National Mental Health Information center. (http://www.mentalhealth.samhsa.gov/publications/allpubs/SMA01-3938/Chapter01.asp).

Bloom, J. D., Williams, M. H., Bigelow, D. A.(2000). The forensic psychiatric system in the United States. International Journal of Law and Psychiatry, 23, 605-613.

Center for Mental Health Services (2001). Mental Health, United States, 2000. Eds: R.W. Manderscheid, M.J. Henderson. DHHS Pub No. (SMA) 01-3537. Washington, DC. (http:// www.samhsa.gov).

Department of Health and Human Services (1999) Mental Health: A report of the Surgeon General. DHSS. U.S. Public Health Service. Pittsburgh.

DHSS (2001). Mental Health: Culture, Race and Ethnicity. DHSS. Maryland. (http://www.surgeongeneral.gov/library).

Geller, J. (2000) The last half-century of psychiatric services as reflected in psychiatric services. Psychiatric Services, 51, 41-67.

Feldman, S. (2003) Reflections on the 40th Anniversary of the US Community Mental Health Centres Act. Australian and New Zealand Journal of Psychiatry, 37, 662-667.

Manderscheid, R. W., Henderson, M. J., Witkin, M. J. et al. (2000) The US Mental Health System of the 1990s. The challenges of managed care. International Journal of Law and Psychiatry, 23, 245-259.

Manderscheid, R. W., Rae, D. S., Narrow, W. E., et al (1993) Congruence of service utilization estimates from the epidemiologic catchment area project and other sources. Archives of General Psychiatry, 50, 108-114.

Uruguay

GENERAL INFORMATION

Uruguay is a country with an approximate area of 176 thousand sq. km. (UNO, 2001). Its population is 3.439 million, and the sex ratio (men per hundred women) is 94 (UNO, 2004). The proportion of population under the age of 15 years is 24% (UNO, 2004), and the proportion of population above the age of 60 years is 17% (WHO, 2004). The literacy rate is 97.3% for men and 98.1% for women (UNESCO/MoH, 2004).

The country is a higher middle income group country (based on World Bank 2004 criteria). The proportion of health budget to GDP is 10.9%. The per capita total expenditure on health is 971 international $, and the per capita government expenditure on health is 450 international $ (WHO, 2004).

The life expectancy at birth is 71 years for males and 79.3 years for females (WHO, 2004). The healthy life expectancy at birth is 63 years for males and 69 years for females (WHO, 2004).

EPIDEMIOLOGY

A nation-wide survey of randomly selected households from urban areas (n=2500 subjects in the age range of 15-65 years) showed that the lifetime, 1-year and 1-month prevalence of use of illicit substances (marijuana, cocaine, inhalants, hallucinogens, etc.) was 4.5%, 1.1%, and 0.7%, respectively. The 1-month prevalence rates for nicotine dependence and alcohol abuse, respectively, was 20% and 19.5%. Age and sex were significantly associated with drug use (Miguez & Magri, 1995). Miguez and Magri (1993) used descriptive anthropological methods to assess drug use among youngsters from high social class and found two clearly defined social-cultural patterns with regard to cannabis and cocaine use. Da Costa e Silva and Koifaman (1998) reported on smoking in Latin American countries including Uruguay. Kohn et al (2001) studied emotional and behavioural disorders among children and sought to establish an association between psychological problems in parents and psychiatric problems in children. Children (n=115) in the 5-15 age-groups from three communities (2 urban and 1 rural) were selected and the mothers were asked to answer the Child Psychiatric Morbidity Questionnaire (QMPI). Both the parents also answered questions from Psychiatric Epidemiology Research Interview Demoralization Scale, CAGE, the Social Support Network Inventory and also questions about their self-perceived mental health. 53% of the children had scores greater than 6 on the QMPI, which indicated the possible presence of behavioural or emotional problems. Fathers' self-perception of emotional problems and mothers' feeling of being demoralized were associated with a greater risk of behavioural or emotional problems in their children. Uruguay has the second highest rate of suicide in Latin America, after Cuba. In 1990, the figures were 10.4/100 000 (16.6/100 000 in men and 4.2/100 000 in women) (WHO, 2000).

MENTAL HEALTH RESOURCES

Mental Health Policy A mental health policy is present. The policy was initially formulated in 1986.
The components of the policy are advocacy, promotion, prevention, treatment and rehabilitation. It was revised in 2003 through a consultative process that involved civil servants, mental health professionals and NGOs. There is no regular budget for its implementation and between 25 to 50% of its original content was put into practice.

Substance Abuse Policy A substance abuse policy is present. Details about the year of formulation are not available. There is no regular budget for its implementation and between 25 to 50% of its original content was put into practice.

National Mental Health Programme A national mental health programme is present. The programme was formulated in 1986. It was revised in 2003. There is no regular budget for its implementation and between 25 to 50% of its original content was put into practice. Its main components are strategy of services reform, promotion and prevention, integration of mental health services in primary care and development of specialized services

National Therapeutic Drug Policy/Essential List of Drugs A national therapeutic drug policy/essential list of drugs is present. It was formulated in 1971.

Mental Health Legislation The mental health law was revised in 2003. It has been implemented less than 10%. It focuses on promotion and prevention, human rights, housing, advocacy, but there is no reference to regulation of mental health services, involuntary treatment and admission and discharge procedures.
The latest legislation was enacted in 2002.

Mental Health Financing There are budget allocations for mental health.
The country spends 8% of the total health budget on mental health.
The primary sources of mental health financing in descending order are tax based, private insurances, social insurance and out of pocket expenditure by the patient or family.
Approximately 4.0% of the budget on mental health is spent on general hospitals, 16.0% in psychiatric hospitals, 40.0% in ambulatory clinics and 40.0% in community care.
The country has disability benefits for persons with mental disorders. Chronic psychosis, mental retardation and dementia are the mental health conditions to be considered a disability for getting public disability benefits. The department in charge is B.P.S.

Mental Health Facilities Mental health is a part of primary health care system. Actual treatment of severe mental disorders is available at the primary level. Less than 25 % of the population is covered by this kind of service. Mental health care in primary health care is provided by primary health care doctors, nurses and psychiatrists. A system of referral is in place.
Regular training of primary care professionals is not carried out in the field of mental health.
There are community care facilities for patients with mental disorders. About 34 multidisciplinary units work for community health. The community care system provides services for up to half of the treated population (preventive/promotion interventions, home interventions, family interventions for 25-50% of the intended population and residential facilities and employment programmes for less than 25%). Vocational training is not provided.

Psychiatric Beds and Professionals

Total psychiatric beds per 10 000 population	5.4
Psychiatric beds in mental hospitals per 10 000 population	4.78
Psychiatric beds in general hospitals per 10 000 population	0.62
Psychiatric beds in other settings per 10 000 population	0
Number of psychiatrists per 100 000 population	22.9
Number of neurosurgeons per 100 000 population	
Number of psychiatric nurses per 100 000 population	0.85
Number of neurologists per 100 000 population	
Number of psychologists per 100 000 population	15.1
Number of social workers per 100 000 population	62

There are many other psychologists working in different sectors. 30% of beds are occupied by long stay patients. More than four-fifths of professionals from various mental health disciplines work in the private sector.

Non-Governmental Organizations NGOs are involved with mental health in the country. They are mainly involved in advocacy, promotion and rehabilitation. These organizations participate in mental health activities related to women, children, consumers and domestic violence.

Information Gathering System There is mental health reporting system in the country. ICD-10 is used for recording purposes. The country has data collection system or epidemiological study on mental health. Service data collection system is conducted for part of the mental health system (public sector) at the 'Dirección de Unidades Asistenciales Especializados' de ASSE. An epidemiological study has been carried out since 1998. Currently, the data for the year 2000 is being compiled.

Programmes for Special Population The country has specific programmes for mental health for minorities, disaster affected population, elderly and children.
There are programmes for women and victims of domestic violence. There is also a programme in the area of treatment and rehabilitation of drug abuse and dependence.

Therapeutic Drugs The following therapeutic drugs are generally available at the primary health care level of the country: carbamazepine, sodium valproate, chlorpromazine, diazepam, haloperidol, lithium, biperiden, levodopa.
The national therapeutic drug policy was adopted in 2001 and revised in 2003. The essential drug list was created in 1971 and revised in 2003.

Other Information

Additional Sources of Information

da Costa e Silva V. L., Koifman, S. (1998) Smoking in Latin America: a major public health problem. Cadernos de Saude Publica., 14 (Suppl. 3), 99-108.

Kohn, R., Levav, I., Alterwain, P., et al (2001) Risk factors for behavioral and emotional problems in childhood: a community study in Uruguay. Pan American Journal of Public Health, 9, 211-218.

Miguez, H., Magri, R. (1995) National study of drug habits in Uruguay. Acta Psiquiatrica y Psicologica de America Latina, 41, 13-23.

Miguez, H. A., Magri, R. (1993) Patterns of drug abuse among youngsters of upper social class. Acta Psiquiatrica y Psicologica de America Latina, 39, 294-300.

WHO, Department of Mental Health (2000) Workshop on the Prevention of Suicide

T–Z

Uzbekistan

GENERAL INFORMATION

Uzbekistan is a country with an approximate area of 447 thousand sq. km. (UNO, 2001). Its population is 26.479 million, and the sex ratio (men per hundred women) is 99 (UNO, 2004). The proportion of population under the age of 15 years is 33% (UNO, 2004), and the proportion of population above the age of 60 years is 7% (WHO, 2004). The literacy rate is 99.6% for men and 98.9% for women (UNESCO/MoH, 2004).

The country is a low income group country (based on World Bank 2004 criteria). The proportion of health budget to GDP is 3.6%. The per capita total expenditure on health is 91 international $, and the per capita government expenditure on health is 68 international $ (WHO, 2004).

The main language(s) used in the country is (are) Uzbek, Russian and Tajik. The largest ethnic group(s) is (are) Uzbek. The largest religious group(s) is (are) Muslim (nine-tenths).

The life expectancy at birth is 65.6 years for males and 70.8 years for females (WHO, 2004). The healthy life expectancy at birth is 58 years for males and 61 years for females (WHO, 2004).

EPIDEMIOLOGY

There is a paucity of epidemiological data on mental illnesses in Uzbekistan in internationally accessible literature. Suicide rates in the former USSR during 1984-1990 varied greatly between different regions. They were reported to be 11.8 per 100 000 inhabitants in Central Asia (Kazakhstan, Kirgizia, Turkmenistan, Uzbekistan and Tajikistan) (Wasserman et al, 1998). Danielov (1975) studied clinical and etiological characteristics of 214 children with mental retardation and found that siblings of a subgroup of these children had an increased rate of mental retardation. In a later study on 150 patients, Danielov and Utin (1988) found a high and approximately equal frequency of mild forms of mental retardation among parents and siblings of mentally retarded probands, which confirms a polygenic model of heredity. Both familial and psychological factors appeared to be involved in the formation of mental retardation.

MENTAL HEALTH RESOURCES

Mental Health Policy A mental health policy is present. The policy was initially formulated in 1993.

Normative acts by the Uzbekistan Ministry of Health have established a voluntary basis for treatment. Provision was made for social and legal assistance, protection by the courts, supervision by the prosecution service and legal aid to protect the legal rights and interests of psychiatric patients. With a view to regulating work with psychiatric patients, the Ministry of Health has issued a number of directives: No. 209 (1991) 'Measures to improve psychiatric care for persons below draft age and of draft age' provides for an increase in the number of psychiatrists working with children and adolescents; No. 303/169 (1994) 'Improving measures to prevent socially harmful activities by psychiatric patients' (with Ministry of Internal Affairs); No. 611 (1994) 'Situation of and prospects for the development of legal psychiatry in the Republic of Uzbekistan'; No. 681 (1993) 'Measures to further improve psychiatric care for the population of Uzbekistan', No. 786 (1996) that confirmed 54 regulations and instructions regulating the activity of psychiatric services; No. 458 (1997) 'Measures to ensure the implementation of decision No. 390 of the Cabinet of Ministers of 6 August 1997 (Measures to improve psychiatric care for the population)'; No. 06-9/125 (1998) 'State norms applicable to medical, pharmaceutical and teaching staff and to the kitchen staff of psychiatric hospitals, departments and wards and psychoneurological dispensaries, departments and practices'; No. 559 (1999) 'Improvement of suicide prevention services in the Republic'; and No. 589 (1999) 'Improvement of psychotherapeutic care for the population'. An annex has been included in the Criminal Code of the Republic of Uzbekistan which provides for heavier penalties for those who involve persons suffering from mental disorders in crimes. The mental health care situation is examined annually by the Ministry of Health. In 2003, the transition of psychiatric services to ICD-10 was completed.

Substance Abuse Policy A substance abuse policy is present. The policy was initially formulated in 2000.

National Mental Health Programme A national mental health programme is absent.

A working group has been set up in the Ministry of Health to prepare a draft national programme for mental health. A 'Plan for the development of the state system of prevention, early detection and rehabilitation of children with mental disorders in order to constitute a healthy generation and reduce the level of mental disorders and disabilities among the Republic's children', is also being drafted as a part of national mental health programme.

National Therapeutic Drug Policy/Essential List of Drugs A national therapeutic drug policy/essential list of drugs is present. Details about the year of formulation are not available.

Mental Health Legislation The Cabinet of Ministers has taken a number of decisions that affect mental health: Decree N° 153 (1997) 'Approval of the list of diseases of public health importance and determination of the benefits to which persons suffering from them are entitled'; Decision No. 390 (1997) 'Measures to improve psychiatric care for the population', which provides for a number of improvements to material and technical facilities, manpower availability, drug supply and social protection for patients, and rehabilitative and residential facilities (however, as the decision was not supported by the requisite funding); and Decree No. 532 (1997) 'Improvement of the system for financing preventive and curative services' that made provision for the free supply of drugs to mental health patients under outpatient treatment and dispensed them from payment for food when hospitalized. The

'Law on social protection for the disabled in Uzbekistan' deals with the occupational rehabilitation of disabled persons, including the mentally disabled, while the Tax Code (1997), introduces tax benefits for firms that employ disabled persons. The comprehensive mental health legislation 'On psychiatric care' was adopted in 2000. In 2000 itself, a supplement to the code of civil procedure entitled 'Compulsory hospitalization in psychiatric establishments' was added. The Mental Health Law provides for the protection of the rights and interests of persons suffering from mental disorders.
The latest legislation was enacted in 2000.

Mental Health Financing There are budget allocations for mental health.
The country spends 4.6% of the total health budget on mental health.
The primary sources of mental health financing in descending order are tax based and out of pocket expenditure by the patient or family.
Funding for psychiatric services has been improving gradually and the shortages in food and drug procurement have been covered. Persons suffering from mental disorders are entitled to benefits such as free nursing care and treatment in psychiatric hospitals as well as free provision of special drugs for out-patients. Funding is also available for rehabilitation workshops for persons suffering from mental disorders. These measures have helped in the reduction of mortality among persons with mental disorders by a factor of 1.4 (from 3497 in 1998 to 2548 in 2003).
The country has disability benefits for persons with mental disorders.

Mental Health Facilities Mental health is a part of primary health care system. Actual treatment of severe mental disorders is available at the primary level. Efforts are being made to reinforce primary level psychiatric services. Psychiatrists hold mental health clinics at general purpose disease prevention and treatment centres for children and adults.
Details about training facilities are not available. On account of the shortage of psychiatrists, general practitioners have been authorized to practice as psychiatrists at the primary care level after completion of a three-month course in psychiatry in the Institute of Further Training for Physicians.
Details about community care facilities in mental health are not available.

Psychiatric Beds and Professionals

Total psychiatric beds per 10 000 population	3.1
Psychiatric beds in mental hospitals per 10 000 population	3
Psychiatric beds in general hospitals per 10 000 population	0.1
Psychiatric beds in other settings per 10 000 population	0
Number of psychiatrists per 100 000 population	3.3
Number of neurosurgeons per 100 000 population	0.9
Number of psychiatric nurses per 100 000 population	7.2
Number of neurologists per 100 000 population	5.9
Number of psychologists per 100 000 population	0.05
Number of social workers per 100 000 population	0.1

There has been a two-fold decline in beds in mental health institutions (from 6.2 per 100 000 population in 1991 to 3.1 in 2003), but an increase in general hospital mental health beds. In order to fill vacant district psychiatrist posts (children's, adolescents' and adults'), a Master's in psychiatry was introduced in higher medical education establishments (in addition to internships).
Standards for the diagnosis and treatment of mental disorders have been developed by specialists and implemented in psychiatric establishments.

Non-Governmental Organizations NGOs are involved with mental health in the country. An NGO named 'Sabr' has started two telephone help lines in Samarkand. Currently it has a staff of 15, including a psychologist, a sociologist, a jurist and a gynecologist. With the financial support from the United States Agency for International Development (USAID), the 'Hamdard' help centre has been operating in the capital of Djizak since 1999. The centre has established partnerships with state institutions, law-enforcement agencies, parliamentary committees and with the mass-media on issues of domestic violence prevention; it also runs training courses on legal aid and support for women, including solitary and elderly women. The centre also operates a telephone helpline which offers anonymous advice during crises in order to prevent suicidal behaviour. In 2002, the Association of Psychiatrists and Drug-abuse Specialists registered with the Uzbekistan Ministry of Justice.

Information Gathering System There is mental health reporting system in the country. The Ministry of Health's directives require the submission of reporting forms (Decree N° 10, 2004 – 'Mental and behavioural disorders' and form N° 38 Hlth – 'Report on the work of the Legal-psychiatric expert committee'). Reporting forms from psychiatric institutions are drawn up at the district level and submitted to the area's principal psychiatric administration (oblast or town). Reports from the areas are received and summarized by the Ministry of Health's Organization and Methods Department and submitted to the Ministry's Data Collection and Analysis Centre and to the Ministry of Macroeconomics. Since this year, reporting forms have been completed using two classifications – ICD 9 & 10.

The country has data collection system or epidemiological study on mental health. According to official figures, in 2003, only about 0.01% of those who were registered with hospitals and clinics had emotional disorders including depression. The attributed prevalence in the community (based on figures of those treated between 1991-2003) for schizophrenia was in the range of 0.226% to 0.336%, for mental retardation in the range of 0.441% to 0.518%, and for all mental disorders 1.245% to1.338%.

Programmes for Special Population The country has specific programmes for mental health for disaster affected population and children. The department responsible for dealing with emergencies has a plan setting out measures and clinical and diagnostic standards for outpatient and inpatient emergency psychiatric care for the population, including care during disasters.
When intrauterine foetal disorders are detected, screening centres provide postnatal monitoring for infants by specialized paediatricians and psychiatrists. Since 1998, an 'infant psychiatry service' has been in place. It operates from maternity hospitals, neonatal departments and paediatric departments. The service detects and treats children principally suffering from residual organic diseases of the central nervous system and convulsive syndromes of diverse etiology and 'transfer disorder' during the neonatal and postnatal period.

Therapeutic Drugs The following therapeutic drugs are generally available at the primary health care level of the country: carbamazepine, amitriptyline, chlorpromazine, diazepam, fluphenazine, haloperidol.
Each year, the list of essential drugs, which includes new atypical anti-psychotics (such as Risperidone) is renewed.

Other Information

Additional Sources of Information

Danielov, M. B., Utin, A. V. (1988) Problem of the etiology of undifferentiated oligophrenia. Zhurnal Nevropatologii i Psikhiatrii Imeni S-S-Korsakova, 88, 78-81.

Danielov, M. B. (1975) Empirical risk of oligophrenia in siblings of proband-oligophrenics in populations with high levels of inbreeding. Genetika, 11, 121-127.

Wasserman, D., Varnik, A., Dankowicz, M. (1998) Regional differences in the distribution of suicide in the former Soviet Union during perestroika, 1984-1990. Acta Psychiatrica Scandinavica, Supplement 394, 5-12.

T–Z

Vanuatu

GENERAL INFORMATION

Vanuatu is a country with an approximate area of 12 thousand sq. km. (UNO, 2001). The country is an archipelago of more than 80 islands. Its population is 0.217 million, and the sex ratio (men per hundred women) is 105 (UNO, 2004). The proportion of population under the age of 15 years is 40% (UNO, 2004), and the proportion of population above the age of 60 years is 5% (WHO, 2004). The literacy rate is 57% for men and 48% for women (UNESCO/MoH, 2004).

The country is a lower middle income group country (based on World Bank 2004 criteria). The proportion of health budget to GDP is 3.8%. The per capita total expenditure on health is 107 international $, and the per capita government expenditure on health is 63 international $ (WHO, 2004).

The main language(s) used in the country is (are) Bislama, English and French. The largest ethnic group(s) is (are) Melanesian. The largest religious group(s) is (are) Presbyterian, and the other religious group(s) are (is) Roman Catholic and Anglican.

The life expectancy at birth is 66.4 years for males and 69.1 years for females (WHO, 2004). The healthy life expectancy at birth is 58 years for males and 59 years for females (WHO, 2004).

EPIDEMIOLOGY

There is a paucity of epidemiological data on mental illnesses in Vanuatu in internationally accessible literature.

MENTAL HEALTH RESOURCES

Mental Health Policy A mental health policy is absent.

Substance Abuse Policy A substance abuse policy is absent.

National Mental Health Programme A national mental health programme is absent.

National Therapeutic Drug Policy/Essential List of Drugs A national therapeutic drug policy/essential list of drugs is present. It was formulated in 1999.

There is a sporadic shortage of essential drugs, but they are available in general.

Mental Health Legislation There is no mental health legislation.

Details about the year of enactment of the mental health legislation are not available.

Mental Health Financing There are no budget allocations for mental health.

Details about expenditure on mental health are not available.

The primary sources of mental health financing in descending order are out of pocket expenditure by the patient or family, private insurances, social insurance and tax based.

Details about disability benefits for mental health are not available.

Mental Health Facilities Mental health is not a part of primary health care system. Actual treatment of severe mental disorders is not available at the primary level. Patients are sent to referral hospitals.

Regular training of primary care professionals is not carried out in the field of mental health. In remote areas, nurses, in the absence of doctors, are given special permission to prescribe medicines if given special training in the discipline. However, there is no nurse who is trained in mental health. Ten nurses have been oriented to mental health through a 3-day training programme in mental health arranged by the Ministry of Health in collaboration with WHO.

There are no community care facilities for patients with mental disorders.

Psychiatric Beds and Professionals

Total psychiatric beds per 10 000 population	0.1
Psychiatric beds in mental hospitals per 10 000 population	0
Psychiatric beds in general hospitals per 10 000 population	0.1
Psychiatric beds in other settings per 10 000 population	0
Number of psychiatrists per 100 000 population	0
Number of neurosurgeons per 100 000 population	0
Number of psychiatric nurses per 100 000 population	0
Number of neurologists per 100 000 population	0
Number of psychologists per 100 000 population	0
Number of social workers per 100 000 population	0

There are no specific psychiatric nurses; general nurses handle patients. Only the referral hospital in the capital offers mental health services.

Non-Governmental Organizations NGOs are not involved with mental health in the country. The Vanuatu Women's Centre provides assistance to victims of domestic violence. It also provides telephone and face-to-face counselling and public education. The Centre for Vanuatu Society for the Disabled provides a day care centre for rehabilitation of disabled children including the mentally challenged ones. It is funded by UNICEF and the Christian Blind Mission of Germany. The Foundation for the People of South Pacific Vanuatu has started a mental health project on youth depression and associated violence with public education and peer support networks as the main components. The Wan Smol Theatre group runs a drop-in centre for youth and provides generic counselling services.

Information Gathering System There is mental health reporting system in the country. Mental disorders are usually reported in the health information.
The country has no data collection system or epidemiological study on mental health.

Programmes for Special Population The country has specific programmes for mental health for disaster affected population. There is a Government disaster management department. All essential services are under it.

Therapeutic Drugs The following therapeutic drugs are generally available at the primary health care level of the country: carbamazepine, phenobarbital, phenytoin sodium, sodium valproate, amitriptyline, chlorpromazine, diazepam, fluphenazine, haloperidol, lithium, carbidopa, levodopa.

Other Information There is an extensive network of primary care, child and maternity clinics, which are all linked with a radiotelephone service.

Additional Sources of Information

T–Z

Venezuela

GENERAL INFORMATION

Venezuela is a country with an approximate area of 912 thousand sq. km. (UNO, 2001). Its population is 26.17 million, and the sex ratio (men per hundred women) is 101 (UNO, 2004). The proportion of population under the age of 15 years is 32% (UNO, 2004), and the proportion of population above the age of 60 years is 7% (WHO, 2004). The literacy rate is 93.5% for men and 92.7% for women (UNESCO/MoH, 2004).

The country is a higher middle income group country (based on World Bank 2004 criteria). The proportion of health budget to GDP is 6%. The per capita total expenditure on health is 386 international $, and the per capita government expenditure on health is 240 international $ (WHO, 2004).

The main language(s) used in the country is (are) Spanish. The largest ethnic group(s) is (are) Mestizo, and the other ethnic group(s) are (is) European and African. The largest religious group(s) is (are) Roman Catholic.

The life expectancy at birth is 71 years for males and 76.8 years for females (WHO, 2004). The healthy life expectancy at birth is 62 years for males and 67 years for females (WHO, 2004).

EPIDEMIOLOGY

Molina et al (2000) conducted autopsies on 611 brains. Out of them 39 showed features of dementia, in which features of vascular dementia were prominent in 33 cases, features of Alzheimer disease in 1 patient and unspecifiable features in 5 cases. Baptista and Uzcategui (1993) studied drug use among medical residents (n=191) using a self-administered questionnaire based on the Spanish version of the DIS. The questionnaire showed a high concordance with the clinical diagnoses and the frequencies of lifetime diagnoses were: tobacco dependence (20.9%), alcohol abuse (11%), alcohol dependence (0.5%), drug abuse (1%) and drug dependence (1%). Baptista et al (1994) also administered the Spanish version of the Diagnostic Interview Schedule (DIS-III-A) to undergraduate medical (n=1013) and pharmacy students (n=426). Substance use disorders were more common in single males. Seale et al (2002) used the Alcohol Use Disorders Identification Test (AUDIT) to interview a randomly selected community sample of indigenous people (n=105) and found that 98% of men and 53% of women had consumed alcohol at some point in their life with 94% of men and 26% of women reporting that they had used it in the last year. Almost 86.5% of men and 7.5% of women were identified as problem drinkers (cut-off score of 8 on AUDIT). Fuentes et al (1998) examined 148 subjects who had entered the emergency room due to lesions caused by aggression, accidents or intoxication and found that one in every four hospital admission for trauma was related to alcohol or drug abuse. A community study utilizing the Self-Rating Depression Scale by Zung (n=3218) found definite clinical depression among 36.8% of the sample (Eblen et al, 1990). Morillo et al (2002) used questionnaires to study erectile dysfunction in men above 40 years of age in Colombia, Ecuador and Venezuela (n=1946) and found that the age-adjusted prevalence of minimal, moderate and complete ED for all three countries was 53.4%, with 19.8% of all men reporting moderate to complete ED. Age was the variable most strongly linked to ED. Comorbid medical conditions like hypertension, prostrate hyperplasia and diabetes and the medications used to treat these conditions were associated with the prevalence of ED. Neehall and Beharry (1993) conducted a 10 month assessment of psychiatric referrals in a hospital. The study revealed that parasuicide was the commonest cause for referral (68%). The commonest disorders were adjustment problems (41%), depression (23%), alcohol dependence (5%) and schizophrenia (5%).

MENTAL HEALTH RESOURCES

Mental Health Policy A mental health policy is present. The policy was initially formulated in 1991.
The components of the policy are promotion, prevention, treatment and rehabilitation. It was revised in 1999. Funds for its implementation have not been earmarked; and between 25 to 50% of its original content has been put into practice.

Substance Abuse Policy A substance abuse policy is present. The policy was initially formulated in 1986. It was revised in 2002. It has a specific budget for its implementation, and is implemented to the extent of 25 to 50%.

National Mental Health Programme A national mental health programme is present. The programme was formulated in 1990. It was revised in 1999. There is no specific budget for its implementation, and it has been implemented to the extent of 10 to 25% by regional authorities. Its main components are strategy of services reform, promotion and prevention, integration of mental health services with primary care and development of specialized services.

National Therapeutic Drug Policy/Essential List of Drugs A national therapeutic drug policy/essential list of drugs is present. It was formulated in 2002.

Mental Health Legislation There is a new code under consideration by the legislature that includes promotion and prevention, human rights, regulation of mental health services, regulation of involuntary treatment, regulation of mental health services, admission and discharge procedures, advocacy and housing.
Details about the year of enactment of the mental health legislation are not available.

Mental Health Financing There are no budget allocations for mental health.
Details about expenditure on mental health are not available.
The primary sources of mental health financing in descending order are tax based, social insurance, out of pocket expenditure by the patient or family and private insurances.
The country has disability benefits for persons with mental disorders. All mental disorders that are associated with severe impairment are considered a disability for getting public disability benefits. Between 25 to 50% of the eligible persons actually receive the benefits. Disability assessment is performed by a multidisciplinary team organized by the Social Security Institute of Venezuela, Instituto Venezolano de los Seguros Sociales (IVSS), which is also responsible for granting disability benefits.

Mental Health Facilities Mental health is a part of primary health care system. Actual treatment of severe mental disorders is not available at the primary level. Less than 25 % of the population is covered by this kind of service. Mental health care is provided by primary health care physicians.
Regular training of primary care professionals is not carried out in the field of mental health.
There are no community care facilities for patients with mental disorders. However, there are some isolated community care facilities in Merida and Guarico states.

Psychiatric Beds and Professionals

Total psychiatric beds per 10 000 population	2.5
Psychiatric beds in mental hospitals per 10 000 population	0.29
Psychiatric beds in general hospitals per 10 000 population	2.23
Psychiatric beds in other settings per 10 000 population	
Number of psychiatrists per 100 000 population	24
Number of neurosurgeons per 100 000 population	
Number of psychiatric nurses per 100 000 population	
Number of neurologists per 100 000 population	
Number of psychologists per 100 000 population	
Number of social workers per 100 000 population	

Country-wide data for personnel is difficult to assess. About 46.5% of beds are occupied by long-stay patients.

Non-Governmental Organizations NGOs are involved with mental health in the country. They are mainly involved in advocacy, promotion, prevention, treatment and rehabilitation. These organizations participate in mental health activities related to women, children, consumers and domestic violence. NGOs are responsible for 30% of all the mental health related activities in Venezuela. Their emphasis is on promotion/prevention and treatment of drug users and victims of domestic violence.

Information Gathering System There is mental health reporting system in the country. ICD-10 criteria are used for recording purposes.
The country has data collection system or epidemiological study on mental health. The epidemiology general department, Dirección General de Epidemiología, is in charge of the data collection system for mental disorders. A service data collection system is conducted for all the mental health system. There is special emphasis in the area of drug abuse.

Programmes for Special Population The country has specific programmes for mental health for disaster affected population and children. There is a National Institute of Child Psychiatry. Due to the disaster of 1999, the plan for psychosocial care and rehabilitation was implemented for victims of disaster.
Also, there are programmes for women and victims of domestic violence.

Therapeutic Drugs The following therapeutic drugs are generally available at the primary health care level of the country: carbamazepine, phenobarbital, phenytoin sodium, diazepam, fluphenazine, haloperidol, lithium.
At present, the essential drug list is being revised to include SSRI's, newer anti-psychotics and other drugs.

Other Information

Additional Sources of Information

Baptista, T., Novoa, D., Hernandez, R., et al (1994) Substance use among Venezuelan medical and pharmacy students. Drug & Alcohol Dependence, 34, 121-127.

Baptista, T., Uzcategui, E. (1993) Substance use among resident doctors in Venezuela. Drug & Alcohol Dependence, 32, 127-132.

Eblen, A.,Vivas, V., Garcia, J. (1990) Prevalence of depression syndrome and its relationship with socioeconomic factors in a population of Valencia City, Carabobo State, Venezuela. Acta Cientifica Venezolana, 41, 250-254.

Fuentes, S. P. D., Medina-Orozco, E., Rojas, M. (1998) Drug consumption prevalence in adult patients attending the emergency room. Salud Publica de Mexico, 40, 234-240.

T–Z

Levine, P. (1996) Developing a community mental health program in the Venezuelan Andes: implications for the international psychosocial rehabilitation. Psychiatric Rehabilitation Journal 19, 23-32.

Molina, O., Cardozo, D., Cardozo, J., et al (2000) Causes of dementia in Maracaibo, Venezuela: a re-evaluation. Revista de Neurologia, 30, 115-117.

Morillo, L.E., Diaz, J., Estevez, E., et al (2002) Prevalence of erectile dysfunction in Colombia, Ecuador, and Venezuela: a population-based study (DENSA). International Journal of Impotence Research, 14, 10-18.

Neehall, J., Beharry, N. (1993) The pattern of in-patient psychiatric referrals in a general hospital. West Indian Medical Journal, 42, 155-157.

Salud Publica de Mexico (2001) 43, 9-16.

Seale, J. P., Seale, J. D., Alvarado, M., et al (2002) Prevalence of problem drinking in a Venezuelan Native American population. Alcohol & Alcoholism, 37, 198-204.

Viet Nam

GENERAL INFORMATION

Viet Nam is a country with an approximate area of 332 thousand sq. km. (UNO, 2001). Its population is 82.481 million, and the sex ratio (men per hundred women) is 99 (UNO, 2004). The proportion of population under the age of 15 years is 30% (UNO, 2004), and the proportion of population above the age of 60 years is 7% (WHO, 2004). The literacy rate is 93.9% for men and 86.9% for women (UNESCO/MoH, 2004).

The country is a low income group country (based on World Bank 2004 criteria). The proportion of health budget to GDP is 5.1%. The per capita total expenditure on health is 134 international $, and the per capita government expenditure on health is 38 international $ (WHO, 2004).

The main language(s) used in the country is (are) Vietnamese. The largest ethnic group(s) is (are) Vietnamese. The largest religious group(s) is (are) Mahayana Buddhist, and the other religious group(s) are (is) Theravada Buddhist.

The life expectancy at birth is 67.1 years for males and 72.2 years for females (WHO, 2004). The healthy life expectancy at birth is 60 years for males and 63 years for females (WHO, 2004).

EPIDEMIOLOGY

McKelvey et al (1993) studied a cohort of 161 Vietnamese Amerasians in Vietnam awaiting settlement in the USA. Ninety-five members of the original cohort were reassessed in Philippines. The researchers used Felsman's 35-item Personal Information Form and the Hopkins Symptom Checklist-25 and found a significant relationship between number of risk factors identified in Viet Nam and symptoms, especially depression, in the Philippines. In a replication sample consisting of 147 Vietnamese Amerasians awaiting relocation, Webb et al (1997) found that the number of risk factors was linearly related to symptoms of both depression and anxiety. There was a decrease in depression and anxiety between the camps in Viet Nam and Philippines. However, these changes were not related to changes in refugee camp conditions or social support within the camp (McKelvey & Webb, 1997a). McKelvey and Webb (1996) found that the prevalence rate of DSM-III psychiatric disorders among Vietnamese Amerasians prior to migration from Viet Nam was lower than previously reported among Vietnamese refugees in the United States and Australia. McKelvey and Webb (1997b) also compared levels of psychological distress in a pre-migratory sample of Vietnamese Amerasians with those in a like-aged, non-migratory sample of Vietnamese living in Ho Chi Minh City, Viet Nam. Subjects were assessed using two measures developed and validated for Vietnamese clinical populations in the United States: the Hopkins Symptom Checklist-25 and the Vietnamese Depression Scale. Amerasians had significantly higher symptom levels on the depression scale of the Hopkins Symptom Checklist-25 but not on the other measures utilized. Amerasians' higher levels of depressive symptoms could reflect their traumatic lives in Viet Nam, but may also reflect acute situational factors or selection bias. Loughry and Flouri (2001) studied emotional and behavioural problems in two groups of children and young adults without parents aged 10-22 years – those who had been repatriated to Viet Nam from camps in Hong Kong and South-East Asia and those who had always remained in Viet Nam. The researchers interviewed 455 subjects of which 238 were refugees using the Achenbach Youth Self-Report, the Cowen Perceived Self-Efficacy scale, a Social Support scale as well as an Exposure to Trauma scale. Results showed that there was no significant difference between the two groups of children on the YSR total score. The former refugee children had significantly lower externalizing scores and failed marginally to report significantly higher internalizing scores than the local children. A significant interaction between the immigration status of the children and the children's subjective perception of their current standard of living explained the differences in the YSR. The study showed that the perceived self-efficacy, number of social supports and experience of social support did not differ between the two groups of children. The authors failed to find any difference in emotional or behavioural pattern among the two groups. There are a large number of studies on Vietnamese refugees settled in different developed countries and on Viet Nam War Veterans. Such studies have not been included in the present discussion. Studies on refugees settled in low-and middle-income countries have been included under the relevant section of those countries.

MENTAL HEALTH RESOURCES

Mental Health Policy A mental health policy is absent.

In 2002, a 'Decision from the Prime Minister' provided for the 'Ratification of the Programme for some Non-Communicable Disease for 2002-2010', which includes mental disorders (epilepsy, depression). Schizophrenia had been included in the priority list of community health programmes earlier. It focuses on prevention and treatment, integration of services at the level of primary care, relevant health education and workforce development at this level and intersectoral collaboration.

Substance Abuse Policy A substance abuse policy is present. The policy was initially formulated in 1993.

National Mental Health Programme A national mental health programme is present. The programme was formulated in 1999. A mental health programme is one of the ten objectives listed in the National Health Programme.

National Therapeutic Drug Policy/Essential List of Drugs A national therapeutic drug policy/essential list of drugs is present. It was formulated in 1980.

Medications approved by the Ministry of Health for people with schizophrenia and epilepsy are routinely available and are free. Medications for other conditions may or may not be available and would not be free.

Mental Health Legislation There is no mental health legislation.
Details about the year of enactment of the mental health legislation are not available.

Mental Health Financing There are budget allocations for mental health.
Details about expenditure on mental health are not available.
The primary sources of mental health financing in descending order are out of pocket expenditure by the patient or family, tax based, social insurance and private insurances.
The Government limits financing to those patients suffering from schizophrenia and epilepsy. For other mental disorders, the patients' families are required to pay for treatment.
The country has disability benefits for persons with mental disorders. Benefits are given by Ministry of Social-Invalid-Labour.

Mental Health Facilities Mental health is a part of primary health care system. Actual treatment of severe mental disorders is available at the primary level. Primary care is provided for maintenance and rehabilitation. Traditional medicines are routinely used for treatment.
Regular training of primary care professionals is not carried out in the field of mental health. All district hospitals and commune health stations have general practitioners. Mental health training for primary care providers has been provided in 7% of communities. A six-month training is provided to the district level physicians and a one-week training to the commune level physicians.
There are community care facilities for patients with mental disorders. Community based mental health care is integrated in the primary care system. Effective psychosocial rehabilitation is still to develop. Proper integration of different facilities is lacking. There is an experimental outpatient psychiatric rehabilitation project funded by the Ha Noi Health Services at one particular hospital. A 50-bed day care/night care psychiatric hospital has been opened. Apart from clinical (e.g. administration of medication on site) and rehabilitative functions (e.g. basic living skills) it has an important training and public education function. Besides this, up to 2-3 patients are allowed to stay overnight if they are in crisis. This helps in prevention/postponement of hospitalization. Three other day care clinics have been established. These clinics are run by district health physicians and nurses who have undergone mental health training under the supervision of psychiatrists. These facilities also cater to children. The health sub-committee of the commune people's committee are informed of the problems in health care follow-up and it plays an active role in convincing families to cooperate with treatment. General physicians either visit patients at their homes or receive these patients at the health centres. There is a monetary incentive for every patient that they attend to.

Psychiatric Beds and Professionals

Total psychiatric beds per 10 000 population	0.63
Psychiatric beds in mental hospitals per 10 000 population	0.59
Psychiatric beds in general hospitals per 10 000 population	0.04
Psychiatric beds in other settings per 10 000 population	0
Number of psychiatrists per 100 000 population	0.32
Number of neurosurgeons per 100 000 population	0.03
Number of psychiatric nurses per 100 000 population	0.3
Number of neurologists per 100 000 population	0.13
Number of psychologists per 100 000 population	0.06
Number of social workers per 100 000 population	0

Most of the personnel work in institutes or hospitals in bigger cities. Out of the 64 provinces and cities in the country, 47 have a psychiatric department in a general hospital and 29 have a psychiatric hospital. However, the level of services and access fall as one moves from province to district to community. Care for chronic patients, including for substance abuse problems is also provided by the Ministry of Labour, Employment and Social Affairs (MOLESA), which provides for about 2000 beds. There are 45 forensic psychiatry beds. Some beds are earmarked for women. There are 2 child and adolescent psychiatrists in the country.

Non-Governmental Organizations NGOs are not involved with mental health in the country. Social organizations like the youth union, the women's union and the union of farmers organize public information sessions twice a month to help families take care of their patients and help the medical staff protect the health of the people. Family associations or clubs exist in big cities.

Information Gathering System There is mental health reporting system in the country.
The country has data collection system or epidemiological study on mental health. Data collection is one of the activities of the national programme of mental health since 1999.

Programmes for Special Population The country has specific programmes for mental health for elderly. There are no special services available.

There is a 20-bedded inpatient child psychiatry unit. This centre also provides outpatient and day care facilities. Child mental health services in a few other cities consist of outpatient and day care centres. The Ministry of Education conducts a health promotion programme in schools where life skills education is provided to children and adolescents. Local women's and youth unions play a role in the psychosocial rehabilitation of adolescents with drug abuse and conduct disorders under the supervision of the district nurse. The Government Programme for drug abuse is under the Ministry of Labour, Invalids and Social Affairs (MOLISA). The MOLISA runs drug abuse treatment services that are not integrated with the general health system. The United Nations International Drug Control Programme (2001-2010) aims at control in supply and demand reduction. This programme is being undertaken with the Youth Union Drugs Project.

Therapeutic Drugs The following therapeutic drugs are generally available at the primary health care level of the country: carbamazepine, phenobarbital, phenytoin sodium, sodium valproate, amitriptyline, chlorpromazine, diazepam, fluphenazine, haloperidol, lithium, biperiden, carbidopa, levodopa.

Other Information Psychiatry was identified as a separate speciality of medicine in 1970. The Russian classificatory system of mental disorders was replaced by ICD system only in 1980.

Additional Sources of Information

Lambert, T., McKenzie, D., Pennella, J. et al (1999) The influence of client's ethnicity on psychotropic medication management in community mental health services. Australian and New Zealand Journal of Psychiatry, 33, 882-88.

Loughry, M., Flouri, E. (2001) The behavioral and emotional problems of former unaccompanied refugee children 3-4 years after their return to Vietnam. Child Abuse & Neglect, 25, 249-263.

McKelvey, R., Sang, D., Tu, H. (1997) Is there a role for child psychiatry in Vietnam? Australian and New Zealand Journal of Psychiatry, 31, 114-119.

McKelvey, R. S., Webb, J. A., Mao, A. R. (1993) Premigratory risk factors in Vietnamese Amerasians. American Journal of Psychiatry, 150, 470-473.

McKelvey, R. S., Webb, J. A., Strobel, R. M. (1996) The prevalence of psychiatric disorders among Vietnamese Amerasians: a pilot study. American Journal of Orthopsychiatry, 66, 409-415.

McKelvey, R. S., Webb, J. A. (1997a) A prospective study of psychological distress related to refugee camp experience. Australian & New Zealand Journal of Psychiatry, 31, 549-554.

McKelvey, R. S., Webb, J. A. (1997b) Comparative levels of psychological distress in a pre-migratory refugee population. Australian & New Zealand Journal of Psychiatry, 31, 543-548.

Webb, J. A., McKelvey, R. S., Strobel, R. (1997) Replication and extension of a risk profile for Amerasian youth. Journal of Traumatic Stress, 10, 645-654.

Yemen

GENERAL INFORMATION

Yemen is a country with an approximate area of 528 thousand sq. km. (UNO, 2001). Its population is 20.732 million, and the sex ratio (men per hundred women) is 103 (UNO, 2004). The proportion of population under the age of 15 years is 48% (UNO, 2004), and the proportion of population above the age of 60 years is 4% (WHO, 2004). The literacy rate is 69.5% for men and 28.5% for women (UNESCO/MoH, 2004).

The country is a low income group country (based on World Bank 2004 criteria). The proportion of health budget to GDP is 4.5%. The per capita total expenditure on health is 69 international $, and the per capita government expenditure on health is 24 international $ (WHO, 2004).

The main language(s) used in the country is (are) Arabic. The largest ethnic group(s) is (are) Arab. The largest religious group(s) is (are) Muslim.

The life expectancy at birth is 58.7 years for males and 62.2 years for females (WHO, 2004). The healthy life expectancy at birth is 48 years for males and 51 years for females (WHO, 2004).

EPIDEMIOLOGY

There is a paucity of epidemiological data on mental illnesses in Yemen in internationally accessible literature. Hassan et al (2002) assessed the effect of khat chewing on mood symptoms in 200 healthy volunteers in a hospital. They used the Hospital Anxiety and Depression Scale to assess symptoms in khat chewing and abstinent arms. More mood symptoms were reported by the group that continued to chew khat.

MENTAL HEALTH RESOURCES

Mental Health Policy A mental health policy is present. The policy was initially formulated in 1986.
The components of the policy are promotion, prevention, treatment and rehabilitation.

Substance Abuse Policy A substance abuse policy is absent.

National Mental Health Programme A national mental health programme is present. The programme was formulated in 1983. The goals of the programme are integration of mental health services into primary care, initiating a school health programme, increasing the number of psychiatric beds in hospitals and providing training facilities.

National Therapeutic Drug Policy/Essential List of Drugs A national therapeutic drug policy/essential list of drugs is present. It was formulated in 1986.

Mental Health Legislation There is no mental health legislation. Islamic laws are used for people with mental illness.
Details about the year of enactment of the mental health legislation are not available.

Mental Health Financing There are budget allocations for mental health.
Details about expenditure on mental health are not available.
The primary sources of mental health financing in descending order are out of pocket expenditure by the patient or family and tax based.
The country has disability benefits for persons with mental disorders. Monthly social benefits may be given to some mentally ill patients.

Mental Health Facilities Mental health is a part of primary health care system. Actual treatment of severe mental disorders is available at the primary level. Primary care is available in some areas only.
Regular training of primary care professionals is carried out in the field of mental health. In the last two years, about 150 personnel were provided training. Medical officers and health workers from rural health facilities and district hospitals and general physicians were trained. Regular in-service training is being provided to nurses.
There are no community care facilities for patients with mental disorders. A community psychiatric care demonstration project has been set up with the help of WHO.

Psychiatric Beds and Professionals

Total psychiatric beds per 10 000 population	1.85
Psychiatric beds in mental hospitals per 10 000 population	1.1
Psychiatric beds in general hospitals per 10 000 population	0.4
Psychiatric beds in other settings per 10 000 population	0.35
Number of psychiatrists per 100 000 population	0.5
Number of neurosurgeons per 100 000 population	0.06
Number of psychiatric nurses per 100 000 population	0.09
Number of neurologists per 100 000 population	0.08
Number of psychologists per 100 000 population	1.2
Number of social workers per 100 000 population	0.04

Some beds have been earmarked for women. The number of beds in prison psychiatric wards have been reduced by two-thirds and psychiatric patients are separated from other inmates in the prison.

Non-Governmental Organizations NGOs are involved with mental health in the country. They are mainly involved in treatment and rehabilitation. The International Committee of the Red Cross has helped in the provision of services and reform in prison psychiatric wards.

Information Gathering System There is mental health reporting system in the country. It is included in the 5 years plan of health reporting.
The country has no data collection system or epidemiological study on mental health.
Rehabilitation centres for mentally challenged individuals are available.

Programmes for Special Population The country has specific programmes for mental health for refugees. There is a mental hospital for women in Sanaa.

Therapeutic Drugs The following therapeutic drugs are generally available at the primary health care level of the country: carbamazepine, phenobarbital, sodium valproate, amitriptyline, chlorpromazine, diazepam, haloperidol.
Yemen follows the WHO Essential Drug List.

Other Information Mental health services were practically non-existent before 1966 and patients used to be kept in prisons. Since then, a lot of improvement has occurred. Hospitals have been built, training provided to different personnel at all levels of care and the administration has been educated about psychiatric illnesses. Different NGOs and WHO helped in building the infrastructure. However, there are some difficulties in the form of inadequate financial support or poor follow-up facilities that have slowed down the implementation of the mental health programme.

Additional Sources of Information

Hassan, N. A., Gunaid, A. A., El Khally, F. M., et al (2002) The effect of chewing Khat leaves on human mood. Saudi Medical Journal, 23, 850-853.

Zambia

GENERAL INFORMATION

Zambia is a country with an approximate area of 753 thousand sq. km. (UNO, 2001). Its population is 10.924 million, and the sex ratio (men per hundred women) is 99 (UNO, 2004). The proportion of population under the age of 15 years is 47% (UNO, 2004), and the proportion of population above the age of 60 years is 5% (WHO, 2004). The literacy rate is 86.3% for men and 73.8% for women (UNESCO/MoH, 2004).

The country is a low income group country (based on World Bank 2004 criteria). The proportion of health budget to GDP is 5.7%. The per capita total expenditure on health is 52 international $, and the per capita government expenditure on health is 27 international $ (WHO, 2004).

The main language(s) used in the country is (are) English. The largest religious group(s) is (are) Christian, and the other religious group(s) are (is) Muslim and Hindu.

The life expectancy at birth is 39.1 years for males and 40.2 years for females (WHO, 2004). The healthy life expectancy at birth is 35 years for males and 35 years for females (WHO, 2004).

EPIDEMIOLOGY

Wapnick et al (1972) reviewed psychiatric diagnoses of a group of female patients admitted in a hospital over 2 consecutive years. The common diagnoses recorded were: depression (26% and 42%) and schizophrenia (14% and 21%). The diagnosis of acute transient psychoses was rare. Kwalambota (2002) assessed the mental health of pregnant women with HIV. 85% of women, who were diagnosed to have HIV during the index hospitalization, showed major depressive episodes and had significant suicidal thoughts, and about 60% showed signs of somatic illness. Those who knew their HIV status before becoming pregnant did not show severe depressive episodes during the index hospitalization but were anxious about the HIV status of their babies. Dhadphale and Shaikh (1983) described an outbreak of epidemic hysteria which was triggered off by a group of girls who were having educational and emotional problems prior to the epidemic. A change in the administrative policy of rigidly segregating the genders apparently prepared an emotionally charged background for the rapid spread of the illness. Rwegellera (1978) examined the records of all suicides and of all open verdicts in Lusaka (Zambia) over a 5-year period. The following suicide rates (per 100 000 of the population per annum) were found: 7.4 for all races (11.3 for males and 3.0 for females), 6.9 for Africans (11.2 for males and 2.2 for females), 12.8 for all Africans above the age of 14 years, and 20.9 for European (20.7 for males and 21.0 for females). In the African population, suicide was associated with gender (males committed suicide five times more often) and age. Hanging was the most common method of suicide by Africans. There was no definite seasonal variation and mental illness and physical diseases were important precipitating factors of suicide. Lin and Ebrahim (1991) studied behaviour patterns among 210 primary school children in the age group of 8-12 years using the Teacher's Rutter Scale and interviews of mothers. The frequency of behaviour disorder was 14.8%with a sex ratio of 1.9:1 (boy:girl). Behaviour disorder was largely associated with the type of school, socio-economic status, mother's occupation, play facilities at home and past history of hospitalization.

MENTAL HEALTH RESOURCES

Mental Health Policy A mental health policy is present. The policy was initially formulated in 2004.
The policy is in the draft form.

Substance Abuse Policy A substance abuse policy is present. The policy was initially formulated in 1998.

National Mental Health Programme A national mental health programme is absent.
It is being formulated using the WHO's Public Mental Health Programme. Priorities for mental health services were outlined by the Ministry of Health in 1979.

National Therapeutic Drug Policy/Essential List of Drugs A national therapeutic drug policy/essential list of drugs is present. It was formulated in 1999.
Psychotropics are in short supply.

Mental Health Legislation The Mental Disorders Act is old and there is a new draft bill.
The latest legislation was enacted in 1951.

Mental Health Financing There are no budget allocations for mental health.
Details about expenditure on mental health are not available.
The primary sources of mental health financing in descending order are tax based, out of pocket expenditure by the patient or family, private insurances and social insurance.
Funds for mental health have been through the basket funds under the Sector Wide Approach.
The country does not have disability benefits for persons with mental disorders. There is a National Disability Act and a National Disability Fund that is available for all persons with disability. However, patients hardly access them. patients who retire on medical grounds are given full benefits. However, it is difficult for the families to receive the benefits due to a shortage of funds.

Mental Health Facilities Mental health is a part of primary health care system. Actual treatment of severe mental disorders is available at the primary level. District hospitals have psychiatric outpatient facilities, and the psychotropic situation has improved in the recent past.
Regular training of primary care professionals is carried out in the field of mental health. In the last two years, about 100 personnel were provided training. Referral system is still a challenge. There is little communication between traditional and orthodox medicine. However, there is good communication between the Ministry of Health and the Mental Health Association, an NGO.
There are community care facilities for patients with mental disorders. Psychiatric units are present in 7 provincial general hospitals. They are managed by clinical officers. Community care is not well developed and is under threat due to the lack of funds. It was started as a pilot project in one particular district with the help of outside funds.

Psychiatric Beds and Professionals

Total psychiatric beds per 10 000 population	0.5
Psychiatric beds in mental hospitals per 10 000 population	0.17
Psychiatric beds in general hospitals per 10 000 population	0.18
Psychiatric beds in other settings per 10 000 population	0.07
Number of psychiatrists per 100 000 population	0.02
Number of neurosurgeons per 100 000 population	0.03
Number of psychiatric nurses per 100 000 population	5
Number of neurologists per 100 000 population	0
Number of psychologists per 100 000 population	0.04
Number of social workers per 100 000 population	0.04

There is a critical shortage of mental health providers. Clinical officers carry out most of the clinical work in psychiatry. They work independently and are registered by the Medical Council of Zambia. And for Zambia, with only one psychiatrist in Government practice, the clinical officers form the backbone of psychiatric practice. There are 154 secure beds for forensic patients. Considering the severe shortage of mental health professionals at all levels, plans are under way to reintroduce pre-service training for primary care professionals in mental health. Many nurses are being recruited for the British NHS.

Non-Governmental Organizations NGOs are involved with mental health in the country. They are mainly involved in advocacy, promotion, prevention and rehabilitation.

Information Gathering System There is mental health reporting system in the country. The mental health reporting system requires to be reviewed to meet the challenges of the health reform programme. Although psychiatric facilities keep records of mental disorders, the ICD 10 criteria has been replaced by the country specific Health Information Management System (HMIS) which limits all types of mental illnesses under one category of 'mental disorders' causing concern among mental health professionals.
The country has data collection system or epidemiological study on mental health. Data are compiled at the main psychiatric hospital and psychiatric units in all provincial general hospitals.
All mental illness together form one rubric.

Programmes for Special Population There are no special programmes.
With the approval of the mental health policy, expectations are high for the development of programmes. Refugees had a trauma programme through UNHCR. The country successfully participated in the two-year WHO-UNDP global initiative on the primary prevention of substance abuse among the young. Currently, it is involved in the five-year Southern African Development Community Network on Drug Use Project.

Therapeutic Drugs The following therapeutic drugs are generally available at the primary health care level of the country: carbamazepine, phenobarbital, phenytoin sodium, sodium valproate, amitriptyline, chlorpromazine, diazepam, fluphenazine, haloperidol, lithium.
The newer anti-psychotics like pimozide are not available. Benzhexol (2mg) is used.

Other Information The overall state of mental health is not adequate from the human resources and services point of view. Health sector reforms in the early 1990s led to downgrading of mental health services. Zambia participated in the European Commission funded Concerted Action Report on Methods for Intervention in Mental Health in Sub-Saharan Africa coordinated by South Bank University of London from 1997-2000.

Additional Sources of Information

Dhadphale, M., Shaikh, S. P. (1983) Epidemic hysteria in a Zambian school: "the mysterious madness of Mwinilunga". British Journal of Psychiatry, 142, 85-88.

Gleisner J. (2002). What causes more destruction, AIDS or aid? Psychiatry in Zambia. Australasian Psychiatry, 10, 166-167.

Kwalombota, M. (2002) The effect of pregnancy in HIV-infected women. AIDS Care, 14, 431-433.

Lin, Y. Q., Ebrahim, G. J., et al (1991) Frequency of behaviour disorder and related factors in school children in Lusaka. Journal of Tropical Pediatrics, 37, 303-309.

Mayeya, J., Chazulwa, R., Mayeya, P.N., et al. (2004) Zambia mental health country profile. International Review of Psychiatry, 16, 63-72.

Rwegellera, G. G., Mambwe, C. C. (1977) Diagnostic classification of first-ever admissions to Chainama Hills Hospital, Lusaka, Zambia. British Journal of Psychiatry, 130, 573-580.

Wapnick, S., Castle, W., Nicholle, D., et al (1972) Cigarette smoking, alcohol and cancer of the oesophagus. South African Medical Journal, 46, 2023-2026.

Zimbabwe

GENERAL INFORMATION

Zimbabwe is a country with an approximate area of 391 thousand sq. km. (UNO, 2001). Its population is 12.932 million, and the sex ratio (men per hundred women) is 99 (UNO, 2004). The proportion of population under the age of 15 years is 42% (UNO, 2004), and the proportion of population above the age of 60 years is 5% (WHO, 2004). The literacy rate is 93.8% for men and 86.3% for women (UNESCO/MoH, 2004).

The country is a low income group country (based on World Bank 2004 criteria). The proportion of health budget to GDP is 6.2%. The per capita total expenditure on health is 142 international $, and the per capita government expenditure on health is 64 international $ (WHO, 2004).

The main language(s) used in the country is (are) English, Ndebele and Shona. The largest religious group(s) is (are) Christian, and the other religious group(s) are (is) indigenous groups.

The life expectancy at birth is 37.7 years for males and 38 years for females (WHO, 2004). The healthy life expectancy at birth is 34 years for males and 33 years for females (WHO, 2004).

EPIDEMIOLOGY

Patel et al (1997, 1998) and Todd et al (1999) developed the Shona Symptom Questionnaire to measure prevalence of common mental disorders (CMD) among African populations. In an unmatched case-control study, they assessed a cohort of 199 cases with CMD recruited from primary health care facilities, traditional practitioners, general practitioners and 197 controls. CMD was significantly associated with female gender, older age, chronicity of illness, number of presenting complaints, beliefs in 'thinking too much' and witchcraft as a causal model, economic impoverishment, infertility, recent unemployment, an unhappy childhood for females, disability, and consultations with traditional medical practitioners and religious priests. The cohort was reassessed after 2 and 12 month. Of the 134 subjects interviewed at both follow-up points, 49% had recovered by 2 months and remained well at 12 months while 28% were persistent cases at both 2 and 12 months. Higher scores on the instrument, a psychological illness model, bereavement and disability predicted a poor outcome at both times. Poorer outcome at 2 month follow-up was associated with belief in witch-craft and an unhappy childhood. Caseness at follow-up was associated with disability and economic deprivation. Onset of new episodes of CMD was recorded in 16% at 2 and 12 months. Higher psychological morbidity scores at recruitment, death of a first-degree relative and disability predicted the onset of CMD at both follow-up points. While female gender and economic difficulties predicted onset at 2 months, belief in supernatural causation was strongly predictive of CMD at 12 months. Caseness at both follow-up points was associated with economic problems and disability. Patel et al (1999) reanalysed five epidemiological data sets from four low to middle income countries (India, Zimbabwe, Chile and Brazil). In all five studies, female gender, low education and poverty were strongly associated with common mental disorders. Broadhead and Abas (1998) found depression and anxiety in 30.8% of 172 randomly selected women in a township. Assessment with the Zimbabwean modification of the Bedford College Life Events and Difficulties Schedule revealed that events like humiliation, entrapment in an ongoing difficult situation and bereavement, which are known to be more depressogenic, were reported much more commonly in this sample compared to a sample in London. Reeler and Immerman (1994) examined the prevalence and factors associated with psychological disorders in Mozambican refugees in Zimbabwe using the SRQ-20. They found that 62% of refugees suffered from psychological disorders. They had multiple somatic complaints and a high suicidal risk. Acuda and Eide (1994) conducted a survey on 2783 secondary school students from randomly selected schools in rural and urban areas using a self-report questionnaire. Drug use was prevalent among the students. The main drugs involved, in descending order, were: alcohol, tobacco, inhalants (solvents), amphetamines and cannabis. Drug use increased with age and involved both sexes, the problem being more acute in the urban schools. Eide et al (1997 a, b) assessed 3061 secondary school children in Zimbabwe, selected by means of a two-stage sample design (first schools and then students registered with them were selected randomly). Standardized procedures were used by trained researchers to collect data. Sensation-seeking, addictive behaviour of significant others (social factors) and global and local cultural orientation (based on choice of media, language and music) explained 29.7% of the variance in dependent drug use. Social variables and global cultural orientation were significantly associated with increased use of cannabis and inhalants.

MENTAL HEALTH RESOURCES

Mental Health Policy A mental health policy is absent.

The mental health policy was developed over a three-year period and it will be officially launched in December 2004.

Substance Abuse Policy A substance abuse policy is absent. The initial formulation of the Zimbabwe National Drug Control Master Plan (substance abuse policy) was in 1999, and it is currently in the Parliament awaiting ratification.

National Mental Health Programme A national mental health programme is present. The programme was formulated in 1984. The national mental health programme was updated in 1996 and is known as National Health Strategic Plan 1997-2007.

National Therapeutic Drug Policy/Essential List of Drugs A national therapeutic drug policy/essential list of drugs is present. It was formulated in 1995.

The first essential drug list was published in 1985. The current list was published in the year 2000. The Zimbabwe National Drug Policy was published in 1995.

Mental Health Legislation There are two recent laws. The Mental Health Act 1996 and the Mental Health Regulation 1999. The latest legislation was enacted in 1996.

Mental Health Financing There are no budget allocations for mental health.
Details about expenditure on mental health are not available.
The primary source of mental health financing is tax based.
The mentally ill are entitled to free health services.
The country has disability benefits for persons with mental disorders. Mental illness falls under the category that qualifies for tax credits.

Mental Health Facilities Mental health is a part of primary health care system. Actual treatment of severe mental disorders is available at the primary level. Primary health care workers have the capacity to handle patients with severe psychosis and refer only those that they feel require specialized services. Most of the rural and district hospitals do not have facilities for inpatient care and only 17 district, provincial and central hospitals have primary care teams.
Regular training of primary care professionals is carried out in the field of mental health. In the last two years, about 2000 personnel were provided training. There are training facilities for nurses, occupational therapists, rehabilitation workers and social workers. All student nurses are supposed to go through a period of training in mental health (4 weeks of theory and 8 weeks of practical experience). Training workshops for mental health are also organized from time to time at the district and provincial level. However, the programme has significant limitations. A system of supervision, referral and back referral has been established in some regions.
There are community care facilities for patients with mental disorders. There is a shortage of material and staff to sustain community care programme.

Psychiatric Beds and Professionals

Total psychiatric beds per 10 000 population	1.2
Psychiatric beds in mental hospitals per 10 000 population	0.9
Psychiatric beds in general hospitals per 10 000 population	0.2
Psychiatric beds in other settings per 10 000 population	0.1
Number of psychiatrists per 100 000 population	0.1
Number of neurosurgeons per 100 000 population	0.07
Number of psychiatric nurses per 100 000 population	4.6
Number of neurologists per 100 000 population	0.009
Number of psychologists per 100 000 population	0.9
Number of social workers per 100 000 population	0.2

There are 221 physiotherapists and 243 rehabilitation technicians who help in mental health. There are 71 occupational therapists.

Non-Governmental Organizations NGOs are involved with mental health in the country. They are mainly involved in advocacy, promotion, prevention, treatment and rehabilitation. NGOs also provide training.

Information Gathering System There is mental health reporting system in the country. Although there is no mention of mental health in the secretaries' annual report, mental health is included in the National Health Profile Annual Report.
The country has data collection system or epidemiological study on mental health. Plans are under way to make the data collection form more user friendly.

Programmes for Special Population There are no special services for these populations. Mental health is integrated into other services and so all types of people benefit.

Therapeutic Drugs The following therapeutic drugs are generally available at the primary health care level of the country: carbamazepine, phenobarbital, phenytoin sodium, amitriptyline, chlorpromazine, diazepam, fluphenazine, haloperidol, biperiden, carbidopa, levodopa.
Benzhexol (5mg) is present. There is a shortage of drugs due to the lack of foreign currency.

Other Information In Zimbabwe, traditional healers have been allowed to form an association of their own through an Act of the Parliament.
The national training programme for registered nurses has been decentralized. In addition to the central hospitals, few rural district hospitals were selected for training, provided they had a separate ward for the care of psychiatric patients.

Additional Sources of Information

Acuda, S. W., Eide, A. H. (1994) Epidemiological study of drug use in urban and rural secondary schools in Zimbabwe. Central African Journal of Medicine, 40, 207-212.

Broadhead, J. C., Abas, M. A. (1998) Life events, difficulties and depression among women in an urban setting in Zimbabwe. Psychological Medicine, 28, 29-38.

Eide, A. H., Acuda, S. W. (1997b) Cultural orientation and use of cannabis and inhalants among secondary school children in Zimbabwe. Social Science & Medicine, 45, 1241-1249.

Eide, A. H., Acuda, S. W., Khan, N., et al (1997a) Combining cultural, social and personality trait variables as predictors for drug use among adolescents in Zimbabwe. Journal of Adolescence, 20, 511-524.

Fidelis, C., Manley, M. (1991). Psychiatry in Zimbabwe. Hospital and Community Psychiatry, 42, 943-947.

Patel, V., Araya, R., de Lima, M., et al (1999) Women, poverty and common mental disorders in four restructuring societies. Social Science & Medicine, 49, 1461-1471.

Patel, V., Todd, C., Winston, M., et al (1997) Common mental disorders in primary care in Harare, Zimbabwe: associations and risk factors. British Journal of Psychiatry, 171, 60-64.

Patel, V., Todd, C., Winston, M., et al (1998) Outcome of common mental disorders in Harare, Zimbabwe. British Journal of Psychiatry, 172, 53-57.

Reeler, A. P., Immerman, R. (1994) A preliminary investigation into psychological disorders among Mozambican refugees: prevalence and clinical features. Central African Journal of Medicine, 40, 309-315.

Todd, C., Patel, V., Simunyu, E., et al (1999) The onset of common mental disorders in primary care attenders in Harare, Zimbabwe. Psychological Medicine, 29, 97-104.

van der Hheide D. H., Gernaat, H. B. P. E. (2001) A psychiatric ward in an African district hospital. Tropical Doctor, 31, 135-138.

Section III

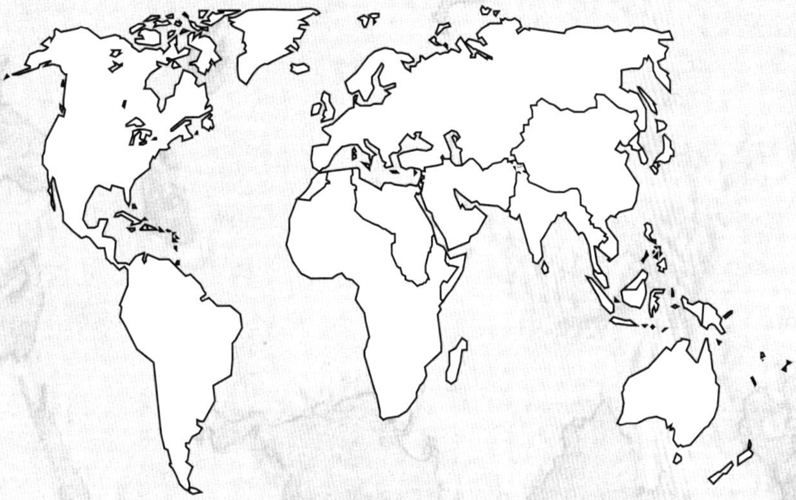

Associate Members, Areas and Territories

American Samoa

GENERAL INFORMATION

American Samoa has an approximate area of 0.2 thousand sq. km. (UNO, 2001). It is an archipelago of 6 islands and 1 atoll. Its population is 0.057 million, and the sex ratio (men per hundred women) is 104 (UNO, 2004). The proportion of population under the age of 15 years is 41% (UNO, 2004). The literacy rate is 98% for men and 97% for women (UNESCO/MoH, 2004). American Samoa is classified as a higher middle income group country (based on World Bank 2004 criteria).
The main language(s) used is (are) Samoan and English. The largest ethnic group(s) is (are) native Samoans who are US nationals (nine-tenths), and the other ethnic group(s) are (is) Caucasian and Tongan. The largest religious group(s) is (are) Christian Congregationalist (half), and the other religious group(s) are (is) Roman Catholic (one-fifth) and other Christian.

EPIDEMIOLOGY

There is a paucity of epidemiological data on mental illnesses in American Samoa in internationally accessible literature. Suicide was responsible for 5% of deaths in the year 2000 (Macdonald, 2004).

MENTAL HEALTH RESOURCES

Mental Health Policy A mental health policy is present. Details about the year of formulation are not available.
The components of the policy are advocacy, promotion, prevention, treatment and rehabilitation.

Substance Abuse Policy A substance abuse policy is present. The policy was initially formulated in 1990.

National Mental Health Programme A national mental health programme is present. The programme was formulated in 1990. A MNH Advisory Council oversees the mental health plan.

National Therapeutic Drug Policy/Essential List of Drugs A national therapeutic drug policy/essential list of drugs is present. It was formulated in 1990.

Mental Health Legislation There is a mental health legislation.
The latest legislation was enacted in 1970.

Mental Health Financing There are budget allocations for mental health.
Details about expenditure on mental health are not available.
The primary source of mental health financing is grants.
There are disability benefits for persons with mental disorders.

Mental Health Facilities Mental health is a part of primary health care system. Actual treatment of severe mental disorders is not available at the primary level. Services are provided only in the general hospital.
Regular training of primary care professionals is not carried out in the field of mental health.
There are no community care facilities for patients with mental disorders.

Psychiatric Beds and Professionals

Total psychiatric beds per 10 000 population	0
Psychiatric beds in mental hospitals per 10 000 population	0
Psychiatric beds in general hospitals per 10 000 population	0
Psychiatric beds in other settings per 10 000 population	0
Number of psychiatrists per 100 000 population	1.5
Number of neurosurgeons per 100 000 population	0
Number of psychiatric nurses per 100 000 population	3
Number of neurologists per 100 000 population	0
Number of psychologists per 100 000 population	0
Number of social workers per 100 000 population	

Mental Health is under the LBJ Hospital which caters to primary care as well as hospitalization needs of mentally ill patients. There is an Acute Care Unit that has 4 rooms including a seclusion unit. If necessary patients are placed in prison cells. There are 5 mental health workers including a psychiatrist who also do follow-up in the community.

Non-Governmental Organizations There are NGOs involved with mental health. They are mainly involved in advocacy and promotion. MOM (Mapusaga O le Mafaufau) consists of mainly family members of mental patients and members of the public and has an alliance with NAMI (National Alliance Mentally Ill), USA. It assists the mental health staff in community care of the mentally ill and also provides support for the families of the mentally ill.

Information Gathering System There is mental health reporting system.
There is no data collection system or epidemiological study on mental health. Some data collection is done by the staff of the Mental Health Unit.

Programmes for Special Population There are specific programmes for mental health for indigenous population, elderly and children.

Therapeutic Drugs The following therapeutic drugs are generally available at the primary health care level: carbamazepine, phenobarbital, phenytoin sodium, sodium valproate, amitriptyline, chlorpromazine, diazepam, fluphenazine, haloperidol, lithium, carbidopa, levodopa.
Benztropine is available. Newer classes of drugs are also available in the unit.

Other Information

Additional Sources of Information

MacDonald, N. C. (2004) Personal Communication (based on records available with WHO Western Pacific Regional Office).

British Virgin Islands

GENERAL INFORMATION

British Virgin Islands has an approximate area of 0.15 thousand sq. km. (UNO, 2001). It is comprised of 60 islands, cays and rocks. Its population is 0.111 million (UNO, 2004). The literacy rate is 97.8% for men and 97.8% for women (UNESCO/MoH, 2004). British Virgin Islands is classified as a high income group country (based on World Bank 2004 criteria). The proportion of health budget to GDP is 0.02%.

The main language(s) used is (are) English. The largest ethnic group(s) is (are) Black (nine-tenths of the population), and the other ethnic group(s) are (is) White, Chinese and Indian. The largest religious group(s) is (are) Christian, and the other religious group(s) are (is) Hindu and Muslim.

The life expectancy at birth is 75.24 years for males and 77.36 years for females (WHO, 2004).

EPIDEMIOLOGY

There is a paucity of epidemiological data on mental illnesses in British Virgin Islands in internationally accessible literature.

MENTAL HEALTH RESOURCES

Mental Health Policy A mental health policy is absent.

Substance Abuse Policy A substance abuse policy is absent.

National Mental Health Programme A national mental health programme is absent.
Components of a mental health programme are available for guidance.

National Therapeutic Drug Policy/Essential List of Drugs A national therapeutic drug policy/essential list of drugs is absent.

Mental Health Legislation In 1985, the Mental Health Ordinance was enacted. Its purpose is to repeal the Female Lunatics (Protection) Act and the Lunacy and Mental Treatment Ordinance and make new provision for the treatment and care of the mentally ill.
The latest legislation was enacted in 1985.

Mental Health Financing There are budget allocations for mental health.
Details about expenditure on mental health are not available.
The primary sources of mental health financing in descending order are tax based, private insurances and out of pocket expenditure by the patient or family.
There are disability benefits for persons with mental disorders. A person unable to work because of mental illness can get social security benefits if they have contributed to the scheme.

Mental Health Facilities Mental health is a part of primary health care system. Actual treatment of severe mental disorders is not available at the primary level. Limited mental health interventions are provided in primary health care.
Regular training of primary care professionals is not carried out in the field of mental health.
There are community care facilities for patients with mental disorders. There is a community mental health center, which provides psychiatric, psychological and nursing services. Home visits and family interventions are done as necessary. Mental health clinics are conducted regularly in the sister islands to other institutions such as prison and home for the elderly.

Psychiatric Beds and Professionals

Total psychiatric beds per 10 000 population	1
Psychiatric beds in mental hospitals per 10 000 population	0
Psychiatric beds in general hospitals per 10 000 population	1
Psychiatric beds in other settings per 10 000 population	0
Number of psychiatrists per 100 000 population	5
Number of neurosurgeons per 100 000 population	0
Number of psychiatric nurses per 100 000 population	20
Number of neurologists per 100 000 population	0
Number of psychologists per 100 000 population	10
Number of social workers per 100 000 population	15

Non-Governmental Organizations There are no NGOs involved with mental health.

Information Gathering System There is mental health reporting system.
There is no data collection system or epidemiological study on mental health.

Programmes for Special Population There are no specific programmes.

Therapeutic Drugs The following therapeutic drugs are generally available at the primary health care level: carbamazepine, phenobarbital, phenytoin sodium, sodium valproate, amitriptyline, chlorpromazine, diazepam, fluphenazine, haloperidol, lithium, biperiden, carbidopa, levodopa.
Many of the newer psychotropics are available for use.

Other Information The basic orientation of psychiatry in British Virgin Islands is towards community care.

Additional Sources of Information

Government document (1985) No 10 of 1985 Mental Health Ordinance, 1985.

La Grenade, L. (1998) Integrated primary Health care. West Indies Medical Journal, 47 (suppl. 4), 31-33.

French Polynesia

GENERAL INFORMATION

French Polynesia is has an approximate area of 4 thousand sq. km. (UNO, 2001). It consists of five scattered archipelagos. Its population is 0.248 million, and the sex ratio (men per hundred women) is 106 (UNO, 2004). The proportion of population under the age of 15 years is 28% (UNO, 2004). The literacy rate is 98% for men and 98% for women (UNESCO/MoH, 2004).
French Polynesia is classified as a high income group country (based on World Bank 2004 criteria).
The main language(s) used is (are) French, Tahitian. The largest ethnic group(s) is (are) Polynesian (seven-tenths), and the other ethnic group(s) are (is) Chinese and French. The largest religious group(s) is (are) Protestant (half), and the other religious group(s) are (is) Roman Catholic (two-fifths).

EPIDEMIOLOGY

There is substantial epidemiological data on mental illnesses in French Polynesia in internationally accessible literature. No attempt was made to include this information here.

MENTAL HEALTH RESOURCES

Mental Health Policy A mental health policy is absent.

Substance Abuse Policy A substance abuse policy is present. Details about the year of formulation are not available.

National Mental Health Programme A national mental health programme is absent.

National Therapeutic Drug Policy/Essential List of Drugs A national therapeutic drug policy/essential list of drugs is absent.

Mental Health Legislation There is a law on alcoholism from 1999. However, details about proper psychiatric laws are not known. Details about the year of enactment of the mental health legislation are not available.

Mental Health Financing There are budget allocations for mental health.
Details about expenditure on mental health are not available.
The primary sources of mental health financing in descending order are tax based and social insurance.
There are disability benefits for persons with mental disorders.

Mental Health Facilities Mental health is a part of primary health care system. Actual treatment of severe mental disorders is available at the primary level.
Regular training of primary care professionals is not carried out in the field of mental health.
There are no community care facilities for patients with mental disorders.

Psychiatric Beds and Professionals

Total psychiatric beds per 10 000 population	2.9
Psychiatric beds in mental hospitals per 10 000 population	2.5
Psychiatric beds in general hospitals per 10 000 population	0.2
Psychiatric beds in other settings per 10 000 population	0.2
Number of psychiatrists per 100 000 population	5
Number of neurosurgeons per 100 000 population	0.4
Number of psychiatric nurses per 100 000 population	9
Number of neurologists per 100 000 population	0.4
Number of psychologists per 100 000 population	12
Number of social workers per 100 000 population	20

There are 3 ergotherapists.

Non-Governmental Organizations There are NGOs involved with mental health. They are mainly involved in treatment and rehabilitation.

Information Gathering System There is mental health reporting system.
There is no data collection system or epidemiological study on mental health.

Programmes for Special Population There are specific programmes for mental health for disaster affected population, elderly and children.

Therapeutic Drugs The following therapeutic drugs are generally available at the primary health care level: carbamazepine, phenobarbital, phenytoin sodium, sodium valproate, amitriptyline, chlorpromazine, diazepam, haloperidol, lithium, carbidopa, levodopa.

Other Information

Additional Sources of Information

Guam

GENERAL INFORMATION

Guam has an approximate area of 0.55 thousand sq. km. (UNO, 2001). Its population is 0.165 million, and the sex ratio (men per hundred women) is 109 (UNO, 2004). The proportion of population under the age of 15 years is 30% (UNO, 2004).The literacy rate is 99% for men and 99% for women (UNESCO/MoH, 2004).

Guam is classified as a high income group country (based on World Bank 2004 criteria).

The main language(s) used is (are) English, Chamorro and Tagalog. The largest ethnic group(s) is (are) Chamorro (almost one-third) and Filipino (almost one-third), and the other ethnic group(s) are (is) Caucasian, Asian and Micronesian. The largest religious group(s) is (are) Roman Catholic.

EPIDEMIOLOGY

There is substantial epidemiological data on mental illnesses in Guam in internationally accessible literature. No attempt was made to include this information here.

MENTAL HEALTH RESOURCES

Mental Health Policy A mental health policy is present. The policy was initially formulated in 1983.
The components of the policy are prevention, treatment and rehabilitation.

Substance Abuse Policy A substance abuse policy is present. The policy was initially formulated in 1983.

National Mental Health Programme A national mental health programme is absent.

National Therapeutic Drug Policy/Essential List of Drugs A national therapeutic drug policy/essential list of drugs is absent.

Mental Health Legislation There is a law on parity in health insurance for mental illness and chemical dependency.
The latest legislation was enacted in 1998.

Mental Health Financing There are budget allocations for mental health.
Details about expenditure on mental health are not available.
The primary sources of mental health financing in descending order are tax based, private insurances, grants, out of pocket expenditure by the patient or family and social insurance.
There are disability benefits for persons with mental disorders. An individual must be certified by a licensed doctor.

Mental Health Facilities Mental health is not a part of primary health care system. Actual treatment of severe mental disorders is not available at the primary level. Psychiatric patients are referred to Government psychiatric set-ups or private psychiatrists.
Regular training of primary care professionals is not carried out in the field of mental health.
Details about community care facilities in mental health are not available. The psychiatric department abides by the legislation PL 17-21 to provide community-based outpatient mental health, alcohol and drug abuse programmes and services for the people.

Psychiatric Beds and Professionals

Total psychiatric beds per 10 000 population	2.2
Psychiatric beds in mental hospitals per 10 000 population	2.2
Psychiatric beds in general hospitals per 10 000 population	0
Psychiatric beds in other settings per 10 000 population	0
Number of psychiatrists per 100 000 population	5
Number of neurosurgeons per 100 000 population	0
Number of psychiatric nurses per 100 000 population	8
Number of neurologists per 100 000 population	1.3
Number of psychologists per 100 000 population	5
Number of social workers per 100 000 population	39

Non-Governmental Organizations There are NGOs involved with mental health in the country. They are mainly involved in advocacy, promotion and prevention.

Information Gathering System There is no mental health reporting system.
There is no data collection system or epidemiological study on mental health. The University of Guam conducted a prevalence study in 2000 on the islands' senior citizen population. It also conducted a study on the prevalence and incidence of mental illness in Guam and submitted a report entitled 'Estimating the prevalence of serious mental illness and serious emotional disturbances: an appraisal survey of mental health service providers in Guam'.

Programmes for Special Population There are specific programmes for mental health for disaster affected population and children. DMHSA follows the 'territorial emergency plan' when serving disaster affected population. DMHSA's child and adolescent unit serves the mental health needs of the youth.

Therapeutic Drugs The following therapeutic drugs are generally available at the primary health care level: carbamazepine, sodium valproate, amitriptyline, chlorpromazine, diazepam, fluphenazine, haloperidol, lithium.

Other Information

Additional Sources of Information

Official Mental Health and Substance Abuse Policy, P.L. 17-21: 83-92. (Government document).

Parity in Health Insurance for Mental Illness and Chemical Dependency. Most Recent Law in the Field of Mental Health, P.L. 24-303. (Government document).

Hong Kong, Special Administrative Region, China

GENERAL INFORMATION

Hong Kong, Special Administrative Region, China has an approximate area of 1 thousand sq. km. (UNO, 2001). It covers Hong Kong island, the Kowloon peninsula and 235 outlying islands. Its population is 7.115 million, and the sex ratio (men per hundred women) is 96 (UNO, 2004). The proportion of population under the age of 15 years is 15% (UNO, 2004). The literacy rate is 96.6% for men and 90% for women (UNESCO/MoH, 2004).
Hong Kong SAR is classified as a high income group country (based on World Bank 2004 criteria). The proportion of health budget to GDP is 2.8%.
The main language(s) used is (are) Chinese (Cantonese) and English. The largest ethnic group(s) is (are) Chinese. The largest religious group(s) is (are) Buddhist, and the other religious group(s) are (is) Taoist and Christian.

EPIDEMIOLOGY

There is substantial epidemiological data on mental illnesses in Hong Kong SARin internationally accessible literature. No attempt was made to include this information here.

MENTAL HEALTH RESOURCES

Mental Health Policy A mental health policy is present. The policy was initially formulated in 1995.
The components of the policy are promotion, prevention and rehabilitation. The policy objective for rehabilitation is to promote and provide such comprehensive and effective measures as are necessary for the prevention of disability, the development of physical, mental and social capabilities of people with disability and the realization of a physical and social environment conducive to meeting the goals of their full participation in social life and development and of equalization of opportunities. Details can be obtained from the website: www.info.gov.hk/hwb. The overall health policy of the HKSAR covers both mental health and physical health. A wide range of services and activities are run to promote mental health in the HKSAR. Rehabilitation services are also provided to mentally ill and mentally handicapped persons.

Substance Abuse Policy A substance abuse policy is present. The policy was initially formulated in 1965. The Government of Hong Kong Special Administrative Region adopts a five-pronged approach to tackle the problem of psychotropic substance abuse which includes legislation and law enforcement, preventive education and publicity, treatment and rehabilitation, research and international cooperation. In view of the rising trend of substance use, a task force on psychotropic substance abuse was set up in early 2000 to recommend measures to more effectively tackle the problem of substance abuse. It comprised of experts from the field of policy making, law enforcement, medicine, social work, education, etc.

National Mental Health Programme A national mental health programme is present. The programme was formulated in 1993.
A wide range of mental health services, including mental health promotion, disease prevention, treatment, rehabilitation and community service is provided by the HKSAR Government in collaboration with non-governmental organizations.

National Therapeutic Drug Policy/Essential List of Drugs A national therapeutic drug policy/essential list of drugs is absent.

Mental Health Legislation There is a mental health ordinance. It was enacted in 1960 and amended in 1999. The amendment was developed after negotiations with community groups. A copy can be downloaded from the website: www.justice.gov.hk/cHome.htm. It facilitates care provision in addition to supervision and control.
The latest legislation was enacted in 1960.

Mental Health Financing There are no budget allocations for mental health.
Details about expenditure on mental health are not available.
The primary sources of mental health financing in descending order are tax based and grants.
Since mental illness and mental handicap are integral parts of disabilities, there is no separate budget line for the mental health programme. The services and programmes pertaining to mental health cut across different policy bureaus and departments.
There are disability benefits for persons with mental disorders.

Mental Health Facilities Mental health is a part of primary health care system. Actual treatment of severe mental disorders is not available at the primary level. Mental disorders are managed at secondary and tertiary level.
Regular training of primary care professionals is carried out in the field of mental health. In the last two years, about 4719 personnel were provided training.
There are community care facilities for patients with mental disorders. The Government provides services within the medical setting like psychiatric wards in the general hospital setting, day hospitals, psychiatric outpatient clinics and aftercare services for discharged patients. The Government has also coordinated and organized intensive public education programmes on mental health and mental illness in public housing estates where community care facilities were to be established. Three community psychiatry teams have been set up to serve defined geographical areas, where they target patients with severe mental illnesses. These provide continuity of care and crisis intervention through domiciliary visits, partnership with other rehabilitation organizations (e.g. advice on management of difficult cases and training of staff) and direct services for the community (e.g. public education, telephone hotlines). The

Government also finances NGOs to provide community-based psychiatric rehabilitation services like day care centres, half-way houses, long-term residential options and sheltered workshops. Social workers are the primary case managers for mental outpatients within the community.

Psychiatric Beds and Professionals

Total psychiatric beds per 10 000 population	7
Psychiatric beds in mental hospitals per 10 000 population	4.5
Psychiatric beds in general hospitals per 10 000 population	2.5
Psychiatric beds in other settings per 10 000 population	0
Number of psychiatrists per 100 000 population	2
Number of neurosurgeons per 100 000 population	0.5
Number of psychiatric nurses per 100 000 population	46.4
Number of neurologists per 100 000 population	0.7
Number of psychologists per 100 000 population	1.4
Number of social workers per 100 000 population	173.5

There are 1059 occupational therapists. The beds refer to mental hospital beds and those available in general hospitals in the public sector. The number of psychologists refer to clinical psychologists working in the Hospital Authority and Department of Health. The figure for social workers is quoted from the Social Worker Registration Board where categorization is based on academic qualifications only, not on the field that they are specialized in.

Non-Governmental Organizations There are NGOs involved with mental health. They are mainly involved in advocacy, promotion, prevention and rehabilitation. NGOs provide a number of residential facilities (half-way houses, hostels, long stay care home), day facilities (activity centres and social clubs) and rehabilitation facilities (sheltered workshops, farms and other supported employment programmes). They have also played a major role in fighting stigma and public opposition to community care of mentally ill patients.

Information Gathering System There is no mental health reporting system. A Centralised Suicide Information System was established in 2002 to register successful and attempted suicide reported by Government departments, schools, hospitals and other agencies. The Central Registry of Drug Abuse established in 1972 monitors the trend and characteristics of drug abuse in Hong Kong. The country has data collection system or epidemiological study on mental health. Data collection is in the form of clinical information system, integrated patient administration system and outpatient appointment system of the Hospital Authority. Mortality data and hospitalization data are also available. Details can be obtained from http://www.info.gov.hk/dh/.

Programmes for Special Population There are specific programmes for mental health for elderly and children. There are services for students and parents of children with developmental problems.
Traditionally child psychiatric services were heavily skewed towards neuropsychiatric and developmental disorders, but with new setups this is changing.

Therapeutic Drugs The following therapeutic drugs are generally available at the primary health care level: carbamazepine, ethosuximide, phenobarbital, phenytoin sodium, sodium valproate, amitriptyline, chlorpromazine, diazepam, haloperidol, lithium, carbidopa, levodopa.
Ethosuximide is used by specialists in hospitals.

Other Information Mental health services in Hong Kong can be divided into the pre-asylum period (1841-1924), the asylum period (1925-1948), the organization period (1948-1965), the initial rehabilitation period (1966-1973), the centralized rehabilitation period (1974-1981) and the civic control versus community care period (1982-1995). Details can be obtained from the work of Yip (1998).

Additional Sources of Information

Abdullah, A. S., Fielding, R., Hedley, A. J. (2002) Patterns of cigarette smoking, alcohol use and other substance use among Chinese university students in Hong Kong. American Journal on Addictions, 11, 235-246.

Chen, C. N., Wong, J., Lee, N., et al (1993) The Shatin community mental health survey in Hong Kong. II. Major findings. Archives of General Psychiatry, 50, 125-133.

Chiu, H. F. K., Lam, L. C. W., Chi, I., et al (1998) Prevalence of dementia in Chinese elderly in Hong Kong. Neurology, 50, 1002-1009.

Chiu, H. F. K., Lam, L. C. W., Pang, A. H. T., et al (1996) Attempted suicide by Chinese elderly in Hong Kong. General Hospital Psychiatry, 18, 444-447.

Lee, D. T. S., Yip, A. S. K., Chiu, H. F. K., et al (2001) A psychiatric epidemiological study of postpartum Chinese women. American Journal of Psychiatry, 158, 220-226.

Leung, S. F., Arthur, D. (2000) The alcohol use disorders identification test (AUDIT): validation of an instrument for enhancing nursing practice in Hong Kong. International Journal of Nursing Studies, 37, 57-64.

Lo, W. H., Leung, T. M. (1985) Suicide in Hong Kong. Australian & New Zealand Journal of Psychiatry, 19, 287-292.

Luk, S. L., Leung, P. W., Bacon-Shone, J., et al (1991) Behaviour disorder in pre-school children in Hong Kong. A two-stage epidemiological study. British Journal of Psychiatry, 158, 213-221.

Pang, A. H. T., Yip, K. C., Cheung, H. K., et al (1997) Community psychiatry in Hong Kong. International Journal of Social Psychiatry, 43, 213-216.

Shek, D. T. L. (1995) Adolescent suicide in Hong-Kong (1980-1991). International Journal of Adolescent Medicine & Health, 8, 65-86.

Tang, O. (1997) General hospital psychiatry in Hong Kong. Hong Kong Journal of Psychiatry, 7, 14-18.

Wong, C. K., Lau, J. T. (1992) Psychiatric morbidity in a Chinese primary school in Hong Kong. Australian & New Zealand Journal of Psychiatry, 26, 459-466.

Wong, V., Lee, P. W., Lieh-Mak, F., et al (1992) Language screening in preschool Chinese children. European Journal of Disorders of Communication, 27, 247-264.

Woo, J., Ho, S. C., Lau, J., et al (1994) The prevalence of depressive symptoms and predisposing factors in an elderly Chinese population. Acta Psychiatrica Scandinavica, 89, 8-13.

Yeung, C. K. (1997) Nocturnal enuresis in Hong Kong: different Chinese phenotypes. Scandinavian Journal of Urology & Nephrology, 183, 17-21.

Yip, K-S. (1998) A historical review of mental health services in Hong Kong (1841 to 1995). International Journal of Social Psychiatry, 44, 46-55.

Yip, P. S., Chiu, L. H. (1998) Teenage attempted suicide in Hong Kong. Crisis: Journal of Crisis Intervention & Suicide, 19, 67-72.

Yip, P. S. (1997) Suicides in Hong Kong, 1981-1994. Social Psychiatry & Psychiatric Epidemiology, 32, 243-250.

Macao, Special Administrative Region, China

GENERAL INFORMATION

Macao, Special Administrative Region, China has an approximate area of 0.02 thousand sq. km. (UNO, 2001). Its population is 0.467 million, and the sex ratio (men per hundred women) is 91 (UNO, 2004). The proportion of population under the age of 15 years is 18% (UNO, 2004). The literacy rate is 95.3% for men and 87.8% for women (UNESCO/MoH, 2004).
Macao SAR is classified as a high income group country (based on World Bank 2004 criteria). The proportion of health budget to GDP is 2.2%.
The main language(s) used is (are) Chinese (Cantonese), Portuguese and English. The largest ethnic group(s) is (are) Chinese (almost 95%), and the other ethnic group(s) are (is) Caucasian.
The life expectancy at birth is 77.2 years for males and 81.5 years for females (WHO, 2004).

EPIDEMIOLOGY

There is a paucity of epidemiological data on mental illnesses in Macao SAR in internationally accessible literature. Da Canhota and Piterman (2001) assessed 386 elderly subjects from general practice clinics using the Hospital Anxiety and Depression Scale (HAD) and clinical records. Nearly 26.2% were found to have depression based on the cut-off score of 11/12 on HAD. Depression was associated with gender (women) and age. The following disorders were common in a treatment setting (n=2726): psychosis (28.7%), neurosis (47.8%), dementia (4.7%) and substance abuse (2.9%) (Department of Psychiatry, 2003).

MENTAL HEALTH RESOURCES

Mental Health Policy A mental health policy is present. The policy was initially formulated in 1994.
The components of the policy are advocacy, promotion, prevention, treatment and rehabilitation.

Substance Abuse Policy A substance abuse policy is present. The policy was initially formulated in 2002. The substance abuse policy is based on 'Controlling Supply and Reducing Demand' (2002 Report on Drug Control in Macao).

National Mental Health Programme A national mental health programme is absent.

National Therapeutic Drug Policy/Essential List of Drugs A national therapeutic drug policy/essential list of drugs is present. Details about the year of formulation are not available.

Mental Health Legislation There is a Mental Health Ordinance.
The latest legislation was enacted in 1999.

Mental Health Financing There are no budget allocations for mental health.
Details about expenditure on mental health are not available.
The primary source of mental health financing is tax based.
The cost of psychiatric drug prescriptions is USD 741 000.00 at an average cost for each patient of USD 271.67 per year.
There are disability benefits for persons with mental disorders.

Mental Health Facilities Mental health is not a part of primary health care system. Actual treatment of severe mental disorders is not available at the primary level. Screening for post-natal depression, treatment of mild psychiatric problems and education programmes in mental health are available at the primary care level.
Regular training of primary care professionals is carried out in the field of mental health. In the last two years, about 40 personnel were provided training.
There are no community care facilities for patients with mental disorders. In 1992, an NGO introduced community psychiatric rehabilitation services under Government financing and technical support.

Psychiatric Beds and Professionals

Total psychiatric beds per 10 000 population	0.7
Psychiatric beds in mental hospitals per 10 000 population	0
Psychiatric beds in general hospitals per 10 000 population	0.7
Psychiatric beds in other settings per 10 000 population	0
Number of psychiatrists per 100 000 population	2.2
Number of neurosurgeons per 100 000 population	1.8
Number of psychiatric nurses per 100 000 population	8.5
Number of neurologists per 100 000 population	9
Number of psychologists per 100 000 population	0.2
Number of social workers per 100 000 population	1.1

There are two other types of mental health workers. Macao completed the psychiatric deinstitutionalization process in 1993. A Government-funded general hospital is the only hospital that provides mental health services. A new purpose-built psychiatric complex with 81 beds has been commissioned recently. The new services include adult, psychogeriatric and forensic inpatient units, a day hospital (45 beds) and outpatient facilities.

Non-Governmental Organizations There are NGOs involved with mental health in the country. They are mainly involved in advocacy, promotion, prevention, treatment and rehabilitation. One NGO is involved in the rendering of community-based psychosocial and vocational rehabilitation services for psychiatric clients. It receives a fixed subsidy of about 2 million at local currency per year granted by the social welfare department.

Information Gathering System There is mental health reporting system.
There is no data collection system or epidemiological study on mental health.

Programmes for Special Population There are specific programmes for mental health for indigenous population and children.

Therapeutic Drugs The following therapeutic drugs are generally available at the primary health care level: carbamazepine, ethosuximide, phenobarbital, phenytoin sodium, sodium valproate, amitriptyline, chlorpromazine, diazepam, fluphenazine, haloperidol, lithium, biperiden, carbidopa, levodopa.
Newer anti-psychotics (e.g. olanzapine and risperidone), anti-depressants (e.g. citalopram, venlafaxine), anxiolytics and hypnotics (e.g. buspirone, zolpidem), anti-epileptics (e.g. lamotrigine, vigabatrin) and other drugs (e.g. rivastigmine) are available. There is no limitation on prescription of atypical anti-psychotics and anti-depressant drugs, and these are free of charge for all psychiatric patients.

Other Information Most of the patients with mental illness and their families are no longer experiencing as much stigma due to the institution of education and public relations activities about mental illness over the last 15 years. However, there are still a significant number of people hesitant to receive psychiatric services.

Additional Sources of Information

Da Canhota, C. M., Piterman, L. (2001) Depressive disorders in elderly Chinese patients in Macau: a comparison of general practitioners' consultations with a depression screening scale. Australian & New Zealand Journal of Psychiatry, 35, 336-344.

Department of Psychiatry, S. Januario Hospital (2003).

New Caledonia

GENERAL INFORMATION

New Caledonia has an approximate area of 19 thousand sq. km. (UNO, 2001). It consists of the main island of New Caledonia, the archipelago of Iles Loyaute, and numerous small, sparsely populated islands. Its population is 0.232 million, and the sex ratio (men per hundred women) is 105 (UNO, 2004). The proportion of population under the age of 15 years is 29% (UNO, 2004). The literacy rate is 96.8% for men and 95.5% for women (UNESCO/MoH, 2004).

New Caledonia is classified as a high income group country (based on World Bank 2004 criteria). The proportion of health budget to GDP is 8.7%.

The main language(s) used is (are) French and Melanesian/Polynesian dialects. The largest ethnic group(s) is (are) Melanesian (two-fifths) and European (two-fifths), and the other ethnic group(s) are (is) Wallisian. The largest religious group(s) is (are) Roman Catholic (three-fifths), and the other religious group(s) are (is) Protestant.

EPIDEMIOLOGY

There is substantial epidemiological data on mental illnesses in New Caledonia in internationally accessible literature. No attempt was made to include this information here.

MENTAL HEALTH RESOURCES

Mental Health Policy A mental health policy is absent.

Substance Abuse Policy A substance abuse policy is present. Details about the year of formulation are not available. There is a programme for alcohol prevention.

National Mental Health Programme A national mental health programme is absent.

National Therapeutic Drug Policy/Essential List of Drugs A national therapeutic drug policy/essential list of drugs is present. Details about the year of formulation are not available.

Mental Health Legislation Details about the mental health legislation are not available.

Mental Health Financing There are budget allocations for mental health.
Details about expenditure on mental health are not available.
The primary sources of mental health financing in descending order are social insurance, private insurances and out of pocket expenditure by the patient or family.
There are disability benefits for persons with mental disorders.

Mental Health Facilities Mental health is a part of primary health care system. Actual treatment of severe mental disorders is available at the primary level.
Regular training of primary care professionals is not carried out in the field of mental health.
There are community care facilities for patients with mental disorders. There are 12 centres for medico-psychiatry and one for alcohol.

Psychiatric Beds and Professionals

Total psychiatric beds per 10 000 population	85.5
Psychiatric beds in mental hospitals per 10 000 population	85.5
Psychiatric beds in general hospitals per 10 000 population	0
Psychiatric beds in other settings per 10 000 population	0
Number of psychiatrists per 100 000 population	9
Number of neurosurgeons per 100 000 population	0
Number of psychiatric nurses per 100 000 population	31.53
Number of neurologists per 100 000 population	1
Number of psychologists per 100 000 population	
Number of social workers per 100 000 population	

The figures for psychiatrists include those of child psychiatrists. Hospital beds include 4.86 places per 10 000 population in traditional therapeutic setting and 3.69 places per 10 000 population in day hospitalization setting.

Non-Governmental Organizations There are no NGOs are involved with mental health.

Information Gathering System There is no mental health reporting system.
There is no data collection system or epidemiological study on mental health. The Central Hospital carried out a study.

Programmes for Special Population There are specific programmes for mental health for disaster affected population and children. Specialized mental health services are also available for adolescents.

Therapeutic Drugs The following therapeutic drugs are generally available at the primary health care level: carbamazepine, ethosuximide, phenobarbital, phenytoin sodium, sodium valproate, amitriptyline, chlorpromazine, diazepam, fluphenazine, haloperidol, lithium, biperiden, carbidopa, levodopa.

Other Information

Additional Sources of Information

Northern Mariana Islands, Commonwealth of the

GENERAL INFORMATION

Northern Mariana Islands, Commonwealth of the has an approximate area of 0.48 thousand sq. km. (UNO, 2001). It includes 14 islands. Its population is 0.077 million, and the sex ratio (men per hundred women) is 92 (UNO, 2004). The literacy rate is 97% for men and 96% for women (UNESCO/MoH, 2004).

It is classified as a higher middle income group country (based on World Bank 2004 criteria).

The main language(s) used is (are) English, Chamorro and Carolinian. The largest ethnic group(s) is (are) Chamorro, Carolinians and other Micronesian, and the other ethnic group(s) are (is) Caucasian, Japanese, Chinese, Filipino, and Korean. The largest religious group(s) is (are) Roman Catholic, and the other religious group(s) are (is) other Christian.

EPIDEMIOLOGY

There is a paucity of epidemiological data on mental illnesses in the Northern Mariana Islands in internationally accessible literature.

MENTAL HEALTH RESOURCES

Mental Health Policy A mental health policy is present. The policy was initially formulated in 1976.
The components of the policy are advocacy, promotion, prevention, treatment and rehabilitation.

Substance Abuse Policy A substance abuse policy is present. The policy was initially formulated in 1976.

National Mental Health Programme A national mental health programme is present. The programme was formulated in 1976.

National Therapeutic Drug Policy/Essential List of Drugs Details about the national therapeutic drug policy/essential list of drugs are not available.

Mental Health Legislation The mental health legislation is entitled 'Involuntary Civil Commitment Act'.
The latest legislation was enacted in 1993.

Mental Health Financing There are budget allocations for mental health.
Details about expenditure on mental health are not available.
The primary sources of mental health financing in descending order are tax based, social insurance, grants, private insurances and out of pocket expenditure by the patient or family.
Funding is mainly tax based and is made available through local funding (Public Law 14-11), Community Mental Health Services Block Grant, Project for Assistance in Transition from Homelessness Block Grant and Substance Abuse Prevention and Treatment Block Grant.
There are disability benefits for persons with mental disorders. An individual must be certified by a licensed psychiatrist to receive disability benefits.

Mental Health Facilities Mental health is a part of primary health care system. Actual treatment of severe mental disorders is available at the primary level. Primary care is available only for stabilized patients after hospital treatment is over.
Regular training of primary care professionals is not carried out in the field of mental health.
There are community care facilities for patients with mental disorders. A community mental health service was established and funded under the country's local fund and US grants.

Psychiatric Beds and Professionals

Total psychiatric beds per 10 000 population	1.4
Psychiatric beds in mental hospitals per 10 000 population	0
Psychiatric beds in general hospitals per 10 000 population	1.4
Psychiatric beds in other settings per 10 000 population	0
Number of psychiatrists per 100 000 population	3
Number of neurosurgeons per 100 000 population	0
Number of psychiatric nurses per 100 000 population	8
Number of neurologists per 100 000 population	0
Number of psychologists per 100 000 population	5
Number of social workers per 100 000 population	9.7

Occupational therapists provide services to children and youth with development disabilities. In addition to registered nurses, 2 licensed practical nurses and 7 nursing assistants are present.

Non-Governmental Organizations There are NGOs involved with mental health. They are mainly involved in advocacy, promotion and prevention.

Information Gathering System There is mental health reporting system.

There is a data collection system or epidemiological study on mental health. Data collection on inpatients and outpatients is done.

Programmes for Special Population There are specific programmes for mental health for disaster affected population and children. The American Red Cross helps disaster affected population. Children and students with special needs are provided services under the public school system special education programme.

Therapeutic Drugs The following therapeutic drugs are generally available at the primary health care level: carbamazepine, ethosuximide, phenobarbital, phenytoin sodium, sodium valproate, amitriptyline, chlorpromazine, diazepam, fluphenazine, haloperidol, lithium, carbidopa, levodopa.
Other drugs like risperidone, clozapine, fluoxetine, venlafaxxine etc. are available.

Other Information

Additional Sources of Information

Commonwealth Health Centre (2000) Purpose and Philosophy.

Tokelau

GENERAL INFORMATION

Tokelau is has an approximate area of 0.01 thousand sq. km. (UNO, 2001). It consists of 3 small atolls. Its population is 0.001 million (UNO, 2004).

Tokelau is classified as a high income group country (based on World Bank 2004 criteria).

The main language(s) used is (are) Tokelauan and English. The largest ethnic group(s) is (are) Polynesian (New Zealand citizens). The largest religious group(s) is (are) Congregational Christian (Church of Samoa, almost three-fourths of the population), and the other religious group(s) are (is) Roman Catholic (one-fourth).

EPIDEMIOLOGY

There is a paucity of epidemiological data on mental illnesses in Tokelau in internationally accessible literature.

MENTAL HEALTH RESOURCES

Mental Health Policy A mental health policy is absent.

Substance Abuse Policy A substance abuse policy is absent.

National Mental Health Programme A national mental health programme is absent.

National Therapeutic Drug Policy/Essential List of Drugs A national therapeutic drug policy/essential list of drugs is present. It was formulated in 1998.

Mental Health Legislation There is no mental health legislation.
Details about the year of enactment of the mental health legislation are not available.

Mental Health Financing There are no budget allocations for mental health.
Details about expenditure on mental health are not available.
The primary source of mental health financing is tax based.
Funding for mental health is supported by New Zealand.
There are no disability benefits for persons with mental disorders. Mental illness is not considered as a criteria for disability.

Mental Health Facilities Mental health is a part of primary health care system. Actual treatment of severe mental disorders is not available at the primary level. Each of the three villages has a small hospital that provides basic primary health care services to its residents. Health services are provided by a small group of nurses who are assisted by locum doctors, usually recruited from New Zealand. When patients have medical conditions that are beyond the expertise of the village health services, they are referred to Samoa or New Zealand for diagnosis and/or treatment.
Regular training of primary care professionals is not carried out in the field of mental health.
There are community care facilities for patients with mental disorders.

Psychiatric Beds and Professionals

Total psychiatric beds per 10 000 population	0
Psychiatric beds in mental hospitals per 10 000 population	0
Psychiatric beds in general hospitals per 10 000 population	0
Psychiatric beds in other settings per 10 000 population	0
Number of psychiatrists per 100 000 population	0
Number of neurosurgeons per 100 000 population	0
Number of psychiatric nurses per 100 000 population	0
Number of neurologists per 100 000 population	0
Number of psychologists per 100 000 population	0
Number of social workers per 100 000 population	0

There is only one medical officer and 4 general nurses to man each of the 3 hospitals on the 3 islands. There are no specific mental hospital or any specific psychiatric beds.

Non-Governmental Organizations There are no NGOs are involved with mental health.

Information Gathering System There is mental health reporting system.
There is no data collection system or epidemiological study on mental health.

Programmes for Special Population No specific programme exists for any special population group.

Therapeutic Drugs The following therapeutic drugs are generally available at the primary health care level: carbamazepine, phenytoin sodium, chlorpromazine, diazepam, fluphenazine, carbidopa, levodopa.
Most drugs are purchased from New Zealand and emergency medicines are obtained from Samoa. All medicines are provided free in primary health care.

Other Information

Additional Sources of Information

Department of Health (2000) Bulk Store Drug Inventory, Drug Order Form. Government of Tokelau – Department of Health.

Wallis and Futuna

GENERAL INFORMATION

Wallis and Futuna has an approximate area of 0.2 thousand sq. km. (UNO, 2001). It includes Ile Uvea (Wallis), Ile Futuna, Ile Alofi, and 20 islets. Its population is 0.014 million (UNO, 2004). The literacy rate is 50% for men and 50% for women (UNESCO/MoH, 2004).

Wallis and Futuna is classified as a high income group country (based on World Bank 2004 criteria).

The main language(s) used is (are) French and Wallisian. The largest ethnic group(s) is (are) Polynesian. The largest religious group(s) is (are) Roman Catholic.

EPIDEMIOLOGY

There is a paucity of epidemiological data on mental illnesses in Wallis and Futuna in internationally accessible literature.

MENTAL HEALTH RESOURCES

Mental Health Policy A mental health policy is absent.

Substance Abuse Policy A substance abuse policy is absent.

National Mental Health Programme A national mental health programme is absent.

National Therapeutic Drug Policy/Essential List of Drugs A national therapeutic drug policy/essential list of drugs is absent.

Mental Health Legislation There is no mental health legislation.
Details about the year of enactment of the mental health legislation are not available.

Mental Health Financing There are no budget allocations for mental health.
Details about expenditure on mental health are not available.
The primary source of mental health financing is grants.
There are no disability benefits for persons with mental disorders. Rehabilitation of mentally ill is included in the mandate of Directorate for Rehabilitation Services under the Ministry of Health, but it is short on financial, human and other resources.

Mental Health Facilities Mental health is a part of primary health care system. Actual treatment of severe mental disorders is available at the primary level. There is one doctor in each primary health centre.
Regular training of primary care professionals is not carried out in the field of mental health.
There are no community care facilities for patients with mental disorders.

Psychiatric Beds and Professionals

Total psychiatric beds per 10 000 population	0
Psychiatric beds in mental hospitals per 10 000 population	0
Psychiatric beds in general hospitals per 10 000 population	0
Psychiatric beds in other settings per 10 000 population	0
Number of psychiatrists per 100 000 population	0
Number of neurosurgeons per 100 000 population	0
Number of psychiatric nurses per 100 000 population	0
Number of neurologists per 100 000 population	0
Number of psychologists per 100 000 population	7
Number of social workers per 100 000 population	0

Non-Governmental Organizations There are no NGOs involved with mental health.

Information Gathering System There is no mental health reporting system.
There is no data collection system or epidemiological study on mental health.

Programmes for Special Population There are no specific programmes for the special populations.

Therapeutic Drugs The following therapeutic drugs are generally available at the primary health care level: carbamazepine, phenobarbital, phenytoin sodium, sodium valproate, amitriptyline, chlorpromazine, diazepam, haloperidol, lithium, levodopa.

Other Information

Additional Sources of Information

West Bank and Gaza Strip

GENERAL INFORMATION

West Bank and Gaza Strip has an approximate area of 6.2 thousand sq. km. (UNO, 2001). Its population is 3.685 million, and the sex ratio (men per hundred women) is 104 (UNO, 2004). The proportion of population under the age of 15 years is 47% (UNO, 2004). The literacy rate is 96.3% for men and 87.4% for women (UNESCO/MoH, 2004).

West Bank and Gaza Strip is classified as a lower middle income group country (based on World Bank 2004 criteria). The proportion of health budget to GDP is 8.6%.

The main language(s) used is (are) Arabic and English. The largest ethnic group(s) is (are) Palestinian Arabs (nine-tenths). The largest religious group(s) is (are) Muslim (four-fifths, predominantly Sunni), and the other religious group(s) are (is) Christians.

EPIDEMIOLOGY

Samour (2002) reported that 69% of postpartum women (n=364) met the criteria for caseness 4 weeks after their delivery when assessed by the Edinburgh Postnatal Depression Scale (EPDS) and that prevalence of depression in these women was associated with political violence and other physical and psychosocial stressors. Qouta et al (1997) found depression, anxiety and paranoia to be more common among subjects who had suffered demolition of their own homes compared to those who had witnessed such acts or controls who had no such experience. Haj-Yahia and Muhammad (2000) reported findings from the Second Palestinian National Survey on wife abuse and battering (n=1334). The experience of abuse explained significant variances in women's low self-esteem, depression and anxiety. Al-Krenawi et al (2001) interviewed 187 women in polygamous marriages using Rosenberg's Self-Esteem Questionnaire and the Brief Symptom Inventory and found greater psychopathology among the senior wives compared to junior wives. Haj-Yahi and Tamish (2001) found similar rates of abuse among female and male undergraduate students (n= 652). Sexual abuse explained between 20.7% and 35.8% of the variance in psychological symptoms. Miller et al (1999) found high rates of conduct disorder, attention deficit-hyperactivity disorders and PTSD among 669 school children in their survey of families living in the Gaza Strip, when they applied the Ontario Child Health Scale (OCHS), the Child Post-Traumatic Stress Reaction Index (CPTS-RI) and the Health Reach Modified War Questionnaire. A significant correlation was found between higher rates of lifetime trauma exposure and higher prevalence rates of mental health problems. Haj-Yahia and Shor (1995), who used the Child Behaviour Checklist in a sample of 150 children from West Bank, also found that exposure to violence and war were related to behavioural problems. Under conditions of high accumulated risk, boys and younger children tended to be affected more. Community context (as indicated by a high or low level of political violence) was a significant factor for girls but not for boys. Kostelny and Garbarino (1994) interviewed mothers of a small group of children and adolescents aged 5-15 years using direct interviews and the Achenbach Child Behaviour Checklist (ACBC). The results showed that younger children suffered more personality and behavioural changes during the Intifada than adolescents did, including sleep disturbances, bedwetting, anxiety and withdrawal. Thabet and Vostanis (1998) interviewed 237 randomly selected children aged 9 to 13 years from 112 schools in Gaza strip. Children completed the Revised Manifest Anxiety Scale and teachers completed the Rutter Scale. Children reported high rates of significant anxiety problems (21.5%), and teachers reported high rates of mental health problems in the children (43.4%). Anxiety problems were associated with age and gender (girls) and living in inner city areas or camps. Low socioeconomic status was the strongest predictor of general mental health problems. Thabet and Vostanis (2000) did a longitudinal assessment of 234 children aged 7-12 years over a one year period using the Child Post Traumatic Stress Reaction Index (CPTS-RI) and the Rutter A2 and B2 Scales for parents and teachers, respectively. The rate of moderate to severe PTSD decreased from 40.6% to 10% over the study period. One-fifth of children were rated above the cut-off for mental health problems on the Rutter A2 (parent) Scales, and one-third of children were above the cut-off on the Rutter B2 (teacher) Scales. The total scores on all three measures had significantly decreased during the 1-year period. The total CPTS-RI score at follow-up was best predicted by the number of traumatic experiences recalled at the first assessment. Barber (1999) conducted a study on 7000 Palestinian families from the West Bank and Gaza Strip. Structural equation analysis of self-reported survey data revealed that Intifada experience increased antisocial behaviour in both male and female children and depression in female children 1-2 years after the end of the Intifada (as adolescents). These behaviours were unrelated to family values, educational values, academic performance or aggression.

MENTAL HEALTH RESOURCES

Mental Health Policy A mental health policy is present. The policy was initially formulated in 2004.

The components of the policy are advocacy, promotion, prevention, treatment and rehabilitation. The Mental Health Plan was made with the assistance of WHO and in consultation with a wide range of stakeholders. It aims to develop a well-coordinated community-based mental health system.

Substance Abuse Policy A substance abuse policy is absent. A High Committee on Drug Issues has been formed under the chairpersonship of the Minister of Social Affairs.

National Mental Health Programme Details about the national mental health programme are not available.

National Therapeutic Drug Policy/Essential List of Drugs A national therapeutic drug policy/essential list of drugs is present. It was formulated in 1999.
Psychotropics are available at the Primary Health Centres. UNRWA and some of the NGOs use essential drug lists.

Mental Health Legislation A workgroup has been formed and comprises members from various stakeholder groups. The major emphasis is on protection of patients' rights.
Details about the year of enactment of the mental health legislation are not available.

Mental Health Financing There are no budget allocations for mental health.
Details about expenditure on mental health are not available.
The primary sources of mental health financing in descending order are tax based, grants, out of pocket expenditure by the patient or family and private insurances.
Mental Health services are free of charge to patients. Psychotropic medication account for 6.42% of the total expenditure on medications.
There are no disability benefits for persons with mental disorders. Rehabilitation of mentally ill is included in the mandate of Directorate for Rehabilitation Services under MoH, but it is short on financial, human and other resources.

Mental Health Facilities Mental health is a part of primary health care system. Actual treatment of severe mental disorders is available at the primary level. Mental health care in primary care is not uniformly developed.
Regular training of primary care professionals is not carried out in the field of mental health. Planned with the help of WHO and the French Government, NGOs and UN agencies (particularly UNICEF) in collaboration with many Ministries run short- and long-term courses on counselling, crisis intervention, nursing and social-work in relation to mental health for health professionals, teachers, parents, adolescents, law enforcement officers etc.
There are community care facilities for patients with mental disorders. The Ministry of Health operates 15 community mental health clinics (CMHC). They are staffed by a psychiatrist and nurses (without specialist training). There is one mental health clinic for children. They provide case management, home visits, school consultation, counselling, public education, emergency and crisis services, substance abuse services, rehabilitation and training, education and research programmes. The Gaza Community Mental Health Programme (GCMHP), an NGO, runs four community mental health clinics. The United Nations Relief and Works Agency (UNRWA) initiated its mental health programme in 1989. It provides services to about 250 patients per week. UNRWA has started day care centres for the disabled. Almost one-third of all mental health patients are seen at the CMHCs.

Psychiatric Beds and Professionals

Total psychiatric beds per 10 000 population	0.91
Psychiatric beds in mental hospitals per 10 000 population	0.87
Psychiatric beds in general hospitals per 10 000 population	0.04
Psychiatric beds in other settings per 10 000 population	0
Number of psychiatrists per 100 000 population	0.6
Number of neurosurgeons per 100 000 population	0.22
Number of psychiatric nurses per 100 000 population	2.2
Number of neurologists per 100 000 population	0.27
Number of psychologists per 100 000 population	1.2
Number of social workers per 100 000 population	3

The other category is mainly composed of school counsellors. In Bethlehem, more than 40% of the beds are earmarked for women. Mental Hospitals offer a certain number of beds for forensic psychiatry. There are no beds earmarked for patients with substance abuse. There are no private mental health beds. The University of Al Quds has introduced a Master's level course in Community Based Mental Health (CBMH) at the School of Public Health in Gaza. Bir Zeit University's postgraduate training programme in Public Health has a mental health module. The Islamic University (in association with the Community Mental Health Services of the Government) offers a Community Mental Health diploma. The Gaza Community Mental Health Programme (NGO) offers a Diploma in Community Mental Health and Human Rights. Intensive in-service professional development programmes are available and participation in continuing professional education is encouraged. Some professionals are sent for advanced courses with the help of WHO and the French, Italian and Egyptian Governments. One forensic psychiatrist is undergoing training overseas.

Non-Governmental Organizations There are NGOs involved with mental health. They are mainly involved in advocacy, promotion, prevention and treatment. Many NGOs are working in West Bank and Gaza. Almost 50 of them employ at least 2 psycho-social/ mental health staff members. Most of them provide counselling and work with specific groups like children, women, drug abusers etc. More than 80% of services offered by NGOs pertains to the urban population. The Gaza Community Mental Health Programme (GCMHP) runs 4 community mental health clinics. It is also involved in public education campaigns, occupational therapy and crisis intervention. Other NGOs offer counselling as a part of other (non-mental health) services. The United Nations Relief

Works Agency (UNRWA) provides counselling and help in supply of medication. UNICEF provides educative and promotive services, and materials for playing, reading, learning and self-expression to children. NGOs provide services to the less seriously ill population. Their services are often directed at specific segments of population like the mentally challenged, psychogeriatric, substance abusers, children, women, political victims, victims of trauma etc. The National Plan of Action for Palestinian Children has a specific website that summarizes information on organizations that specifically aim to address the psychosocial needs of children (http://www.npasec.org/DisplayOrg.asp).

Information Gathering System There is mental health reporting system.
There is data collection system or epidemiological study on mental health.

Programmes for Special Population There are specific programmes for mental health for disaster affected population, indigenous population, elderly and children.
Specific services for children include one outpatient child mental health clinic (2 days/week) in Gaza and four psychiatric beds in Gaza Mental Hospital. A school health programme provides integrated management of childhood illnesses and promotion of health including mental health (under the Health Promotion and Education Directorate). UNRWA also identifies and manages children suffering from mental retardation and disabilities. Refugees are cared for particularly by the UNRWA, and disaster affected population are often the focus of NGOs and UN agencies. But in a situation where facing trauma is almost a norm, the whole population may be said to be disaster affected. UNICEF provides educational and promotion services and materials for children.

Therapeutic Drugs The following therapeutic drugs are generally available at the primary health care level: carbamazepine, phenobarbital, phenytoin sodium, sodium valproate, amitriptyline, chlorpromazine, diazepam, fluphenazine, haloperidol, lithium, carbidopa.
Other drugs like benzhexol, clozapine and cloimipramine are included in the essential drug list.

Other Information

Additional Sources of Information

Al-Krenawi, A., Graham, J., Izzeldin, A. (2001) The psychosocial impact of polygamous marriages on Palestinian women. Women & Health, 34, 1-16.

Barber, B. K. (1999) Political violence, family relations, and Palestinian youth functioning. Journal of Adolescent Research, 14, 206-230.

Gaza Community Mental Health Program, Annual Reports 1994-2003.

Giacaman, R. (2004) Psychosocial/ Mental Health Care in the Occupied Palestinian Territories: the Embryonic System. Birzeit:Institute of Community & Public Health, Birzeit University.

Haj-Yahia, M. M. (2000) Implications of wife abuse and battering for self-esteem, depression, and anxiety as revealed by the Second Palestinian National Survey on Violence against Women. Journal of Family Issues, 21, 435-463.

Haj-Yahia, M. M., Shor, R. (1995) Child maltreatment as perceived by Arab students of social science in the West Bank. Child Abuse & Neglect, 19, 1209-1219.

Haj-Yahia, M. M., Tamish, S. (2001) The rates of child sexual abuse and its psychological consequences as revealed by a study among Palestinian university students. Child Abuse & Neglect, 25, 1303-1327.

Kostelny, K., Garbarino, J. (1994) Coping with the consequences of living in danger: the case of Palestinian children and youth. International Journal of Behavioral Development, 17, 595-611.

Miller, T., el-Masri, M., Allodi, F., et al (1999) Emotional and behavioural problems and trauma exposure of school-age Palestinian children in Gaza: some preliminary findings. Medicine, Conflict & Survival, 15, 368-378.

Ministry of Health. Mental health and mental disorders. In: National Strategic Health Plan, Palestine 1999-2003.

Ministry of Health. Mental Health Services, Palestinian Ministry of Health, Annual Reports 1994-2003.

Ministry of Health. Palestinian Ministry of Health, Annual Report 1994-2003.

Ministry of Planning and International Cooperation. (1999) National plan for action for Palestinian children. Agenda for social renewal. Revised and Updated 1999-2001.

Murad, I., Gordon, H. (2002) Psychiatry and the Palestinian population. Psychiatric Bulletin, 26, 28-30.

National Authority Bulletin, Palestine 2004.

Palestinian Central Bureau of Statistics (2003) Health Survey Main Findings.

Qouta, S., Punamaeki, R.-L., El Sarraj, E. (1997) House demolition and mental health: victims and witnesses. Journal of Social Distress & the Homeless, 6, 203-211.

Samour, A. M. (2002) Prevalence and risk factors of postpartum depression in Gaza Strip. Gaza Strip: Al Quds University.

Thabet, A. A., Vostanis, P. (1998) Social adversities and anxiety disorders in the Gaza Strip. Archives of Disease in Childhood, 78, 439-442.

Thabet, A. A., Vostanis, P. (2000) Post traumatic stress disorder reactions in children of war: A longitudinal study. Child Abuse & Neglect, 24, 291-298.

WHO. Country projects: selected cases. West bank and Gaza Strip :improving mental health policy and service delivery. http://www.who.int/mental_health/media/en/country%20Report%20compiled_WHA.pdf

WHO EMRO. World Health Day 2001. http://www.emro.who.int/mnh/whd/CountryProfile-PAhtm.

Atlas Resources

The Mental Health Atlas-2005 data are also available free-of-charge on the internet. The web-based format is designed to make the information more dynamic and interactive. The site allows the user to view and analyse data at the country, region, or world level, and to create maps, tables and diagrams in ways corresponding to individual research needs. The Mental Health Atlas-2005 website can be accessed at:

http://www.who.int/mental_health/evidence/atlas/index.htm

OTHER PUBLICATIONS OF INTEREST:

ATLAS: Mental Health Resources in the World 2001, Order no. 1930191

ATLAS: Country Profiles on Mental Health Resources 2001, Order no. 1930192

ATLAS: Country Resources for Neurological Disorders 2004, ISBN 92 4 1 156283 8

ATLAS: Child and Adolescent Mental Health *(in preparation)*

ATLAS: Epilepsy *(in preparation)*

ATLAS: Intellectual Disabilities *(in preparation)*

ATLAS: Psychiatric Training (WPA and WHO) *(in preparation)*

ATLAS: Role of Nurses in Mental Health Care (ICN and WHO) *(in preparation)*

ATLAS: Substance Abuse *(in preparation)*

To order WHO Publications or get additional information,
consult the following website or send an email to: bookorders@who.int
http://bookorders.who.int/bookorders/index.htm